**Recent Developments in Non-ruminant Nutrition**

# Recent Developments in Non-ruminant Nutrition

*Editors*

PC Garnsworthy

J Wiseman

*School of Biosciences, University of Nottingham*

NOTTINGHAM
University Press

Nottingham University Press
Manor Farm, Main Street, Thrumpton
Nottingham, NG11 0AX, United Kingdom

NOTTINGHAM

First published 2006


**British Library Cataloguing in Publication Data**
Recent Developments in Non-ruminant Nutrition:
I. Garnsworthy, Philip C. II. Wiseman, J.

ISBN 1-904761-34-8

*Disclaimer*

Every reasonable effort has been made to ensure that the material in this book is true, correct, complete and appropriate at the time of writing. Nevertheless the publishers, the editors and the authors do not accept responsibility for any omission or error, or for any injury, damage, loss or financial consequences arising from the use of the book.



Typeset by Nottingham University Press, Nottingham
Printed and bound by Cromwell Press Ltd, Trowbridge, Wiltshire

# CONTENTS

# INTRODUCTION

The University of Nottingham UK has been organising annual Feed Conferences since 1967; each year papers presented are published in the proceedings 'Recent Advances in Animal Nutrition'. These texts are considered to be extremely informative reviews of high scientific quality, which are of direct relevance to the animal feed industry worldwide. In response to demand, collections of papers from these proceedings, grouped according to species, have been published in one volume under the 'Recent Developments' title. Previous titles have included 'Ruminants', 'Pigs' and 'Poultry', and they have received much acclaim from research workers, teachers, students advisors and, ultimately, the industry itself. It has now been decided that to publish a series of papers under the 'Non-Ruminant' title would be very opportune.

The opening chapters deal with pigs. Traditionally diet formulation was based on total amino acid content but, with increasing emphasis on precision, feed compounders are examining alternative approaches. The paper on amino acid digestibility in formulation of diets for pigs provides a useful review of a complex subject. With the European Union ban on feed-grade antibiotic growth promoters (AGPs) introduced in January 2006, there is much interest in gastro-intestinal matters; these are covered in the paper on gut health and immunity in young piglets. The theme of health is continued with a consideration of post weaning multisystemic wasting syndrome, a condition which has ravaged the pig industry in many countries. Subsequent chapters deal with the breeding animal. Sow herd replacement rates are frequently high and possible reasons for this are dealt with in nutritional influences on lifetime performance of the sow. Pregnant sows are frequently fed below ad libitum levels, which can create problems associated with poor gut fill that may have welfare implications. A nutritional solution is discussed in feeding gestating sows with high fibre diets. Finally, the role of fatty acids is becoming increasingly topical and is covered in fatty acids and reproduction in the pig.

The next section covers poultry. Nutrition often considers rapidly growing birds with little emphasis on the newly hatched chick. The chapter on early nutrition in young poultry is a timely reminder of the importance of the first few days of life. The environmental impact of animal production enterprises is increasingly important and ways of reducing this are very topical; the paper on phytase in poultry nutrition addresses one particular nutrient, phosphorus, whose release into the environment may be reduced considerably. Further considerations of this approach are dealt with in endogenous enzymes as pro-nutrients in broiler diets followed by a further discussion on the importance of microbial phytase in broiler nutrition. Modern broilers are invariably fed diets of high nutrient and energy concentration, and the consequences, in terms of performance and carcass quality, are covered in the chapter on high energy diets for poultry. The most important energy-yielding component of poultry diets is starch and its value is considered in kinetics of starch digestion in broilers. On-farm nutritional strategies for optimising broiler nutrition are covered in putting poultry nutrition into practice. The final paper in the section discussed the laying hen and egg quality by examining natural pigments

The third section commences with companion animals, the nutrition of which is assuming greater importance in many developed countries. Three papers cover nutrient requirements of grazing horses, speciality diets for horses and equine nutrition, as those involved in the equine sector are moving towards a greater understanding of the scientific principles. Cats and dogs are considered in the chapter on companion animal nutrition.

The next section covers subjects of general interest and starts with three papers with a general theme of animal health. The first considers the immune system and productivity of animals, the second nutrition and immunity in farm animals, and the third bacteriological aspects of antibiotics and their alternatives. The subsequent paper covers the topical area of roles of plant extracts in non-ruminants as industry searches for more natural solutions of problems of gut health.

The concluding papers again deal with subjects which are occupying the minds of scientists and the industry. The subject of GMOs is never far from centre stage and one aspect covered is effects of processing on DNA fragmentation in animal feeds. Finally, the book returns to the theme of environmental impact by considering feed composition and environmental pollution.

J Wiseman
PC Garnsworthy

1

# AMINO ACID DIGESTIBILITY IN FORMULATION OF DIETS FOR PIGS: PRESENT INTEREST AND LIMITATIONS, FUTURE PROSPECTS

B. SÈVE and V. HESS
*Station de Recherches Porcines F35590 Saint-Gilles, France*

## Introduction

It is well established that there is no amino acid (AA) absorption from the large intestine. Furthermore, the microflora present will metabolise some of the undigested AAs there, which will not accordingly appear in the faeces. Therefore, the nutritional availability of AAs is primarily determined by their digestibility measured at the end of the small intestine, i.e. at the ileum, giving the definition of "ileal digestibility". A number of organisations have published such figures for the main foodstuffs used in pig feeding. This chapter deals with the meaning and the reliability of these figures. First, the different expressions of ileal digestibility (apparent *vs.* true or standardised values) and implications are discussed. Second, the limits of the available information in terms of the factors affecting within-foodstuff variability of ileal digestibility results in relation to experimental conditions (animal parameters) and feed components or processing will be considered. Then, the experimental evidence for the advantage of using ileal digestible rather than total supplies of AAs in diet formulation will be reviewed. Finally, the availability of ileal digestible AAs for tissue metabolism will be discussed. Among the factors affecting this availability, the impact of indigestible endogenous protein losses specifically induced by feed components will be emphasised.

## Measurement and expression of ileal digestibility

The *apparent digestibility* may be measured either with total recovery of ileal flow from pigs fitted with ileo-rectal anastomosis (IRA), or from determination of the concentration of an indigestible marker, generally chromic oxide, in a sample of ileal digesta from pigs fitted with cannulae. Comparison of the two techniques has shown differences in opposite directions (Köhler *et al* 1990;

Leterme *et al* 1990) or very similar figures (Yin *et al* 1993). Different IRA techniques have been compared, sometimes showing differences between the end-to-end technique involving isolation of the large intestine and the end-to-side technique involving a risk of contamination of the ileal digesta with residual contents from the colon and hence with its microflora. This generally affected the digestibility of non-starch polysaccharides to a greater extent than that of AAs. The same observations were made with or without conservation of the ileo-caecal valvula (Laplace *et al* 1994).

Apparent digestibility does not take into account the endogenous or exogenous origin of the indigestible nitrogen (N) or AA. Total indigestible N or AA related to a particular foodstuff may be assumed to be proportional to the dry matter intake of this foodstuff. If the diet used for the measurements contains other ingredients, the amount of indigestible N or AA generated by the dry matter of these ingredients should be estimated. Then, calculation of the indigestible N or amino acid from the tested foodstuff should be made "by difference", i.e. by discounting this fraction. This should apply in the case of substitution of the tested foodstuff for a basal diet, regardless of whether the latter contains protein or not. It is important to be aware that measurement of the apparent digestibility of protein-rich foodstuffs often involved dilution with protein-free ingredients and that, generally, no correction for losses associated with these ingredients was made. As a consequence, apparently digestible N or AA contents of protein-rich foodstuffs may be underestimated and not additive with contents determined for low-protein foodstuffs. Such corrections were made for the apparent digestibilities published together with standardised digestibilities in recent French tables (INRA-AFZ, 2004).

A number of experiments (e.g. Fan *et al* 1994) have shown that the apparent digestibility, even correctly calculated, increased with the level of protein or AA in the foodstuff. This observation gave rise to some concern about possible underestimation of true AA availability from low-protein foodstuffs through apparent digestibility. The variation of apparent digestibility according to the level of protein was consistent with the hypothesis of a *'basal endogenous loss'* proportional to total dry matter intake (DMI) rather than proportional to protein intake (Figure 1.1). The relative importance of the basal endogenous loss decreases compared to that proportional to protein intake when the foodstuff protein content increases. It may be considered as a part of body protein expense independent of feed components and close to losses measured with a maize-starch-based protein-free diet. On this basis, it was proposed to "standardise" the apparent digestibility into *'true digestibility'*, discarding the basal endogenous loss, measured with a protein free diet, from the apparently indigestible fraction.

AA Ileal True Digestibility (ITD) =

AA Ileal Apparent Digestibility (IAD)

\+ basal endogenous loss per kg DMI/foodstuff AA content per kg DMI

This expression of digestibility gives an estimate of amino acid availability independent of the foodstuff protein content.

Conversely, when it is possible to find a dietary factor explaining the variation of true digestibility, the relevance of the assumption of a basal endogenous loss may be established

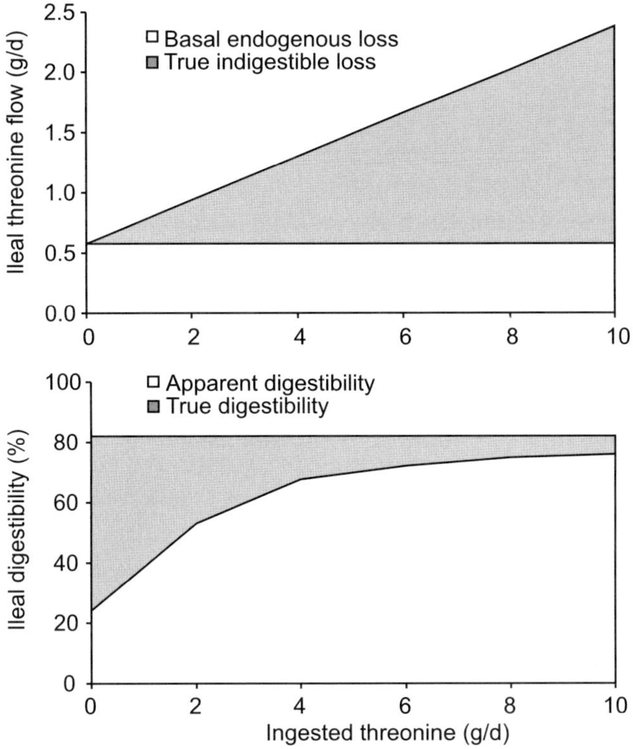


**Figure 1.1**. Effect of dietary amino acid content on the ileal flow and the digestibility of this amino acid (example threonine).

if a negative constant term could be shown to be significant in the model. This was demonstrated through modelling the apparent digestibility of threonine, serine and glycine from wheat meal by-products (Table 1.1) according to their acid detergent fibre (ADF) content (Sève *et al* 1994a).

The true digestibility concept is particularly well adapted to measurements made with dilution of a single protein foodstuff with protein-free ingredients. In such a situation, Furuya and Kaji (1991) have shown that the apparently digestible AA content of a barley-soybean meal diet calculated from the apparent digestible contents measured with two separate single foodstuff diets, without correction for the contribution of protein free ingredients, did not provide additive data. In contrast, true digestible contents were additive (Table 1.2).

**Table 1.1** MODELLING APPARENT ILEAL DIGESTIBILITY (AID, %) IN WHEAT-MEAL CO-PRODUCTS (SÈVE *et al.*, 1994)

| | | | |
|---|---|---|---|
| AID Thr = 84.4(±2.7) | - | 1.14(±0.13) x ADF/Thr | $R^2$ = 0.92; RSD = 2.8; n = 8. |
| AID Thr = 94.3(±3.1) | - | 1.02(±0.08) x ADF/Thr | |
| | - | 41.0(±11.3) / Thr | $R^2$ = 0.98; RSD = 1.7; n = 8. |
| AID Ser = 89.6(±2.6) | - | 1.18(±0.17) x ADF/Ser | $R^2$ = 0.89; RSD = 2.8; n = 8. |
| AID Ser = 100.8(±3.1) | - | 0.97(±0.10) x ADF/Ser | |
| | - | 61.7(±15.5) / Ser | $R^2$ = 0.97; RSD = 1.5; n = 8. |
| AID Gly = 91.0(±3.5) | - | 7.0(±1.0) x ADL/Gly | $R^2$ = 0.90; RSD = 3.1; n = 8. |
| AID Gly = 104.9(±5.3) | - | 6.8(±0.7) x ADL/Gly | |
| | - | 79.6(±27.4) / Gly | $R^2$ = 0.96; RSD = 2.1; n = 8. |

Thr = threonine, Ser = serine, Gly = glycine, ADF = acid detergent fibre, ADL = acid detergent lignin, g/100 g dry matter.

**Table 1.2** COMPARISON OF THE MEASURED DIGESTIBILITY (%) VALUES OF A BARLEY-SOYBEAN MEAL DIET TO THOSE CALCULATED FROM MEASUREMENTS MADE ON THE SINGLE FOODSTUFFS DIETS (FURUYA and KAJI 1991)

| *Diet* / *Amino acid* | *Digestibility* | *Barley* | *Soybean meal* | *Barley + soybean meal* | |
|---|---|---|---|---|---|
| | | | | *Measured* | *Calculated* |
| Threonine | Apparent | 51 | 69 | 71 | 63 |
| | True | 75 | 81 | 82 | 79 |
| Lysine | Apparent | 55 | 80 | 78 | 73 |
| | True | 75 | 87 | 86 | 84 |

In best-cost formulation with a given feed matrix, the apparent and true digestible AA data will lead to the same diet composition with the condition that the requirement for true digestible AA is higher than the requirement for apparent digestible AA by an amount corresponding to the basal endogenous loss.

## Variability of the basal endogenous loss and of the ileal digestibility

True digestibility values are dependent on the choice of an estimate for the basal endogenous loss of each AA. The use of a protein-free diet was criticised but, under certain conditions, it is probably the most appropriate means of representing the obligatory digestive expense of AA by the pig (see the discussion by Sève and Henry 1996). It was concluded, from an initial study, that basal endogenous losses are proportional to dry matter intake (DMI) with the condition that feed intake is higher than 70 g DMI per unit metabolic weight (Mariscal-Landin *et al* 1995).

This was confirmed in a more recent study showing, in addition, that the basal loss of N or AA per kg DM intake decreased with the weight of the pig (Hess and Sève 1999). The evidence that fibre increased the basal endogenous loss measured with a protein-free diet (Mariscal-Landin *et al* 1995) raised some concern about its postulated independence of dietary components. However, this response was at a plateau at 30-34g crude fibre/kg, very close to the level used in standard diets, and it may be assumed that this level of fibre allows optimal functioning of the digestive tract, together with satisfactory feed intake. On this basis, it is possible to recommend that the basal endogenous loss be measured with a maize-starch-based protein-free diet enriched with about 40g purified paper cellulose/kg. Nevertheless it is important to mention that, at constant live weight and feed intake, the individual quantitative and qualitative (AA pattern) variations remain high (Hess and Sève 1999). In addition, basal endogenous losses as well as digestibility data may be affected by unidentified genetic or environmental parameters associated with the site of measurement (Table 1.3). Altogether these observations imply that, as far as possible, the basal endogenous loss and apparent digestibility should be assessed on the same pigs at similar live weight. It is interesting to note that digestibility differences between sites seem more important with foodstuffs of low digestibility suggesting that health status could be involved in these variations.

**Table 1.3** EFFECT OF THE SITE OF MEASUREMENT ON THE TRUE DIGESTIBILITY (%) OF THREONINE AND LYSINE FROM THREE DIFFERENT FOODSTUFFS (SÈVE *et al.*, 2000)

| *Sites* | *Threonine* | | | *Lysine* | | |
|---|---|---|---|---|---|---|
| | *Barley* | *Pea* | *Soybean meal* | *Barley* | *Pea* | *Soybean meal* |
| 1 | 61 | 79 | 86 | 67 | 85 | 91 |
| 2 | 67 | 83 | 89 | 72 | 90 | 92 |
| 3 | 69 | 80 | 88 | 70 | 86 | 90 |

Within the same type of foodstuff, large variations of digestibility may be associated with specific features such as fibre concentration, anti-nutritional factor contents, heat treatment etc (Table 1.4).

For example, in wheat-meal co-products, AA digestibility may be predicted as a function of acid detergent fibre (ADF) expressed in g per g AA or of the proportion of total N associated with neutral detergent fibre (NDF). Similar results were obtained with soybean meal. Tannin content could be a good predictor for sorghum seeds, but content of anti-trypsin factors is a poor predictor for pea seeds. For animal meals, "Carpenter" lysine (with free ε-amino groups) or in vitro digestibility (from protease action) could be used.

**Table 1.4** EXAMPLES OF PREDICTION OF ILEAL DIGESTIBILITY (%) OF LYSINE FROM DIFFERENT FOODSTUFFS (SÈVE 1994)

| | | | | |
|---|---|---|---|---|
| Wheat milling co-products | (n = 11) | CUDv Lys = 97.5 | - 1.19 ADF/Lys[1] | $R^2 = 0.84$ |
| Pea | (n = 5) | CUDv Lys = 90.6 | - 1.31 antitrypsin factor | $R^2 = 0.67$ |
| Sorghum | (n = 4) | CUDv Lys = 73.2 | - 19.1 tannins | $R^2 = 0.95$ |
| Meat meals | (n = 5) | CUDv Lys = 13.3 | + 0.75 Carpenter lysine[2] | $R^2 = 0.99$ |
| Miscellaneous meat meals | (n = 10) | CUDv Lys = 40.7 | + 0.45 Carpenter lysine[2] | $R^2 = 0.49$ |
| Miscellaneous meat meals | (n = 10) | CUDv Lys = 10.5 | + 0.94 N solubilised in vitro | $R^2 = 0.57$ |
| | | CUDv Lys = 25.4 | + 0.65 N solubilised in vitro + 0.25 Lys liberated in vitro | $R^2 = 0.71$ |

[1]ADF/Lys = Van Soest dried acid detergent residue (% of dry matter), g/g lysine.
[2]Lysine with free epsilon-amino group (% total lysine), determined according to Roach *et al.*, (1967).

## Advantage of ileal digestible AA vs. total AA in pig diet formulation

Only relatively few experiments have directly shown the advantage of measuring digestibility at the ileum instead of faecal level or even the advantage of ileal digestible vs. total AA in the formulation of diets for pigs (Wiseman *et al* 1991; Buracewska and Buracewski 1997). For example, the latter authors have shown that the additional industrial amino acids required to meet pig requirements on a digestible instead of total supply basis improved growth performance and nitrogen retention (Table 1.5). Other experiments were less successful (Fuller *et al* 1981; Buracewska *et al* 1999). Some of the experimental failures may be ascribed to inadequate supplies of AA considered as second limiting.

**Table 1.5** ADVANTAGE OF TAKING IN ACCOUNT THE ILEAL DIGESTIBLE AA INSTEAD OF TOTAL AA FOR SUPPLEMENTATION OF A DIET BASED ON BARLEY, WHEAT, SOYBEAN MEAL AND RAPESEED MEAL (BURACEWSKA AND BURACEWSKI 1997)

| *Basis of formulation* | *Ileal digestible AA* | *Total AA* |
|---|---|---|
| Average daily gain, g/d | 756 | 780 |
| Feed conversion ratio | 2.15 | 2.07 |
| Nitrogen retention[1], g/d | 19.4 a | 20.7 b |

[1] Means followed by different letters, within the same row, differ ($P < 0.05$)

As a matter of fact, the use of ileal digestible AA has rapidly developed in commercial pig diet formulation. In this respect, in EU countries, the trend to impose, by law, reductions of dietary N supply was a strong incentive. This is because dietary N reduction gives more importance, firstly to the fraction of dietary protein provided by cereal grain protein of lower digestibility compared to protein-rich foodstuffs such as soybean meal and, secondly, to industrial free amino acids that are assumed to be 100 % digestible and available (Table 1.6).

**Table 1.6** DECREASE IN AA ILEAL DIGESTIBILITY ASSOCIATED WITH REDUCTION OF PROTEIN CONTENT IN A DIET BASED ON BARLEY, WHEAT AND SOYBEAN MEAL

| *Crude protein (%)* | *17* | *13* |
|---|---|---|
| Digestibility of | | |
| Lysine | 90 | 86 |
| Methionine | 90 | 89 |
| Threonine | 89 | 86 |
| Tryptophan | 89 | 87 |

## Availability of ileum digestible amino acids for tissue metabolism

Three main objections have been raised on the value of ileal digestibility as an estimate of the availability for tissue metabolism.

Firstly, a number of experiments have suggested that free AA could not be considered 100 % available since, due to more rapid absorption than protein-bound AA, they could be oxidised in the liver rather than used for protein synthesis. In this respect, Batterham (1984) reported that supplemental free lysine in a deficient diet was more efficient when meal frequency increased from 1 to six times a day (Table 1.7). Such a risk is certainly higher when pigs are fed at restricted levels but, in commercial herds, feeding pigs ad libitum reduces the problem.

**Table 1.7** EFFECT OF MEAL FREQUENCY ON THE UTILISATION OF DIETARY ADDITIONAL L-LYSINE (BATTERHAM 1984)

| *Feeding frequency (F) meal/d* | *L-lysine addition (L) (g/kg)* | *Average daily gain (g/d)* | *Feed conversion ratio* |
|---|---|---|---|
| 1 | 0 | 435 | 3.09 |
| 1 | 2 | 491 | 2.75 |
| 2 | 0 | 446 | 3.09 |
| 2 | 2 | 530 | 2.57 |
| F x L interaction | | $P < 0.01$ | $P < 0.05$ |

Secondly, even when feeding pigs every third hour, Batterham *et al* (1990) have shown lower efficiency of ileal digestible lysine when it came from meat meal and cottonseed meal rather than from soybean meal (Table 1.8). Because other AAs were less affected than lysine, these authors suggested that the heat treatment applied to these foodstuffs could induce variations in AA availability undetectable by ileal digestibility. It is well known that under these circumstances, lysine may be absorbed under chemical forms unavailable for tissue metabolism. This was probably true in the case of overheated fishmeal (Wiseman *et al* 1991). However the latter data showed, at least, that the decrease in performance due to overheating was much higher when formulation was made on the basis of ileal digestible rather than total AA (Table 1.9). Overheating of pea seeds also affected the efficiency of ileal digestible lysine (Van Barneveld 1994). Therefore, in severely heated foodstuffs, the ileal digestibility of lysine probably overestimates its true availability. Moughan and Rutherford (1996) proposed determining the digestibility of reactive lysine, i.e. lysine that can be guanidinated into homoarginine.

**Table 1.8** EFFICIENCY OF ILEAL DIGESTIBLE AMINO ACIDS FROM DIFFERENT FOODSTUFFS IN PIGS FED AT 3 H INTERVALS (BATTERHAM *et al.*, 1990)

| *Foodstuff* | *Cottonseed meal* | *Meat meal* | *Soybean meal* |
|---|---|---|---|
| Average daily gain, g/d | 377 | 492 | 541 |
| Feed conversion ratio | 3.5 | 2.6 | 2.3 |
| Lysine retained/ileal digestible lysine | 0.36 | 0.60 | 0.75 |

**Table 1.9** EFFECT OF THE HEAT TREATMENT OF FISHMEAL ON PIG WEIGHT GAIN (g/d), ACCORDING TO THE BASIS OF FORMULATION (WISEMAN *et al.*, 1991)

| *Fishmeal heat treatment* | *Untreated* | *130 ° C* | *160 °C* |
|---|---|---|---|
| Basis of formulation | | | |
| Total AA | 497 | 473 | 318 |
| Ileal digestible AA | 466 | 498 | 406 |
| | Interaction heat treatment x basis of formulation, P = 0.072 | | |

The third objection relates to the fact that, at the ileal level, total endogenous protein losses largely exceed basal losses. It means that the "true" indigestible N or AA fraction is made of two parts, both proportional to the tested protein intake, as has been shown with a soy protein isolate (Figure 1.2). The first part results from incomplete digestion of dietary protein, corresponding to its *'real' digestibility*. The second part results from undigested additional secreted protein, termed the *'specific endogenous loss'* (Sève and Henry 1996). Taking into account the basal endogenous loss leads to calculation of the *true digestibility*. Taking in account the specific endogenous loss leads to calculate

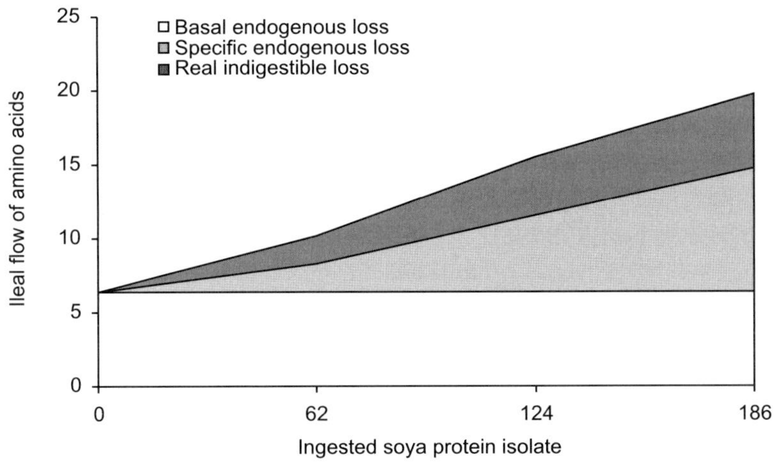


**Figure 1.2** Partition of the true indigestible amino acids from a soya protein isolate into a real indigestible fraction and the specific endogenous losses (Sève *et al.*, 1994b)

the *real digestibility*. These terms were clearly defined by Low (1982). At the 9th International Symposium on Digestive Physiology in Pigs, a group of experts was appointed to redefine digestibility terminology in a technical note. "Standardised digestibility" will replace "true digestibility" and "true digestibility" will replace "real digestibility". With the two examples shown in Table 1.10 involving peas (Huisman *et al* 1992) and soy protein isolate (Sève *et al* 1994b), it is clear that the impact of the specific endogenous loss on the apparent digestibility may exceed that of the basal endogenous loss.

**Table 1.10** SPECIFIC COMPARED TO BASAL ENDOGENOUS LOSSES IN PROPORTION TO N OR AA CONTENT WITH TWO DIFFERENT FOODSTUFFS (SÈVE and HENRY 1996)

| *Foodstuff*<br>*Unit Item* | *Frijaune pea*<br>*g/100 g N* | *Soy protein isolate*<br>*g/100g AA* |
|---|---|---|
| Apparent digestible | 74.1 | 89.3 |
| *Basal endogenous loss* | *7.8* | *3.5* |
| True digestible | 81.9 | 92.8 |
| *Specific endogenous loss* | *11.0* | *4.5* |
| Real digestible | 92.9 | 97.3 |
| | Huisman *et al* 1992 | Sève *et al* 1994 |

Using $^{15}N$ labelled diets, the existence of a specific endogenous loss in excess of the basal loss has been confirmed (Hess 1999) through measurements of higher endogenous amino acid losses with diets based on wheat, wheat middling and different varieties of pea seeds, than with protein-free diets (Table 1.11). In those examples, there was an indication that a higher real digestibility may be associated with a higher stimulation of endogenous losses. However, not surprisingly, the highest real digestibility of pea protein was obtained with "micro" grinding of the Solara seeds, leading to particle size around 30-40 μm, without any increase in endogenous losses. Micro grinding probably caused

**Table 1.11** ILEAL ENDOGENOUS LOSSES AND REAL DIGESTIBILITY (%) WITH WHEAT AND WHEAT MIDDLING (EXPERIMENT 1) AND DIFFERENT VARIETIES OF PEA SEEDS, ONE OF THEM MICRO-GROUND (EXPERIMENT 2) (HESS 1999)

| *Diets* | | *Expt 1* | | | *Expt 2* | *Peas* | | |
|---|---|---|---|---|---|---|---|---|
| | *Protein free* | *Wheat* | *Wheat middling* | *Protein free* | *Solara* | *Solara micro* | *Eiffel* | *Madria* |
| Threonine: | | | | | | | | |
| Endogenous | | | | | | | | |
| Ileal loss, g/kg | 0.5 a | 0.7 b | 0.8 b | 0.6 a | 0.9 b | 0.8ab | 1.3c | 1.4 c |
| Real digestibility | | 88 a | 93 a | | 80 c | 90 a | 84 b | 78 c |
| Lysine: | | | | | | | | |
| Endogenous | | | | | | | | |
| Ileal loss, g/kg | 0.4 a | 0.5 a | 0.7 b | 0.4 a | 0.4 a | 0.6ab | 1.1 c | 0.8bc |
| Real digestibility | | 81 b | 89 a | | 83 c | 95 a | 87 b | 80 c |

Means followed by different letters, within the same row and the same experiment, differ ($P < 0.05$)

disruption of the seed cells making all their protein content directly accessible to proteases and almost totally digestible.

It was postulated that higher endogenous losses involved additional urinary N losses (Huisman *et al* 1993; Grala *et al* 1994, 1999) as a result of decreased efficiency of ileal digestible amino acids. Assuming that dietary ideal protein is the limiting factor, the impact of these endogenous losses on the requirement for N may be estimated through partition of the real digestible N (Nr) into two fractions. The first one corresponds to the total cost of the ileal flow of total endogenous N (Ne), obtained with the efficiency Ke. The second one corresponds to the total cost of other body N retention (Nb), obtained with the efficiency Kb:

$$Nr = Ne/Ke + Nb/Kb \quad (1.1)$$

Ke and Kb can be calculated directly from this model or from a regression of body N retention on the endogenous loss, both expressed per g of really digested N:

$$Nb/Nr = -(Ne/Nr)(Kb/Ke) + Kb \quad (1.2)$$

If $Ke < 1$ ($1/Ke > 1$) the total cost of total endogenous loss $Ne/Ke$ will be higher than the loss itself and the difference $Ne/Ke - Ne = Ne(1/Ke - 1)$ will represent its metabolic cost.

This was confirmed with diets based on peas differentially stimulating the endogenous losses (Figure 1.3). The regression showed a linear decrease in body N retention with the increase in endogenous loss. Ke was estimated at 0.45, i.e., about half the value of Kb (0.82). Therefore, the total cost of the endogenous loss was about twice the loss itself and, consequently, the metabolic cost was of the same magnitude as the loss.

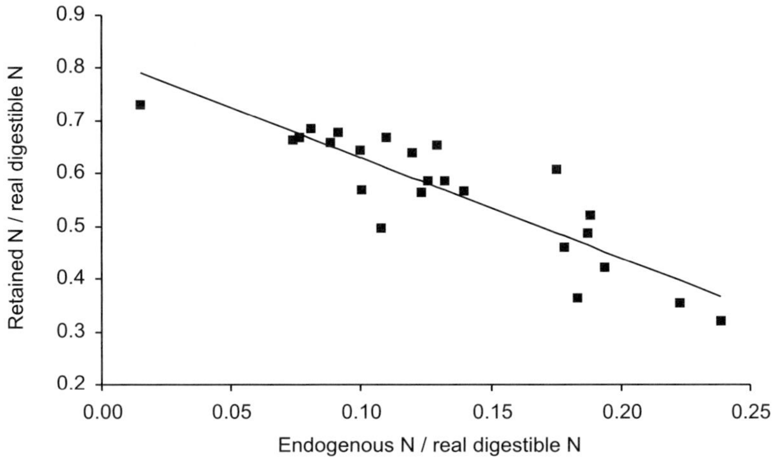


**Figure 1.3** Linear reduction of N retention according to N endogenous losses both expressed per g real digestible N ($Y = 0.82 - 1.90X$, $R^2 = 0.81$) (Hess, 1999)

On this basis, availability criteria can be derived from digestibility criteria. The apparent available N will be derived from the real digestible N by removal of the total cost of the endogenous loss

$$\text{Apparent Available N} = \text{Real digestible N} - \text{Ne/Ke} \quad (1.3)$$

Since Real Digestible N = Apparent digestible + Ne, then

$$\text{Apparent Available N} = \text{Apparent digestible N} - \text{Ne}(1/\text{Ke} - 1) \quad (1.4)$$

But, for the same reasons as explained earlier, a true available N content that ignores the basal endogenous loss (Nbe) may be defined and only takes into account the specific endogenous loss Nse = Ne –Nbe. While the apparent available N derives from the apparent digestible N by removal of the metabolic cost of total endogenous loss (equation 1.4), the true available N content is derived from the true digestible content by removal of the metabolic cost of the specific endogenous losses:

$$\text{True Available N} = \text{True digestible N} - \text{Nse}(1/\text{Ke} - 1) \quad (1.5)$$

This implies that a similar relation to the one defined between apparent and true digestible N can be found between the apparent and true available N:

$$\text{Apparent Available N} = \text{True available N} - \text{Nbe/Ke} \qquad (1.6)$$

where Neb/Ke, the total cost of the basal endogenous loss should be considered as part of the N requirement to be met with the true available N supply.

In the pea experiments, despite supplementation of the diets with DL methionine and L-tryptophan, dietary protein AA did not really match the ideal protein profile. In fact, in terms of ileal digestible AA per unit of net energy, threonine was the first limiting factor for N retention. Therefore, it was assumed that the efficiencies Ke and Kb determined for N applied to threonine and that threonine true availability could be derived from threonine true digestibility using equation 1.5 (Table 1.12).

**Table 1.12** TRUE DIGESTIBILITY (%) AND TRUE AVAILABILITY (%) OF THREONINE IN PEA SEEDS (HESS 1999)

| *Diet* | *Solara* | *Solara micro* | *Eiffel* | *Madria* |
|---|---|---|---|---|
| True digestibility | 75 b | 87 a | 73 b | 67 c |
| True availability | 68 b | 83 a | 58 c | 51 c |

Means followed by different letters, within the same row, differ ($P < 0.05$)

The two criteria did not classify the pea varieties in the same way. The Eiffel cultivar did not differ from the Solara cultivar in terms of threonine true digestibility. But, due to higher endogenous losses, threonine availability was significantly lower for Eiffel than for Solara. Therefore, these data clearly confirmed that variations in the endogenous output might cause deviations of ileal digestibility from availability values.

## Conclusions

Altogether, the available literature allows the conclusion that the true, also termed "standardised", ileal digestible AA provides a reasonably good estimation of available AA in protein sources commonly used in pig feeding. However, attention should be paid to the reliability of published apparent digestibility values, which may provide non-additive digestible AA contents, depending on the way the measurement and calculation was made. In addition, considering the variability of ileal digestibility, it is important firstly to have measurements made at different sites and, secondly, to correct the apparent digestibility into true digestibility using basal endogenous losses corresponding, at least, to this site and, at best, to the individual pigs. Furthermore, the standard error of the estimates should be reported in published digestibility tables, so that users can take it in account in their foodstuff composition matrix and formulate their diets safely. For the near future, the identification of predictors and the implementation of in vitro methods, remain important challenges for research.

Nevertheless, it is important to be aware that there are some limitations to the use of ileal digestibility as an estimate of the availability of AA for tissue metabolism. Kinetic effects on the utilisation of free vs. protein-bound amino acids have been mentioned, although this drawback seems to be overcome in ad libitum fed pigs. The risk of a deviation of true digestibility from true availability is more important, particularly for lysine, in foodstuffs submitted to severe heat treatment. It will require the development of correction methods. Finally, it is clear that specific endogenous losses, by increasing the requirement for the limiting amino acid, reduce the provision by some foodstuffs of ileal digestible AA for carcass tissue maintenance and growth, and decrease their efficiency. A new availability criterion derived from true digestibility, taking in account the metabolic cost of the specific endogenous loss, can be proposed. In the future, more attention should be paid to the factors affecting the endogenous losses of protein in the whole digestive tract.

The proposed correction of AA digestibility for endogenous losses and their metabolic cost was validated on ileorectomised pigs. Validation on intact pigs requires measurements in the large intestine; no reliable figures are available at present.

## References

Batterham, E.S. (1984) Utilization of free lysine by pigs. *Pigs News Information*, **5**, 85-89.

Batterham, E.S., Andersen, L. M., Baigent, D.R., Beech, S.A. and Elliott, R. (1990a) Utilization of ileal digestible amino acids by pigs: lysine. *British Journal of Nutrition*, **64**, 679-690.

Buracewska, L. and Buracewski, S. (1997) Nutritional effects in pigs fed diets supplemented with amino acids according to the requirement based on their total or ileal digestible content. In *Digestive Physiology in Pigs*, pp. 387-390. Edited by J.P. Laplace, C. Février, and A..Barbeau. Proceedings of the 7th International Symposium, St-Malo, France, May 26-28 1997, EAAP Publication n°88, INRA, Paris, France.

Buracewska, L., Wasilewko, J., Fandrejewski, H., Zebrowska, T. and Han, I.K. (1999) Formulation of pig diets according to ileal digestible amino acid content. *Livestock Production Science*, **59**, 13-24.

Fan, M.Z. and Sauer, W.C. (1994) Digestibility in pigs: effect of dietary amino acid level. Journal of Animal Science, **72**, 2851-2859.

Furuya, S. and Kaji, Y. (1991) Additivity of the apparent and true digestible amino acid supply in barley, maize, wheat or soya bean based diets for growing pigs. *Animal Feed Science and Technology*, **32**, 321-331.

Grala, W., Jansman, A.J.M., van Leeuwen, P., Verstegen, M.W.A., Huisman, J. and Gdala J. (1994) Nitrogen excretion by pigs fed different diets balanced for the apparent ileal digestible protein content. In *Proceedings of the 6th International Symposium on Digestive Physiology in Pigs (Bad Doberan, 4-6th October 1994)*, vol. I, pp. 83-85. Edited by W.B. Souffrant and H. Hagemeister Ed., EAAP Publication No. 80. Forschungsinstitut für die Biologie landwirtschaftlicher Nutztiere, Shriftenreihe 3, Dummerstorf, Germany.

Grala, W., Verstegen, M.W.A., Jansman, A.J.M., Huisman, J., van Leeuwen, P. and Tamminga, S. (1999) Effects of ileal endogenous losses and dietary amino acid supplementation on nitrogen retention in growing pigs. *Animal Feed Science and Technology*, **80**, 207-222.

Hess, V. (1999) Disponibilité vraie des acides aminés et impact des pertes endogènes spécifiques selon la source de protéines alimentaire chez le porc. *Ph.D. thesis*, 168 pp. Rennes University, France.

Hess, V and Sève, B. (1999) Effect of body weight and feed intake level on basal endogenous losses in growing pigs. Journal of Animal Science, **77**, in press.

Huisman, J., Heinz, T.H., Van Der Poel, A.F.B., Van Leeuwen, P., Souffrant W.B. and Verstegen M.W.A. (1992) True protein digestibility and amounts of endogenous protein measured with the $^{15}$N-dilution technique in piglets fed on peas (Pisum Sativum) and common beans (Phaseolus Vulgaris). *British Journal of Nutrition*, **68**, 101-110.

Huisman, J., Verstegen, M.W.A., van Leeuwen, P. and Tamminga S. (1993) Reduction of N pollution by decrease of the excretion of endogenous N in pigs. In *Nitrogen flow in pig production and environmental consequences*, pp.55-61. Edited by M.W.A. Verstegen, L.A. den Hartog , G.J.M van Kempen and J. H. M. Metz, EAAP Publication n° 69, Pudoc, Wageningen, Netherlands.

Köhler, T., Mosenthin, R., Verstegen, M.W.A., Huisman, J., Den Hartog, L.A. and Ahrens, F. (1992) Effect of ileo-rectal anastomosis and post-valve T-caecum cannulation on growing pigs. 1. Growth performance, N-balance and intestinal adaptation. *British Journal of Nutrition*, **68**, 293-303.

INRA-AFZ (2004) *Tables of Composition and Nutritive Value of Feed Materials.* Edited by D. Sauvant, J-M Perez and G. Tran. Wageningen Academic Publishers, Wageningen.

Laplace, J.P., Souffrant, W.B., Hennig, U., Chabeauti, E. and Février, C. (1994)

Measurement of precaecal dietary protein and plant cell wall digestion in pigs; comparison of four surgical procedures. *Livestock Production Science*, **40**, 313-328.

Leterme, P., Théwis, A., Beckers, Y. and Baudart, E. (1990) Apparent and true ileal digestibility of amino acids and nitrogen balance measured in pigs with ileo-rectal anastomosis or T-cannulas, given a diet containing peas. *Journal of the Science of Food and Agriculture*, **52**, 485-497.

Low, A.G. (1982) Digestibility and availability of amino acids from feedstuffs for pigs: a review. *Livestock Production Science*, **9**, 511-520.

Mariscal-Landin, G., Sève, B., Colléaux, Y. and Lebreton, Y. (1995) Endogenous amino nitrogen, collected from pigs with end-to-end ileorectal anastomosis is affected by the method of estimation and altered by dietary fiber. *Journal of Nutrition*; **125**, 136-146.

Moughan, P.J. and Righerford, S.M. (1996) A new method for determining digestible reactive lysine in foods. *J. Agric Food Chem.* **44**, 2202-2209.

Sève, B. (1994) Alimentation du porc en croissance: intégration des concepts de protéine idéale, de disponibilité digestive des acides aminés et d'énergie nette. *INRA Production Animale*, **7**, 275-291.

Sève, B., Mariscal-Landin, G., Février, C. and Lechevestrier, Y. (1994a) Prédiction de la digestibilité iléale des acides aminés chez le porc: Le cas des issues de blé. *Journées de la Recherche Porcine en France*, **25**, 259-266.

Sève, B., Mariscal-Landin, G., Colléaux, and Lebreton, Y. (1994b) Ileal endogenous amino acid and amino sugar flows in pigs fed graded levels of protein or fibre. In *Proceedings of the 6th International Symposium on Digestive Physiology in Pigs (Bad Doberan, 4-6th October 1994)*, vol. I, pp. 35-38. Edited by W. B. Souffrant and H. Hagemeister, EAAP Publication No. 80, Forschungsinstitut für die Biologie landwirtschaftlicher Nutztiere, Shriftenreihe 3, Dummerstorf, Germany.

Sève, B. and Henry Y. (1996) Protein utilization in non ruminants. In *Protein Metabolism and Nutrition,* pp. 59-82. Edited by A.F. Nunes, A.V. Portugal, J. P. Costa, J.R. Ribeiro. Proceedings of the 7$^{th}$ International Symposium, Vale de Santarém - Portugal 24-27 May 1995, EAAP-Publication n°81,. Estaçao Zootecnica, Santarém, Portugal.

Van Barneveld, R.J. (1993) Effect of heating proteins on the digestibility, availability and utilisation of lysine by growing pigs. *Ph.D. Thesis*, 221 pp, University of Queensland, Australia.

Wiseman, J., Jagger, S., Cole, D.J.A. and Haresign, W. (1991) The digestion and utilization of amino acids of heat-treated fish meal by growing/finishing pigs. *Animal Production*, **53**, 215-225.

Yin, Y.-L., Huang, R.-L. and Zhong, H.-Y. (1993). Comparison of ileorectal anastomosis and the conventional method for the measurement of ileal digestibility of protein sources and mixed diets in growing pigs. Animal Feed Science and Technology, **42**, 297-308.

*This paper was first published in 2000*

2

# GUT HEALTH AND IMMUNITY IN YOUNG PIGLETS

M VARLEY[1] and B MILLER[2]
[1]*SCA Nutrition, Dalton, Thirsk, North Yorkshire, YO7 3HE, UK*
[2]*University of Bristol, Langford House, Langford, Bristol BS40 5DU, UK*

## Introduction

The young pig at birth is immunologically naive having received no maternally derived antibodies across the placenta and it has not, at this time, established the ability to generate its own immunoglobulins. Throughout the next few days and weeks, the piglet acquires the ability to protect itself from pathogenic invasion in a number of separate and important ways.

Initially, the neonate must suckle the sow to receive passive protection from the high concentration of maternal immunoglobulins in the colostrum. These pass immediately into the piglet's blood stream across the gut wall whilst the gut is 'open' in the first 24 hours after birth. This provides systemic protection for the next 2-4 weeks of life; the level and length of this protection is directly proportional to the level of ingestion of colostrum.

Subsequently, from the moment of birth onwards, the piglet is exposed to the same pathogenic environment as the sow and the active immune system of the piglet gradually becomes 'educated' to respond by producing appropriate immune responses to these challenges. This second level of immunological protection over the early weeks of life also progressively becomes stronger and ultimately replaces passive protection from maternal antibodies.

It is also evident that the so-called non-specific immunological mechanisms gradually increase in functionality over the early days of life and these in effect are the front-line defences that will eliminate the bulk of pathogenic challenge before the programmed humoral and cell-mediated systems are brought into play. All of these functions coupled with the infection pressure that the young piglet is exposed to mediate the gut health status of the growing piglet.

The achievement of a high level of gut health, where the gut lumen and gut lining conditions are stable and the mucosal system is in equilibrium with the gut microbiotica, is crucial if neonatal and post-weaned piglets are to survive and grow rapidly towards the relative safety of maturity. In their 'natural' state piglets are not fully weaned until about 16 weeks of age and the whole process allows a steady transition to full immunological and nutritional independence (Held & Mendl 2001). In commercial practice the whole process is reduced to a single event at 3-4 weeks of age and this inevitably leads to many of the on-farm disease situations that develop.

The purpose of this chapter is to focus on those factors that can influence gut health in the young neonatal and post-weaned piglet and to explore the practical implications of these phenomena.

## Basic immunological principles

The basic immune system of the piglet is present at birth in that it has much of the cellular machinery available to mount immune responses. It is questionable, however, that the regulatory control mechanisms are so fully developed and thus piglets are at risk of not mounting an appropriate immune response.

Protective immune responses themselves arise from specific pathogenic challenges via the various routes of infection (dermal contact, inhalation, ingestion etc). Antibody molecules or immunoglobulin proteins are produced in response to this challenge and these bind directly to the various antigenic sites on pathogens, or indirectly on infected cells. This either helps neutralise or inactivate the pathogen. It is also important to remember that this mechanism is only one arm of the immune repertoire.

Cell-mediated immunity is also extremely important and the programmed T lymphocytes that contain large numbers of binding sites on their cell surfaces are highly potent immune factors. Not only do they bind to pathogenic antigens but they can also produce substances (cytokines) that directly kill pathogens. In addition, some cytokines have regulatory functions to act in a catalytic way during an immune response (T helper cells) or to shut down the response (T suppressor cells).

The regulatory functions in many ways are as important as the effector functions that kill bacterial and viral particles. Any inappropriate immune responses associated with prolonged action will be damaging to the animal's own tissues, due to the vast array and amounts of immune substances generated. This is what happens in allergic or hypersensitivity reactions.

All of these elements of the immune response work in close harmony to register a challenge, react to it appropriately, eliminate the cellular debris and then return quickly to quiescence. In reality this may not always work as efficiently as it should do and some disease situations are caused by the immune system itself. What is also clear is that the immunological education process necessary to programme this system is very delicate and there are key phases in the life of the animal when the correct signals are required. The neonatal phase is an important one in this respect.

## Gut development

There have been some excellent reviews on the developmental stages in gut development by Sangild, (2001) and by Stokes *et al.* (2001), but it is pertinent here to summarise the major changes that affect gut health.

### FOETAL STAGE

The development of the gut itself, from the late foetal stages onwards, moves very quickly from phase to phase. Some of these developmental changes are gene-driven, but environmental factors are at least as important. Reviews in this area have recently been prepared by Kelly and King (2001) and by Bailey *et al.* (2001) and attention will only be given to the major points.

The development of the cellular layers within the gut wall, from mid gestation onwards, shows rapid change. In particular the villus structures are important because of the enterocyte cells on their surfaces that are responsible for nutrient absorption; they are the ultimate interface between the internal environment (self) and the external environment (pathogenic challenge, food antigens and commensal bacteria).

As early as day 35, primitive villi appear on the foetal gut wall and, by day 110 of gestation, these are normal. Crypt development also begins by day 60 of gestation and is complete by full term. The foetus depends on parenteral nutrition for its growth and development, but foetuses also ingest about 20% of their body weight of amniotic fluid. There is a very low turnover of enterocyte cells during the foetal stages and oxygen uptake into the gut lining is at a relatively low level. It is probable that, if oxygen uptake is impeded further (perinatal stress), then this can adversely affect gut development through the neonatal stages and potentially could affect the predisposition of the post-weaning piglet to diarrhoea.

### POST NATAL PRE-SUCKING

In the first few hours after birth, the neonatal piglet incurs a profound change in its environment. In addition to the rigors of temperature change and the initiation of respiration, it is also in direct immediate and intimate contact with every pathogen that is present in the local environment. Most piglets will die within hours of birth under this challenge unless they can utilise their gene-driven instincts to move to the udder, locate a teat and ingest colostrum.

## POST-NATAL POST-SUCKING

The only way that fragile neonates can survive is to suckle very quickly and very effectively. This not only repletes the liver of vital glycogen and maintains metabolic homeostasis, but also helps to support thermoregulation in the first critical hours. Furthermore, survival prospects are directly proportional to the level of colostrum acquisition. At some point between 6 and 24 hours after birth, the gut wall can no longer absorb intact immunoglobulins (Igs), lymphocytes and growth factors (gut closure). There are considerable variations in suckling behaviour in the early days and weeks. In studies (M. Varley; unpublished), 5% of all viable piglets born did not suckle at all during the first 24 hours and, for those that did, Ig intake varied from about 2000 to 20,000 mg over the first 24 hours of life.

## POST-NATAL POST-CLOSURE

Following gut closure, immunoglobulins are used progressively in the process of immune defence and blood concentrations progressively fall. If early suckling is ineffective, Ig concentrations fall quickly to a level where systemic disease overtakes the piglet. During lactation, the piglet receives enteric protection from the IgA immunoglobulins present in milk.

There are also very rapid changes in the gut wall itself in relation to milk intake. The villus structures grow and the enterocytes, together with other cell types, change progressively over a 2-week period from immature to fully functional and mature. The intake achieved per piglet largely drives these changes. There are also crucial growth factors in colostrum, and in milk, such as epidermal growth factor (EGF) and TGFa (transforming growth factor), that are powerful agents for stimulating development. The insulin-like growth factors IGF-1 and IGF-2 are also known to be present in colostrum and milk in variable amounts that influence GIT (gastro-intestinal tract) development. There is, in addition, a GLP-2 peptide (glucagon like peptide), produced by the ileal-L cells, which also may be an important signal in GIT growth stimulation.

The gut is hence protected to a high degree by passive signals derived from milk at this time. It seems that piglets can be exposed to a very high level of infection pressure at this time, but they do not succumb to infection because of this passive protection. It is also likely that this infection pressure is absolutely necessary to allow immunological education and to set up the appropriate array of lymphocytes and Igs so that the piglet, at a much later stage, can survive independent of its dam.

## MID / END OF LACTATION

By mid lactation, gut development of the piglet is still directly influenced by the overall level of nutrient intake and the array of milk proteins and peptides. By this stage, however, the gut lining has a complex microflora consisting of about 500 species of bacteria, viruses and other microorganisms (Hillman, 2001). Exposure to this microflora enables the expression of all the genes involved in immunological defence. On the bacterial cell surfaces various glycans, oligosaccharides, proteins and lipids are expressed, which are antigenic determinants. The mucosal immune system gradually learns to generate appropriate and relevant molecules to deal in different ways with these antigens, but this is not a rapid and immediate process.

By the end of lactation (21-28 days) the healthy piglet gut has a very stable microbiotica, which is kept in balance by both the supply of IgA from the sow and also by the increasing supply of immuno-reactive cells and molecules from the piglets' own resources (active immunity). This latter system however may be far from mature, even by 28 days of age.

## POST-WEANING

Immediately after weaning there are significant changes and challenges for the young piglet and these are probably just as acute as the post-natal challenges. The IgA support from the sow is withdrawn and the environment changes (farrowing house to weaner house), which means new pathogens, new thermal environment and new nutrition; there is a tremendous opportunity for the prevailing microbial flora to develop in an adverse way for the piglet. Bacteria such as pathogenic *E.coli* strains tend to proliferate quickly, to the detriment of the more commensal and protective types, such as *lactobacillus* strains.

The outcome of these changes is that the rate of migration of enterocytes from the base of the villi to the tips is increased significantly and the length of the villous structures themselves is reduced. This has deleterious implications for nutrient absorption and feed intake capacity, so many piglets are pre-disposed to acute diarrhoea. Figure 2.1 illustrates how villus height and crypt depth change within hours of weaning. These observations have been repeated at many other laboratories around the world (Pluske *et al.*, 1996; van Beers-Schreurs 1996; Nabuurs, 1991; Hampson *et al.*, 1986)

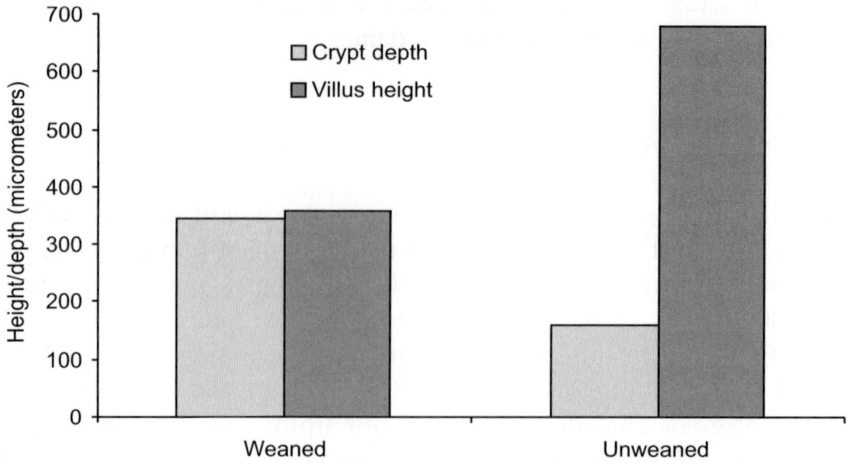


**Figure 2.1** The effect of weaning on villus height and crypt depth (Miller *et al.*, 1986)

It is possible, by careful environment and nutritional management, to maintain feed intake after weaning, but the villus structures take 7 to 10 days to recover their height and function.

There are, therefore, some important developmental phases that the gut structure must undergo during the early weeks of life if a normal healthy gut is to be sustained. Some of this is timed development under genetic control, but undoubtedly much of it is controlled by exposure to various environmental factors, including pathogens.

## Mucosal immunity and the young piglet

The mucosal immune system in the gut requires initiation and immunological education in the early weeks of life if the piglet is to reach a mature healthy state as quickly as possible. Whilst systemic or blood-borne immunity receives initial promotion from colostral antibodies, the gut wall (which is a major interface between the animal and its external environment) requires a separate route for protection. The mucosal immune system has evolved to provide this protection.

Milk contains IgA and other classes of antibodies throughout lactation and these, as they pass onto the gut mucosal surfaces, provide a constant protective barrier to pathogenic invasion. They can bind and inactivate antigens directly and the IgA molecules are protected from proteolysis by their dimer structure and the so-called J chain protein that connects the two main chains.

There is also a very rapid transfer of antigen-programmed lymphocytes from the gut wall of the sow directly to the mammary gland itself, where they produce relevant immunoglobulins that are immediately available to the suckling piglet. This is known as the gut-mammary link. This very elegant biological defence system ensures also that whatever the sow is exposed to by ingestion is very rapidly translated into the correct neutralising antibody proteins that appear quickly in the milk and hence give the right array of protective immunoglobulins on the piglet's gut wall.

As time progresses up to weaning, whilst the piglet receives this defence package, the gut wall is exposed to these same antigens and the active mucosal system gradually gathers the ability (immunological education) to generate its own antibody molecules in the gut wall.

There are a number of specialised lymphoid areas and cell types in the gut mucosal layer and attached to the small intestine (Peyer's Patches, M cells) that facilitate these functions, and these systems are now well understood. Basically, any antigen recognized by the gut wall is transported across the wall itself and presented by the M cells to the lymphoid cells within a Peyer's patch. This stimulates the generation of programmed lymphocytes (T & B) that are in turn delivered back to the gut wall and lodge in the *lamina propria* tissue layer. These immunologically programmed cells proliferate and accommodate the gut lining in this way and can produce rapid IgA responses or T cell reactions as principal effector functions that control the gut microbiotica in a beneficial way for gut health.

## DEVELOPMENTAL STAGES AND MUCOSAL IMMUNE FUNCTION

In the same way that the general immune system and the gut itself undergo distinct developmental stages, the mucosal immune system also has timed elements that are gene driven and there are also antigen driven developments that are time-independent. The B & T lymphocyte cell lines that lodge in the *lamina propria*, for example, double in number over the first four weeks of life. This is also a period when mature regulatory T cell function is developing.

In the neonatal period, generally, there are very few lymphocytes in either epithelial or *lamina propria* regions of the intestine. There are also no Peyer's Patches at this early stage. Over the period from birth to 14 days of age, the intestine is rapidly colonised with lymphocytes but not CD4+ (helper) cells or CD8+ (effector) cells. Peyer's Patches develop to 'normal' by 15 days of age. Between 14 and 28 days of age, the intestinal mucosa becomes colonised with CD4+ T cells in the lamina propria. CD8+ cells however are still absent at this time. Small numbers of B cells begin to appear (IgM producing) during this period.

From 35 days of age onwards, CD8+ cells begin to appear in intestinal epithelium and the basement membrane. In the crypt area many IgA+ B cells are evident. It is not until the piglet is 7 weeks of age that the immunological architecture can be considered fully mature. It is therefore self-evident that the practice of weaning at 3 weeks of age involves removing an immunologically compromised piglet from its main source of protection, the sow. Weaning later at even 28 days of age means a better chance of avoiding gut health problems due to immuno-incompetence.

## IMMUNO-REACTION VERSUS IMMUNO-REGULATION

Any food antigens passing through the gut during the processes of digestion and absorption can generate similar mucosal responses to those described above. If the mucosal system reacted in this way to every single food protein and food particle, the immune system would be overwhelmed with activity and a disease situation would probably result from this overreaction. Miller *et al.* (1994) and Wilson *et al.* (1989) carried out much work in this area and this programme is still continuing (Bailey *et al.,* 2001) to understand these mechanisms.

In order to offset these effects, the gut from birth onwards must learn, and continue to learn, what is a harmless food or commensal bacterial antigen (which must be ignored) and what is a potentially harmful pathogenic antigen towards which a vigorous immune response must be brought to bear. The phenomenon of immune tolerance is an important component of this learning development. If intimate presentation of antigen is made to the gut wall at the right stage of development (neonatal stage) then a variety of mechanisms are initiated such as the generation and recruitment of T suppressor cell lines that close down future reactions to these antigens before they waste resources and do damage. There are a number of such regulatory mechanisms that are extremely important in allowing the animal to express responses to pathogens whilst leaving alone the normal food proteins and other antigenic particles.

The neonatal period is a time when the gut is particularly sensitive to this immunological tolerogenesis process. The piglet can therefore be exposed to a whole host of food substances and learns not to react to them, whilst the gut is effectively protected by the passive IgA delivered via colostrum and milk. The process of immuno-regulation, however, continues throughout life and, for some food antigens, constant exposure may be required if immune tolerance is to be maintained. Immune tolerance to antigens can be induced in a number of ways, but the two principal components are high zone tolerance, where the gut or other mucosal surface is challenged with a very sudden high level of exposure to antigen, and low zone tolerance, where a smaller dose is given and maintained over a very prolonged period.

Much work has been carried out in this area using the young piglet as a model. Miller *et al.* (1984 1986) have suggested that at weaning, piglets are highly predisposed to hypersensitivity reactions against their feed ingredients, which induce acute diarrhoea and high mortality rates. In commercial practice, much post-weaning enteric disease may well be ascribed to reactions of this kind. Producers overcome this problem by offering a creep feed in the correct way to ensure that sufficient food antigen is given over a long period, from about 7 days of age to weaning at 21-28 days of age. Tolerance is achieved before weaning and the piglet subsequently has no problems. This latter strategy may be the preferred option in most cases because of the added benefits of a significantly better weaning weight, which may be increased by 1 kg when a good quality creep feed is used (Varley and Cole, 2000) and because of the enhancement of the enzyme system before the piglet is weaned. The only problem is ensuring sufficient creep intake, which can be difficult when weaning as young as 21 days.

Clearly the mucosal immune system is in a delicate balance before and after weaning; the balance between immuno-reaction (to pathogens) and immuno-regulation can be influenced by management and nutritional practices.

## The neonatal piglet and colostrum

There are a number of pitfalls for the piglet in this overall system where immunological protection may fail. Lack of sufficient colostrum initially represents a major source of variation in the later functionality of the system. Moreover, a lack of the relevant antigenic signals or stimulation may also be a prelude for immunological incompetence at a later stage. The piglet probably requires a steady exposure to antigens (pathogens, commensals and food antigens) throughout lactation, at a time when it has profound gut immunological protection from milk, if it is to survive the later weeks.

The neonatal hours and days are particularly crucial, in both the establishment of immuno-regulation machinery and in the acquisition of passive protection, for immediate and long-term survival prospects.

Work carried out in the 1980s (Varley, Maitland & Ross, 1986; Varley, Maitland & Towle, 1986; Varley, Wilkinson & Maitland, 1987), using colostrum-deprived piglets reared under aseptic conditions from birth onwards, showed that where colostrum is not ingested by the neonatal piglet, not only are the immediate health and survival prospects of that piglet compromised, but the long-term prospects for normal immunological development are impaired for a very prolonged period (See Figure 2.2). These piglets were reared in a highly biosecure environment for the first two weeks of life and were then transferred to more conventional flat-deck cages, but still in very high hygiene conditions. They were not exposed to piglets reared normally until six weeks of age. On transfer to conventional grower/ finisher accommodation, there was a very high level of morbidity and mortality until slaughter at 90 kg. It seemed that, despite even long-term exposure to a conventional pig unit environment, the mature immune systems in these colostrum-deprived pigs could not yield the necessary responses. In part, of course, these observations were due to lack of antigenic challenge, but the lack of colostrum signals (growth factors, Igs) appeared to be an overriding component that was missing.

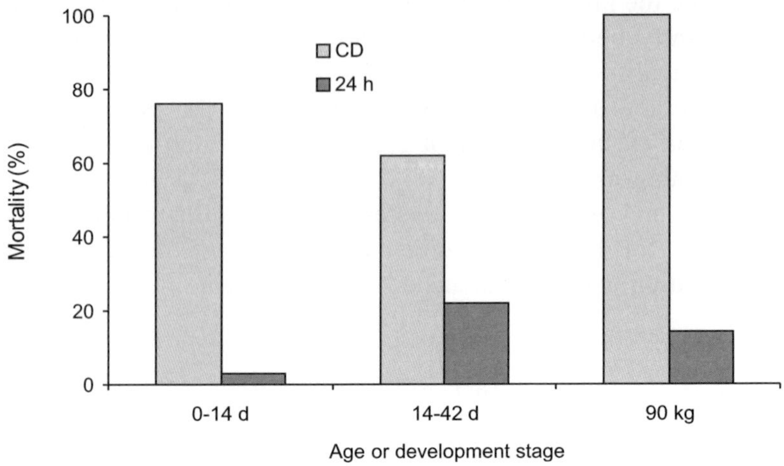


**Figure 2.2** The effect of weaning at birth with no colostral ingestion (colostrum deprived - CD) or 24 h of suckling on mortality to 90 kg (Varley, Maitland and Ross, 1986)

It might be speculated that, under more normal farming conditions, many of the enteric diseases that are seen could be due to variations in colostrum delivery (and ingestion) and to inappropriate immunological development in very early life.

Weaning is a significant immunological event for piglets. In the wild, weaning is a prolonged process of transition, but in commercial practice it is carried out abruptly between 3 to 4 weeks after birth, when the active protective mechanisms are still under construction. At a stroke, the supply of protective IgA immunoglobulins is withdrawn and the piglet is transferred to new accommodation and mixed into a new social group. The stress of weaning in its own right induces a depletion of the ability to mount immune responses (Blecha & Kelley, 1981). The piglet is also faced with the added problem of adapting quickly to a new programme of nutrition, usually in the form of a dry feed. It may not have encountered this before and it also has to find and learn to use a novel drinking system before it dehydrates.

There is good evidence that all of these facets of the weaning event have a serious deleterious effect on the gut wall (Kelly & King 2001, Bailey *et al.*,

2001) and, as a consequence, the cellular machinery of the mucosal immune system. The combined effects of stress and food withdrawal cause a much more rapid migration of the enterocytes on the villi structures on the gut wall. This leads to impaired villi function because they are reduced significantly in height, with an associated depression in mean crypt depth. This is also associated with a reduction in mucosal immune function and gut health suffers the consequences. The bacterial colonies on the gut wall change in favour of a pathogenic flora and the animal develops diarrhoea.

## Feeding practices

The foregone discussion suggests that there are some tactics that can be used commercially or nutritionally to alleviate the worst effects of these phenomena. Weaning later, for example, can allow a greater level of passive gut protection and ensures that the piglet's own active mechanisms are at the highest level possible before it has to cope independently. There is good evidence that both humoral and cell-mediated immune mechanisms are depressed when early weaning takes place (Varley, 1995; Blecha & Kelley 1981). Figure 2.3 presents data from work using a phytahaemaglutinin skin test to assess the activity of the cell-mediated immune system of pigs at 42 days of age, after weaning at 10, 20, 30 and 40 days of age. Clearly, cell-mediated immunity was progressively depressed as weaning age decreased.

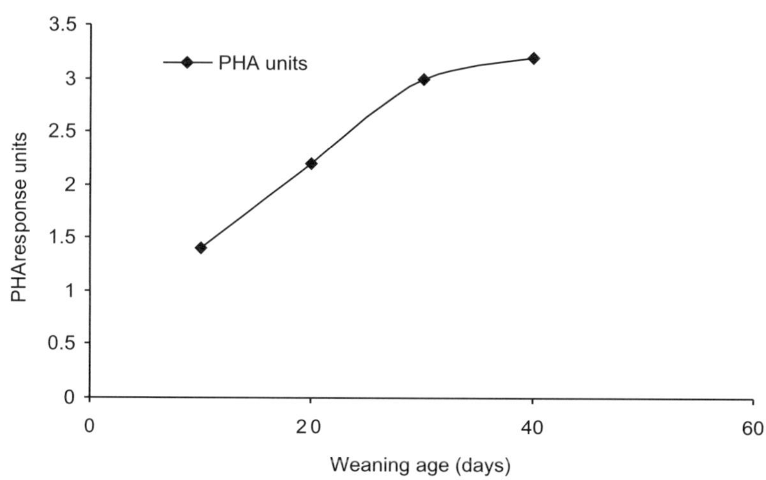


**Figure 2.3** The influence of weaning age on cell-mediated immunity (Varley 1995)

The nutritional package itself is also important. If the enzyme and immunological system has been primed by an effective pre-weaning feeding regime (creep feed), it is more likely that the animal will successfully make the transition from pre to post-weaning.

The post-weaning diet itself is also a prime factor. Protective proteins and a highly digestible energy source in the form of pre-cooked cereals and refined milk proteins can be built into the feeding regime to go towards substituting for the withdrawal of antibody support from the sow. There is also no doubt that the prevailing level of health status on a particular farm is very important because this reduces the overall burden on the immune system and gives a better chance to acquire appropriate immunological education before being swamped by pathogenic challenge. Koutos and Klasing (2001), for example, showed that when the immune system is activated by antigenic challenge, up to 6% of feed energy is diverted towards the immunological reaction. With multiple challenges that exist on some farms, it is obvious that this will severely affect food conversion and growth performance, even if disease is not evident.

The absolute level of feed (energy/protein) intake is also a key factor in achieving a high order of gut health after weaning. The work on villus function in the young piglet has shown how these structures are affected by the weaning event. It has also been shown (Pluske *et al.,* 2001) that this effect can be reduced significantly if feed energy intake can be maintained or increased (Figure 2.4). Moreover, the use of milk proteins in the post-weaning diets rather than alternative (vegetable) proteins can also reduce the worst effects of villus depression. Feed intake is notoriously variable in the post-weaned piglet and there is an urgent need to understand why this is so.

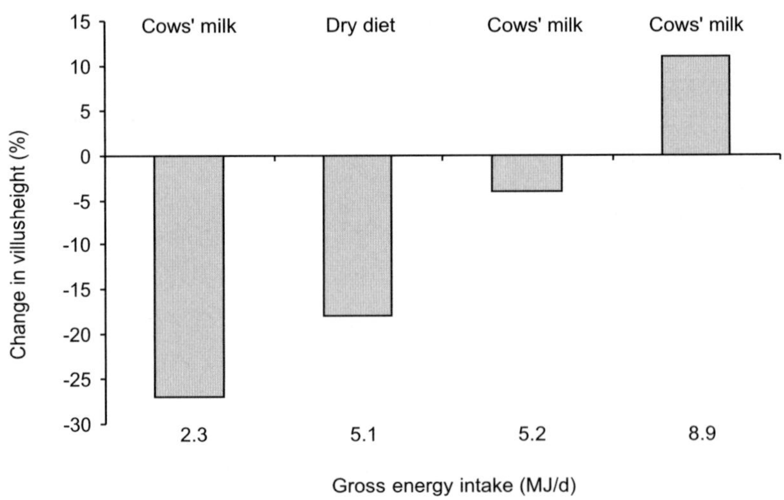


**Figure 2.4** The effect of feed energy intake and source of dietary protein on villus height after weaning (Pluske 1996)

## Conclusions

In conclusion, it is clear that the links between nutrition, immunology and gut health status are profound. Gut health is intimately connected to nutrient absorption efficiency across the gut wall and, as a consequence, food conversion efficiency and growth. In the past, antibiotics have been used to control gut microflora, gut health and growth, but the current socio-political environment increasingly precludes their use. Other tools are available for use in this context, such as acidulants, probiotics and prebiotics, and there are various immuno-stimulatory compounds that can augment mucosal reactions and control gut health. Undoubtedly, these will all be used widely in the future, but more basic research is required to understand their functions to a higher degree and to be able to predict more accurately the likely outcomes when they are used on farms. Subsequently, it will be possible to increase on-farm piglet performance and health to a much higher order than that achieved at the present time.

## References

Bailey, M., Vega-Lopez, M.A., Rothkötter, H-J., Bland, P.W., Miller, B.J. and Stokes, C.R. 2001. Enteric immunity and gut health. In *The Weaner Pig: Nutrition and Management.* M. A. Varley and J. Wiseman. CABI Publishing. UK. pp 207-222.

Blecha, F. and Kelley, K.W. 1981. Effects of cold and weaning stressors on the antibody-mediated immune response of pigs. *Journal of Animal Science* **53**: 439-447.

Bruininx, E.M.A.M., van der Peet-Schwering, C.M.C and Schrama, J.W. Individual feed intake of group-housed weaned pigs and health status. In *The Weaner Pig: Nutrition and Management.* ed. M. A. Varley and J. Wiseman. CABI Publishing. UK. pp 113-122.

Held, S. and Mendl, M. 2001. Behaviour of the young weaner pig. . In *The Weaner Pig: Nutrition and Management.* ed. M. A. Varley and J. Wiseman. CABI Publishing. UK. pp 273-298.

Hampson, D.J. and Kidder, D.E. 1986. Influence of creep feeding and weaning on brush border enzyme activities in the piglet small intestine. *Research in Veterinary Science* **40**: 24-31.

Hillman, K. (2001) Bacteriological aspects of the use of antibiotics and their alternatives in the feed of non-ruminant animals. In *Recent Advances in Animal Nutrition - 2001* (Eds. P.C. Garnsworthy and J. Wiseman), pp 107-134. Nottingham University Press, Nottingham.

Kelly, D and King, T.P., 2001. Digestive physiology and development in pigs. In *The Weaner Pig. Nutrition and Management.* ed. M. A. Varley and J. Wiseman. CABI Publishing. UK. pp 179-206.

Koutos, E.A. and Klasing, K.C. 2001. Interactions between the immune system, nutrition and productivity of animals. In *Recent Advances in*

*Animal Nutrition - 2001* (Eds. P.C. Garnsworthy and J. Wiseman), pp 173-190. Nottingham University Press, Nottingham.

Miller, B.J., Newby, T.J., Stokes, C.R. and Bourne, F.J. 1984. Influence of diet on post-weaning malabsorbtion and diarrhoea in the pig. *Research in Veterinary Science*. **36**: 187-193.

Miller, B.J., James, P.S., Smith, M.W. and Bourne, F.J. 1986. Effect of weaning on the capacity of pig intestinal villi to digest and absorb nutrients. *Journal of Agricultural Science* Cambridge **107**: 579:589.

Miller, B.G., Whittemore, C.T., Stokes, C.R and Telemo, E. 1994. The effect of delayed weaning on the development of oral tolerance to soyabean protein in pigs. *British Journal of Nutrition* **71**: 615-625.

Nabuurs, M.J.A. 1991. Etiologic and pathogenic studies on post-weaning diarrhoea. PhD dissertation. State University Utrecht, The Netherlands

Pluske, J.R., Williams, I.H. and Aherne, X. 1996. Villous height and crypt depth in piglets in response to increases in the intake of cows' milk after weaning. *Animal Science* **62**:145-158.

Pluske, J.R., Kim, J.C., McDonald, D.F., Pethick, D.W. and Hampson, D.J. 2001. Non-starch polysaccharides in the diets of young weaned piglets. In *The Weaner Pig. Nutrition and Management.* ed. M. A. Varley and J. Wiseman. CABI Publishing. UK. pp 81-112.

Sangild, P.T. 2001. Transitions in the life of the gut at birth. . In *Digestive Physiology of Pigs*. Ed. J.E Lindberg and B. Ogle. CABI Publishing. UK. pp 3-17.

Stokes, C.R., Bailey, M. and Haverson, K. 2001. Development and function of the pig gastrointestinal immune system. In *Digestive Physiology of Pigs*. Ed. J.E Lindberg and B. Ogle. CABI Publishing. UK. pp 59-66.

Van Beers-Schreurs, H.M.G. 1996. The changes in the function of the small intestine of weaned piglets. PhD dissertation, Faculty of Veterinary Medicine, Utrecht University, The Netherlands.

Varley, M.A. 1995. The effects of weaning age on cell-mediated immunity in weaned piglets. University of Leeds Project 1995.

Varley, M.A and Cole, M.A. 2000. Reaping returns from higher weaning weights. *Pig World*. August 2000. **48** (8) 2-3.

Varley, M.A., Maitland, A. and Ross, L.N. 1986. The performance of piglets weaned at birth or one day of age and the use of oral vaccines against E. coli antigens. *Livestock Production Science* **15**: 83-95.

Varley, M.A., Maitland, A. and Towle, A. 1986. Artificial rearing of piglets: the administration of two sources of immunoglobulins after birth. *Animal Production* **43**:121-126.

Varley, M.A., Wilkinson, R.G. and Maitland, A. 1987. Artificial rearing of baby piglets: the effect of colostrum on survival and plasma concentrations of IgG. *British Veterinary Journal* **143**: 369-378.

Wilson,. A.D., Stokes, C.R. and Bourne, F.J. 1989. Effect of age on absorption and immune responses to weaning or introduction of novel dietary antigens in pigs. *Research in Veterinary Science* **46**:180-186.

*This paper was first published in 2002*

3

# POST WEANING MULTISYSTEMIC WASTING SYNDROME (PMWS) IN PIGS

A. GRESHAM
*Veterinary Laboratories Agency, New Haw, Addlestone, Surrey, KT15 3NB, UK*

## Introduction

Post weaning multisystemic wasting syndrome (PMWS) is the name given to a wasting disease of weaned pigs, which was first identified in Western Canada in 1991 (Harding, 1996). PMWS commonly occurs in 6-14 week old pigs and is clinically characterised particularly by wasting leading to cachexia, dyspnoea, lymph node enlargement, diarrhoea, cutaneous pallor and jaundice. PMWS is associated with variable but sometimes high levels of morbidity and mortality. PMWS has now been reported in many pig-producing countries around the world (Table 3.1) but at present in 2001 it is of particular significance in Western Europe. Due to the high and protracted levels of morbidity and mortality, PMWS is of particular economic importance. In 2001 the aetiology, pathogenesis and many other aspects of PMWS have yet to be fully understood but there are now strong indications that infection with a porcine circovirus type 2 (PCV-2) is central to the development of this disease.

Recent experience in several countries, but especially in France, has indicated that improvements in basic management and hygiene on affected farms may greatly reduce the incidence of disease associated with PMWS.

## Background

Although the syndrome of PMWS was first identified in 1991, it was not until PCV-2 was first identified (Mehan *et al.*, 1998) and tests were developed for this virus, that associations between PCV-2 and PMWS were possible. These associations have evolved gradually. Some of this evolution may have been delayed by problems in differentiating PMWS from other diseases, in particular

**Table 3.1** COUNTRIES IN WHICH PMWS AND PDNS HAVE BEEN REPORTED WITH REFERENCES TO INDICATE THE SOURCE OF THE REPORT

| *Country* | *PMWS reported* | *PDNS reported* |
|---|---|---|
| Argentina | | +(42) |
| Australia | | +(9) |
| Austria | + (63) | |
| Belgium | +(17) | |
| Canada | + (25) | +(28) |
| Chile | | +(53) |
| Czechoslovakia | +(16) | |
| Denmark | + (6) | |
| France | + (40) | |
| Germany | + (31) | |
| Greece | + (36) | |
| Hungary | +(34) | |
| Ireland | + (72) | +(28) |
| Italy | +(46) | +(64) |
| Japan | + (61) | |
| Lithuania | + (54) | |
| Mexico | +(79) | |
| Netherlands | +(17) | |
| Poland | +(55) | |
| South Korea | + (10) | |
| South Africa | | + (80) |
| Spain | + (67) | +(66) |
| Taiwan | + (17) | |
| Thailand | +(63) | |
| United Kingdom | + (33) | +(70) |
| United States of America | + (13) | +(56) |

from porcine reproductive and respiratory syndrome (PRRS) which, after it was first identified in the USA in 1987 to 1988, has been a very commonly diagnosed infectious cause of post weaning disease and death in pigs in many countries. However, further problems that were identified following the development of tests for PCV-2 were: 1) the understanding that PCV-2 infection is already widespread in pigs in several countries (where testing has been carried out) (Allan and Ellis, 2001). This includes some countries where PMWS is not a major problem. 2) The understanding, from retrospective testing, that PCV-2 has been present in some pig populations around the world for many years before PMWS was identified. (Table 3.2). But the reality of PMWS in the last few years is that epizootics of a recognisable and severe new disease syndrome have occurred, and this has spread with all the characteristics of an infectious disease. This disease has been especially severe in Western European

**Table 3.2** YEAR OF FIRST IDENTIFICATION OF PMWS, PDNS AND RETROSPECTIVE IDENTIFICATION OF PCV-2 IN COUNTRIES AS INDICATED WITH REFERENCES TO INDICATE THE SOURCE OF THE REPORT RELATING TO THE IDENTIFICATION OF PCV-2

| *Year* | *Identification of PCV-2 infection* | *Identification of PMWS* | *Identification of PDNS* |
|---|---|---|---|
| 1973 | Northern Ireland (82) | | |
| 1974 | | | |
| 1975 | | | |
| 1976 | | | Chile |
| 1977 | | | |
| 1978 | | | |
| 1979 | | | |
| 1980 | | | |
| 1981 | | | |
| 1982 | | | |
| 1983 | | | |
| 1984 | | | |
| 1985 | Canada (48), Japan (61) | | |
| 1986 | England (30), Spain (59) | | |
| 1987 | | | England, Netherlands |
| 1988 | | | |
| 1989 | | | |
| 1990 | | | Northern Ireland |
| 1991 | Germany (63) | Canada | Scotland |
| 1992 | Denmark (6) | | |
| 1993 | USA (71) | | |
| 1994 | | | |
| 1995 | | France | Canada |
| 1996 | | USA | Spain |
| 1997 | | Spain | France, USA |
| 1998 | | Austria, Denmark, Germany, Ireland, Italy, Netherlands, Northern Ireland | |
| 1999 | | England, Japan, Korea, Portugal, Taiwan | |
| 2000 | | Greece | |
| 2001 | | Czechoslovakia, Mexico, Poland, Scotland | |

countries including the United Kingdom (primarily England and excluding Northern Ireland, Scotland and Wales), Spain, France, Italy, Germany and the Netherlands. In these countries and particularly in England, Spain and the Netherlands, PMWS has been closely associated with epizootics of porcine dermatitis and nephropathy syndrome (PDNS) in finishing pigs, and it appears

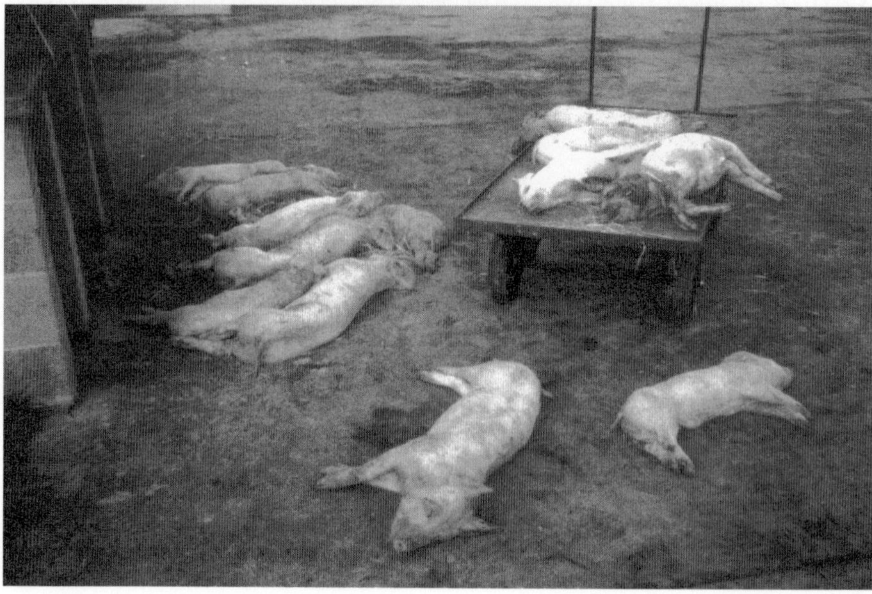

**Figure 3.1** PMWS. A day's mortality on one farm.

that these diseases are linked (Gresham *et al.,* 2001). Although the cause of PDNS remains unclear, epizootic PDNS is clinically different (if only in incidence) from a sporadic disease consistent with PDNS that was first described by Morales and Guzman (1976) in Chile. The term 'porcine dermatitis and nephropathy syndrome' was first used by Smith *et al.* (1993) to describe outbreaks of PDNS that had been recognised since 1987 in England, Wales and Scotland. PDNS has now been reported from many countries around the world (Table 3.1). Between 1993 and 1998, an annual average of nine incidents of sporadic PDNS were recorded in England, Wales and Scotland by the Veterinary Laboratories Agency (VLA) and the Scottish Agricultural Colleges (SAC).

In the UK, PMWS was first reported in 1998 in Northern Ireland (Spillane, Kennedy, Mehan and Allan, 1998). In the autumn of 1999 many outbreaks of PMWS, often coupled with epizootics of PDNS, were identified in East Anglia and in the south east and south west of England (Gresham *et al.,* 2000), (Table 3.3). In December 1999 and April and December 2000 the VLA carried out three surveys of Veterinary Practitioners in England and Wales to indicate the prevalence and incidence of PMWS and PDNS.

The cumulative results of these three surveys are indicated in Table 3.4. By mid-December 2000 the reports from Veterinary Practitioners indicated that

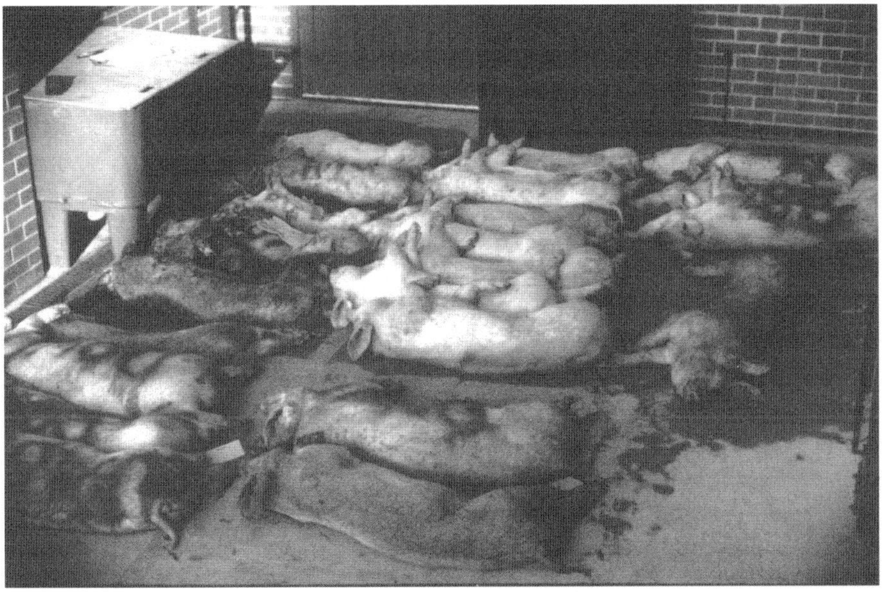

**Figure 3.2** PDNS. Dead pigs from several farms collected for post mortem examination.

**Table 3.3** DIAGNOSES (SEPARATE FARM INCIDENTS) OF PMWS (IN ENGLAND ONLY) AND PDNS (IN GB) RECORDED BY VLA AND SAC BETWEEN 1993 AND 2000

| *Year* | *Diagnoses of PMWS* | *Diagnoses of PDNS* |
|---|---|---|
| 1993 | Nil (not recorded) | 12 |
| 1994 | Nil (not recorded) | 23 |
| 1995 | Nil (not recorded) | 5 |
| 1996 | Nil (not recorded) | 6 |
| 1997 | Nil (not recorded) | 1 |
| 1998 | Nil (not recorded) | 7 |
| 1999 | 10 | 22 |
| 2000 | 70 | 86 |

PMWS and PDNS had affected between 75 and 80% of herds in the Eastern Region of England. In England and Wales as a whole, a total of 796 herds (between 18 and 20% of pig holdings with >100 sows and/or >200 growers according to the 1999 census) had been affected.

The case fatality reported in incidents of PMWS in England ranged from <1% to 100% in some batches of pigs, but with an average of between 10 and 15%. The case fatality reported in incidents of PDNS in England ranged from <1% to 100% in some batches of pigs, but with an average of between 5 and 10%.

**Table 3.4** NUMBER OF PIG HOLDINGS* IN ENGLAND AND WALES ON WHICH PMWS AND/OR PDNS WAS REPORTED BY VETERINARY PRACTITIONERS BETWEEN 1/8/99 AND 10/12/00

| *Region* | *No of pig holdings** | *No of holdings on which PMWS reported between 1/8/99 and 10/12/00* | *No of holdings on which PDNS reported between 1/8/99 and 10/12/00* |
|---|---|---|---|
| North East | 95 | 0 | 0 |
| North West including Merseyside | 233 | 1 | 2 |
| Yorkshire and Humberside | 1384 | 12 | 8 |
| East Midlands | 425 | 4 | 6 |
| West Midlands | 327 | 0 | 5 |
| Eastern | 1107 | 278 | 417 |
| South East | 336 | 9 | 123 |
| South West | 589 | 21 | 21 |
| Wales | 77** | 0 | 0 |
| **Totals** | **4573**** | **325** | **471** |

(* Number of pig holdings with >100 sows and/or >200 growers according to the 1999 census. **The number of pig holdings for Wales was not given for the 1999 census. The figure of 77 is from the 1998 census).

Currently (Autumn 2001), PMWS has only been recorded on one farm in Scotland. Between August 1999 and December 2000 pigs on only three farms were reportedly diagnosed with PDNS. Within these herds, only 0.5 per cent of pigs were affected with PDNS (Thomson *et al.*, 2000; Gresham and Thomson, 2001). Currently, the prevalence and incidence of PMWS and PDNS in the UK is unclear. To date further surveys have not been possible due to the effects of the outbreak of foot and mouth disease, which occurred in the UK from February 2001. Even so, there are now indications of spread of PMWS and PDNS to other parts of England, particularly into Yorkshire and Humberside.

The effects of widespread and severe PMWS and PDNS in England have had significant regional and national effects on the pig industry. The increased post weaning morbidity and mortality affected production at farm, regional and national levels leading to knock-on effects on abattoirs and retailers. PMWS and PDNS have also affected pig welfare and disrupted the sale of breeding stock. Most importantly, the clinico-pathological similarities of both PMWS and PDNS to African swine fever (ASF) and classical swine fever (CSF) led to serious concerns regarding ASF and CSF (Done, 2001). This is of major significance considering the recent epizootic of CSF in Europe and the smaller outbreak of CSF in East Anglia in the autumn of 2000.

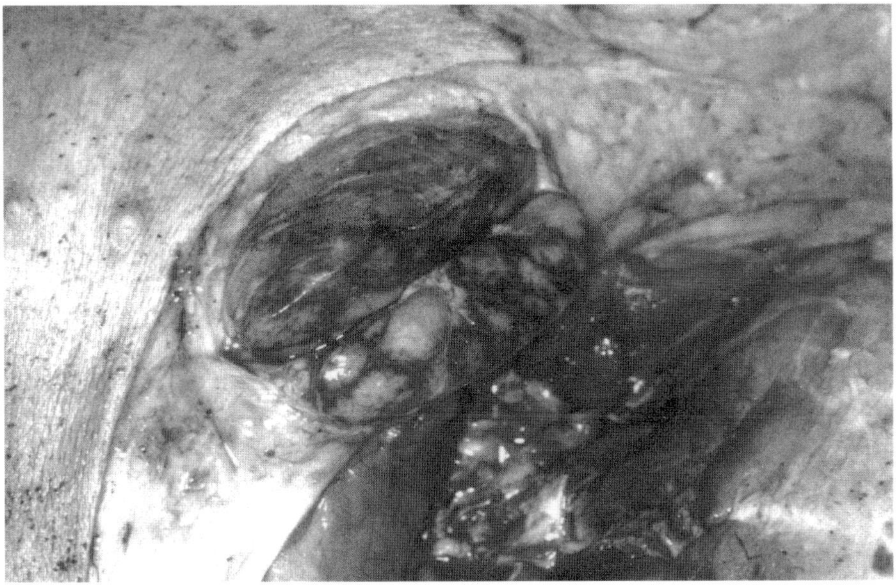

**Figure 3.3** PDNS. Enlargement and haemorrhage of a superficial inguinal lymph node. This appearance is consistent with possible swine fever.

Experience of individual outbreaks of PMWS and of the general spread of this disease in England has indicated a possible feed association but this is far from proven and farm trials involving feed changes have had only limited effects on controlling the disease. In addition, a case-control study (Cook *et al.*, 2001) carried out on breeder-finisher farms in England and Wales did not indicate an association with mouldy feed nor with mycotoxins. However, on many farms, the application of management techniques that reduce stress and infection pressure have significantly reduced the incidence of disease associated with PMWS. Even so, a full understanding of the disease and complete control has not yet been achieved.

There are, therefore, a number of fundamental questions that remain to be answered:

a If PCV-2 is the aetiological agent causing PMWS, is it the same PCV-2 that has been identified retrospectively in samples before the PMWS epizootics occurred or is it a new strain?

b. If it is the same PCV-2 that was identified retrospectively, why is PMWS spreading like a new disease?

c. Even if it is or is not the same strain of PCV-2, what causes pigs to develop PMWS? Is it PCV-2 infection alone or are other infections or non-infectious environmental/infectious/management/nutritional factors required?

d. Why are so many outbreaks of PMWS so severe (in terms of morbidity and mortality)?

e. Why are so many outbreaks of PMWS so protracted (often up to 18-24 months)?

f. How are PMWS and PDNS linked?

## Aetiology

According to Krakowka *et al.* (2000), Koch's postulates have been fulfilled for PCV-2 as the sole cause of PMWS in gnotobiotic pigs. This is now widely accepted. However Krakowka *et al.* (2000) also concluded that exposure of piglets to undefined environmental factors and/or infectious agents that facilitate stimulation of the piglet's immune system may be necessary, in conjunction with exposure to PCV-2, to produce clinical disease.

In 1974 a circovirus, which is now termed porcine circovirus type 1 (PCV-1), was identified as a contaminant of a pig kidney cell line (Tischer *et al.*, 1974). PCV-1 is considered non-pathogenic in pigs and is thought to be widespread in pig populations in many countries around the world (Allan and Ellis, 2001). It was against the historical background of the recognition of PCV-1 that, in 1998, PCV-2 was first reported to have been isolated in Canada from lesions of pigs affected with PMWS (Mehan *et al*, 1998). Shortly after this, isolates of PCV-2 were made from pigs affected with PMWS in many countries, and further reports of PMWS were made from more countries around the world (Table 3.2). PCV-2 has also been reported to be associated with congenital tremor type AII (Hines and Lukert, 1994), foetal myocarditis and abortion (West *et al.*, 1999), proliferative necrotising pneumonia Harding (2001), and PDNS (Segales *et al.,* 1998).

Both PCV-1 and PCV-2 are small (17nm) non-enveloped DNA viruses containing a single-stranded circular genome. Circoviruses have been identified in other animal species including chicken infectious anaemia virus (CIAV) in domestic fowl, psittacine beak and feather disease virus (PBFDV) in psittacines, and pigeon circovirus (PiCV) in pigeons. While the virions of PCV-1 and PCV-2, PBFDV and PiCV are of similar size, CIAV is slightly larger at 25 – 26.5 nm. Although these viruses all have similar protein components and nucleic acid characteristics, there are also several specific differences in the protein and nucleic acid characteristics of CIAV in particular. Accordingly CIAV has been assigned to a new genus named *Gyrovirus* within the Circovirus family. PBFDV and PCV-1 and PCV-2 are members of the genus *Circovirus.* PiCV is currently classified as an unassigned member of the Circovirus family

(Todd, 2000, Todd, 2001). Circoviruses are recognised in a number of other avian species but these will not be discussed here.

Information available on the biophysical properties of PCV-2 virus indicates that it is highly resistant to heating, freezing, exposure to ultraviolet light and chemical disinfectants (Krakowka *et al.,* 2000) and it is likely that PCV-2, as other circoviruses, will persist for long periods in the environment (Todd, 2000).

## Epizootiology and pathogenesis

Serological surveys have indicated wide seroprevalence of PCV-2 infection in several countries and, where possible, retrospective testing has indicated that this has been present for some years - well before PMWS was identified. Retrospective serological testing has been reported from Northern Ireland, Canada, Japan, Spain, Germany, Denmark and the USA, and retrospective in-situ hybridisation on paraffin-fixed material from England (Table 3.3). In particular, whereas PMWS was first identified in Northern Ireland in 1998, retrospective serology indicated that PCV-2 infection was present in the pig population there at least as long ago as 1973 (Walker *et al.*, 2000).

In England, PMWS spread between herds with the features of an infectious disease. The means of spread of PMWS between individual pigs and herds remains unclear, but clinical observations in outbreaks of natural disease indicate that both vertical and horizontal transmission are likely.

In England, the initial dissemination of PMWS and PDNS in the autumn of 1999 appeared to largely follow the movement of pigs from affected herds. Disease associated with PMWS and PDNS was particularly severe on rearing and finishing units operated by large integrated pig producing companies. On these rearing and finishing units, pigs from multiple sources were mixed together. When pigs from affected farms were not placed on these units, in some, but not all cases, the incidence of PMWS and PDNS was reduced. This indicated that the main means of transmission is by movement of pigs from one affected farm to another.

Lateral transmission of PMWS, from affected herds into unaffected pig herds without any pig movements between the two, has also been reported. Many of these sites are either outdoor herds or straw barns, where there is no control over bird movements. Veterinary practitioners in England are now generally of the opinion that birds are probably a significant (mechanical) vector of PMWS.

Although PCV-2 was reported to have been identified in semen (Larochelle *et al.*, 2000), in this and subsequent reports, the virus has not been proven to be viable or infectious. PMWS has not been shown to be spread through the use of artificial insemination (AI), but anecdotal information from Great Britain (GB) has recently indicated that this has in fact probably occurred. The detection of PCV-2 by PCR in semen (and serum) over a three-month period in one boar has now been reported (Le Tallec *et al.,* 2001), indicating that prolonged excretion of PCV-2 in semen may occur.

Both diseases have been reported from all management systems, although those with multiple sourcing of piglets at weaning seem most at risk. Experience in the field indicates that transmission of PMWS seems more likely in young piglets. The incidence of disease is apparently reduced if mixing of pigs is delayed as far as possible until about 10-12 weeks of age, although this was not confirmed by a recent case-control study carried out in breeder-finisher herds in England and Wales (Cook *et al*, 2001). This case-control study did however confirm a common observation on farms - that both PMWS and PDNS often occur in large herds, and in herds that are close (less than three kilometres) to others. The case-control study also indicated that PMWS and PDNS are more commonly observed in herds that have a high intake of gilt replacements.

It has been found possible to control PMWS and PDNS in some continuous-flow finishing units; by identifying the source of pigs that are introducing the problem and eliminating them from the site. This suggests that incoming pigs from some farms seed the infection into the herd. The possibility of vertical transmission (such as may occur for example through persistently viraemic piglets that were infected *in utero)* underlying this problem has been reported by workers in several countries. These include Spain (Segales, 1999), France (Madec *et al.*, 2000), Canada (Clark, 2000) and Northern Ireland (Ellis and Allan, 2000). Indeed, *in-utero* infection of foetuses between days 32 and 114 of gestation has now been reported (Ohlinger *et al.*, 2000). Natural vertical transmission (by *in-utero* infection) of PCV-2 infection has been associated with foetal myocarditis and abortion (West *et al*, 1999).

The involvement of vertical transmission has also been investigated in some herds in England by recording disease in pigs that are marked at birth (for example by tagging piglets with the sow number). The results of these investigations are not yet available. Litter and parity effects have not been reported in all incidents but clearly unless piglets are marked and recorded when they become affected or die and if detailed examinations are not carried out, a litter or parity effect may not be recognised. Litter effects reported from Spain (Marco, 2001) and France (Guillaume, 2001) were not reported to occur in succeeding litters of sows that produced affected progeny in a previous litter.

Experimentally, in one study, lesions consistent with PMWS and maximum viral load were identified at about 20 days post infection (PI) (Magar, Larochelle, Thibault, and Lamontagne, 2000). This information, coupled with field studies where clinical signs of PMWS commonly occurs in pigs aged between six and 16 weeks of age, suggests that in some pigs, infection may occur later after weaning or possibly that lesions may take more than three weeks to develop. In addition, in experimental studies, PCV-2 infection has been detected in tissues of infected pigs for long periods. Magar *et al.* (2000) report detection of infection up to 34 days PI but, interestingly, Bolin, Stoffregen, Nayar and Hamel, 2001) report that infrequently infection may be detected even until 125 days PI. They point out that this suggests that even adult pigs may be carriers of PCV-2. The report by Le Tallec *et al.* (2001) of the detection of viraemia of three months duration in a boar indicates that this is likely to be the case. The report by Le Tallec *et al.* (2001) refers to the detection of PCV-2 by PCR in serum; it may be that if whole blood is tested, the duration of detectable viraemia may be even longer. Allen (2001) rightly questioned whether in this case the PCR detected infectious virus or just viral DNA.

In the field it is well recognised that PMWS is not always clinically apparent even when PCV-2 infection is present (Krakowka *et al.*, 2000) even on a national basis (for example in Scotland (Thomson *et al.*, 2000), or Denmark (Hassing *et al.,* 2001). It therefore appears that PCV-2 infection alone is not the sole cause for PMWS. Immunosuppression associated with B lymphocyte depletion has been reported in pigs affected with PMWS (Shibuhara, Sato, Ishikawa and Kadota, 2000). Experimental work, coupled with field observations, now indicates that secondary infection with other agents including bacteria, viruses and mycoplasma may precipitate clinical PMWS in a pig infected with PCV-2. Krakowka *et al.* (2000) reported that 'activation of the immune system is the pivotal event in the production of wasting disease in pigs affected with PCV-2'. Ellis and Allan 2000) concluded that "exposure of piglets to undefined environmental factors and/or infectious agents that facilitate stimulation of the piglets immune system may be necessary, in conjunction with exposure to PCV-2, to produce clinical disease." Although PMWS can be reproduced experimentally by infection of pigs with PCV-2 alone (Bolin *et al*, 2001), there are a number of reports where the reproduction of clinical PMWS has required co-infection with other agents such as porcine parvovirus (Allan *et al.,* 1999) and PRRS virus (Allan *et al.*, 2000). In some (but not all) naturally occurring outbreaks, the administration of inactivated *Mycoplasma hyopneumoniae* vaccines to unweaned and weaned pigs has been reported to have been a significant predisposing factor in the development of PMWS after weaning. Kyriakis *et al.* (2001) suggested that the wider use of strongly immunogenic vaccines in pigs in recent years may have predisposed pigs to the development of disease associated with PCV-2 infection.

These experimental and field observations are consistent with the effects of the control measures propounded by a number of authors, which have culminated in the so-called "French 20 Point Plan" (Madec *et al.,* 2001). These control measures reduce stress and infection pressure on young pigs, but interestingly these are not effective on all affected farms. Clearly this may be because the control measures were not fully applied but may also be due to the presence of other predisposing factors not covered by the plan. Overall, the experimental and field observations together indicate that PCV-2 causes immune dysfunction and that clinical PMWS occurs due to antigenic challenge which may be associated with a variety of secondary infections or non-infectious factors such as administration of inactivated vaccines.

The epizootiology and pathogenesis of PDNS is unclear. Pathologically this is consistent with a systemic immune-complex disease. Segales et al, (1998) reported the identification of PCV-2 infection in pigs affected with PDNS. As mentioned above, Gresham *et al* (2001) reported links between PMWS and PDNS. Thomson *et al.* (2001a,b) reported that *P.multocida* infection might play a significant role in the aetiology and pathogenesis of PDNS.

## Comparisons with circovirus infections in chickens, psittacines and pigeons

The results of experimental work and lessons from natural outbreaks of PMWS as outlined above suggest that PMWS is due to infection with PCV-2 or a new strain of PCV-2 or other micro-organisms or other factors possibly acting in combination with this virus. This situation is not without precedent in that the effects of CIAV infection in chickens may be clinically very variable (Von Bulow and Schat, 1997) and outbreaks of CIA may follow a similar but shorter, pattern to that seen with PMWS in pigs. According to Von Bulow and Schat (1997), in chickens "the outcome of CIAV infection is influenced by a number of viral, host and environmental factors", and uncomplicated CIAV infection, especially if caused by horizontal infection, may result in nothing more than slightly increased mortality and transient poor performance of affected flocks. Therefore, it could even go unobserved in commercial settings. This is occurring with PCV-2 and PMWS in pigs on some farms. Von Bulow and Schat (1997) also state that maternal immunity confers almost complete protection against CIA but that this may be partly overcome, for example, by immunosuppression due to other viral infections (such as reovirus and Marek's disease virus) or chemically (such as with betamethasone). They also state that in field infections, environmental and other factors causing a decrease in immunocompetence have been suspected to enhance CIAV pathogenicity. Von Bulow and Schat (1997) also state that virulence of the strain and the infectious dose may be particularly important. This point is of interest in that Liu, Wang, Willson and Babiuk, (2000) reported that the development of PMWS in pigs might require "a certain amount of PCV-2". In other words a high infectious dose of PCV-2 may be required to cause the development of PMWS. Von Buloo and Schat (1997) also describe age dependent immunity to CIA, which develops rapidly during the first week of life and becomes complete by three weeks of age or even earlier. This depends on the virulence of the infecting strain although importantly development of age resistance may be delayed by immunosuppression; for example by simultaneous infection with another virus such as infectious bursal disease virus. CIAV infection of embryos occurs through semen from infected cocks (Hoop, 1993).

PBFD also exhibits some notable characteristics in that it too shows a significant degree of age susceptibility. Although some older birds (up to about three years of age) do develop PBFD, it is suspected that these birds were infected at a younger age but have carried the infection latently until clinical disease develops. In PBFD, varied susceptibility of different psittacine species is a prominent feature (Ritchie, 1995). Breed susceptibility is suspected in PMWS (Madec, 2001). In contrast to present experience with PCV-2 infection in pigs and with CIAV infection in chickens, as indicated above, prolonged latent infection with PBFDV is reported to occur in some psittacine birds infected as chicks (Ritchie, 1995). However, in both CIAV and PBFD, in hens infected as adults, latent infection does not appear to occur. In parallel with CIAV in chickens, PBFD in psitticines, and PiCV infection in pigeons, immunosuppression is reported as a feature of PMWS in pigs. Also, severe disease associated with infection with a variety of secondary micro-organisms is reported to be a feature of clinical disease associated with all four viruses: PCV-2 in pigs, CIAV in chickens, PBFDV in psitticines and PiCV in pigeons. In pigeons, the maturation of the immune system appears to be a significant physiological event associated with apoptotic death of lymphocytes; apoptosis may be important in the pathogen of PiCV (Abadie *et al.*, 2001). This is interesting considering that pigs develop PMWS at 6-12 weeks of age, but in pigs it is not until 12 weeks of age that lymphocyte and cell mediated immunity matures (Done, 1988).

## Possible involvement of feed factors

In searching for possible underlying environmental/nutritional or management factors in the development of PMWS and PDNS, experience in England indicates, but by no means proves, a possible feed association with these diseases. As mentioned above, the case-control study (Cook *et al*, 2001) carried out on breeder-finisher farms in GB did not indicate an association with feed nor with mycotoxins.

However, serious outbreaks of PMWS and epizootic PDNS (which appear to be related -see clinical signs later) first appeared primarily in East Anglia but also in the South East and South West of England in the autumn of 1999. The reason for this and the timing of the appearance of these diseases is still unclear but this was linked to the poor wheat harvest associated with the wet summer in East Anglia in 1999. It has also been suggested that this may relate to mycotoxicosis and particularly to ochratoxicosis, but there is currently insufficient information to support or deny this hypothesis. Some possible supporting evidence for an association with mycotoxins was provided by Henry (2001), who quoted reports by Smith and Abramson that in western parts of Canada epidemics of head blight associated with *Fusarium graminearum* have occurred in wheat and barley in the last 10 years. In this respect it is possibly relevant that PMWS was first identified and reported by Harding (1996) in pigs in western Canada. In this part of Canada pigs are fed on rations based on cereals rather than maize as in other parts of Canada and most of the USA. The outbreaks of PMWS in GB in the autumn of 1999 were also temporally linked to the licensed use of strobilurin fungicides on cereals. In the UK strobilurin fungicides were used to a limited extent in 1997, more widely in 1998, and then used on almost all cereal crops in 1999 and 2000. Considering possible involvement of mycotoxins, the use of strobilurin fungicides is especially noteworthy. This is because when some strobilurin fungicides are used without concurrent application of triazole fungicides, mycotoxin concentrations - especially those produced by fusarium moulds - may increase (Simpson *et al.,* 2001). This is particularly problematical as the standing cereal crop and harvested grain may appear to the naked eye to be of reasonable quality although significant concentrations of mycotoxin may be present. This is also compounded by the fact that in GB only limited testing for mycotoxins in cereals used for animal feed stuffs is routinely carried out. As a result - because 1) cereal producers are not required to provide information on fungicide use, 2) cereals from different suppliers are generally mixed by feed compounders, 3) most commercial pigs farms buy in specialist rations for weaned pigs (rather than produce them from home-produced cereals) - it is very difficult to prove cause and effect by using epidemiological techniques. A further result is that it is difficult to provide an indication of what experimental studies, if any, should be carried out to test these hypotheses.

Even so, due to suspected feed associations, a number of feed trials have been carried out in affected pig herds in England. Unfortunately many of these trials have not been properly constructed nor controlled and the results have not been adequately reported. However, in a feed trial on one farm, where feed wheat of poor quality was replaced with food grade (milling) wheat combined with the use of a clay based mycotoxin binder, the incidence of PMWS decreased significantly. In particular, the acute presentation associated with severe pulmonary oedema was reduced. Whether the disease that was controlled in this case was PMWS or a directly mycotoxin- related disease was not clear. Unfortunately this was not a controlled trial and to the author's knowledge this has not been repeated on other farms.

According to Blanchard (2000) attention to hygiene, management and nutritional management are required to control PMWS and PDNS. The nutritional controls relate specifically to cereal quality, mycotoxins (if suspected), factors predisposing to gastric ulceration, diet, palatability, digestibility and feed additives. The use of immunofacilitators may in fact be counterproductive.

There are also indications of possible feed involvement in other countries. For example in France, when attempting to control outbreaks of PMWS, attention to possible feed-related factors is considered to be very important (Guillaume, 2001). Particular points involved are:

1. To use a high quality weaner ration of known composition.
2. To use heat-processed flour (the heat processing is considered to be a decontamination procedure).
3. To use preventive treatments for mycotoxins (such as mycotoxin binders).
4. To use organic acids in feed.
5. To use enzymes in feed and supplement vitamins A, C and E
6. To ensure that drinking water is of adequate quality.

In Spain (Marco, 2001), feed factors that are addressed are:

a) Using feed of high quality both in palatability and digestibility.
b) Making 'sure' that mycotoxins are not present. In case of doubt the addition of a 'capturing' substance (such as a mycotoxin binder) could be beneficial.

## Clinical signs

The clinical signs of PMWS show a reasonably precise age distribution. Adults, unborn and unweaned pigs are generally clinically unaffected although, as mentioned above, there have been reports of an association of PCV-2 infection with abortion and mycarditis, congenital tremor type AII, sow abortion and mortality syndrome, proliferative necrotising pneumonia, and PDNS. In some cases transient postweaning diarrhoea occurs. The main clinical presentation in PMWS usually occurs in pigs from between five to six and up to 14 weeks of age, with disease peaking at about 9-10 weeks of age. At this time there is often rapid loss of condition in a number of pigs with cutaneous pallor and generalised illthrift. While many pigs affected with PMWS show cutaneous pallor, not all are anaemic. Anaemia, when present, is commonly microcytic and hypochromic and is associated with blood loss due to gastric ulceration; in some pigs the erythrocytic indices are consistent with a dyshaemopoietic anaemia. Some pigs, including some in good condition, appear dyspnoeic. This is associated with interstitial pneumonia and sometimes with severe pulmonary oedema. Hepatogenous jaundice may occur.

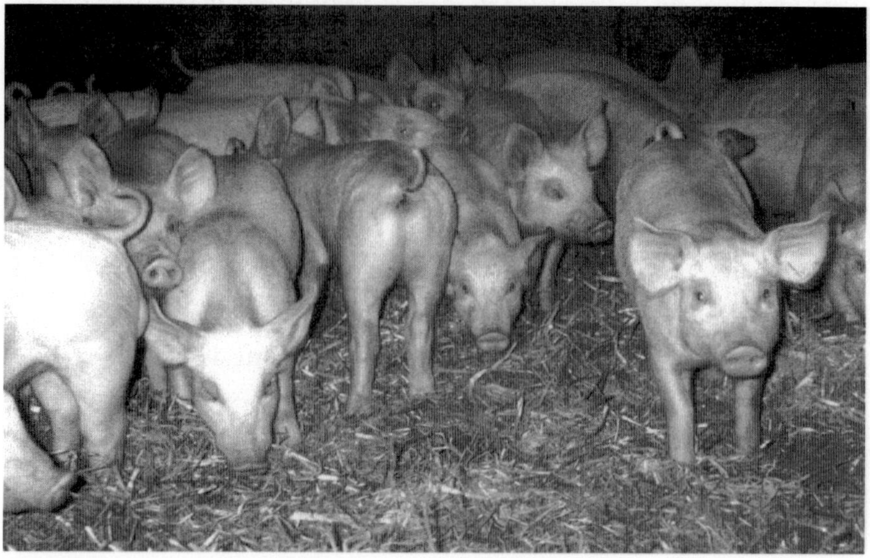

**Figure 3.4** PMWS. Note the variable condition and especially the poor condition of the pig in the centre of the group

The lymph nodes of affected pigs are frequently significantly enlarged and the subcutaneous lymph nodes are often palpable. Some pigs also show neurological signs, particularly ataxia, but whether this is just a result of cachexia is unclear. In addition to these signs, other infectious diseases present on the farm may become clinically more overt. Diarrhoea and pneumonia are frequently obvious. For example, the case-control study mentioned above indicated a positive association with salmonellosis. Glasser's disease (*Haemophilus parasuis* infection), enzootic pneumonia (*Mycoplasma hyopneumoniae* infection), pasteurellosis, and meningitis and septicaemia associated with *Streptococcus suis* infection, are also commonly identified. In outbreaks of PMWS, postweaning mortality rises significantly (always in excess of 3%), but this often averages between 8% and 20% and in some cases may be much higher. Finisher herd mortality also increases, typically to between 5% and 10% but some of this is often associated with PDNS. The growth rate of affected pigs is often significantly reduced. Overall growth rate and appetite may be reduced (Richardson, 2001), but on some affected farms this actually increases in the remaining pigs; possibly as a result of lower stocking density and reduced competition.

## Pathology

The gross and microscopic lesions of PMWS and PDNS are indicated in Tables 3.5 and 3.6. The main pathological lesions in pigs affected with PMWS are severe

**Table 3.5** GROSS POST MORTEM LESIONS SEEN IN PIGS AFFECTED WITH PMWS IN THE UK SINCE SEPTEMBER 1999

| | |
|---|---|
| Skin | Pallor. Icterus. |
| Lymph nodes | Enlarged nodes. Homogeneous pale oedematous cut surfaces Particularly inguinal, mesenteric, renal, bronchial and mediastinal. |
| Lungs | Non-collapsed. Firm, rubbery. Mottled surfaces. In severe cases, scattered red-brown areas. Atelectatic or consolidated cranial/middle lobes. |
| Liver | Yellow/orange. Mild to moderate mottling. Diffuse atrophy. Interlobular connective tissue prominent. |
| Kidney | No lesions or diffusely scattered white foci with oedema of peripelvic connective tissue or grossly enlarged, oedematous or waxy. |
| Spleen | Enlarged sometimes congested. |
| Stomach | Ulcers *pars oesophagea*. Oedema and petechial haemorrhage of stomach wall. |
| Intestine | Fluid-filled, thin-walled. Oedema of wall of caecum and colon. Focal necrosis of colonic mucosa. |

**Table 3.6** GROSS POST MORTEM LESIONS SEEN IN PIGS AFFECTED WITH EPIZOOTIC PDNS IN THE UK SINCE SEPTEMBER 1999

| | |
|---|---|
| Carcases | Acute, usually good condition. Subacute/chronic, fair to poor condition |
| Skin lesions | Typically over perineal area of hind quarters, limbs and dependent part of the abdomen, thorax and ears. In severe cases the flanks and thorax may also be involved. In these cases subcutaneous and intracutaneous oedema and generalised oedema is also present. Red to purple macules may coalesce to form plaques. May become brown or black within 2-3 days. May resolve with or without scarification in 2-3 weeks. Rarely whole body. General pallor in some pigs. |
| Kidneys | Pale, focal lesions in kidney (60%)Consistently kidneys are enlarged, sometimes haemorrhage and oedema. In chronic cases, kidneys enlarged, pale and fibrous. |
| Joints | May be excess joint fluid, particularly in hind limb joints. |
| Lymph nodes | In acute, enlarged several times compared to normal with interfollicular and subcapsular haemorrhage. May be oedematous. In subacute/chronic may be slightly enlarged/haemorrhagic. Inguinal, subiliac, renal and tracheobronchial nodes particularly. |
| Oedema | May be present in subcutaneous locations, in pleural, peritoneal and pericardial cavities. May be oedema in the spiral colon or mesentery and may be severe. |
| Haemorrhages | Any mucosal or serosal surfaces, also lymph nodes.May be extensive pleural haemorrhages or into pulmonary parenchyma |
| Ulceration | Particularly at the ileocaecocolic junction. Occasionally gastric *pars oesophagea*. |

systemic lymphadenopathy, particularly affecting the mesenteric, renal, inguinal and broncho-mediastinal lymph nodes. Affected lymph nodes may become significantly enlarged, even to four times normal size. The cut surfaces of affected lymph nodes are generally pale and oedematous. Sometimes petechial haemorrhages are scattered throughout. After several weeks, lymph nodes reduce in size and atrophy, and necrotic zones may be present. This is often especially prominent in mesenteric lymph nodes. The spleen, Peyer's patch, and the tonsils are similarly affected.

The histopathological lesions are variable, but severe lymphocytic degeneration and depletion is often seen. The reduced lymphocyte density is often apparent to the naked eye in stained histological preparations. There is loss of B cells particularly around lymphocyte follicles, and additional loss of parafollicular T cells. Subsequently there is expansion of parafollicular areas containing T cells. In early lesions, clusters of densely stained amphophilic, predominantly intracytoplasmic, inclusions of variable size, are present. In many cases, where much cellular loss occurs, inclusions may be scattered free in the tissue. Subsequently a granulomatous reaction occurs and macrophage syncytia may be present; sometimes in large numbers. The lymphocyte population gradually returns but the lymph node structure appears disorganised. Similar changes are found in other lymphoid tissues including the tonsil, spleen and Peyer's patch.

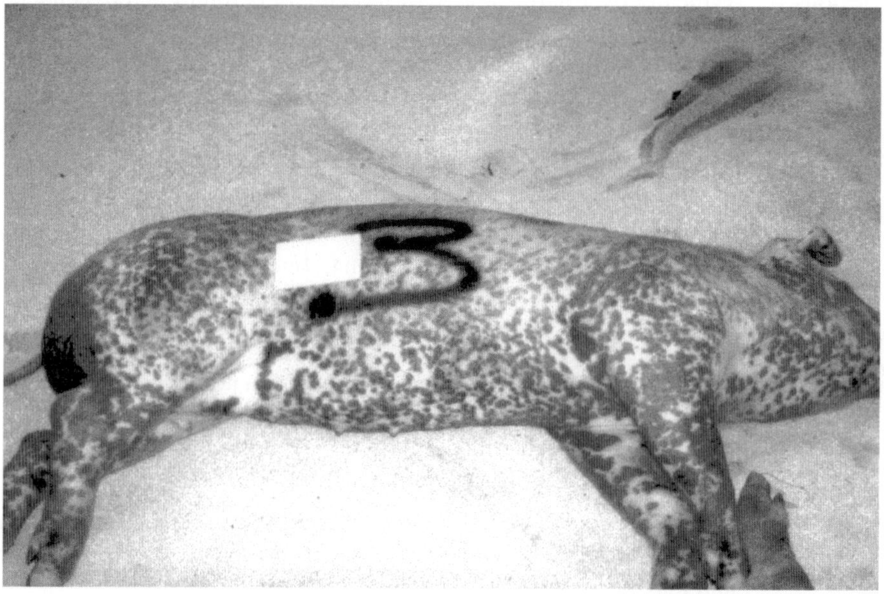

**Figure 3.5** PDNS. Extensive cutaneous purpura. Note – the purpura is rarely this extensive.

## Diagnosis

A diagnosis of PMWS is based on the history, clinical signs, gross and histopathological findings, and identification of PCV-2 infection in association with the lesions of PMWS. In general, a history of prolonged and raised postweaning mortality, occurring primarily between six and ten weeks of age, is suggestive. PCV-2 may be demonstrated in the lesions of affected pigs by immunocytochemistry and in-situ hybridisation. Serology and simple virus detection (such as by polymerase chain reaction (PCR)) are of questionable use for routine diagnostic purposes at present due to the wide prevalence of PCV-2 infection and also due to the persistence of the virus in infected pigs.

## Treatment and control

Currently there are no commercially available veterinary medicinal products, which are recommended for the treatment of PMWS and PDNS. Serotherapy using serum taken from blood collected from slaughter-weight pigs on the farm of origin has, in some incidents led to a significant reduction in mortality associated with PMWS in France (Ferreira *et al.,* 2001). This is now becoming more widely favoured by producers in England. The serum is administered to weaned pigs either by subcutaneous or intra-peritoneal injection. Treatment and control of concurrent susceptible bacterial and mycoplasmal infection is important. As regards PDNS, the prophylactic antibiotic treatment of pigs in anticipation of developing PDNS may be beneficial (Thomson *et al*, 2001a). Immune stimulation is positively contraindicated (Kyriakis *et al*, 2001). The use of non-steroidal anti-inflammatory drugs may reduce the mortality rate in pigs severely affected with PDNS (Douglas, 1999). From mid-2000, management controls for PMWS have been widely developed in several countries. These have culminated in the so-called "French 20 Point Plan" (Madec *et al*, 2001), which is shown in Table 3.7. In effect the controls incorporated in the 'French 20 point plan' will reduce stress and secondary infections. Other control measures proposed by a number of advisers are shown in Table 3.8.

## Hypotheses and conclusions

### HYPOTHESES

Overall, it is tempting to theorise that PMWS is probably occurring as the result of both vertical and horizontal infection of pigs with a new or variant

**Table 3.7** THE "FRENCH 20 POINT PLAN" (COURTESY OF F. MADEC)

| | |
|---|---|
| **Farrowing** | |
| 1 | All-in/all-out and empty pit and clean and disinfect between batches. |
| 2 | Wash sows and treat for parasites before farrowing. |
| 3 | Limit cross-fostering to that which is really necessary within 24 hours of farrowing. |
| **Post-weaning** | |
| 4 | Small pens (<13 pigs) and solid partitions. |
| 5 | Empty pit and clean and disinfect, sticking to strict all-in/all-out. |
| 6 | Lower stocking density (3 pigs per sq m = 0.33 sq m per pig). |
| 7 | Increased space at the feeder at least 7cm/piglet. |
| 8 | Improved air quality. |
| 9 | Improved temperature control. |
| 10 | No mixing of batches. |
| **Grower/Finisher Stage** | |
| 11 | Small pens, small partitions. |
| 12 | Empty pit, clean and disinfect and maintain strict all-in/all-out policy |
| 13 | No mixing of pigs from the post-weaning pens. |
| 14 | No re-mixing between finishing pens. |
| 15 | Lower stocking density at least 0.75 sq m per pig. |
| 16 | Improved air quality and temperature. |
| **In Addition …** | |
| 17 | Appropriate vaccination programme. |
| 18 | Sensible flow within buildings (air and animals). |
| 19 | Strict hygiene in practices such as (nail and teeth clipping, injections and so forth). |
| 20 | Early removal of sick pigs to a hospital room or euthanasia. |

strain of PCV-2. Vertical infection probably occurs as a result of infection of a gilt or sow naïve to PCV-2 infection. Vertical infection is probably occurring primarily before the age of development of foetal immunocompetence. Persistent infection will be of particular significance in adults.

Post-natally, there is probably age dependent immunity developing from about six weeks of age but this is probably not completely developed until about 12 weeks of age or more (this is the age at which the pig's immune system is fully matured). Passive immunity is probably partially protective until about six weeks of age. In parallel with CIAV in chickens it is likely that other virus infections, in particular PRRSV, and nutritional and environmental factors, such as immunosuppressive effects of mycotoxins, when coupled with heavy PCV-2 infection may lead to the development of clinical disease.

**Table 3.8** ADDITIONAL CONTROL MEASURES FOR PMWS

1. Use correct management and nutrition to achieve optimum birth and weaning weights.
2. Colostrum – Adjust management and nutrition as necessary to optimise lactation by the sow, especially colostrum production and let-down. Where possible, manage farrowings to optimise colostrum intake by all new-born piglets.
3. Injectables – Use one needle to remove injectable preparations from containers and another to inject pigs. When injecting piglets use a needle for a maximum of only one litter. When injecting older pigs use a new needle for all adults and growing and finishing pigs at least up to 12 weeks of age.
4. Vaccines – avoid administration of vaccines to weaned pigs at or shortly after weaning (delay at least 7-10 days; for example until six weeks of age if weaning at 3-4 weeks of age).
5. Where possible wean later (as late as is practicable on the farm involved).
6. Avoid mixing litters at weaning.
7. Cleansing and disinfection – PCV-2 is likely to be as persistent as other circoviruses such as CAIV so it is important to clean thoroughly. Disinfectants known to be active against circoviruses (Royer, Nawagitgul, Paul, and Halbur, 2000) should be used.
8. Feed - Use a high quality weaner ration of known composition.
   Use preventive treatments for mycotoxins (such as mycotoxin binders).
   Use organic acids in feed.
   Use enzymes in feed and supplement with vitamins A, C and E
9. Ensure that water provided is of satisfactory quality.
10. Take replacements as weaners and ensure thorough exposure to herd infections before service.
11. Do not take replacements nor semen from herds where the health status is imbalanced, and, especially if it has recently broken down with PMWS

The clinical signs of PMWS are probably due to immunosuppression caused by PCV-2 infection coupled with severe secondary infections. Particularly severe outbreaks in some areas are likely to be associated with feed-related factors such as mycotoxins – this may be due to seasonal effects and changes in fungicide use.

The peak of disease after six to nine months in many affected herds is possibly consistent with a flush of disease due to vertical transmission through infection of naïve gilts and sows. The prolonged duration of some reported outbreaks (18 months to two years in some cases) is possibly consistent with resulting weight of virus infection present particularly in farrowing and weaner accommodation (both first and second stage - up to about 30 kg live weight or 10 weeks of age) coupled with at least some persistently or chronically infected pigs. It is likely that PCV-2 infection is transmitted in natural service and by AI.

In instances where the disease is predominantly occurring in progeny of older sows this may be due to introduction of infection into a naïve herd by replacements. In other words, most younger replacements will be immune and their progeny will be least affected. In other situations, where younger sows are affected, disease may occur through the introduction of naïve gilts into a heavily infected herd.

The reason why CIAV disease can be controlled more effectively in chickens is because of the higher standards of hygiene which are possible in chicken production (egg laying and broiler production) aided primarily by all-in all-out production systems. There is also the clear benefit of effective CIAV vaccines.

It is likely that PDNS is the result of systemic immune-complex vasculitis occurring due to infection with other micro-organisms, such as Gram-negative bacteria, in pigs affected with PMWS in which immune dysfunction has occurred due to PCV-2 infection.

## Conclusions

PMWS and epizootic PDNS are now highly important diseases of pigs resulting in significant economic loss. PCV-2 infection appears central to the development of both PMWS and PDNS. The pathogenesis of both PMWS and PDNS is still unclear, but it is likely that environmental, infectious and managemental factors are important in the development of clinical disease. Experience in England indicates that feed factors are particularly important and that mycotoxins may be involved, but at present these suspicions are unproven. Further epidemiological studies, for example on the temporal and spatial nature of outbreaks of PMWS and PDNS, are needed to give a better indication of the predisposing factors involved, and so to give firmer pointers for more specific lines of research into these diseases.

## Acknowledgements

The author acknowledges the assistance of Prof. S. Done in the compilation of the tables of pathological lesions (Tables 3.5 and 3.6). The permission of Dr F. Madec to reproduce the details of the 'French 20 point plan' (Table 3.7) is gratefully acknowledged.

## References

Abadie, J., Nguyen. F., Groizeleau, C., Amenna, N., Fernandez, B., Guereaud,

C., Guigand, L., Robart, P., Lefebvre, B. and Wyers, M. (2001) *Avian Pathology*, **30**, 149-158.

Allan, G. (2001) Comments in discussion at *International Conference on ssDNA viruses of Plants, Birds, Pigs and Primates*, St Malo, France.

Allan, G. and Ellis, J. (2001) Journal *of Veterinary Diagnostic Investigation*, **12**, 3-14.

Allan, G., Kennedy, S., McNeilly, F., Foster, J., Ellis, J., Krakowka, S., Meehan, B. and Adair, D. (1999) *Journal of Comparative Pathology*, **121**, 1-11.

Allan, G., McNeilly, F., Ellis, J., Krakowka, S., Meehan, B., McNair, I., Walker, I. and Kennedy, S. (2000) *Archives of Virology*, **145**, 2421-2429.

Allan, G., McNeilly, F., Meehan, B., Kennedy, S., Mackie, D., Ellis,J., Clark, E., Espuna, E., Saubi, N., Riera, P., Botner, A. and Charreyre, C. (1999) *Veterinary Microbiology*, **66**, 115-123.

Blanchard, P. (2000) *Pig Farming*, **48**, (11), 22-24.

Bolin, S., Stoffregen, W., Nayar, G. and Hamel, A. (2001) *Journal of Veterinary Diagnostic Investigation*, **13**, 185-194.

Cameron R. (1999). Diseases of the skin. In: *Diseases of Swine*, 8$^{th}$ edition, pp 941-958. Edited by Straw, B., D'Allaire, S., Mengeling, W. and Taylor, D. Iowa State University Press, USA.

Choi, C., Chae, C. and Clark, E. (2000) *Journal of Veterinary Diagnostic Investigation*, **12**,151-153

Clark, E. (2000) Personal communication.

Cook, A. Wilesmith, J., Pascoe, S. and Gresham, A. *The Pig Journal,* **48**, 53-60.

Daft, B., Nordhausen, R., Latimer, K. and Niagro, F. (1996) *Proceedings of the 39$^{th}$ Meeting of the American Association of Veterinary Laboratory Diagnosticians*, **39**, 32

Done, S. (1988) *The Pig Veterinary Society Proceedings*, **20**, 31-60.

Done, S. (2001) *State Veterinary Journal*, **11**, 12-16.

Douglas, R. (1999) Personal communication.

Dubansky, V., Drabek, J. (1999) *Veterinarstvi*, **49**, (5),193-194.

Ellis, J. and Allan, G. (2000) *Procedings of Merial PMWS Symposium, International Pig Veterinary Society Conference,* Melbourne Australia,3-19.

Ferreira, D., Sansot, B. and Laval, A. (2001) *Proceedings of International Conference on ssDNA viruses of Plants, Birds, Pigs and Primates*, St Malo, France, 144.

Gresham, A., Jackson, G., Giles, N., Allan, G., McNeilly, F. and Kennedy, S. (2000) *Veterinary Record*, **146**, 143

Gresham, A., Allan, G., McNeilly, F. and Kennedy, S. (2001) *The Pig Journal*, **47**, 155-159.

Gresham, A. and Thomson, J. (2001) *Veterinary Record*, **148**, 387.

Guillaume, J-M. (2001a). *Proceedings of Conference on PMWS and PDNS*, Stoneleigh, England, Published on the internet: www.thepigsite.com

Guillaume, J-M. (2001a). Unpublished. Comments at *Conference on PMWS and PDNS*, Stoneleigh, England.

Harding, J., (1996) *Proceedings of the Western Canadian Association of Swine Practitioners Meeting*, 21.

Harding, J. (2001) Comments attributed to Clarke, E. in *Proceedings of International Conference on ssDNA viruses of Plants, Birds, Pigs and Primates*, St Malo, France, 67-68.

Hassing, A., Botner, A., Ladekjaer-Mikkelsen, A., Baekbo, P., Jorsal,S. and Bille-Hansen, V. (2001) *Proceedings of International Conference on ssDNA viruses of Plants, Birds, Pigs and Primates*, St Malo, France, 93.

Helie, P., Drolet, R., Germain, M-C. and Bour-Gault, A. (1995) *Canadian Veterinary Journal*, **36**, 150

Henry, W. (2001) *Feed International*, September 2001, 34-36.

Higgins, R., O'Toole, D., Clark, E., West, K., Wells, G., Blackburn, P. and Cundall, C. (2000) *Proceedings of the American Association of Veterinary Laboratory Diagnosticians*. **43**, 9.

Hinrichs, U., Ohlinger, V., Pesch, S. et al (1999) *Tieraerztl Umsch*, **54**, 255-258.

Hoop, R. (1993) *Veterinary Record*, **133**, 551-552.

Kennedy, S., Allan, G., McNeilly, F., Adair, B., Hughes, A. and Spillane, P. (1998) *Veterinary Record,* **142**, 495 – 496.

Kiss, I., Kecskemeti, S., Tuboly, T., Bajmocy, E. and Tanyi, E. (2000) *Acta Vet Hungarica*, **48**, (4), 469-475.

Krakowka, S., Ellis, J., McNeilly, F., Ringler, D., Rings, D. and Allan, G. (2000), *Veterinary Pathology*, **38**, 31-42.

Kyriakis, S., Kennedy, S., Saoulidis, K., Lekkas, S., Miliotis, C., Balkamoutos, G. and Papoutis, P. (2000) *Proceedings of 16th International Pig Veterinary Society Conference*, Melbourne, Australia, 633.

Kyriakis, S., Saoulidis, K., Lekkas, S., Miliotis, C. Papoutis, P. and Kennedy, S. (2001) *Proceedings of International Conference on ssDNA viruses of Plants, Birds, Pigs and Primates*, St Malo, France, 141.

Larochelle, R., Bielanski, A., Muller, P. and Magar, R. (2000) *Proceedings of 16th International Pig Veterinary Society Conference*, Melbourne, Australia, 580.

Le Tallec, B., Pozzi, N., Blanchard, P. Mahe, D., Jestin, A. and Guerin, B. (2001) *Proceedings of International Conference on ssDNA viruses of Plants, Birds, Pigs and Primates*, St Malo, France, 120.

LeCann, P., Albina, E., Madec, F., Cariolet, R. and Jestin, A. (1997) *Veterinary Record* , **141**, 660.

Liu, Q., Wang, L., Willson, P. and Babiuk, L. (2000) *Journal of Clinical Microbiology*, **38**, (9), 3474-3477.

Machuca, M., Segales, J., Idiart, J., Sanguinetti, H. and Perfumo, C. (1999) *Pathologia y deteccion de circovirus porcino*, (Enc Nac de Pat Vet (ENAPAVE).

Madec, F. (2001) Comments in discussion at International Conference on ssDNA viruses of Plants, Birds, Pigs and Primates, St Malo, France.

Madec, F., Eveno, E., Morvan, P., Hanon, L., Blanchard, P., Cariolet, R., Amenna, N., Morvan, H., Truong, C., Mahe, D., Albina, E. and Jestin, A. (2000) *Livestock Production Science*, **63**, 223-233.

Madec, F., Rose, N., Eveno, E., Morvan, P., Larour, G., Jolly, J. Le Diguerher, G., Cariolet, R., Le Dimna, M., Blanchard, P., and Jestin, A. (2001) *Proceedings of International Conference on ssDNA viruses of Plants, Birds, Pigs and Primates*, St Malo, France, 86-88.

Maecato, P., Sidoli, L., Mandrioli, L., Della-Salda, I., Cerati, C, and Rolla, G. (1999) *Atti della Societa Italiana di Patologia ed allvamento dei Suini*, 1999 XXV Meeting Annuale, Brescia, Italy, pp 107-124.

Magar, R., Larochelle, R., Thibault, S. and Lamontagne, L. (2000) *Journal of Comparative Pathology*, **123**, 258-269.

Magar, R., Muller, P. and Larochelle, R. (2000) *Canadian Journal of Veterinary Research*, **64**, 184-186.

Marco, E. (2001) *Proceedings of Conference on PMWS and PDNS*, Stoneleigh, England, Published on the internet: www.thepigsite.com

Marco, E. (2001a). Unpublished. Comments at *Conference on PMWS and PDNS*, Stoneleigh, England.

Mehan, B., Mcneilly, F., Todd, D., Kennedy, S., Jewhurst, V., Ellis, J., Hassard, L., Clark, E., Haines, D. and Allan, G. (1998) *Journal of General Virology*, **79**, (9), 2171-2179.

Morales, G. and Guzman, V. (1976) *Proceedings of the 4th International Pig Veterinary Congress*. June 22-24, Ames, Iowa, 121

Ohlinger, V., Schmidt, U. and Pesch, S. (2000) *Proceedings of 16th International Pig Veterinary Society Conference*, Melbourne, Australia, 577.

Pejsak, Z. (2000) *Zycie-Weterynaryjne*, **75**, (11), 575-579.

Ramos-Vara, J., Duran, O., Render, J. and Craft, D. (1997), *Veterinary Record*, **141**, 479-480.

Richardson P (2001). *Proceedings of Conference on PMWS and PDNS*, Stoneleigh, England, Published on the internet: www.thepigsite.com

Ritchie, B. (1995) Psittacine Beak and Feather Disease. In *Avian viruses, Function and Control*. pp 223-252. Wingers Publishing, Inc, Lake Worth, Florida, USA.

Rossell, C., Segales, J., Rovira, A. and Domingo, M. (2000) *Veterinary Record*, **146**, 591-592.

Royer, R., Nawagitgul, P., Paul, P. and Halbur, P. (2000) *Proceedings of the 31st Meeting of the American Association of Swine Practitioners*, Indianapolis, Indiana, 45

Sato, K., Shibahara, T., Ishikawa, Y., Kondo, H., Kubo, M. and Kadota, K. (2000) *Journal of Veterinary Medical Science*, **62**, 627-633.

Segales, J. (1999) Unpublished. Comments at *Pig Health Conference* (Sponsors Elanco Animal Health and PIC). Market Bosworth, England. 1st December 1999.

Segales, J. and Domingo, M. (1999) *Proceedings of Pig Health Conference* (Sponsors Elanco Animal Health and PIC). Market Bosworth, England. 1st December 1999.

Segales, J. and Domingo, M. (2000) *Proceedings of Merial PMWS Symposium, International Pig Veterinary Society Conference*, Melbourne, Australia, 21-31.

Segales, J., Domingo, M. and Latimer, K. (1998) *Proceedings of the 15th meeting of the International Pig Veterinary Society*, Birmingham, England, **2**, 215.

Segales, J., Piella, J., Marco, E. and Domingo, M. (1996) *Proceedings of the 14th meeting of the International Pig Veterinary Society*, Bologna Italy, **14**, 709.

Segales, J., Sitjar, M., Domingo, M., Dee, S., Del Pozo, M., Noval, R., Sacristan, C., De las Heras, A., Ferro, A. and Latimer, K. (1997) *Veterinary Record*, **141**, 600-601.

Shibuhara, T., Sato, K., Ishikawa, Y. and Kadota, K.(2000) *Journal of Medical Science*, **62**, (11), 1125-1131.

Simpson, D., Weston, G., Turner, J. Jennings, P. and Nicholson, P. (2001) *European Journal of Plant Pathology*, **107**, 421-431.

Smith, W., Thomson, J. and Done, S. (1993) *Veterinary Record*, **13**, 47.

Sorden, S. (2000) *Swine Health and Production*, **8**, 133-136.

Spillane, P., Kennedy, S., Meehan, B., Allan, G. (1998) *Veterinary Record*, **143**, 511-512..

Thomson, J., Smith, W., Allan, G., McNeilly, F., McVicar, C. (2000) *Veterinary Record*, **146**, 651-652.

Thomson, J., Henderson, L., Meikle, C. and MacIntyre, N. (2001a) *Veterinary Record*, **148**, 282-283.

Thomson, J., MacIntyre, N., Henderson, L. and Meikle, C. (2001b) *Veterinary Record*, **149**, 412-417.

Tischer, I. Rasch, R. and Tochtermann, G. (1974) Zentralbe Bakteriol Org A. **226**, 153-167.

Todd, D. (2000) *Avian Pathology*, **29**, 373-394.

Todd, D. (2001) *Proceedings of International Conference on ssDNA viruses of Plants, Birds, Pigs and Primates*, St Malo, France, 81.

Trujano, M., Iglesias, G., Segales, J. and Palacios, J. (2001) *Veterinary Record,* **148**, 792.

Van Halderen, A., Bakker, S., Wessels, J., Van der Lugt, J. (1995) *Tydskrif van die Suid Afrikaanse veteriner Mediese Vereniging*, **66**,108

Von Bulow, V. and Schat, K. (1997) Chicken Infectious Anaemia. In *Diseases of Poultry*, pp 739-756. Edited by B. Calnek. Iowa State University Press, Ames, Iowa, USA.

Walker, I., Konoby, C., Jewhurst, V., McNair, I., McNeilly, F., Meehan, B., Cottrell, T., Ellis, J. and Allan, G. (2000) *Journal of Veterinary Diagnostic Investigation*, **12**, 400-405.

West, K., Bystrom, J., Wojnarowicz, C., Shantz, N., Jacobson, M., Allan, G., Haines, D., Clark, E., Krakowka, S., McNeilly, F., Konoby, C., Martin, K. and Ellis, J. (1999) *Journal of Veterinary Diagnostic Investigation*, **11**, 530-532.

*This paper was first published in 2002*

4

# NUTRITIONAL INFLUENCES ON LIFETIME PERFORMANCE OF THE SOW

B.P. Gill
*Meat and Livestock Commission, Milton Keynes, UK*

## Introduction

During the last 30 years, there has been progress in both the development and practical implementation of nutritional and feeding strategies to enhance sow productivity and avoid loss of body condition over consecutive parities. This has been coupled with improvements in housing, husbandry and welfare standards. Thus endemic cases of poor sow physical condition, such as the so- called 'thin sow syndrome' widely reported in the 1960's (Maclean, 1968) have virtually disappeared from UK farms.

It is now recognised that modern lean genotypes are far more sensitive to nutritional mismanagement then their predecessors which had ample fat reserves at the start of their breeding life to buffer them against quite extreme shortfalls between nutrient demand and supply. Indeed an accepted strategy was to deplete such fat reserves progressively over consecutive parities, a strategy that would fail for lean young modern sows.

In the main, nutritional and feeding strategies for modern genotypes have been developed to increase nutrient intake during lactation and correct losses in body tissue reserves during the following pregnancy. The benefits of using a high nutrient concentration (protein and energy) diet during lactation followed by a diet balanced in favour of energy relative to protein during pregnancy have been demonstrated under both applied research (O'Dowd *et al.*, 1997) and field conditions (MLC, 1999). Thus the dual diet system is now gradually becoming an accepted norm for feeding sows on UK farms.

Despite these advances, there remains considerable scope for improving sow productivity by reducing inefficiency and losses during her lifetime performance. In this chapter it is not the purpose to consider where such improvements could be made as a number of comprehensive reviews and texts on this subject have been published. The objective is to focus on the problem of premature disposal of young sows and the consequences for lifetime performance of nutritional strategies aimed at enhancing longevity.

## Premature culling: scale, reasons and economic impact

Farm data recording services and surveys of commercial farms indicate that premature disposal of young sows continues to be a problem in countries with modern pig producing systems (Table 4.1). Although the productive life span of sows in such countries is below the suggested optimum of about 3 years (or 7 to 8 litters/sow lifetime), there are some notable differences. For example in the USA, which has seen a recent and rapid expansion of large-scale industrialised systems of production, average life span is particularly short at under 22 months. On the other hand, in Britain, where welfare legislation has banned the close confinement of pregnant sows, average productive life span is nearly 30 months. Nevertheless, the life span of most sows on commercial farms is disappointingly short, given that the pig is renowned for its high fertility and fecundity. An indication of the gap between actual and biological potential can be found within survey data collected from commercial herds.

**Table 4.1** AVERAGE SOW LIFETIME PRODUCTIVITY IN BRITAIN AND SOME MAJOR PIG PRODUCING COUNTRIES

| | *Britain*[4] | *USA*[3] | *France*[1] | *Netherlands*[2] |
|---|---|---|---|---|
| Lifetime sow productivity | | | | |
| Productive life span (years) | 2.4 | 1.8 | 2.0 | 2.3 |
| Litters per sow lifetime | 5.4 | 4.2 | 4.2 | 4.6 |
| Piglets weaned per sow lifetime | 52.8 | 36.8 | 37.6 | 39.3 |
| Annual replacement rate (%) | 42 | 56 | 50 | 43 |

(Source[1,2,3,4]: Dagron and Aumaitre, 1979; Kroes and Male, 1979; Lucia *et al.*, 1999; MLC, 1999)

For example, in a recent US survey of about 9,400 sows in 29 herds over 5 years, the maximum lifetime output was recorded from 2 sows which weaned 122 pigs each over 11 parities (Lucia *et al.*, 1999). The average productivity in these herds was less than a third of what appears to be biologically possible. In summary, average sow productivity on farms is most certainly below what is biologically possible and is between 50% and 70% of the suggested commercial target of 75 to 80 piglets weaned per sow lifetime.

## Reasons for the premature disposal of young sows

Although caution is required in the comparison of the recorded reasons for sow culling between different sources and countries over different years, reproductive failure is a consistent and major reason for the disposal of sows across all parities (Table 4.2). Thus nearly a third of all sows were culled due to a failure to show oestrus and failure to conceive after insemination.

**Table 4.2** REASONS (IN %) FOR CULLING SOWS FROM COMMERCIAL HERDS (ALL PARITIES)

| | *Britain*[4] | *USA*[3] | *France*[1] | *Netherlands*[2] |
|---|---|---|---|---|
| Reproductive failure | | | | |
| Failure to conceive | 19.8 | - | 31.0 | 25.2 |
| No oestrus | 5.9 | - | 5.4 | 9.0 |
| Total | 25.7 | 29.6 | 36.4 | 34.2 |
| Low productivity | | | | |
| Old age | 25.4 | - | 27.2 | 11.0 |
| Small litters | 7.9 | 9.4 | 4.0 | 6.2 |
| Health/physical damage | 7.7 | 18.7 | - | 16.0 |
| Mothering ability | 5.6 | 8.8 | 8.4 | 13.9 |
| Lameness/leg weakness | 6.5 | 11.0 | 8.8 | 10.5 |
| Death | 10.7 | 10.7 | 6.5 | - |
| Aborted | 2.5 | 5.0 | 2.8 | - |
| Miscellaneous | 8.0 | 6.6 | 5.9 | 8.2 |

(Source[1,2,3,4]: Dagron and Aumaitre, 1979; Dijkhuizen *et al.*, 1989; Stein *et al.*, 1990; MLC, 1999)

Analyses of within parity culling pattern (see for example Figure 4.1) suggest that proportionally reproductive failure is particularly high in young sows, accounting for between 40% and almost 50% of all first litter culls (Dagron and Aumaitre, 1979; Dijkhuizen *et al.*, 1989; Stein *et al.*, 1990). Reproductive failure tends to persist over the second and even third parity, followed by a decrease reaching about 20% for culls in parity 7 and beyond (Dagron and Aumaitre, 1979; Dijkhuizen *et al.*, 1989). As with reproductive failure, lameness and leg weakness appears to afflict the younger sow, accounting for nearly 15% of first and second litter culls in several surveys (e.g. Dagron and Aumaitre, 1979; D'Allaire, Stein and Leman, 1987; Dijkhuizen *et al.*, 1989; Stein *et al.*, 1990). With advancing parity reproductive failure and leg weakness are replaced by old age and reduced litter viability and performance as the major reasons for the disposal of older multiparous sows.

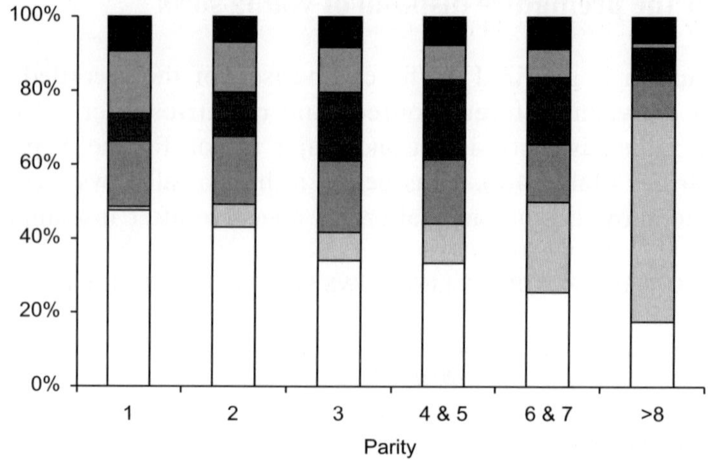


**Figure 4.1** Relative importance of culling reasons across parities in commercial herds (☐ Reproductive failure; ■ Low productivity; ■ Health/physical damage; ■ Mothering ability; ☐ Lameness; ■ Other) After Dijhuizen *et al.* (1989)

## Economic impact

The economic impact of culling an individual sow from a commercial herd will depend on many factors including the difference between replacement cost and the cull value. It is generally accepted that, where production is based on achieving several consecutive litters from each sow, premature disposal from the herd will result in a cost disadvantage. However, if the value of the carcass from a gilt slaughtered after weaning her first litter was closer to that of a bacon pig, then production based on the so-called once bred gilt system has considerable economic attraction. This is because efficiency is greatly enhanced by sharing maintenance between growth and pregnancy in a reproductively functional yet a rapidly growing young animal. Unfortunately there is a continued reluctance in the market towards paying a higher value for carcasses from first litter gilts, despite work showing a lack of difference in the quality of meat produced from bacon pigs and once-bred gilts (Ellis *et al.*, 1996). This is increasingly exasperating with the increasing volume of pig meat entering the catering and processing sectors where at the consumer level it would be difficult to differentiate between meat produced from a once-bred gilt and that from a finished pig.

Records from commercial herds have been analysed to compare the economic impact of culling according to parity and reason for disposal. Using an economic index based on opportunity cost of a deferred replacement, Dijkhuizen *et al.* (1989) ranked the reasons for disposal according to cost burden (see Table 4.3). It is not surprising that the reasons with the highest index value are those conditions which more readily afflict the younger sow.

**Table 4.3** REPLACEMENT COST INDEX (ADJUSTED TO 100) ACCORDING TO SPECIFIC REASONS FOR CULLING SOWS FROM COMMERCIAL HERDS

| *Reason for culling* | *Index*[a] |
|---|---|
| Reproductive problems | 15 |
| Failure to conceive | 14 |
| No oestrus | 17 |
| Low productivity | 2 |
| Old age | 1 |
| Small litter | 3 |
| Health and physical damage | 13 |
| Mothering ability | 8 |
| Lameness and leg weakness | 17 |
| Other | 11 |

(After: Dijkhuizen *et al.* 1989)
[a]Higher value indicates increased cost

The wastage of young females is further highlighted by the parity profile analysis of the culled population from commercial herds. In four surveys, first litter gilts accounted for about 21% of all culls, or nearly 1 in 5 of the culled females were once-bred gilts (Dagron and Aumaitre, 1979; Kroes and Male, 1979; Dijkhuizen *et al.*, 1989; Stein *et al.*, 1990). There was remarkable consistency in this figure between the different studies. In two studies where maiden gilts were included in the cull population, these animals accounted for 16 and 19% of the culls (D'Allaire *et al.*, 1987; Lucia *et al.*, 1999). The parity profile of sows remaining in herds with a high annual replacement rate is inevitably skewed towards a higher proportion of younger animals which have yet to reach their optimum litter productivity. For example, in 85 herds classified as low, medium or high in annual culling rate (31 v 43 v 55% respectively), first and second litter sows accounted for 27, 36 and 44% of the farrowings respectively (Kroes and Male, 1979). Thus in herds with a high replacement rate, a greater proportion of the piglet yield is derived from young sows, which are at greater risk from reproductive failure. Dijkhuizen *et al.* (1989) concluded that premature disposal was equivalent to about 16% of income on commercial pig farms.

## Aetiology of reproductive failure

There is often a temptation to over-play the role of nutrition in every aspect of pig science on the basis that feed accounts for between 50 and 70% of the total cost of production. The significance of nutritional factors in the aetiology of reproductive failure and lameness has to be balanced against other causes and reasons for this problem. For example, Muirhead and Alexander (1997) suggested that the problem of anoestrus in gilts was largely due to a failure of the stockperson to recognise, detect or check for oestrus. In a field study, it was found that one third of anoestrus gilts examined at slaughter had been cycling, one third were pregnant and only one third were actually anoestrus.

Although the premature disposal of young sows is a major problem on many commercial farms throughout the world, there is a surprising lack of published epidemiological information on the aetiology of reproductive failure, the major reason for culling first and second litter sows. It is therefore difficult to establish the extent to which nutrition and nutritional management contribute to the problem of reproductive failure and in turn lifetime influences on the performance of young sows. The causes of lameness, which also afflict growing pigs for meat production have received greater attention (e.g. Nakano, Brenan and Aherne, 1987).

In an attempt to position nutrition in the aetiology of reproductive failure, a subjective score has been used to compare the relative importance of nutrition against other causes of this problem under commercial conditions (see Table 4.4). Whilst this is very much a personal analysis and is open to criticism, the major causes of reproductive failure are most likely to be environmental components and shortfalls in the training of inexperienced stock workers (English *et al.*, 1998). Nutritional influences are therefore unlikely to play a major role in bringing about a premature loss of reproductive function in the young sow, unless an essential micronutrient has been accidentally excluded from an otherwise balanced diet.

**Table 4.4** SUBJECTIVE RATING OF THE REASONS FOR PREMATURE REPRODUCTIVE FAILURE IN COMMERCIAL HERDS

| *Causes of premature reproductive failure* | *Rating*[a] |
|---|---|
| Poor environment | |
| Lighting | *** |
| Feeding method | *** |
| Watering | *** |
| Hygiene | *** |
| Temperature control | **** |
| Flooring | **** |
| Aerial pollutants | * |
| Stockworker inexperience | ***** |
| Seasonal infertility (indoor/outdoor) | **/**** |
| Boar stimulation and infertility | *** |
| Genetic abnormalities | * |
| Infectious disease | * |
| Nutrition | * |

[a]Rating: * = not very important to ***** = very important cause

## Recommended nutritional management of the replacement gilt

The effort in generating a genetically improved F1 gilt commands a significant premium above the commercial value of a gilt finished for slaughter. Although commercial producers have continued to invest in acquiring this genetic premium, there is a lack of published recommendations or guidance in the form of manuals, on the management of replacement gilts after they have been delivered to the farm. This includes scientific recommendations for nutrient requirements to optimise lifetime reproductive performance. For example in the Nutrient Requirements of Pigs (ARC, 1981), it was suggested that there was insufficient evidence from trials with potential breeding females to indicate whether their protein requirements up to the time of their first mating were different from those of growing females intended as meat animals. In the more recent North American equivalent of this publication, the National Research Council (NRC, 1998) recommended that developing gilts should be fed *ad libitum* to about 100 kg body weight after which they should be restricted to achieve the desired weight at the time of breeding. However, no rationale is provided for this advice nor any indication of what the desired weight should be or how it could be ultimately achieved.

Targets for age, weight and body fatness at first service are available in the published literature. Whittemore (1998) has placed importance on the need to achieve adequate stores of fat at the start of the breeding life and has recommended a backfat depth in excess of 18 mm (>17% body lipid) at this stage. A target weight of around 130 kg and an age of 220 days at first mating are suggested for optimum subsequent fertility and longevity. An outline of the nutritional strategy to achieve these targets is based on a combination of reduced protein levels in the diet to limit lean gain and encourage fat deposition and feed restriction to restrain growth and allow attainment of maturity. Although the consequences of this approach for lifetime performance are not discussed, the author has cautioned that low protein rearing may be counter-productive as protein status may be of equal importance to fat status in determining age at first conception and in its success. Similar emphasis on achieving adequate levels of fatness and targets for weight and age (18 to 19 mm, 130 to 140 kg and 220 to 230 days) at first mating have been recommended by Close and Challinor (1996).

Although advice in delaying first mating until about 220 to 230 days of age to allow further development of physiological and reproductive maturity seems sensible, data from commercial herds indicate a contrary relationship between age at first mating and longevity. In two large scale surveys of commercial farms, both longevity and economic performance improved with a decrease in the age of gilts at first conception (Schukken *et al.*, 1994; Culbertson and Mabry, 1995).

Advice focusing on the importance of achieving adequate fat stores at the point of first service is founded on good evidence which shows that there is a conflict between intensive selection for reduced fatness and reproductive function/performance in the sow (e.g. Nelson *et al.*, 1990; MLC, 1991; Gaughan *et al.*, 1995; Kerr and Cameron, 1995). However, there are potential risks in the extrapolation of results from such selection studies to the development of nutritional strategies that aim to encourage fat deposition in genetically determined high lean animals. Taking the work of Gaughan *et al.* (1995) as an example, an advantage of an extra 8 piglets weaned per lifetime in gilts with 18.5 mm of backfat at selection was shown over those with only 12.2 mm. A possible conclusion from this could be that lifetime productivity could be enhanced by increasing backfat depths in genetically lean gilts from 12 to about 19 mm at selection through nutritional strategy. Whether this is possible and the effect on lifetime reproductive performance in attempting to achieve such a target could challenge such assumptions.

## Research on nutritional influences on lifetime performance of the sow

Studies seeking to establish nutritional influences on lifetime performance are extremely costly since large numbers of animals per treatment are required and records of individual sow performance over several parities are essential if sound conclusions are to be drawn from the results. There may be significant nutrition-genotype interactions, which makes direct comparison of similar studies difficult if genotypes with different potentials for fat and lean deposition are used. Thus such research should consider evaluation of body composition to allow baseline comparisons and also at critical stages of reproduction, since nutrition, maternal body composition and reproductive function and performance are inextricably linked. Consequently nutritional research in sows has in the main focused on selected stages of the reproductive cycle, such as the effect of nutrient intake in lactation on litter growth rate. The potential residual impact of previous nutrition and the influence of the nutritional treatments on the ensuing and subsequent parities are often ignored.

## Research methodology

Experiments on either short-term or lifetime responses in reproductive performance to nutritional influences are usually based on the following approaches to modifying the animal's nutritional status:

1. Changing the daily feed allowance (gross supply).
2. Changing the demand (e.g. artificial reduction or increase in size of the litter suckled by lactating sows).
3. Modifying the balance between energy and ideal protein in the diet.
4. Altering the levels of specific ingredients in the diet that may affect reproductive function (e.g. vitamins, trace elements, fatty acids and fibre type).

In some investigations, nutritional stress is either augmented or attenuated by applying the treatments (e.g. changing supply and demand) to populations of animals with low and high levels of body reserves (e.g. fat) at the start of the experiment (e.g. Yang *et al*., 1989). It is not within the scope of this chapter to review the large number of scientific papers based on different approaches to investigating nutritional influences on reproductive performance. The aim will be to highlight some of the major findings, where appropriate referring to relevant studies as background knowledge. The subject of specific dietary factors which are of importance to reproductive function deserves a separate review and will not be considered here.

## Influence of nutrient supply and demand on reproductive performance

### UTERINE ENVIRONMENT

There is a general acceptance that the established conceptus is reasonably well protected from quite adverse influences resulting from maternal nutritional deprivation. Although pregnancy under such circumstances may be successfully concluded, there may be long-term adverse effects on the fertility and fecundity of the female offspring. This is possible since, in mammals, development of the pituitary, oogenesis and histogenesis of the uterus in the conceptus are initiated prenatally. Thus if ovarian development in the foetus is compromised by shortfalls in uterine nutrient supply due to poor maternal nutrition, then such effects may carry forward in the form of sub-optimal reproductive performance in the next generation. The work of Jensen *et al.* (1983) suggests that such influences may exist, since it was found that gilts with the heaviest birth weights went on to produce a higher number born in their first litter, but such effects were not seen in the size of the second litter. However, uterine nutritional influences on the reproductive potential of the offspring have not been well researched in the pig.

## Postnatal growth and development

Understanding of potential nutritional influences during postnatal growth and development on the subsequent reproductive performance of female littermates is also very limited. The piglet following birth to about 3 weeks of age is almost entirely dependent on the supply of nutrients and water by the lactating sow. Thus shortfalls in both the quantity and quality of the milk supply may adversely influence the subsequent reproductive performance of the female offspring, as well as its growth potential.

The positive influences of an adequate milk supply on both pre-weaning growth and subsequent reproductive performance of female littermates were demonstrated by Jensen *et al.* (1983), where an increase in gilt weaning weight was associated with an increase in numbers born alive in her first litter. Nelson and Robison, (1976b) manipulated the competition for maternal milk by altering the number of piglets suckled to either 6 or 14 from birth to weaning at 8 weeks. Gilts nursed under more privileged conditions (6 per litter) were about 4.5 kg heavier at weaning and went onto to produce increased number born alive in their first litter (8.71 v 7.53) resulting from a higher ovulation rate (12.96 v 11.95 corpora lutea). In a similar study, Martin and Crenshaw (1989) found that gilts nursed over a 4 week lactation in a reduced litter size of 6, compared with 12, subsequently had a higher ovulation rate (16.6 v 14.1 corpora lutea), but this did not translate into increased number born alive. The benefit to early reproductive performance in female offspring suckled under favourable conditions of milk supply have been demonstrated in other species such as mice (Nelson and Robison, 1976a).

These studies indicate that the nutrition of gilts during the sucking stage can influence their subsequent reproductive performance. There appears to be a positive association between high pre-weaning growth rate and ovulation rate and the size of the first litter produced by female littermates.

## Beyond weaning to puberty

The influence of nutritional supply beyond weaning on age, weight and body condition at puberty in the female has received much interest in all species including the pig (Kirkwood *et al.*, 1987). In pigs, weight and age at puberty can have a potential impact on the economics of production in relation to culling, reproductive performance during the first litter and lifetime productivity. Thus there have been many studies on determining the effects of different feeding levels during the rearing stage on age and weight at puberty. However, nutritional supply is likely to interact with many other factors which influence the attainment of puberty and such factors make direct comparison of different studies extremely difficult. Some of these factors are summarised below.

1. Initial age, weight and body condition of the gilt at which different levels of feed restriction are applied in the rearing stage.
2. Previous nutritional history.
3. Health status.
4. Genotype.
5. Extreme difference in feeding level studied.
6. Intensity and duration of feed restriction.
7. Nutrient composition of the diet fed.
8. Boar stimulation.
9. Group v individual penning.
10. Relocation of animals during the course of the study.

Whilst taking account of the varying conditions under which different studies have been conducted, the results suggest that puberty is only noticeably delayed when feed restriction (equivalent to between 0.5 and 0.88 of *ad libitum* intake) is either initiated or applied during early growth (approximately <50 kg body weight) (Friend, 1976; Etienne *et al.*, 1983; Hartog and Noordeweir, 1984; Kirkwood, 1985; Lunen and Aherne, 1987; Beltranena *et al.*, 1991; Cozler*et al.*, 1998). In some studies the impact of feed restriction (0.6 of semi-*ad libitum* level) has been proportionally greater in reducing body weight than substantially increasing age at puberty (Hartog and Noordeweir, 1984). This suggests that physiological maturity, which is time dependent, is of greater importance to the attainment of puberty than body weight *per se*. Nutrient restriction applied after about 50 kg body weight appears to have a limited or no influence on age at puberty, although body weight is still reduced (Etienne *et al.*, 1983; King, 1989; Newton and Mahan, 1992; Klindt *et al.*, 1999).

In summary, studies on the influence of nutrition on the attainment of puberty suggest that reproductive development is more sensitive to a restriction in nutrient supply during early growth.

## Influences of feed supply before first service on ovulation rate, embryonic mortality and litter size

The underlying mechanisms by which nutritional environment within the uterus and during nursing influence the subsequent reproductive performance of the female offspring are poorly understood. In the studies of Nelson and Robison (1976b) and Martin and Crenshaw (1989), gilts nursed in reduced litter sizes had increased ovulation rates but there was a lack of consistency in the benefit to numbers born alive because of differences in embryonic mortality.

A reduction in feed supply before and up to puberty has been associated with a decreased ovulation rate at the first observed oestrus. The difference in ovulation rate between full-fed and restricted gilts has been found to increase with the advance in oestrus number (Hartog, 1984; Beltranena *et al*., 1991). In a review of 22 trials evaluating the effects of feed allowance over 30 to 75 days before ovulation rate was measured, an average ovulatory response of an additional 1.2 ova was observed at the higher level of feed intake (25 v 37 MJ DE/day) (Anderson and Melampy, 1972). However, the high variability in ovulation rate and the limited number of gilts in many studies does not allow for statistical confidence in the effects of nutrient supply on the number of ova shed, irrespective of trends. Although ovulation rate tends to increase with increased level of feeding during the rearing stage, this advantage often fails to translate into increased number born alive because of natural adjustments through embryonic mortality and still births (Hartog, 1984).

The possibility of increasing ovulation rate by increasing the plane of nutrition shortly before mating in gilts previously offered restricted levels of feed has continued to attract interest. This so-called flush feeding is anticipated to increase the number of oocytes shed either equivalent to or in excess of those produced by gilts reared under *ad libitum* feeding. In the studies of Etienne *et al*. (1983) and Beltranena *et al*. (1991), flushing either before or after the first oestrus increased ovulation rate in restrict-fed gilts to a level similar to that found in *ad libitum* fed gilts. Thus flushing did not give an additional bonus in the number of ova shed in gilts previously reared under restricted feeding. Moreover the benefit in increased ovulation rate from flushing and *ad libitum* feeding over restricted feeding was lost by day 105 of pregnancy through increased embryonic mortality in flushed gilts and increased foetal losses in *ad libitum* fed gilts. Thus by day 105 of pregnancy, Etienne *et al*. (1983) found that gilts carried a similar number of foetuses irrespective of differences in nutritional management before mating at first oestrus. More recently, Klindt *et al*. (1999) were unable to increase ovulation rate by flushing gilts following restricted feeding (0.74 of *ad libitum* intake from 13 to 25 weeks of age or about 44 to 103 kg). Although gilts reared on *ad libitum* feeding had a higher ovulation rate, by day 30 of pregnancy the number of live embryos did not differ from those found in flushed gilts.

The existence of a positive influence of increased feed supply before mating (1.15 v 3.5 kg/day over an entire oestrus cycle preceding mating) on both ovulation rate and embryonic survival in Meishan gilts has been reported in the studies of Ashworth *et al*. (1999). However, a ration of 1.15 kg per day is a severe level of restriction and it could be argued that normal reproductive function in a highly prolific and fecund breed is compromised by under-nutrition rather than enhanced by feed allowances closer to voluntary intake. For example, Mburu *et al.* (1998) found that food deprivation lasting for 48 hours after ovulation reduced embryonic cleavage rate and the number of accessory spermatozoa in the zona pellucida of the fertilised ova. There were also a greater number of food-deprived sows with degenerative embryos.

## Pregnancy

The use of concentrated cereal-based diets necessitates restriction of feed intake during pregnancy to avoid excess weight gain and adverse consequences for subsequent reproductive performance. The difference between daily feed allowance and the appetite potential of pregnant sows has led to investigations on the use of high-fibre low-density diets to satisfy hunger and thus enhance sow welfare. Such an approach has proved commercially unsuccessful because of increased cost and operational difficulties in handling bulky fibrous feeds and the increased volume of manure from using such materials. Thus commercial feeds for dry sows continue to be based on the use of dry high-energy cereal and protein-rich ingredients that require increased precision of feeding level. The adverse influences on reproductive performance of either under- or over-supplying feed to pregnant sows are well known and have been the subject of previous reviews (e.g. Einarsson and Rojkittikhun, 1993; Dourmad *et al.*, 1994). Problems identified with over supply in previous studies (e.g. excessive weight gain, increased risk of lameness together with reduced intake and increased weight loss in lactation and extended weaning to rebreeding interval) probably apply to current genotypes. However, it is worth noting that the levels of allowance which were considered 'high' some 20 and even 10 years ago would be approaching those currently used to retain sows in satisfactory body condition. Certainly the mature weight of breeding pigs has progressively increased with continued selection for increased lean content in slaughter pigs marketed at a fixed weight of between 95 and 100 kg. As a consequence, the young sow will continue to demonstrate a high potential for maternal lean gain over parities 1 to 3 ultimately reaching mature weight well beyond the average age at disposal. Farm records indicate a progressive increase in the amount of feed used per sow per year (Gill, 1996) and the higher requirements associated with increased mature weight will have certainly made a contribution to this trend.

Although studies on gross feed supply will continue to redefine the level at which elements of sow productivity are optimised, genetic selection has generated new nutritional challenges by pushing together lean growth, leanness and reproduction within the same timeframe. Thus the balance between energy and ideal protein in the diet, together with the level of daily supply have to be considered against the requirements and consequences for growth and reproduction in young lean sows.

## Influences from changing the balance of energy and ideal protein in the diet

Opportunities for manipulating the balance between energy and protein intake in the offspring, to determine subsequent influences on reproductive performance, are limited before weaning and more so before birth. The impact of restricting protein intake, under non-limiting levels of energy supply, during foetal and postnatal growth on reproductive function has not been widely researched.

## Post weaning

In many of the previous studies based on altering feed supply during rearing, it has not been possible to dissociate the effects of protein and fat gain on the attainment of puberty and reproductive performance in the young gilt. Differential manipulation of lean is better achieved through changing ideal protein content in the diet whilst attempting to achieve comparable levels of energy content and intake. The rationale is that by limiting the amount of essential amino acids available for lean tissue growth, metabolisable energy must be diverted to the accretion of fat reserves.

It is worth noting that the recent studies using this technique were designed to promote fat deposition in lean genotypes before mating and during first pregnancy (Gill, 1996; O'Dowd *et al.*, 1997) rather than to investigate a potential relationship between lean growth and reproduction. However, the early results from the large-scale study established by the Meat and Livestock Commission (MLC) in 1995 on the control of lean growth during rearing and pregnancy (see Figure 4.2) and complementary work at the Scottish Agricultural College places new concerns over the adverse effects of this strategy on early reproductive performance. In the MLC trial, a 50% reduction in the lysine: energy ratio of diets fed *ad libitum* to gilts from about 35 kg body weight reduced maternal body weight and increased backfat at mating, but age at first oestrus and mating was delayed by 11 days Table 4.5 (Gill, 1996). Subsequent analysis of first litter data showed that gilts fed a series of diets with a high ratio of lysine: energy during rearing and pregnancy produced the largest first litters Table 4.6 (Gill and Taylor, 1999).

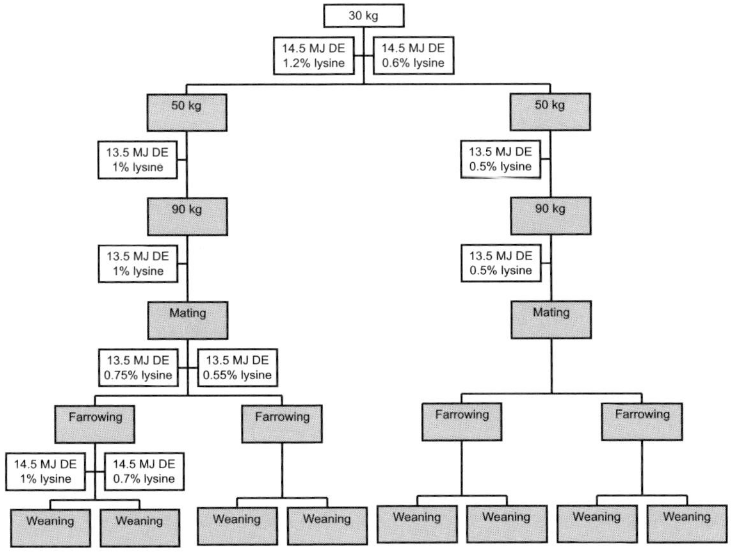


**Figure 4.2** Nutritional pathways of Large White x Landrace gilts fed series of diets differing in lysine: energy ratios from about 30 kg to completion of the first parity in the MLC Stotfold trial. (After: Gill 1996)

**Table 4.5** INFLUENCE OF HIGH V LOW LYSINE TO ENERGY BALANCE IN DIETS FED DURING THE REARING STAGE ON AGE AT FIRST OESTRUS AND AGE, WEIGHT AND CARCASS BACKFAT THICKNESS AT MATING IN LARGE WHITE X LANDRACE GILTS

| *Lysine: Energy ratio in diet* | *High* | *Low* | *s.e.d.* | *P* |
|---|---|---|---|---|
| *From serially slaughtered gilts* | | | | |
| n | 8 | 8 | | |
| Weight at mating (kg) | 133 | 113 | 7.8 | * |
| Carcass P2 at mating (mm) | 11.9 | 15.6 | 1.83 | P=0.06 |
| *Gilts remaining in herd* | | | | |
| n (interim analysis) | 40 | 40 | | |
| Age at first oestrus (days) | 164 | 176 | 5.0 | * |
| Age at mating (days) | 220 | 233 | 5.1 | ** |
| Weight at mating (kg) | 136 | 125 | 3.3 | *** |

(After: Gill 1996 and 1999)

The studies by Cia *et al.* (1998) showed that gilts reared on low-lysine diets had increased latency to exhibit oestrus, reduced ovulation rate and a lower incidence of spontaneous second oestrus, following treatment with exogenous gonadotrophin at 160 days of age. Recently Crisol *et al.* (1997) were able to

TABLE 4.6 FIRST LITTER PERFORMANCE OF LARGE WHITE X LANDRACE GILTS ACCORDING TO NUTRITIONAL PATHWAY (SEE FIGURE 10.2) FROM 30 KG TO WEANING

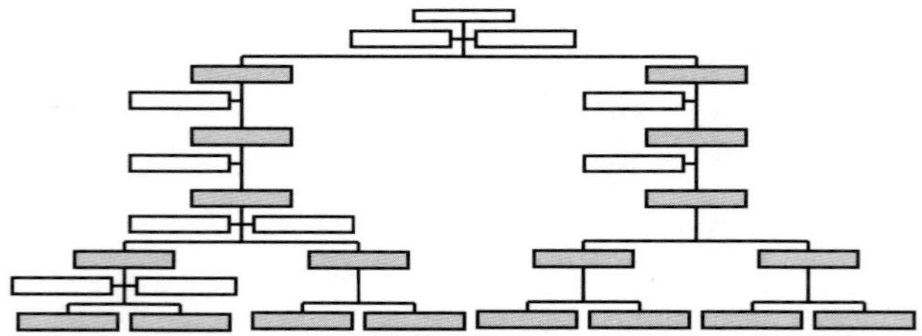

| | | | | | | | | | *Significance*[b] | | | | | | |
|---|---|---|---|---|---|---|---|---|---|---|---|---|---|---|---|
| | | | | | | | | | *R* | *P* | *L* | *RxP* | *RxL* | *PxL* | *RxPxL* |
| *At farrowing* | | | | | | | | | | | | | | | |
| Born alive | 10.6 | | 9.1 | | 9.9 | | 9.5 | | NS | * | - | NS | - | - | - |
| Total born | 11.5 | | 10.1 | | 10.6 | | 10.4 | | NS | * | - | NS | - | - | - |
| Birth weight (kg) | 1.37 | | 1.37 | | 1.38 | | 1.42 | | NS | NS | - | NS | - | - | - |
| *At weaning* | | | | | | | | | | | | | | | |
| Number of gilts | 28 | 29 | 27 | 25 | 29 | 32 | 30 | 29 | | | | | | | |
| Number weaned | 10.5 | 10.3 | 10.2 | 9.7 | 10.1 | 10.2 | 9.9 | 10.7 | NS | NS | NS | NS | 0.10 | NS | NS |
| Weaning weight (kg) | 6.4 | 5.8 | 6.2 | 6.0 | 6.0 | 6.2 | 6.5 | 6.0 | NS | NS | * | NS | NS | NS | 0.06 |

(After: Gill 1999)

[a] See Figure 10.2 for details of treatments

[b] R = Effect of rearing diet, high v low lysine (30 kg to mating)

P = Effect of pregnancy diet, high v low lysine

L = Effect of lactational diet, high v low lysine

RxP = Interaction between rearing and pregnancy diets

RxL = Interaction between rearing and lactational diets

PxL = Interaction between pregnancy and lactational diets

RxPxL = Interaction between rearing, pregnancy and lactation diets.

reverse the negative effects of protein restricted growth on ovulation rate (first and second oestrus) by increasing ideal protein intake and thus growth rate 5 days before induction of puberty with exogenous gonadotrophins (PG600) at 180 days of age.

These recent studies are now clearly showing that lean growth before puberty and during the first and perhaps the second parity in young sows cannot be separated from reproduction. Nutritional influences which promote the high growth potential of modern lean genotypes are also those which promote optimum reproductive function at the first and possibly the second litter. Once the risk of mismatch between ideal protein supply and the requirements for lean deposition disappear as the animal approaches mature weight, then the adverse influences of a restricted protein supply on reproductive performance will greatly diminish.

## Lifetime influences of early nutrition

Amongst the many studies on the influence of nutrition before puberty on reproduction in the gilt, there have been very few which have carried on to investigate residual effects on lifetime sow performance. However, the evidence from these trials is both disappointing in that nutrition during the rearing stage offers limited scope for greatly enhancing lifetime reproduction, but reassuring in that nutritional attenuation of pre-pubertal growth appears to have no serious lasting effects after the first litter. Where early reproductive function has been compromised either through protein or feed restriction, this can be reversed over a relatively short period by increasing nutrient supply (Beltranena *et al.*, 1991; Crisol *et al.*, 1997).

## Feeding level during rearing

Whilst litter size averaged over several parities seems generally unaffected by feeding intensity over the rearing stage, gilts with excessive weight gains before first service are more likely to be prematurely culled for lameness and may thus have reduced life-time productivity (Jongbloed *et al.,* 1984; Sorensen *et al.*, 1993).

## Protein/energy balance

The MLC gilt rearing study is based on altering growth and body composition at first mating through the manipulation of dietary energy and ideal protein balance under *ad libitum* feeding rather than through feed allowance. It is not possible to establish if protein restriction during the rearing stage and in first pregnancy will significantly influence lifetime sow performance since the trial is due for completion in 2001. However, there are some similarities with trials based on altering feed allowances, in that the feeding of a series of diets with higher ideal protein: energy ratios during rearing promoted higher weight gains (Gill, 1996) but increased the risk of premature culling for lameness (Gill and Taylor, 1999). On the other hand protein restriction increased the proportion of first litter sows culled for reproductive failure (Figure 4.3).

Thus there appears to be a conflict between the need to avoid lameness and enhance early reproductive performance in relation to nutritional management of growth before first service.

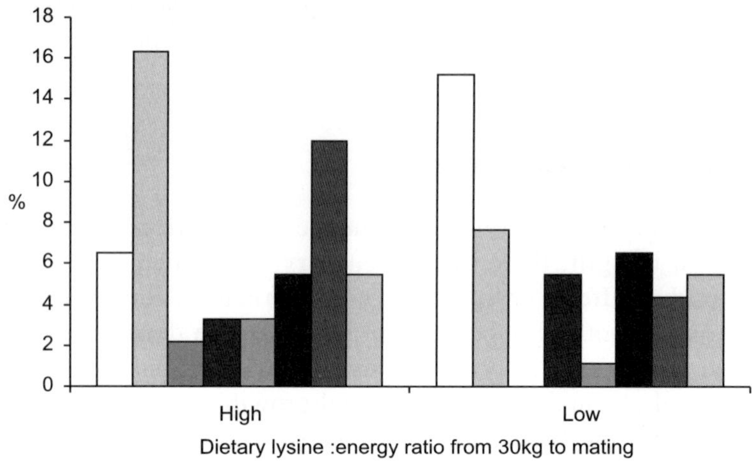


**Figure 4.3** Reasons for gilts failing to produce a viable first litter in the MLC Stotfold trial (□ Rep. failure; □ Legs; ■ Not standing to boar; ■ Died; □ Health; ■ Other; ■ Poor milker; □ Unknown) (After: Gill 1999)

Results from analysis of body composition of gilts fed diets containing high v low lysine: energy ratios, in a factorial sequence over rearing (about 35 kg to first mating), pregnancy and lactation, are summarised in Figures 10.4a to 10.4f. It is worth noting that it was not possible to achieve a target backfat thickness of 19mm at first mating despite *ad libitum* access, during the entire rearing stage, to diets restricted by 50% in ideal protein (lysine) content. Gilts fed the lysine-restricted diets during rearing, pregnancy and lactation had the lightest and fattest (lipid/protein ratio) maternal bodies after weaning their first litter. It remains to be seen if differences in maternal size and composition at the end of the first parity are associated with differences in lifetime productivity.

Figures 4.4a to 4.4f Numbers and body composition of F1 Large White x Landrace gilts serially slaughtered from the MLC Stotfold gilt trial (see Figure 4.2 for experimental design).

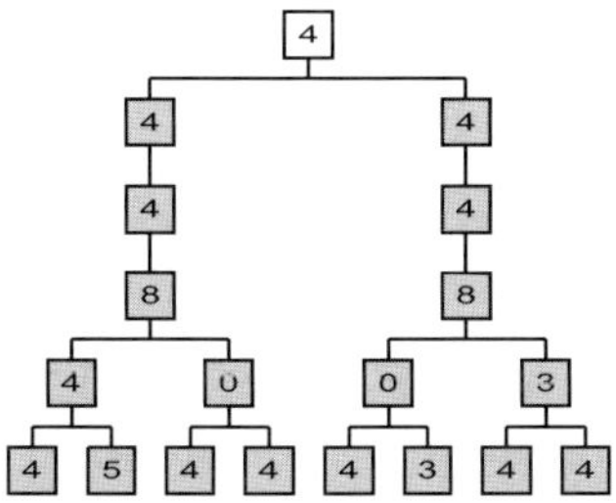


**Figure 4.4a** Number of gilts slaughtered

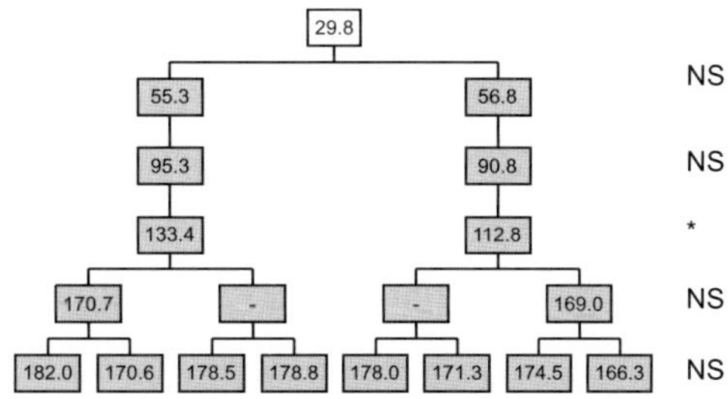


**Figure 4.4b** Live weight (kg)

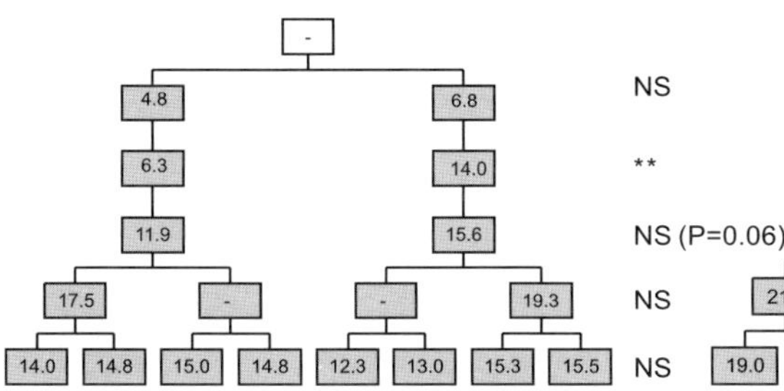


**Figure 4.4c** Carcass backfat P2 (mm)

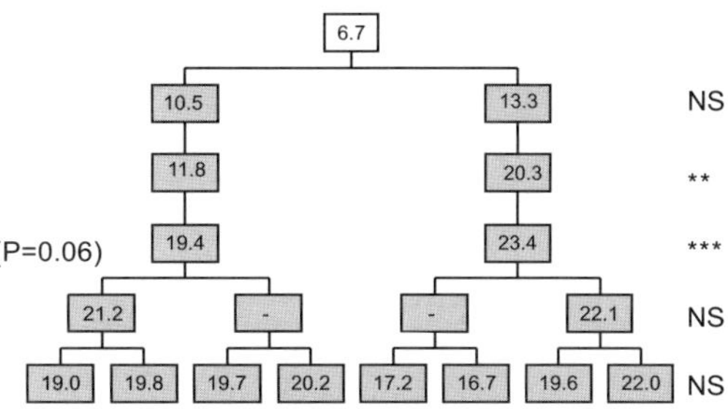


**Figure 4.4d** Body lipid (%)

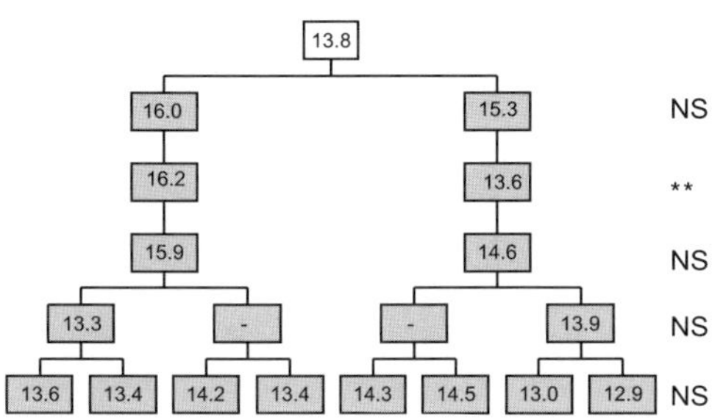


**Figure 4.4e** Body protein (%)

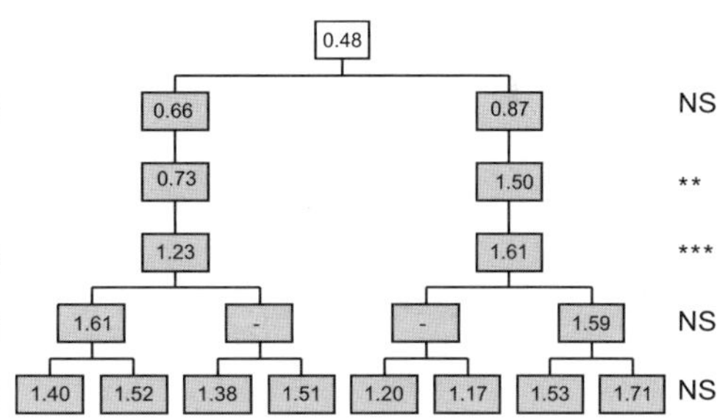


**Figure 4.4f** Body lipid:protein ratio

## Longer-term trials and lifetime performance

The influence on sow performance of nutritional treatments applied before first mating and consecutively over subsequent parities has been investigated in a number studies. However, few studies have concluded by examining lifetime performance.

Several studies based on feeding level have failed to influence litter size averaged over several parities (Hoppe *et al.*, 1990; Simmins *et al.*, 1992; Coffey *et al.*, 1994), though where intake during pregnancy has been excessively restricted, piglet birth weights have decreased and litters per sow lifetime have been reduced through increased culling (Elsley *et al.*, 1969; Young *et al.*, 1990).

Earlier co-ordinated trials designed to establish protein requirements over consecutive parities found no appreciable benefits in litter productivity and performance by increasing dietary protein content during lactation (Greenhalgh *et al.*, 1977; Mahan, 1979). Thus for simplicity, the use of a single diet with a similar level of energy and protein for both pregnancy and lactation was recommended. It is interesting to note that in the studies of Greenhalgh *et al.* (1977) there was a positive linear response in numbers born alive in the first litter to ideal protein intake during pregnancy. There was also a positive response in maternal growth in first pregnancy to increased levels of protein intake. It is possible that the origin of these responses is not dissimilar to those reported in recent investigations on protein restriction in modern genotypes (Gill, 1996; Cia *et al.*, 1998; Gill and Taylor, 1999) and that continued selection for increased leanness has just made it more apparent. The results of a further co-ordinated trial from the Rowett Research Institute showed that there was potential merit from using different protein levels in pregnancy and lactation with respect to litter growth rate but not litter size over three parities (Greenhalgh *et al.*, 1980). As intensive selection for lean content accelerated in commercial breeding companies, the benefits to sow lifetime productivity from using a two-diet system became clear in the results of renewed research at Aberdeen (O'Dowd *et al.*, 1997). In this study the feeding of a high concentration lactating diet (14.8 MJ DE, 9.5 g lysine per kg) coupled with a diet to promote fat reserves in pregnancy (13.0 MJ DE, 4.5 g lysine per kg) reduced the proportion of animals failing to produce three litters (0.17 v 0.30) and culled for reproductive failure (0.03 v 0.11). Over recent years the two diet system has become increasingly adopted to enhance sow productivity on commercial farms in the UK.

## Lactational feeding strategies

Nutritional influences during lactation are pivotal to the successful rebreeding of young sows. It is probable that the greater benefit from using a two-diet system comes from preventing excessive mobilisation of maternal tissues through feeding a high-concentration lactating diet (Hoste *et al.*, 1994). It is beyond the scope of this chapter to consider in depth the subject of nutritional requirements and influences during lactation on sow lifetime performance. Much of what has been considered in previous reviews (Cole, 1989; Edwards, 1998) will remain relevant to current pig production although it is likely that the challenge of increasing nutrient intake during lactation will become greater with the increasing demands on highly prolific lean genotypes.

An area which holds future potential is that of liquid-feeding using sensor technology that allows lactating sows to feed on demand without the problem of rejected feed turning stale and suppressing appetite. Liquid-feeding also increases producer accessibility to a wider range of ingredients which occur in liquid form and to improve nutritional value through enzyme treatment. Currently there is a lack of controlled research on the liquid-feeding of lactating sows and this is needed to substantiate anecdotal evidence of 15% improvements in dry matter intake and pig weaning weights on commercial farms using such systems.

## Conclusions

Premature culling of young sows due to reproductive failure has remained a serious problem in the pig industry in many countries over many years. Failure to show oestrus, conceive and rebreed are the major reasons for the early disposal of sows due to reproductive problems. Lameness in young sows is another significant cause of wastage. It is often tempting to over-state the role of nutrition and genetics in bringing about premature reproductive failure. Many other factors are involved and some of them will have a much greater contribution than nutritional effects. These include the quality of the environment under which gilts and young sows are housed and the experience of stockpeople in managing replacement gilts to produce their first litter and successfully rebreed for their second.

Recommended targets for body fatness at first mating may have to be revised against the response of modern lean genotype to nutritional influences and their requirements to achieve optimum lifetime performance. Evidence from recent research indicates the increasing importance of protein supply in relation to growth during the rearing and the first parity and early reproductive function and performance. It seems that nutritional influences which promote the high growth potential of modern lean genotypes are also those which promote optimum reproductive function at the first and possibly the second litter. However, the increased risk of lameness by promoting high growth rates will need to be managed through higher standards of housing and husbandry and possibly thorough genetic selection.

Nutrition during lactation, particularly during the first and second parity, will remain pivotal to successful rebreeding and lifetime productivity. Liquid-feeding technology offers increased scope for enhancing the nutritional status of young lactating sows, whereby body weight losses could be reduced and the chances of rebreeding improved. However, this requires research so that the benefits can be quantified.

Trials designed to establish the effects of nutrition or feeding strategies on the lifetime performance of sows should include a cost-benefit analysis. The economic value of improved lifetime sow productivity must be greater than the cost of achieving the increased output.

Improving reproductive efficiency will remain a challenge and this will require a holistic multidisciplinary approach, bringing together research teams including nutritionists and reproductive physiologists. Eventually the benefits of research should be transferred to the industry, perhaps by adopting a blueprint approach which has proved successful in the uptake of new technologies and research on meat quality.

## References

Anderson, L.L. and Melampy, R.M. (1972) Factors affecting ovulation rate in the pig. In: *Pig Production* pp 329-366. Edited by D.J.A. Cole. Proceedings of the 18th Easter School in Agricultural Science, University of Nottingham. Butterworths, London.

ARC. (1981) The nutrient requirements of pigs. Commonwealth Agricultural Bureaux, Slough, UK.

Ashworth, C.J., Antipatis, C. and Beattie, L. (1999) Effects of pre- and post-mating nutritional status on hepatic function, progesterone concentration, uterine protein secretion and embryonic survival in Meishan pigs. *Reproduction, Fertility and Development Fertility* **11**:67-74.

Beltranena, E., Aherne, F.X., Foxcroft, G.R. and Kirkwood, R.N. (1991) Effects of pre- and post- pubertal feeding on production traits at first and second estrus in gilts. *Journal of Animal Science* **69**: 886-893.

Cia, M.C., Edwards, S.A., Glasgow, V.L., Shanks, M. and Fraser, H. (1998) Modification of body composition by altering the dietary lysine to energy ratio during rearing and the effect on reproductive performance of gilts. *Animal Science* **66**: 457-463.

Close, W.H. and Challinor, C.H. (1996) Good management will secure your gilt investment. Pigs. Society of Feed Technologists, Coventry. pp 4.

Coffey, M.T., Diggs, B.G., Handlin, D.L., Knabe, D.A., Maxwell, C.V., Noland, P.R., Prince, T.J. and Gromwell, G.L. (1994) Effects of dietary energy during gestation and lactation on reproductive performance of sows: A cooperative study. *Journal of Animal Science* **72**: 4-9.

Cole, D.J.A. (1989) Nutritional strategies to optimise reproduction in pigs. Proceedings of the *Third International Conference on Pig Reproduction*, University of Nottingham, Sutton Bonington, pp. 67-82.

Cozler, Y.L., David, C., Beaumal, V., Hulin, J.C., Neil, M. and Dourmad, J.Y. (1998) Effect of feeding level during rearing on performance of Large White gilts. Part 1: Growth, reproductive performance and feed intake during the first lactation. *Reproduction Nutrition Development 38*: 363-375.

Crisol, M., Edwards, S.A. and English, P.R. (1997) Short and long term effects of protein nutrition on reproduction in gilts. Proceedings of the Winter Meeting, Scarborough.

Culbertson, M.S. and Mabry, J.W. (1995) Effect of age at first service on first parity and subsequent lifetime sow performance (Annual Report 1995 ). University of Georgia, Athens, USA.

Dagron, J. and Aumaitre, A. (1979) Sow culling: Reasons for and effect on productivity. *Livestock Production Science* **6**: 167-177.

D'Allaire, S., Stein, T.E. and Leman, A.D. (1987) Culling patterns in selected Minnesota swine breeding herds. *Canadian Journal of Veterinary Research* **51**: 506-512.

Dijkhuizen, A.A., Krabbenborg, R.M.M. and Huirne, R.B.M. (1989) Sow replacement: A comparison of farmer's actual decisions and model recommendations. *Livestock Production Science* **23**: 207-218.

Dourmad, J.Y., Etienne, M., Prunier, A. and Noblet, J. (1994) The effect of energy and protein intake of sows on their longevity: A review. *Livestock Production Science* **40**: 87-97.

Edwards, S.A. (1998) Nutrition of the rearing gilt and sow. *Progress in Pig Science*, Nottingham University Press, pp. 361-382.

Einarsson, S. and Rojkittikhun, T. (1993) Effects of nutrition on pregnant and lactating sows. *Journal of Reproduction and Fertility Supplement* **48**: 229-239.

Ellis, M., Fowler, V.R., Franklin, M.F., Wood, J.D. and Varley, M.A. (1996) The influence of feeding regimen and lactation length on growth, carcass characteristics and meat quality of once-bred gilts. *Animal Science* **62**: 561-576.

Elsley, F.W.H., Bannerman, M., Bathurst, E.V., Bracewell, A.G., Cunningham, J. M.M., Dodsworth, T.L., Dodds, P.A., Forbes, T.J. and Laird, R. (1969) The effect of level of feed intake in pregnancy and in lactation upon the productivity of sows. *Animal Production* **11**: 225-241.

English, P.R., McPherson, O., Tarocco, C., Bertaccini, F., Deligeorgis, S.G. and Vidal, J.M.(1998) Evaluation of training methodologies, motivational influences and staff and enterprise development for pig industry workers in Scotland, Greece, Spain, Italy and Norway. Proceedings of the 15th International Pig Veterinary Society Congress, Nottingham University Press, pp. 15.

Etienne, M., Camous, S. and Cuvillier, A. (1983) Effect of feed restriction during growth on puberty and reproductive performance in gilts. *Reproduction Nutrition Development* **23**: 309-319.

Friend, D.W. (1976) Nutritional effects on age at puberty and plasma amino acid level in Yorkshire gilts and on chemical composition, nucleic acid, fatty acid and hydroxyproline contents of the uterus. *Journal of Animal Science* **43**: 404-412.

Gaughan, J.B., Cameron, R.D.A., Dryden, G.M. and Josey, M.J. (19950 Effect of selection for leanness on overall reproductive performance in Large White sows. *Animal Science* **61**: 561-564.

Gill, B.P. (19960 The nutritional management of gilts to enhance lifetime productivity. Pigs. *Society of Feed Technologists*, Coventry, pp. 12.

Gill, B.P. and Taylor, L. (1999) The nutritional management of gilts to enhance lifetime productivity: second progress report on the Stotfold gilt trial - body composition and first litter performance. Pigs. Society of Feed Technologists, Coventry, pp. 14.

Greenhalgh, J.F.D., Baird, B., Grubb, D.A., Done, S., Lightfoot, A.L., Smith, P., Toplis, P., Walker, N., Williams, D. and Yeo, M.L. (1980) Coordinated trials on the protein requirements of sows: 2. A comparison of two levels of dietary protein in gestation and four in lactation. *Animal Production* **30**: 395-406.

Greenhalgh, J.F.D., Elsley, F.W.H., Grubb, D.A., Lightfoot, A.L., Saul, D.W., Smith, P., Walker, N., Williams, D. and Yeo, M.L. (1977) Coordinated trials on the protein requirements of sows: 1. A comparison of four levels of dietary protein in gestation and two in lactation. *Animal Production* **24**: 307-321.

Hartog, L.A. den (1984) The effect of energy intake during rearing on reproductive traits in gilts. *Netherlands Journal of Agricultural Science* **32**: 281-292.

Hartog, L.A. den and Noordeweir, G.J. (1984) The effect of energy intake on age at puberty in gilts. *Netherlands Journal of Agricultural Science* **32**: 263-280.

Hoppe, M.K., Libal, G.W. and Wahlstrom, R.C. (1990) Influence of gestation energy level on the production of Large White x Landrace. *Journal of Animal Science* **68**: 2235-2242.

Hoste, S., O'Dowd, S., Francis, M.J.H., Mercer, J., Fowler, V.R. and Edwards, S.A. (1994) The effects of diet nutrient density during lactation on the reproductive performance of gilts of lean genotype. Proceedings of the 45th Annual Meeting, European Association of Animal Production, Edinburgh.

Jensen, P., Nielsen, H.E. and Danielsen, V. (19830 The influence of birth weight on the reproductive performance of gilts (Internal Communication No. 484/1983): National Institute of Animal Science, Foulum, Denmark.

Jongbloed, A.W., Diepen, J.T.M. and Hopman, L.C.C. (1984) The influence of energy level during rearing of breeding sows on longevity and lifetime production (Internal Report No. 169). Lelystad: Institute for livestock feeding and nutrition research (IVVO).

Kerr, J.C. and Cameron, N.D. (1995) Reproduction performance of pigs selected for components of efficient lean growth. *Animal Science* **60**: 281-290.

King, R.H. (1989) A note on the effects of nutrient intake during the later stages of rearing and early reproductive life on the subsequent reproduction efficiency of gilts. *Animal Production* **48**:241-244.

Kirkwood, R.N. (1985) Nutrition and sow productivity. Proceedings of the Sixth Western Nutrition Conference, Winnipeg, pp. 88-109.

Kirkwood, R.N., Cumming, D.C. and Aherne, F.X. (1987) Nutrition and puberty in the female. Proceedings of the Nutrition Society **46**: 177-192.

Klindt, J., Yen, J.T. and Christenson, R.K. (1999) Effect of prepubertal regimen on reproductive development of gilts. *Journal of Animal Science* **77**: 1968-1976.

Kroes, Y. and Male, J.P.V. (1979) Reproductive lifetime of sows in relation to economy of production. *Livestock Production Science* **6**: 179-183.

Lucia, T., Dial, G.D. and Marsh, W.E. (1999) Estimation of lifetime productivity of female swine. *Journal of American Veterinary Medicine Association* **214**: 1056-1059.

Lunen, T.A.V. and Aherne, F.X. (1987) Effect of long-term restriction on age at puberty of gilts. *Canadian Journal of Animal Science* **67**: 797-801.

Maclean, C.W. (1968) The thin sow problem. *The Veterinary Record*: 308-316.

Mahan, D.C. (1979) Effect of dietary protein sequence on long-term sow reproductive performance. *Journal of Animal Science* **49**: 514-521.

Martin, R.E. and Crenshaw, T.D. (1989) Effect of postnatal nutritional status on subsequent growth and reproductive performance of gilts. *Journal of Animal Science* **67**: 975-982.

Mburu, J.N., Einarsson, S., Kindahl, H., Madej, A. and Rodriguez-Martinez, H. (1998) Effects of post-ovulatory food deprivation on oviductal sperm concentration, embryo development and hormonal profiles in the pig. *Animal Reproduction Science* **52**: 221-234.

MLC. (1991) Stotfold Pig Development Unit, First Trial Results. Meat and Livestock Commission, Milton Keynes.

MLC. (1999) Pig Yearbook 1999. Meat and Livestock Commission, Milton Keynes.

Muirhead, M.R. and Alexander, T.J.L. (1997) Managing pig health and the treatment of disease. A reference for the farm. First Edition. 5M Enterprises Ltd.

Nakano, T., Brenan, J.J. and Aherne, F.X. (1987) Leg weakness and osteochondrosis in swine. *Canadian Journal of Animal Science* **67**: 883-901.

Nelson, A.H., Mabry, J.W., Benyshek, L.L. and Marks, M.A. (1990) Correlated responses in reproduction, growth and composition to selection in gilts for extremes in age at puberty and backfat. *Livestock Production Science* **24**: 237-247.

Nelson, R.E. and Robison, O.W. (1976a) Effects of postnatal litter size on reproduction of female mice. *Journal of Animal Science* 42: 824.

Nelson, R.E. and Robison, O.W. (1976b) Effects of postnatal maternal environment on reproduction of gilts. *Journal of Animal Science* **43**: 71-76.

Newton, E.A. and Mahan, D.C. (1992) Effect of feed intake during late development on pubertal onset and resulting body composition in crossbred gilts. *Journal of Animal Science* **70**: 3774-3780.

NRC. (1998) Nutrient requirements of swine. 10th Edition. National Academy Press, Washington.

O'Dowd, S., Hoste, S., Mercer, J.T., Fowler, V.R. and Edwards, S.A. (1997) Nutritional modifications of body composition and the consequences for reproductive performance and longevity in genetically lean sows. *Livestock Production Science* **52**: 155-165.

Schukken, Y.H., Buurman, J., Huirne, R.B.M., Willemse, A.H., Vernooy, J.C. M., Broek, J.v. d. and Verheijden, J.H.M. (1994) Evaluation of optimal age at first conception in gilts from data collected in commercial herds. *Journal of Animal Science* **72**: 1387-1392.

Simmins, P.H., Edwards, S.A., Spechter, H.H. and Riley, J.E. (1992) Lifetime performance of sows given different rearing and pregnancy feeding regimes. *Animal Production* **54**: 457A.

Sorensen, M.T., Jorgensen, B. and Danielsen, V. (1993) Different feeding intensity of young gilts:effects on growth, milk yield, reproduction, leg soundness and longevity (Internal Communication 14/1993): National Institute of Animal Science, Foulum, Denmark.

Stein, T.E., Dijkhuizen, A., D'Allaire, S. and Morris, R.S. (1990) Sow culling and mortality in commercial swine breeding herds. *Preventive Veterinary Medicine* **9**: 85-94.

Whittemore, C.T. (1998) The Science and Practice of Pig Production. Second Edition. Blackwell Science Ltd.

Yang, H., Eastham, P.R., Phillips, P. and Whittemore, C.T. (1989) Reproductive performance, body weight and body condition of breeding sows with differing body fatness at parturition, differing nutrition during lactation, and differing litter size. *Animal Production* **48**: 181-201.

Young, L.G., King, G.J., Walton, J.S., McMillan, I., Klevorick, M. and Shaw, J. (1990) Gestation energy and reproduction in sows over four parities. *Canadian Journal of Animal Science* **70**: 493-506.

*This paper was first published in 2000*

5

# FORMULATING FEEDS FOR SOWS – FEEDING GESTATING SOWS WITH HIGH FIBRE DIETS

R.DURÁN GIMÉNEZ – RICO
*Technical Department, Trouw Nutrition España, Nutreco, Ronda de Poniente, 9, 28760, Tres Cantos, Madrid, Spain*
*Current address: Danisco Animal Nutrition, Reyes Católicos, 6, OF.1A 28220, Majadahonda, Spain*

## Introduction

*"Prediction is very difficult, especially about the future"* (Niels Bohr)

Hunger in pregnant sows is considered a major welfare problem, especially in the Northern European countries. Pregnant sows are fed restrictively; the biggest effect of feeding during pregnancy is on the body weight of the sow and excessive dietary energy intake leads to heavier sows with increased maintenance requirements. Furthermore, those animals might show a decrease feed intake in the following lactation and, most probably, an excessive loss of body condition at weaning. On the other hand, under-feeding should be avoided, as this is associated with a risk of impairing reproductive performance and poor body condition. Pregnant sows are fed once or twice per day and, with these allowances, their maintenance requirements and those necessary to support a small amount of maternal growth and the growth of conceptus are met. However, these conditions might not fulfil the feeding motivation needs of these animals; this means that satiety level is not reached and sows will develop stereotyped activities (Meunier-Salaün, 1999). The latter are characterised by behavioural patterns performed repetitively in a fixed order and without any evident function. Abnormal behaviours (including stereotypes) are indicators of poor welfare (Vestergaard, 1997).

Fibre is suggested as a means of increasing bulkiness of the diet and acts as an energy diluent. The influence of fibre in the diet will depend on the inclusion rate, the type of fibre used and the non-starch polysaccharide (NSP) content. Increased bulkiness may be beneficial in pregnant sows that are currently fed well below their appetite potential. In this way, the utilisation of fibre in diets for pregnant sows and the improvement of their welfare by means of a reduced stereotypic behaviour observed in some recent studies (Brouns, 1994, 1995; Vestergaard, 1997; Ramonet, 1999) has gained popularity in countries such as The Netherlands and Denmark. The former decided to make it compulsory to formulate diets for pregnant sows with a minimum of 140 g CF/kg diet or 340 g OOS("Overige Organische Stoff", or Other Organic Material) / kg diet. Within the Dutch Agricultural Legislation of September 1998, a list of fibre-containing ingredients was included as possible materials for feeding to pregnant sows ("Varkensbesluit", Sept., 1998). Moreover, the above mentioned 140 g CF/kg level was also adopted as a way of enabling the formulation of complete diets without the need for extra dry or green roughage.

At the same time, the new evaluation system of net energy for sows (Noblet, 1993-1994) was the subject of study by the main feed compound industries in The Netherlands: a useful link between fibre-containing ingredients – new NE system for sows – and welfare of sows was established.

This chapter describes a detailed programme of work conducted by Nutreco in the Netherlands. The overall objective was to obtain a practical solution to feeding pregnant sows high levels of fibre without impairing reproductive performance.

## Utilisation of energy from ingredients

The Gross Energy (GE) of ingredients is not fully available to animals. Part of that energy is lost in faeces, in urine and in gaseous products resulting from fermentation in the hindgut. The final metabolic utilisation of the energy from feed implies also a loss of energy called heat increment. Different ratios are calculated in order to appreciate the efficiencies at each level. Mean energy losses, expressed as proportion of GE, together with mean efficiencies, were proposed by Noblet (1994) (Figure 5.1).

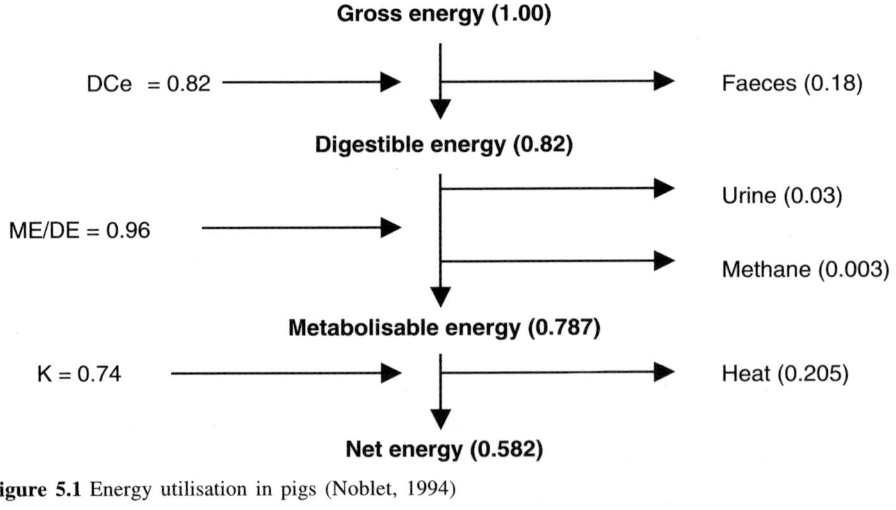


**Figure 5.1** Energy utilisation in pigs (Noblet, 1994)

For most pig diets, the coefficient of energy-digestibility (DCe) varies between 0.70 and 0.90 (Noblet, 1996); for individual ingredients, variations are greater (0 to 1.00). These variations are due to differences in faecal digestibility of the constituents of organic matter. Starch and sugars, both soluble carbohydrates, are highly digestible (>0.95); protein and crude fat between 0.60 and 0.95, while most of the variation in DCe is associated with the presence of fibre, referred to subsequently as OOM (from the Dutch OOS).

## OOM DEFINITION

OOM is a dietary category that includes all carbohydrates, including lignin, but with the exception of starch and sugar. Essentially, OOM represents that proportion of a feed and/or ingredient that might be potentially fermented in the hindgut, or even partially fermented in the lower parts of the small intestine (e.g. OOM from sugar beet pulp).

Though seen as an artefact, OOM is defined as (OM – CP – EE – Starch – Sugar), where OM=organic matter; CP = crude protein; EE = ether extract. It has become a practical tool for formulating high-fibre diets for gestating sows (SRC, Nutreco 1997-2000) while designing and performing the trials on sow feeding. Differences between the NSP and OOM contents of several feedstuffs are shown in Table 5.1.

**Table 5.1** COMPARISON OF CRUDE FIBRE (CF) AND NON-STARCH POLYSACCHARIDE (NSP) CONTENTS OF SOME COMMONLY USED INGREDIENTS (G/KG DM; LONGLAND AND LOW, 1995). OOM VALUES IN G/KG DM (CVB, 1999 AND CVB VERKORTE TABEL, 1994)

| | *CF* | *NSP* | *OOM* |
|---|---|---|---|
| Barley | 53 | 147 | 221 |
| Wheat bran | 85 | 360 | 474 |
| Soya hulls | 354 | 868 | 758 |
| Soyabean meal | 85 | 190 | 284 |
| Rapeseed meal | 120 | 286 | 392 |
| Sugar beet pulp | 174 | 635 | 736 |
| Citrus pulp | 118 | 415 | 600 |
| Wheat straw | 400 | 632 | 877 |

Differences in NSP and OOM are as predicted if fibre is defined in accordance with Low (1985), who described fibre as "the non-starch polysaccharides (NSP) plus lignin". In other words, OOM is the NSP plus the lignin content of a given ingredient or complete feed.

## DIGESTIVE UTILISATION OF FIBRE

In agreement with Noblet and Shi (1993), the digestibility coefficient of energy in diets decreased linearly when the NDF content increased. According to the previous definition of OOM, the neutral detergent fibre (NDF) fraction is included in OOM; therefore, it is assumed that the more OOM in the diet, the less digestible it becomes for pigs. Additionally, sows showed a higher capacity to digest fibrous diets than growing pigs (Shi and Noblet, 1993). The cell wall components present in the dietary fibre fraction (NDF or NSP or OOM) show much lower digestibility coefficients than other components of ingredients or diets. Ramonet (1999, Table 5.2) showed differences in DC of fibre between growing pigs and sows for various ingredients. While the NDF fraction of sugar beet pulp is well digested by both pigs and sows, the difference for maize fibre was 0.42. Pectins in sugar beet pulp are water soluble and more digestible than lignin, in which maize fibre is very rich. Consequently, variability in DCe for different ingredients is associated with fibre origin as well as cell wall content (lignin content).

**Table 5.2** COEFFICIENT OF DIGESTIBILITY OF FIBRE FRACTIONS IN GROWING PIGS AND SOWS (ADAPTED FROM RAMONET, 1999)

| | *Wheat bran* | | *Maize fibre* | | *Sugar beet pulp* | |
|---|---|---|---|---|---|---|
| | *Pig* | *Sow* | *Pig* | *Sow* | *Pig* | *Sow* |
| NDF | 0.48 | 0.51 | 0.39 | 0.81 | 0.84 | 0.89 |
| ADF | 0.26 | 0.33 | 0.38 | 0.82 | 0.89 | 0.92 |
| NDF–ADF | 0.58 | 0.62 | 0.38 | 0.82 | 0.88 | 0.93 |
| Cellulose | 0.25 | 0.32 | 0.38 | 0.82 | 0.87 | 0.91 |
| NSP | 0.46 | 0.54 | 0.36 | 0.82 | 0.89 | 0.92 |

NDF = neutral-detergent fibre; ADF = acid-detergent fibre; NSP = non-starch polysaccharides.

The major site of fibre digestion is the large intestine, in which microbial fermentation takes place. The volatile fatty acids produced here, as a result of fermentation processes, can meet between 0.05 and 0.25 of the energy needs of pigs. The proportions of volatile fatty acids produced in the large intestine can be modified by fibre level. In accordance with results of Noblet and Shi (1993), and also with those presented in Table 5.2, a higher contribution of fibre to the final energy utilisation of pigs can be assumed when considering sows.

## ENERGY VALUE FOR SOWS

In 1997, a programme was started to investigate digestibility of feed ingredients for sows. Twenty-five ingredients were evaluated. Barley was considered as the reference ingredient; therefore its faecal-energy digestibility was determined three times by including it in the basal diet at 980 g/kg. The remaining 24 ingredients were mixed at different inclusion rates in combination with the basal diet (barley+ marker + premix) and their digestibility coefficients were calculated by difference from the one measured for barley (average of three determinations; 0.835 ± 0.0082). The inclusion levels (g/kg) of the ingredients in the basal diet ranged from 250 (citrus pulp, soya hulls, lucerne) to 400 (wheat bran, sugar beet pulp, soyabean meal). Diets were evaluated with non-pregnant sows fed 2 kg daily, in two feeds, for 15 days (10 days acclimatisation; 5 days total faecal collection).

## RESULTS AND FURTHER APPROACH (Net Energy for sows: NEsows).

Data for DCe are presented in Table 5.3, in comparison with data published by Noblet (1997).

**Table 5.3** COEFFICIENT OF DIGESTIBILITY OF GROSS ENERGY IN 11 FEED INGREDIENTS GIVEN BY INRA (NOBLET, 1997) AND SRC (1998, INTERNAL COMMUNICATION)

| | *Growing pigs* | *Sows* | *Sows (SRC)* |
|---|---|---|---|
| Wheat | 0.875 | 0.892 | 0.908 |
| Barley | 0.826 | 0.835 | 0.836 |
| Maize | 0.889 | 0.916 | 0.917 |
| Peas | 0.808 | 0.871 | 0.908 |
| Soyabean meal | 0.845 | 0.894 | 0.914 |
| Wheat bran | 0.585 | 0.646 | 0.712 |
| Maize gluten feed | 0.686 | 0.755 | 0.716 |
| Sugar beet pulp | 0.698 | 0.764 | 0.795 |

For a given ingredient, energy digestibility is higher as live weight increases and as feeding level falls (Noblet, 1997). Growing pigs might represent finishing pigs, but they do not represent sows. The DE data obtained were converted to NE using the conversion factors identified in Figure 5.1, with an assumption that NE was 0.77 of ME (Table 5.4).

The NE values for sows proposed by Noblet (1997) differ slightly from those proposed by SRC (1998) when considering cereals. However, differences already existed between values given by CVB (1998) and Noblet (1997).

**Table 5.4** NE VALUES (MJ/KG) PROPOSED FOR SOWS (SRC, 1998)

| | *NE pigs (CVB, 1998)* | *NE sows (SRC, 1998)* | *NE sows (Noblet, 1997)* |
|---|---|---|---|
| Wheat | 9.76 | 9.91 | 11.02 |
| Barley | 9.13 | 9.13 | 10.28 |
| Maize | 10.70 | 10.01 | 11.33 |
| Peas | 9.38 | 9.92 | 10.25 |
| Soyabean meal | 8.06 | 9.98 | 9.43 |
| Wheat bran* | 5.97 | 7.77 | 7.89 |
| Maize gluten feed | 6.93 | 7.82 | 7.44 |
| Sugar beet pulp | 9.02 | 8.68 | 8.28 |

(*):NE sows = (DCe Wheat bran / DCe Barley) * NE pigs Barley

The conclusion from this phase of the programme was that DE values obtained for growing- finishing pigs will underestimate the energy contribution of a number of raw materials currently used in practical formulations of diets for sows. Therefore, for NE (and also for DE), it is advisable to assign two energy values to each ingredient: NEpigs and NEsows.

## EFFECT OF FIBRE ON WELFARE

A comprehensive review on the effect of fibre on welfare of gestating sows was recently published by Meunier-Salaün (1999). The current chapter will summarise the major findings and present additional data from Roelofs (1998).

Stereotypies can be described as regularly repeated movements that are identical and without any obvious function (Ödberg, 1978, cited by Roelofs, 1998). A stereotypic behaviour develops as follows:

1. Environmental factors cause frustration;
2. It results in a burning "desire" to do something;
3. This leads to obvious behaviour, but this behaviour is not fulfilling;
4. The behaviour is repeated;
5. The behaviour becomes automated, simplified and inherent.

Stereotypies probably arose from the behaviour that was typical at the outset (in this case, lack of feed). It is not impossible that, in performing these ritual behaviours, the animal helps to lessen the seriousness of the frustration. However, animals that show stereotypic behaviour have serious welfare disorders. It is beneficial for the individual animal to express stereotypies because it is a compromise for what they are missing (more feed in order to chew...). Nevertheless, for the whole system, it is a sign that animal welfare is seriously compromised (Vermeer, 1997).

The pig possesses considerable drives both to forage for feed over long periods of time (and distances) and to manipulate thoroughly what it finds in its mouth. The natural situation can be contrasted with modern systems of production where the full daily allowance is provided in a trough and can be consumed in a feeding time of 20 minutes or less (Roelofs, 1998). This shows that it is impossible for sows to perform their natural behaviour in modern systems of production. In other words, the low current feeding level of pregnant sows is probably related to the stereotypic behaviour of sows housed in tethers and/or cages.

Vestergaard (1997), Ramonet (1999) and Meunier-Salaün (1999) have recently published very convincing data showing the benefit of dietary fibre on the welfare of pregnant sows. The figures presented here are from the results of Roelofs (SRC, 1998). The objective was to study the effect of feeding high-fibre diets, combined with different feed presentations, on the stereotypic behaviour of mature non-pregnant Hypor sows. Twenty sows, varying from the third to the eleventh parity, were fed during two periods of three weeks a diet containing either a standard (65 g CF/kg) or high level of fibre (155 g CF/kg), in pellet or meal form. The total daily intake of energy was calculated to be the same for both diets (maintenance level). Daily allowances of the standard and the high-fibre diets were, respectively, 2.0 kg and 2.4 kg. Feed was delivered once per day during a three-week experimental period (two weeks of adaptation). The animals were closely observed for five days, during the last week, from 7.30 a.m. until 10.00 a.m. Eating time (total time eating the feed allowance) increased with the high-fibre diet (P=0.001). It took approximately 2.4 minutes/kg longer (5 minutes extra/daily allowance) to consume the high-fibre feed. When the standard diet was compared with the high-fibre diet, active behaviour decreased by 13% (P=0.003) with the high-fibre diet, lying behaviour increased by 15% (P=0.009; Figure 2) and oral stereotypic behaviour decreased by 10% (P=0.007). When the pellet form was compared with the meal form, active behaviour decreased by 5% (P=0.027) with the meal form and lying behaviour decreased by 16% (P=0.002; Figure 5.3). The meal form showed the largest differences between the two fibre levels.

These results indicate that high-fibre diets may have beneficial effects on the welfare of sows.

The sows fed on the standard diet were more active and spent less time lying down than the sows fed on the high-fibre diet (Table 5.5), confirming the observations of other authors (Broom and Potter, 1984; Robert, *et al.*, 1993; Haaksma, 1994; Brouns, *et al.*, 1994; Ramonet, *et al.*, 1997). This increase in resting time and decrease in active behaviour for the sows fed on the high-fibre diet has been associated

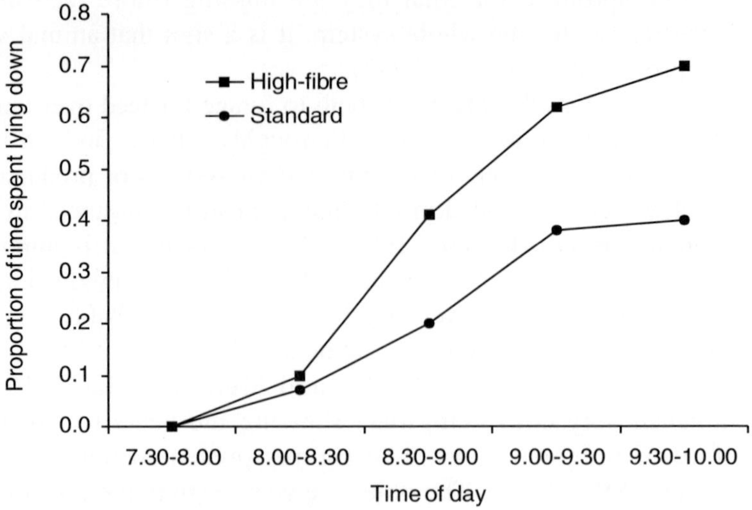


**Figure 5.2** Effect of dietary fibre on sow behaviour

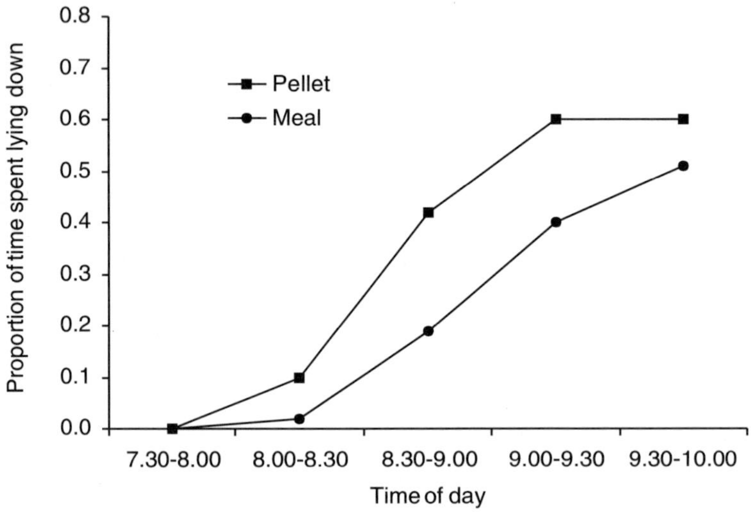


**Figure 5.3** Effect of diet form on sow behaviour.

with a decrease in feeding motivation, as a consequence of gut fill (probably due to the fibre content of feed) controlling appetite. However, feeding motivation will only stop if the diet fulfils the minimal metabolic needs of the animal (Robert, *et al*, 1993).

**Table 5.5** EFFECT OF DIET ON SOW BEHAVIOUR: PROPORTION OF TIME SPENT ON VARIOUS ACTIVITIES (8.00 – 10.00 A.M.) (ROELOFS, 1998)

| | *Standard* | | *High fibre* | | |
|---|---|---|---|---|---|
| *Behavioural category* | *Mean* | *S.E.* | *Mean* | *S.E.* | *P* |
| Oral stereotypic | 0.65 | 0.259 | 0.55 | 0.278 | 0.007 |
| Stereotypic lying | 0.18 | 0.240 | 0.24 | 0.268 | 0.077 |
| Stereotypic standing/sitting | 0.47 | 0.324 | 0.31 | 0.267 | <0.001 |
| Stereotypic 'rooting' | 0.20 | 0.179 | 0.18 | 0.109 | NS |
| Active | 0.86 | 0.182 | 0.73 | 0.270 | 0.003 |
| Lying | 0.30 | 0.296 | 0.45 | 0.282 | 0.009 |

It was interesting to note the effect when pellet and meal feeding were compared (Table 5.6), possibly associated with physical characteristics of the food and their influence on eating behaviour. The meal form may not have provided enough oral stimulation (a minimum chewing activity) and this might have led to increased feeding motivation and increased restlessness. It was concluded, however, that neither feed form was adequate in terms of satisfying foraging behaviour, and therefore improving welfare. Although sows fed the pellet form spent a greater proportion of their time lying down (0.45 vs 0.29), they also performed more stereotypic activities while seated/lying (0.28 vs 0.13). However, it is presumed that when the sows lie down, they feel calmer and welfare is improved.

**Table 5.6** EFFECT OF DIET FORM ON SOW BEHAVIOUR: PROPORTION OF TIME SPENT ON VARIOUS ACTIVITIES (8.00 – 10.00 A.M.) (ROELOFS, 1998)

| | *Pellet* | | *Meal* | | |
|---|---|---|---|---|---|
| *Behavioural category* | *Mean* | *S.E.* | *Mean* | *S.E.* | *P* |
| Oral stereotypic | 0.60 | 0.277 | 0.59 | 0.270 | NS |
| Stereotypic lying | 0.28 | 0.268 | 0.13 | 0.220 | <0.001 |
| Stereotypic standing/sitting | 0.32 | 0.279 | 0.46 | 0.315 | <0.001 |
| Stereotypic 'rooting' | 0.21 | 0.171 | 0.17 | 0.118 | NS |
| Active | 0.82 | 0.227 | 0.77 | 0.247 | 0.027 |
| Lying | 0.45 | 0.289 | 0.29 | 0.285 | 0.002 |

It could be concluded that high-fibre diets have a positive, though variable, effect on welfare in three ways: decreasing oral/rooting activity, reducing total activity and increasing lying time. The latter effect might be variable, but it was assumed to reduce stereotypic behaviour. Feed form had no clear effect, although differences in oral stereotypic behaviour were greater between the two CF levels when the sows were fed in meal form (differences of 0.17 vs 0.03); which, although not significantly different, indicated a clear trend (Table 5.7).

**Table 5.7** INTERACTION BETWEEN FEED FORM AND CF LEVEL ON BEHAVIOUR OF MATURE SOWS: PROPORTION OF TIME SPENT ON VARIOUS ACTIVITIES (8.00 – 10.00 A.M.) (ROELOFS, 1998)

| | *Pellet form* | | | | *Meal form* | | | |
|---|---|---|---|---|---|---|---|---|
| | *Standard CF* | | *High CF* | | *Standard CF* | | *High CF* | |
| | *Mean* | *S.E.* | *Mean* | *S.E.* | *Mean* | *S.E.* | *Mean* | *S.E.* |
| Oral stereotypic | $0.61^{ac}$ | 0.291 | $0.58^{ab}$ | 0.265 | $0.68^{c}$ | 0.222 | $0.51^{b}$ | 0.288 |
| Lying | $0.39^{ac}$ | 0.293 | $0.51^{a}$ | 0.276 | $0.20^{b}$ | 0.268 | $0.38^{c}$ | 0.275 |
| - Stereotypic | $0.26^{a}$ | 0.266 | $0.31^{a}$ | 0.270 | $0.10^{b}$ | 0.184 | $0.17^{b}$ | 0.249 |
| - Passive | $0.13^{a}$ | 0.180 | $0.21^{ab}$ | 0.254 | $0.10^{a}$ | 0.160 | $0.22^{b}$ | 0.225 |
| - sham chewing | $0.25^{a}$ | 0.266 | $0.29^{a}$ | 0.265 | $0.10^{b}$ | 0.179 | $0.16^{c}$ | 0.249 |

$^{a,b,c}$: Different superscripts in the same row indicate differences among treatments ($p<0.10$).

## AD LIBITUM FEED INTAKE

Gestating sows are fed below their maximal feed-intake capacity, thus it is well accepted that their natural rooting and chewing behaviour is not fully expressed, which compromises welfare. On the other hand, sows cannot be fed *ad libitum,* as this would not allow maintenance of optimum body condition and live weight to be achieved during gestation. This would result in reproductive failures due to lower feed intake during lactation, excessive weight loss at weaning and an increased interval from weaning to oestrus. Sows are currently fed in tethered in cages; in this way, feeding to achieve defined body condition is not a real challenge for the farmer, other than time taken to distribute the daily allowances. However, in many European countries concerns about animal welfare have already been reflected by legislation. Countries like the UK, The Netherlands and others ban the use of tether and stall housing for dry sows. One existing clause in European legislation has major implications for sow feeding practice: EU directive 91/630 on The Welfare of Pigs states that *"all pigs must be provided with a diet appropriate to their age, weight and behavioural and physiological needs, to promote a positive state of health and well-being"*. The *"Codes of recommendations for the welfare of livestock, pigs*"(UK, 1994), *"Act on indoor keeping of gestating sows and gilts"* (Denmark, 1994) or the *"Varkensbesluit"* (The Netherlands, 1994), are clear and well defined examples of a commitment towards an improved welfare of pigs and sows. In September 1998, in The Netherlands, a minimum level of either 140 g CF/kg or 340 g OOM/kg of diet became compulsory when feeding gestating sows with no access to any other fibre source (also clearly defined by law in their quality and quantities/sow/day) additional to the daily standard diet allowance.

The same EU directive, 91 630/EU, states that from the 1st of January 2006 keeping dry sows in tethers will not be allowed. They can be kept in pens (limited space and movement) or in groups. Expensive housing designs, which offer individual feeding facilities in group-housing systems, have been developed to prevent aggression due to feed competition. However, the problem still exists and sows still suffer from hunger express stereotypic behaviours.

Both the need to feed *ad libitum* in order to reduce the development of stereotyped oral behaviour and the need to house sows in groups make the utilisation of high fibre diets an interesting approach to feeding dry sows. Moreover, precise nutritional evaluation of the fibre-like ingredients will allow nutritionists to formulate the most appropriate diets for these animals.

When diets were offered *ad libitum*, Brouns *et al.* (1995) showed how, depending on the NSP/OOM origin, the effect varies considerably, especially in the case of sugar beet pulp; levels of unmolassed sugar-beet pulp as high as 650 g/kg were used. This could be a simple effect of reduced palatability, as the organoleptic properties of such a diet may be very different from those of wheat, maize or barley-based diets. However, the other diets used could be also considered to have low palatability (Table 5.8): diets formulated with barley straw, oat husks, malt culms, rice bran or wheat bran were also extremely high in CF or NSP/OOM.

**Table 5.8** MEAN VOLUNTARY FEED INTAKE (LAST TWO WEEKS OF EXPERIMENTAL PERIOD) OF DIETS BY GESTATING SOWS (BROUNS *et al.*, 1995).

| | *Inclusion level (g/kg)* | *DE (MJ/d)** | *VFI (kg/d)** | *CF (g/d)* | *OOM (g/d)* | *DOOM (g/d)*** |
|---|---|---|---|---|---|---|
| Sugar beet pulp | 650 | 18 | 2.3 | 294 | 1060 | 867 |
| Straw | 360 | 42 | 6.4 | 1029 | 2450 | 802 |
| Oat husks | 370 | 58 | 7.7 | 1088 | 3047 | 809 |
| Malt culms | 460 | 52 | 6.8 | 624 | 2171 | 797 |
| Rice bran | 610 | 52 | 7.6 | 1485 | 2810 | 806 |
| Wheat bran | 670 | 54 | 7.1 | 590 | 2204 | 738 |

*: $p<0.001$.
**: DOOM refers to the digestible (fermentable) OOM.

Materials particularly high in soluble fibres (sugar beet pulp) had the greatest effect on restricting feed intake. According to a number of Danish studies (National Committee for Pig Breeding, Health and Production, Annual Report, 1998) the long-term feeling of satiety is achieved by means of dry complete feed, with large amounts of sugar beet pellets, or wet complete feed with sugar beet waste or maize silage. The awareness of the adverse effects of hunger on abnormal behaviour, competition for food and overall aggression has led to attempts to devise practical and cheap systems whereby group-housed pregnant sows could be fed *ad libitum*. The system has been proven to be effective when based on diets with a high inclusion of sugar beet fibre (Noordman, 1999): results from the survey on 37 Dutch farms with this *ad libitum* system concluded, among other things, that the mean gestational feed intake was 3.5 kg/sow/day (sugar beet pulp-based). Because the energy content was calculated to be approximately 10.7 MJ DE/kg, sows would have eaten on average 37.5 MJ DE/d, which matches the 35 MJ DE /d of standard feed (2.7 kg/d) given to sows on some reference farms. The report commented on the possibility that water holding capacity and the viscosity properties of sugar beet pulp could explain these effects.

There seems to be a relationship between daily intake of DOOM and total feed consumption (Table 5.8): in other words, once a sow has consumed a certain quantity of DOOM (750-900 g/d), maximum intake capacity is also attained. In this way, by including high amounts of soluble fibre (thus high amounts of DOOM) in the diet, voluntary feed intake might be "naturally" restricted (Figure 5.4).

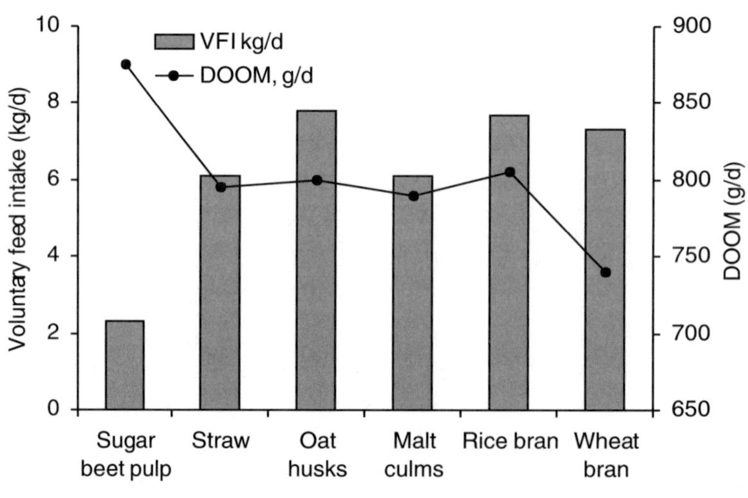


**Figure 5.4** VFI (kg/d) and DOOM (g/d) from Brouns *et al.* (1995).

A number of experiments with mature barrows were conducted at the Nutreco experimental research unit in The Netherlands. Recent results showed a similar trend to those observed by Brouns *et al.* (1995). The combination of sugar beet pulp (400 g/kg diet) and citrus pulp (200 g/kg diet) gave intakes of 2.28 kg/d and 765 g DOOM/d, whereas intakes of 2.82 kg/d and 760 g DOOM/d were observed when citrus pulp (400 g/kg), combined with soya-bean hulls (200 g/kg), was offered *ad libitum* to mature entire males (194 kg live weight) kept in groups of five animals per pen. The difference was not significant (p=0.13), but suggest a requirement for a certain amount of fermentable fibre (DOOM) before the animal stops eating when offered free access to feed.

## Reproductive performance with high-fibre diets

The high intake capacity of dry sows limits any attempts at offering a conventional diet *ad libitum* because of concomitant obesity. However, diets with a high inclusion level of fibrous ingredients (soluble fibre type) might be able to restrict nutrient intake to acceptable levels. Moreover, the interest in fibrous ingredients – especially in The Netherlands - for gestating-sow diets has increased for three reasons already mentioned: firstly, Dutch regulations (September 1998) established a minimum level of 140 g CF/kg (or 340 g OOM/kg) in all gestation diets (a trend that might be followed in other EU countries); secondly, the low nutrient requirements of gestating sows make the use of bulky diets diluted with fibrous ingredients possible and economically attractive, while minimizing feed restriction, thus improving welfare; thirdly, during the past decade, research performed by INRA in France indicated that high-fibre raw materials are more efficiently utilised by sows when compared with growing-finishing pigs. Therefore, because of the higher digestibility and utilization of dietary fibre in sows, there seems to be a great potential for using various fibrous feeds.

Introduction of high-fibre feeds, especially those high in soluble fibre (those that are readily fermented: sugar beet pulp, citrus pulp), during gestation seems practical because no adverse effects on reproductive performance (i.e., pigs farrowed, birth weight, mortality) were observed (Varel and Yen, 1997). Even slight improvements were observed in some studies (Matte *et al.*, 1994): indeed, the use of bulky diets diluted with fibrous ingredients has beneficial effects on body condition and on some measures of reproductive performance in sows. The growth of the litter was increased by approximately 20% during the second parity when a bulky diet, based on wheat bran and maize cobs, was fed to sows during the first and second parities. This improvement may be linked to the beneficial effect of this diet on sow well-being, which was also reported.

In previous experiments, Robert and Matte (1993) found an increase of 12.8% (more than 3 hours/d) in resting time, and a reduction of at least 50% in incidence of stereotypies during the second gestation was observed when the same diet was fed. This altered behaviour could have decreased the energy requirements for maintenance and consequently left more energy available for sow and conceptus growth.

Furthermore, positive effects on development of the digestive tract could be expected which, in turn, could increase voluntary feed intake capacity of sows during subsequent lactation. Voluntary feed intake of sows during lactation is frequently insufficient to meet nutrient demands for maintenance and maximal milk production. Insufficient feed intake during lactation results in sows losing large amounts of weight. Excessive weight loss has been associated with several common reproductive problems, including an increased interval from weaning to oestrus (King and Williams, 1984 cited by Noblet *et al.*, 1998) and reduced litter size in subsequent litters (Kirkwood *et al.*, 1987, cited by Williams, 1998). The effect of *ad libitum* feeding on the gastrointestinal tract of young sows has been examined (National Committee for Pig Breeding, Health and Production, Annual Report 1998, Denmark). Although no data are given in the report, they reported a difference in the weight of stomach, small and large intestines plus rectum from five young sows fed with an ordinary feed mix, compared with the weight of the gastrointestinal tract from five young sows fed given a diet containing large amounts of sugar feed waste.

Vestergaard (1997) showed that when nutritional requirements were met, sows had a large capacity to increase their total feed intake during pregnancy, without influencing on body weight and litter size (Tables 5.9 and 5.10). Dietary fibre increased the gut fill of sows, leading to a greater live-weight gain during pregnancy, but also to a larger weight loss at farrowing, when a standard lactation diet was offered. Thus, the true body-weight gain was the same for all three groups of sows.

**Table 5.9** CHEMICAL ANALYSIS AND CALCULATED NET ENERGY CONTENT OF DIETS (VESTERGAARD, 1997)

| | *Standard* | *SBP*[1] | *Mixed*[2] | *Lactation* |
|---|---|---|---|---|
| Dry Matter (DM; g/kg) | 889 | 888 | 891 | 884 |
| Crude Protein (g/kg DM) | 154 | 158 | 144 | 203 |
| Ether Extract (g/kg DM) | 55 | 55 | 62 | 75 |
| Crude Fibre (g/kg DM) | 46 | 127 | 135 | 36 |
| Net Energy (MJ/kg DM) | 9.03 | 8.49 | 6.72 | 9.88 |

[1] SBP: 500 g sugar beet pulp + 315 g barley
[2] Mixed : 415 g barley + 150 g grass meal + 150 g wheat bran + 200 g oat hulls.

Feed intake during pregnancy (kg/d) was highest for the mixed diet and lowest for the standard diet. However, net energy intake (MJ/d) was the lowest for the sugar beet pulp diet. Mean piglet weight at birth was lower for the sugar beet pulp diet but, at weaning, the mean weights of piglets were the same for all three treatments (Table 5.10). According to these results, it is possible to feed pregnant sows with high levels of fibre; the sows showed capacity to reach the same energy intake without detrimental effects on performance.

**Table 5.10** EFFECT OF THREE DIETS (TABLE 9) ON INTAKE AND REPRODUCTIVE PERFORMANCE (VESTERGAARD, 1997)

| | *Standard* | *SBP* | *Mixed* | *P-value* |
|---|---|---|---|---|
| Feed Intake during gestation | | | | |
| - mean for three cycles (kg) | 281.1[a] | 289.7[b] | 368.2[c] | <0.001 |
| - mean for three cycles (MJ NE) | 2296[a] | 2216[b] | 2282[a] | <0.001 |
| Feed intake during lactation | | | | |
| - mean for three cycles | 1450[a] | 1528[b] | 1438[a] | 0.002 |
| Performance (mean of three cycles) | | | | |
| - pregnancy live-weight gain (kg) | 58.7[a] | 61.6[a] | 67.9[b] | <0.001 |
| - live-weight loss at farrowing (kg) | 21.4[a] | 26.7[b] | 25.9[b] | <0.001 |
| - live-weight loss during lactation (kg) | 8.0 | 6.3 | 8.0 | 0.270 |
| Litter performance (mean of three cycles) | | | | |
| - number of piglets born alive | 10.8 | 10.9 | 10.7 | 0.860 |
| - number of piglets weaned | 9.5 | 9.3 | 9.3 | 0.900 |
| - live weight at birth (kg) | 1.62[a] | 1.47[b] | 1.65[a] | <0.001 |
| - live weight at weaning (kg) | 8.4 | 8.1 | 8.4 | 0.550 |
| - litter weight at weaning (kg) | 77.2 | 73.7 | 75.8 | 0.350 |

[a,b,c] means in same row with different superscripts bare significantly different.

A similar experiment (Durán, 1998) was conducted to measure the effect of bulky diets, based on soluble fibre (163 g CF/kg with sugar beet pulp, 450 g/kg and soyabean hulls, 200 g/kg) or insoluble fibre (170 g CF/kg with grass meal, 230 g/kg, wheat bran, 100 g/kg, lucerne, 60 g/kg and straw, 80 g/kg), compared with a standard diet (70 g CF/kg), on performance of sows during gestation and their following lactation. Though no significant differences were found, the trends were similar to those observed by previous researchers (Matte, 1994, Vestergaard, 1997, Ramonet, 1999). Results shown in Table 5.11 were obtained from 93 Hypor sows fed with the diets described; a standard vs. two bulky ones – insoluble and soluble fibre types. Mean feed allowances were 2.4, 3.0 and 2.9 kg respectively, leading to similar intakes of NE (21MJ/d), more than 325 g CP/d and around 10 g ileal-digestible lysine/d; sufficient to meet maintenance requirements and allow for maternal gain and conceptus growth.

**Table 5.11** PERFORMANCE OF SOWS FED ON DIETS DIFFERING IN FIBRE CONTENT, WITH SIMILAR INTAKES OF NET ENERGY (DURÁN, 1998)

| | *Standard diet* | *Insoluble-fibre diet* | *Soluble-fibre diet* |
|---|---|---|---|
| Parity number | 3.9 | 4.6 | 4.5 |
| Initial weight (kg) | 193.4 | 190.8 | 186.5 |
| Live-weight gain during gestation (kg) | 51.1 | 49.6 | 54.1 |
| Net maternal gain during gestation (kg) | 34.0 | 32.1 | 37.7 |
| [1]NEpigs intake (MJ/d) | 21.0 | 21.0 | 21.0 |
| [1]NEsows intake (MJ/d) | 22.3 | 23.7 | 23.2 |
| Lactation | | | |
| - live-weight loss (kg) | -15.2 | -15.9 | -17.5 |
| - litter birth weight (kg) | 17.5 | 17.2 | 16.5 |
| - litter live-weight gain after 24 days (g/d) | 2332 | 2269 | 2269 |
| - Feed intake during lactation (kg/d) | 7.6 | 7.6 | 7.8 |

[1] NEpigs and NEsows: net energy values for growing pigs or sows, as given in Table 5.4.

Fibre-based diets were efficiently used by multiparous sows, but there was no positive effect of fibre on litter birth weight due to, as suggested by Matte (1994), an energy-sparing effect of fibre in the feed. However, there was a higher net weight gain in those sows fed the soluble fibre. It is debatable whether differences in weight arose from an increased hind-gut mass (weight), a gut-fill effect of diet (larger amounts of digesta in the hind-gut), or to an "extra energy intake" by the fibre-fed sows because of the higher intake of energy when the latter was expressed as NE sows (previously defined). Litter performance, birth weight, growth rate and weaning weight did not differ among treatments. Although sows fed the soluble fibre showed a higher feed intake during lactation, this was not reflected in any litter improvement.

## Conclusions

It is possible to improve the welfare of sows by correct feeding of fibrous ingredients, without impairing reproductive performance.

It may be predicted that although this practice is already being used in some countries, the utilization of fibrous diets for gestating sows will keep increasing across the rest of the EU members.

## Acknowledgements

I am grateful to all the staff at SRC, especially Jos Weerts, who taught me all that is not in the books about management and feeding of sows: *Hartelijk bedankt Jos !!*. Also to Yannick Ramonet and Rosil Lizardo, from INRA: *merci beaucoup !!*. Thanks to C. van der Peet-Schwering, from Rosmalen.

## References

Broom, D.M. and Potter, M.J., (1984) In: Factors affecting the occurrence of stereotypes in stall-housed dry sows. J. Unshelm, G. van Putten and K. Zeeb (Editors), Proceedings of the International Congress on Applied Ethology in Farm Animals. pp. 229-231. Kiel, Germany. KTBL, Germany.

Brouns, F., Edwards, S.A. and English, P.R. (1994) Effect of dietary fibre and feeding system on activity and oral behaviour of group housed gilts. *Applied Animal Behaviour Science*, **39,** 215-223.

Brouns, F., Edwards, S.A. and English, P.R. (1995) Influence of fibrous feed ingredients on voluntary intake of dry sows. *Animal Feed Science and Technology*, **54,** 301-313.

CVB, Veevoedertabel 1998 (1998).

CVB, Veevoedertabel 1999 (1999).

CVB, Verkorte tabel 1994 (1994). Centraal Veevoederbureau, cvb-reeks no. 15, August 1994.

Durán, R. (1998) Effect of bulky diets based on beet pulp/soyabean hulls or grass/straw on gestation performance of sows and their subsequent lactation . *Report S0297 – 03. SRC, Nutreco.*

Haaksma, J. (1994) Bietenpulp: Voederwaarde en het effect op het gedrag bij varkens. *Bergen op Zoom (Instituut voor rationele suikerproduktie).*

Longland, A.C. and Low, A.G. (1995) Prediction of the energy value of alternative feeds for pigs. In *Recent Advances in Animal Nutrition - 1995*, pp 187-209. Edited by P.C. Garnsworthy and D.J.A. Cole. Nottingham University Press, Nottingham.

Manteca, J. (1998) El bienestar animal en la granja del 2000. *II Jornadas Técnicas de porcino de Nanta, S.A.*

Matte, J.J., Robert, S., Girard, C.L., Farmer, C. and Martineau, G.-P. (1994) Effect of bulky diets based on wheat bran or oat hulls on reproductive performance of sows during their first two parities. *Journal of Animal Science,* **72**, 1754-1760.

Meunier – Salaün, M-C. (1999) Fibre in diets of sows. In *Recent Advances in Animal Nutrition - 1999*, pp 257-273. Edited by P.C. Garnsworthy and J. Wiseman. Nottingham University Press, Nottingham.

National Committee for Pig Breeding, Health and Production, Annual Report, 1998.

Noblet , J. Etienne, M. and Dourmad, J.-Y. (1998) *Energetic efficiency of milk production.* The Lactating sow, Wageningen Pers, 1998, pp: 113-130

Noblet, J. (1996) Digestive and metabolic utilization of dietary energy in pig feeds: comparison of energy systems. In *Recent Advances in Animal Nutrition - 1996*, pp 207-232. Edited by P.C. Garnsworthy, J. Wiseman and W. Haresign. Nottingham University Press, Nottingham.

Noblet, J. (1997) Two energy values for each ingredient. *Pig International,* **27,** *no.10, 25-26.*

Noblet, J. and Shi, X.S. (1993) Comparative digestible of energy and nutrients in growing pigs fed ad libitum and adult sows fed at maintenance. *Livestock Production Science*, **34,** 137-152.

Noblet, J. and Shi, X.S. (1994) Effect of body weight on digestive utilization of energy and nutrients and diets in pigs. *Livestock Production Science, 37, 323-338.*

Noordman, M. (1999) Onbeperkt voeren van dragende zeugen. *Hendrix UTD VSN*

Ramonet, Y. (1999) *Réponses comportementales, digestives, hormonales et métaboliquesá la restriction énergétique chez la truie gestante: effects d´une incorporation de fibres alimentaires dans la ration.* Thesis, University of Rennes.

Ramonet, Y.; Meunier-Salaün, M-C.; Dourmad, J.Y. (1997) Effets d'une incorporation de parios végétales dans la ration alimentaire sur l'activité comportementale des truies gestantes. *Journées Rech. Porcine en France,* ***29,*** *167-174.*

Robert, S., Matte, J.J., Farmer, C., Girard, C.L. and Martineau, G.-P. (1993) High fibre diets for sows: effects on steretypies and adjunctive drinking. *Applied Animal Behaviour Science,* **37**, 297.

Roelofs, J. (1998) Effect of feed form and crude fibre level on the oral stereotypic behaviour of tethered sows. *Report S1197 – 02. SRC, Nutreco.*

Shi, X.S. and Noblet, J. (1993) Contribution of the hindgut to digestion of diets in growing pigs and adult sows: effect of diet composition. *Livestock Production Science*, **34,** 237-252.

Van der Peet-Schwering, C. (2000) *The use of welfare diets during gestation.* Nutrition of sows during gestation and lactation. Wageningen, Tuesday March 28, 2000.

Varkensbesluit (1994). Helpdesk Dierenwelzijn sector Varkenshouderij Nr 5.

Vermeer, H.M.; Ekkel, E.D.; Groot, J.S.M. de; Klooster, C.E. van 't; Peet, G.F.V. Van der Swinkels, J.W.G.M (1997), Welzijn van varkens: van verzorgingsvoorschriften naar verzorgingsmaatregelen. *Proefverslag nummer P1.173, Rosmalen, Nederland.*

Vestergaard, E-M. (1997) Phd Thesis: *The effect of dietary fibre on welfare and productivity of sows.* Institut for Husdyrbrug og Husdyrsundhed, Veterinary School, Copenhagen, Denmark.

Vestergaard, E-M. and Danielsen, V. (1998) Dietary fibre for sows: effects of large amounts of soluble and insoluble fibres in the pregnancy period on the performance of sows during three reproductive cycles. *Animal Science,* **68**, 355-362.

Williams, I.H. (1998) Nutritional effects during lactation and during the interval from weaning to oestrus. In *The Lactating Sow*, pp: 159-181. Wageningen Pers, Wageningen.

*This paper was first published in 2001*

6

# FATTY ACIDS AND REPRODUCTION IN THE PIG

JOHN A. ROOKE[1], ELIZABETH M. FERGUSON[1], ANNA G. SINCLAIR[1] AND BRIAN K SPEAKE[2]
[1]*Sustainable Livestock Systems, SAC, Craibstone Estate, Aberdeen AB21 9YA*
[2]*Animal Health Centre, SAC, Auchincruive, Ayr KA6 5HW*

## Introduction

Sow productivity is comprised of various components that determine the number of piglets attaining slaughter weight per annum. As far as direct effects of reproduction are concerned, the main factors involved are ovulation rate of the sow, successful fertilisation, the extent of pre and post natal mortality and parturition-rebreeding interval. In quantitative terms, ovulation and fertilisation is about 90% successful as judged by first service returns (MLC, 2001) and is therefore much less of a problem than in the dairy industry. Mortality between birth and weaning is around 10% of pigs born alive (MLC, 2001). Ante-natal mortality is more difficult to estimate, about 1 piglet / litter is borne dead or mummified (9% of pigs borne alive, MLC 2001) but this will only represent a small fraction of ante-natal mortality. Pope (1994) estimated a mortality of 27% before day 35 of pregnancy. There is therefore scope for improvement in all aspects of reproductive performance. The correct nutrition of the sow and to a lesser extent the boar has a major effect on reproductive success of the sow; however ration formulation has to date correctly focussed on major dietary constituents and trace elements and vitamins. Less attention has been paid to the type and quantities of fatty acids in the diet and their influence on reproductive success.

### FATTY ACIDS

Apart from the general importance of dietary fat as a concentrated energy source, nutritionally fatty acids are important as a source of essential fatty acids. The structure of fatty acids will be described using the following nomenclature with linoleic acid, 18:2 n-6, as an example where: 18 (left of the colon) denotes the number of carbon atoms in the fatty acid; 2 (right of the colon), the number of double bonds in the carbon chain and n-6 the position of the first double bond counting from the methyl end of the carbon chain. The essentiality of fatty acids in mammalian nutrition is determined by the absence of the desaturase enzymes necessary to introduce double bonds between the methyl end of the fatty acid carbon chain and the n-9 position. Thus there are two functionally important series of polyunsaturated fatty acids (PUFA), which contain their first double bond at the n-3 and n-6 positions respectively and therefore must be supplied in the diet. The 18 carbon fatty acids, 18:2 n-6 and 18:3 n-3 (linolenic acid) are the parent compounds from which all other metabolically important fatty acids are synthesised. The biological importance of the essential fatty acids resides in the longer chain PUFA that can be synthesised from the 18 carbon fatty acids.

## BIOSYNTHESIS OF FATTY ACIDS

The structure and common names of the important fatty acids and their biosynthetic routes are given in Figure 6.1. The key points to note from Figure 6.1 are:

- that both series of fatty acids are substrates for the same desaturase and elongase enzymes involved in synthesis of the long chain PUFA.
- n-3 and n-6 fatty acids cannot be inter-converted.
- it is generally accepted that the rate-limiting step in the pathway is the first desaturation step catalysed by delta 6 desaturase.

Recently Sprecher (2000) showed that the biosynthetic pathway for the 22-carbon chain PUFA given in Figure 6.1 is more complex. Figure 6.2 shows that two elongation steps generate a 24-carbon fatty acid, which is the substrate for delta 6 desaturase. The 24-carbon fatty acid is then degraded to the 22-carbon fatty acid. This degradation by beta-oxidation takes place in the peroxisome of the cell rather than in the endoplasmic reticulum, the site of chain elongation and desaturation. This physical separation of oxidation from elongation and desaturation may in part explain the relative inefficiency of synthesis of 22:6 n-3 (docosahexaenoic acid) from 18:3 n-3 when compared with 20:5 n-3 (eicosapentaenoic acid, Wood and Enser, 1997; Rooke *et al.*, 2000). Peroxisomal beta-oxidation also provides a basis for the retro-conversion of, for example, 22:6 n-3 to 20:5 n-3 and shows in general that PUFA metabolism is more complex than the simple synthesis of a PUFA followed by its degradation, as there may be limited degradation and re-synthesis for all long chain PUFA (Sprecher, 2000). The entire pathway described by Sprecher (2000) is active in the piglet liver at 14 days of age (Li *et al.*, 2000); however, no synthesis of 22:6 n-3 from 20:5 n-3 could be detected in the foetal piglet liver.

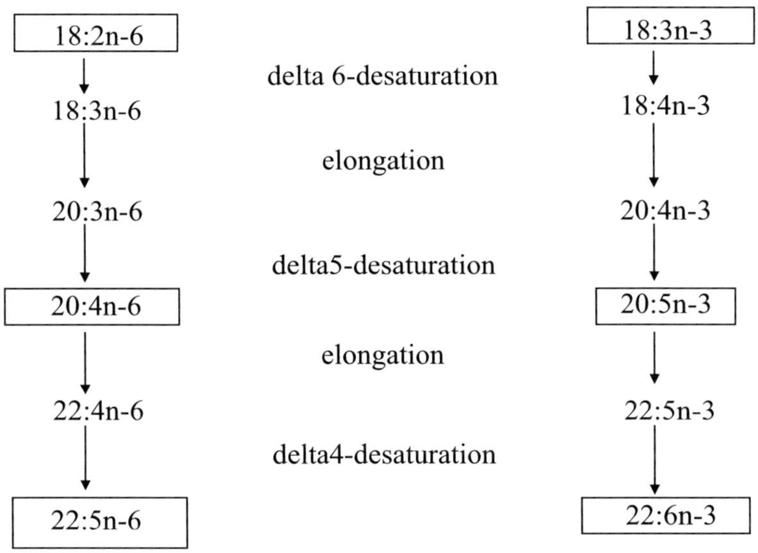


18:2n-6 Linoleic acid
18:3n-3 Linolenic acid
20:4n-6 Arachidonic aicd
20:5n-3 Eicosapentaenoic acid
22:5n-6 Docosapentaenoic acid
22:6n-3 Docosahexaenoic acid

**Figure 6.1** "Standard" biosynthetic pathway for long chain PUFA from 18:2 n-6 and 18:3 n-3. (Common names for fatty acids given below biosynthetic pathway).

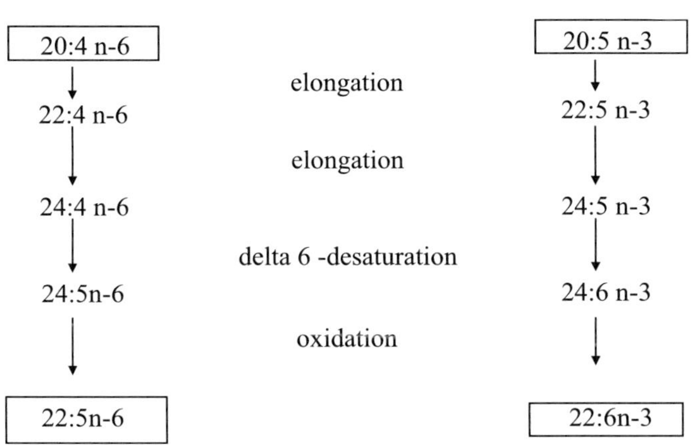


**Figure 6.2** Revised biosynthetic pathway for 22 carbon PUFA from 20 carbon PUFA (Sprecher, 2000)

ESSENTIAL FATTY ACID REQUIREMENTS

Requirements for fatty acids (Agricultural Research Council, 1981; National Research Council, 1998) include requirements for n-6 fatty acids as 18:2 n-6 but, while acknowledging the essentiality of the n-3 series, do not quantify the requirement for these fatty acids either because of a lack of information (Agricultural Research Council, 1981) or the assumption that normal diets provide an adequate supply (National Research Council, 1998). This is in contrast to the situation in human nutrition (Simopoulos *et al.*, 2000), where adequate intakes have been defined for both 18:2 n-6 and 18:3 n-3, with minimum inclusion rates specified for 20:5 n-3 and 22:6 n-3. Additional recommendations have been made for 22:6 n-3, for intakes by pregnant mothers and to be supplied in infant formulae, thus recognising the conditional essentiality of 22:6 n-3 during pregnancy to ensure adequate supplies to the developing foetus. In addition, an upper limit has been recommended for inclusion of 18:2 n-6, recognising the potential adverse effects of an excess of 20:4 n-6 (arachidonic acid) and its metabolic derivatives (Whelan, 1996). Current diets for pregnant sows, being based on cereal products, contain proportionately more n-6 fatty acids than n-3 fatty acids and, in addition, little or no n-3 acids in the form of 20:5 n-3 and 22:6 n-3. Typically ratios of n-6 to n-3 fatty acids are greater than 8, a value considered unbalanced in human nutrition. Therefore, the starting point for considering the effects of different fatty acids on reproduction in the pig is that current diets may be sub-optimal in terms of both the balance of essential fatty acids and in specific dietary fatty acids supplied.

This chapter will discuss possible mechanisms whereby changing the fatty acid composition of the diet influences reproductive performance and then relate these mechanisms, where possible, to practical examples. However, in many cases, potential mechanisms of action of fatty acids in relation to reproductive performance have been described using laboratory animal species and information is scarce or lacking in the pig; although it will be necessary to extrapolate between species, caution should be exerted in so doing. Furthermore, a large body of the available information on the pig has involved supplementation of the diet with lipid-containing materials and therefore it is difficult to separate specific effects of fatty acids from effects of energy supplementation *per se*.

## Underlying mechanisms

At the cellular and molecular level, there are several possible mechanisms that explain effects of different fatty acids on whole-animal responses. Although these will be described separately, in reality there are interactions between mechanisms. Changes in dietary fatty acids may:

- Influence the fatty acid composition of specific cell types that rely for optimum function on high concentrations of specific fatty acids.
- Change the pattern of lipid-derived biologically active products such as the eicosanoids.
- Modify gene expression by changing receptor activity, modifying intra-cellular signalling pathways or the intra-cellular signals themselves.

## FATTY ACID COMPOSITION OF SPECIFIC TISSUES

In the pig, in common with most mammals, the lipids of brain, retina and spermatozoa contain substantially higher proportions of 22:6 n-3 than other tissues (see review by Leskanitch and Noble, 1999). There is substantial deposition of 22:6 n-3 in brain and retina during late pregnancy and experimental models have shown that a deficiency of dietary 22:6 n-3 leads to visual impairment (Neuringer *et al.,* 1984) and changes in brain function (Innis, 2000a). The requirement for 22:6 n-3 in the neurones of the brain, rod outer segments of the retina and the tail phospholipids of sperm for optimum function is still to be completely elucidated (see review by Speake et al., 2003). However, biophysical studies are beginning to suggest mechanisms. The 22:6 n-3 acyl side chains in cell membranes containing 22:6 n-3 rich lipids are highly flexible and able to convert rapidly from an extended to a looped conformation. This endows membranes containing 22:6 n-3 with high levels of flexibility, compressibility and elasticity. Using reconstituted membranes containing rhodopsin, the pigment in the retina whose photo-activation is the first step in light detection, it has been shown that the conformational change which rhodopsin undergoes upon activation is facilitated most effectively by phospholipids containing 22:6 n-3. This attribute of 22:6 n-3 is derived from the flexible nature of 22:6 n-3 side chains, which allow the membranes to accommodate the changes in rhodopsin conformation. Other stages of the visual transduction pathway which involve protein-protein as well as protein-lipid interactions are facilitated by 22:6 n-3 containing phospholipids and these types of mechanism may explain the importance of 22:6 n-3 in neural transmission.

## LIPID-DERIVED BIOLOGICALLY ACTIVE COMPOUNDS

A principal function of 20:4 n-6 synthesised from 18:2 n-6 is as a substrate for the synthesis of prostaglandins and other eicosanoid mediators whose major function is to modulate the intensity of the inflammatory reaction (Calder, 2002). Prostaglandins and other eicosanoids are synthesised from phospholipid-bound 20:4 n-6 by cycloxygenase and lipoxygenase after its release from the phospholipids principally by phospholipase $A_{2.}$ The prostaglandin products from 20:4 n-6 are prostaglandins of the 2 series, which include prostaglandins $F_{2\alpha}$ and $E_2$ and have particular importance in luteolysis, whether it occurs at the end of the oestrous cycle or at the end of pregnancy (Abayasekara and Wathes, 1999). As in the biosynthesis of PUFA, n-3 fatty acids, particularly 20:5 n-3, are also substrates for the enzymes involved in the biosynthesis of prostaglandins, but produce prostaglandins of the 3 series, which are generally considered to be less biologically active than prostaglandins derived from 20:4 n-6. In addition, feeding 20:5 n-3 decreases the amounts of 20:4 n-6 in membranes and 20:5 n-3 also inhibits phospholipase $A_2$ mediated release of 20:4 n-6 from phospholipids and competitively inhibits the activity of cycloxygenase and lipoxygenase (Figure 6.3). The net effect of 20:5 n-3 is therefore to reduce 20:4 n-6 mediated prostaglandin production. The biological effects in any given tissue system will depend on the relative potency of tissue-specific prostaglandins produced. This is of particular importance in luteolysis in the pig, where prostaglandin $F_{2\alpha}$ is luteolytic whilst prostaglandin $E_2$ is luteotrophic and therefore any changes in the net luteolytic signal may depend on the relative potencies of 3-series prostaglandins. In addition, it is relevant to note that, both *in vitro* and *in vivo*, increasing the n-3 fatty acid content of the diet suppresses production of the cytokine, tumour necrosis factor $\alpha$, which acts synergistically with prostagladin $F_{2\alpha}$ in causing functional luteolysis in the pig (Wuttke *et al.*, 1998).

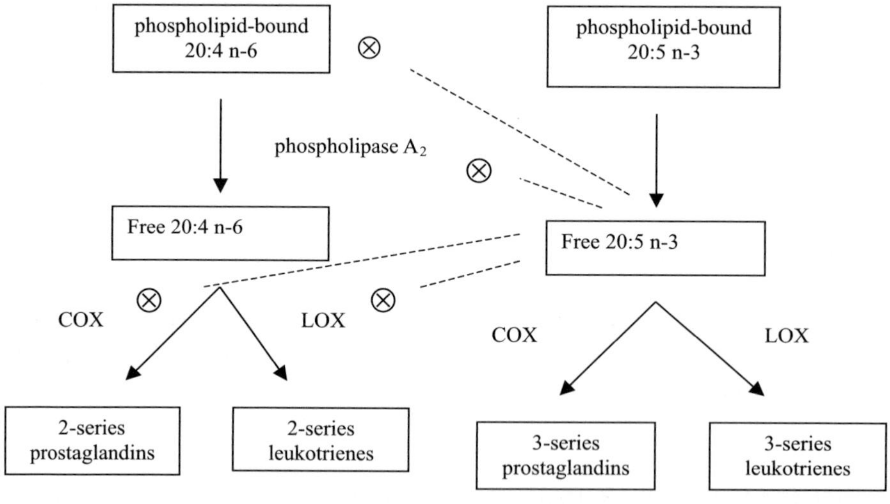


**Figure 6.3** Biosynthesis of prostaglandins and leukotrienes from 20:4 n-6 and 20:5 n-3 showing points where 20:5 n-3 inhibits biosynthesis from 20:4 n-6. (COX, cyclooxygenase; LOX lipoxygenase).

## MODIFICATION OF GENE EXPRESSION

Fatty acids are not only components of biological membranes and substrates for eicosanoid production, but are involved in modification of gene expression. It is well-established that PUFA down-regulate genes involved in both lipogenesis and glycolysis in a tissue and fatty acid specific manner (Raclot and Oudart, 1999). However, the effects of PUFA on gene expression are more general, with n-3 fatty acids modulating inflammatory reactions by suppressing gene expression (Calder, 2002). Fatty acids may modify gene expression in several ways, considered later.

## MEMBRANE FLUIDITY

By changing membrane fluidity, the activity of receptors may be altered. Although there is considerable inter-species variation, insulin receptor activity is influenced by membrane fluidity. In the mini-pig, fed either maize or Menhaden fish oil, there were significant relationships between membrane fluidity and insulin binding (Bhathena *et al.*, 2001).

## SECOND MESSENGERS

Derivatives of membrane phospholipids are components of intracellular second messages, e.g. inositol triphosphate and diacylglyceride generated by the activity of phospholipase C on phosphatidyl inositol. In the pig, supplementation of the diet with fish oil increased n-3 fatty acids in cardiac myocytes and these changes resulted in reduced inositol triphosphate release and protein kinase C activity (which is initiated by diacyl-glycerol) (Nair *et al.*, 2000; 2001).

## NUCLEAR RECEPTORS AND TRANSCRIPTION FACTORS

The best well-documented effects of fatty acids on gene expression are their interactions with nuclear receptors and transcription factors. This is a rapidly developing area of research and the number of factors whose activity is regulated by fatty acids is increasing. Jump (2002) reviewed recent research on liver gene expression and listed four families of transcription factors (peroxisome proliferator activated receptor α (PPAR), liver X receptor α, sterol regulatory element binding proteins and hepatic nuclear factor-4α) which are targets for fatty acids or their metabolites and which affect the expression of genes directly related to lipid metabolism. In addition, the effects of polyunsaturated fatty acids on immune function may be mediated by regulation of the activity of nuclear factor kappa ß (Calder, 2002). Clearly, the relevance of studies on rat liver to reproductive tissues in the pig is questionable, but the above would at least suggest that effects of fatty acids on gene expression relevant to reproduction in the pig will be complex and mediated through a variety of mechanisms and factors. There is limited evidence that expression of genes involved in lipid metabolism in the pig is influenced by dietary fatty acids. For example, the transcription factors PPARγ and CCAAT/enhancer binding protein α (Ding and Mersmann, 2001) are expressed in porcine adipose tissue and their mRNA levels were enhanced by 18:1 n-9 (oleic acid).

## Responses to different fatty acids

In contrast to the effects of fat supplementation, especially in the neonatal period (Pettigrew, 1981), there is a limited literature from which reproductive responses to diets differing in fatty acid composition can be assessed; in many cases measurement of responses in reproductive terms was not the primary objective of the study and numbers of sows used were too few for reliable production results. For example, there are many studies in which the bottle-fed piglet has been used to evaluate the effects of different formula milks for human consumption on, for example, brain development (for review, see Innis, 2000b). In general, where vegetable oils and animal by-products such as lard have been evaluated, no differences have been observed. Malm *et al.* (1976) fed lard or maize oil throughout pregnancy and lactation and found no differences in performance. Farnworth and Kramer (1988; 1989) fed sows tallow or soya-bean oil from day 57 of pregnancy and, although fatty acid composition of piglet carcasses differed, again there were no differences in piglet weight or litter size. More recently Gerfault *et al.* (1999; 2000) fed diets containing copra oil, sunflower oil, lard or an isoenergetic diet based on starch to sows throughout pregnancy and lactation and followed the offspring to slaughter at 100 kg weight. Although differences in fatty acid composition were observed in the offspring and in the number of adipocytes / g adipose tissue, no differences in performance were observed. A common feature of the oils used in the above studies was that they contained no long chain PUFA and would not have reduced the ratio of n-6 to n-3 PUFA from values commonly observed in pig diets. It is against this background that the effects of long chain n-3 PUFA on reproductive performance in the pig will be reviewed with a focus on research conducted at SAC.

## MALE REPRODUCTIVE PERFORMANCE

Boar spermatozoa, in common with other mammalian sperm phospholipids, contain very high concentrations of 22-carbon fatty acids, 22:6 n-3 and 22:5 n-6 (docosapentaenoic acid; Paulenz *et al.*, 1995; Leskanitch and Noble, 1999; Rooke *et al.*, 2001a). The significance of long chain PUFA for sperm function is discussed more fully elsewhere (Speake *et al.*, 2003). The proportions of 22:6 n-3 and 22:5 n-6 are reciprocally related and the ratio of 22:6 n-3 to 22:5 n-6 is inversely related to the age of the boar (Speake *et al.*, 2003) and the presence of 22:5 n-6 probably reflects either a sub-optimal supply to, or synthesis of, 22:6 n-3 within the testis. When marine oils were added to the diet of boars, consistent increases in 22:6 n-3 and decreases in 22:5 n-6 concentrations in sperm fatty acids were observed (Paulenz *et al.*, 1995; Penny *et al.*, 2000; Rooke *et al.*, 2001a); the time scale of this change was consistent with that of *de novo* spermatogenesis. Although Paulenz *et al.* (1995) observed no benefits in sperm quality or reproductive performance, more recent studies have observed positive effects (Table 6.1) on sperm quality (Penny *et al.*, 2000; Rooke *et al.*, 2001a) and boar performance (Penny *et al.*, 2000). The concentrations of viable sperm / ml ejaculate were increased, as was motility and the proportion of sperm with a normal acrosome which, in the study reported by Penny *et al.* (2000), was reflected in an increase in the numbers of piglets born alive per 100 services. It should be noted that no corresponding data exist for 18:3 n-3 and so, at present, it is not possible to differentiate between a sub-optimal supply of n-3 acids in general or 22:6 n-3 in particular as the basis for the responses described.

**Table 6.1** RESPONSES OF WORKING BOARS TO DIETARY SUPPLEMENTATION WITH TUNA ORBITAL OIL

| *Study* | *Penny et al., 2000* | | *Rooke et al., 2001a* | |
|---|---|---|---|---|
| *Diet* | *Control* | *Tuna oil*[1] | *Control* | *Tuna oil*[2] |
| Sperm concentration (x $10^8$ / ml) | 5.0 | 5.8*** | 2.0 | 4.1NS |
| Sperm viability (% alive) | 78 | 88* | 71 | 80** |
| Motile sperm (%) | | | 72 | 77** |
| Normal acrosome (%) | | | 45 | 54*** |
| Piglets born alive / 100 services | 84.6 | 95.4*** | | |

[1] Diet supplemented with tuna orbital oil, vitamin E and selenium

[2] Diet supplemented with 30 g tuna orbital oil /kg

Superscripts denote supplemented diet significantly different (*, P<0.05; **, P<0.01; ***, P<0.001) from control diet.

## FEMALE REPRODUCTIVE PERFORMANCE

Before considering the underlying hypothesis that addition of long chain n-3 PUFA to the diet of the sow during critical stages of development would improve piglet viability, there is some limited evidence that addition of PUFA to the diet of the sow prior to and during the peri-ovulatory period might increase conception rate and early foetal survival. Perez-Rigau *et al.* (1995) added 40 g/kg of either coconut oil (medium chain fatty acids), soya-bean oil (mainly 18:2 n-6) or menhaden fish oil (20:5 n-3 and 22:6 n-3) to the diet of gilts prior to service and continued until slaughter between days 37 to 45 post-service. The same protocol was also followed using third parity sows. Overall, menhaden oil improved the number of live foetuses (68 %, as a percentage of corpora lutea) compared with a starch-based isoenergetic control diet (63%), with the soya-bean and coconut oils having no effect. However, results were variable and responses were less marked in multiparous sows than in gilts. Possible reasons for the difference between gilts and multiparous sows may have been the length of feeding periods prior to service (sows (approximately 5 d) less than gilts (approximately 28 d) and probably greater adipose tissue reserves of 22:6 n-3 since sows with no previous exposure to fish oil feeding have approximately 0.5 g 22:6 n-3 / 100g total fatty acids in their subcutaneous tissue (Rooke *et al.*, 2000). Kojima *et al.* (1997) reported that feeding gilts a preparation derived from a mould (*Mucor circinelloides*) containing high concentrations of 18:3 n-6 (gamma linolenic acid), thereby bypassing the rate-limiting step in PUFA biosynthesis, improved ovulation rate and embryo morphology when compared with diets containing safflower (18:2 n-6) and perilla (18:3 n-3) oils. However, these data must be treated with caution as the diets were not isoenergetic and the mould preparation was ill-defined containing, for example, substantial quantities of vitamins.

## EFFECT OF MARINE OILS ON FEMALE REPRODUCTION

As noted earlier, typical diets fed to pregnant sows may not be optimally balanced in their fatty acid profile, certainly when current recommendations for human nutrition are considered. Brain development in the piglet is quantitatively important *in utero* between days 60 and term. Therefore, optimising supply of long chain n-3 PUFA for brain development may improve piglet viability at birth. A series of studies has recently been carried out at Aberdeen to investigate this issue. These studies had two parts: a series of detailed studies, using relatively small numbers of multiparous sows to provide guidance on how to optimise fatty acid deposition in the tissues of new-born piglets and a commercial-scale study to investigate the effect of long chain n-3 PUFA on piglet mortality and associated measurements.

At the outset, a practical problem was evidence that transfer of fatty acids across the porcine placenta was limited in late pregnancy (Thulin *et al.*, 1989, Ramsay *et al.*, 1991), recently confirmed by Pere (2001), who reported concentrations of free fatty acids in umbilical blood were three times lower than in maternal blood and extraction efficiency (umbilical arterio-venous difference) by the piglet was 7.8%. However, an initial experiment in which tuna orbital (30g/kg) or soya-bean oils were fed to the sow from day 90 of pregnancy (Rooke *et al.* 1998) showed that n-3 fatty acid, particularly 22:6 n-3, content of piglet tissues at birth was increased, with corresponding decreases in n-6 acids, particularly 20:4 n-6, in response to tuna oil feeding. Thus, albeit with a low efficiency of transfer (~ 5%) from diet to foetal tissues, 22:6 n-3 contents of brain and retina could be increased by adding long chain n-3 PUFA to the maternal diet. Further experiments (Rooke *et al.*, 2000, 2001b,d) have shown that in terms of changes in piglet tissue fatty acids at birth, feeding marine oils from day 60 of pregnancy produced similar responses to feeding for all of pregnancy. Addition (17.5 g/kg) of 18:3 n-3 (from linseed oil) to the maternal diet throughout pregnancy was compared with 22:6 n-3 (and 20:5 n-3) from tuna orbital oil (Rooke *et al.*, 2000) and showed (Table 6.2) that 18:3 n-3 was relatively ineffective in modifying piglet tissue long chain n-3 PUFA composition. Estimates showed that 18:3 n-3 increased brain long chain n-3 PUFA 0.17 fold the values obtained with supplying pre-formed acids, a value similar to that reported (0.24) by Arbuckle and Innis (1992) for formula-milk-fed piglets. It is important that the correct amounts of n-3 fatty acids are fed as negative effects have been observed when high concentrations of dietary fish oils have been used (Innis, 2000b), including reduced brain weights in formula-fed piglets (Arbuckle *et al.*, 1991) and reduced infant growth (Carlsson *et al.*, 1992; 1993). In the human, the depression in growth was more closely correlated with a depression in 20:4 n-6 status than with an increase in 22:6 n-3. Therefore, the optimum amount of dietary long chain n-3 PUFA for the pig was assessed (Rooke *et al.*, 2001d) by feeding increasing amounts of fish oil from day 60 of pregnancy and piglet responses were assessed by changes in brain weight and fatty acid composition (Figure 6.4). The optimum inclusion of fish oil was 10g oil / kg diet, which corresponded to 6g / sow / day of 20:5 n-3 and 22:6 n-3 together (total intake 2.5 kg/day) or 0.6 % DE intake. In summary, these experiments would suggest that to obtain optimum responses in piglet tissue at birth, pre-formed long chain n-3 PUFA should be included in the maternal diet from at least day 60 of pregnancy and comprise 0.6% DE intake.

Although the number of sows used in the above experiment was too small to assess piglet mortality, a variety of relevant measurements were made. Given the differing experimental objectives, results (Table 6.3) were, not surprisingly, variable, but there were indications of positive effects of added n-3 PUFA. Therefore, a larger trial was carried out under commercial conditions (Rooke *et al.*, 2001c).

**Table 6.2** CHANGES IN FATTY ACID COMPOSITION (G/100G TOTAL FATTY ACIDS) IN PIGLET TISSUES AT BIRTH IN RESPONSE TO FEEDING THE SOW DIFFERENT OILS (ROOKE *et al.*, 2000)

| | *Oil* | | |
|---|---|---|---|
| *Fatty acid* | *Maize* *18:2 n-6* | *Linseed* *18:3 n-3* | *Tuna* *20:5 n-3 + 22:6 n-3* |
| Cord plasma | | | |
| 18:3 n-3 | 0.4 | 0.6 | 0.5 |
| 20:5 n-3 | 1.2[a] | 1.7[b] | 2.2[c] |
| 22:6 n-3 | 1.4[a] | 1.7[a] | 2.4[b] |
| Liver | | | |
| 18:3 n-3 | 0.2[a] | 0.5[b] | 0.2[a] |
| 20:5 n-3 | 0.5[a] | 1.2[b] | 2.5[c] |
| 22:6 n-3 | 4.9[a] | 5.5[a] | 8.2[b] |
| Brain | | | |
| 18:3 n-3 | <0.1 | 0.1 | <0.1 |
| 20:5 n-3 | <0.1[a] | <0.1[a] | 0.2[b] |
| 22:6 n-3 | 13.3[a] | 13.4[a] | 15.6[b] |

Means in same row with different superscripts are significantly different.

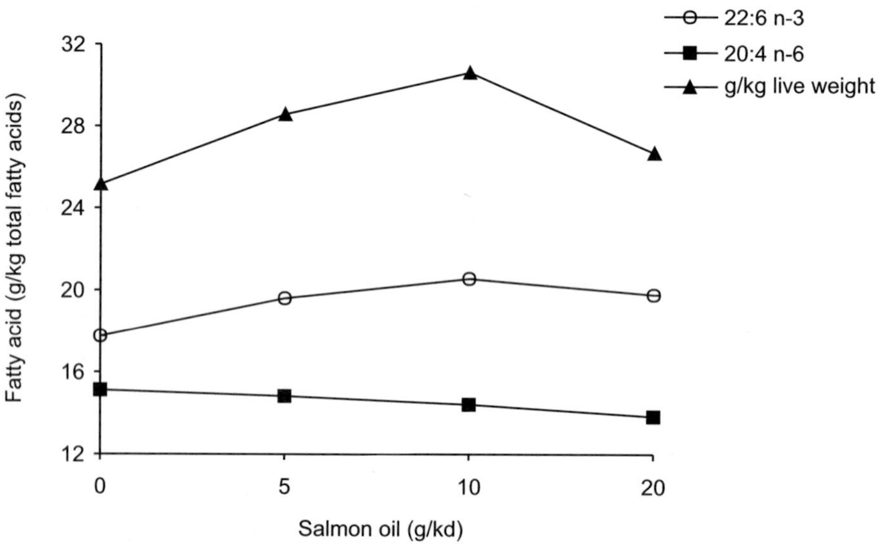


**Figure 6.4** Effects of including increasing amounts of long chain n-3 PUFA (g salmon oil/kg diet) on brain weight (g/kg live weight) and brain 20:4 n-6 and 22:6 n-3 concentrations (g/kg total fatty acids). (Rooke *et al.*, 2001d).

**TABLE 6.3** RESPONSES OF PIGLETS TO FEEDING FISH OILS TO THE SOW DURING PREGNANCY

| | *Experiment* | | | |
|---|---|---|---|---|
| | *1* | *2* | *3* | *4* |
| Brain weight | ++ | + | + | ++ quadratic |
| Udder seeking | o | n | ++ | n |
| Growth | | | | |
| Suckling | n | o | ++ | n |
| Post-weaning | n | + | ++ | n |

Experiment: 1, Rooke *et al.* (1998); 2, Rooke *et al.* (2000); 3, Rooke *et al.* (2001b); 4, Rooke *et al* (2001d).
Key to codes: n, not measured; o, no response; +, response (non-significant); ++, significant response.

Sows (approximately 100 / treatment) were fed diets containing 16.5 g salmon oil /kg, essentially replacing vegetable oil throughout pregnancy and lactation. The increased gestation length when salmon oil was fed (Table 6.4) was similar to that noted by Edwards and Pike (1997) when a fishmeal containing n-3 fatty acids was fed to pregnant sows. The extension of gestation length was probably caused by decreases in 2-series prostaglandin production by feeding the salmon oil noted in other studies with piglets (Fritsche *et al.*, 1993; Huang and Craig-Schmidt 1996). The lower piglet birth-weight when salmon oil was fed did not result in adverse litter performance, as weaning weights did not differ. However, pre-weaning mortality was reduced when salmon oil was fed. Figure 6.5 shows this reduction was largely caused by a reduction in the number of piglets crushed by the sow. As Edwards and Pike (1977) also found that feeding 50 g/kg fishmeal during pregnancy reduced mortality, the results with salmon oil suggest that it was the oil content of the fishmeal which was the causative factor reducing mortality. The reductions in mortality in Table 6.4 were independent of factors such as birth weight known to influence pre-weaning mortality.

## MISCELLANEOUS

Other fatty acids fed to the sow during pregnancy have improved post-natal performance. Medium–chain triglycerides fed to the sow during late pregnancy and early lactation improved pre-weaning mortality of piglets (Azain, 1993). The underlying mechanisms compared with long chain fatty acids, e.g. more rapid digestion and absorption, complete oxidation and entry to the

**Table 6.4** EFFECTS OF FEEDING LONG CHAIN N-3 PUFA AS FISH MEAL OR FISH OIL ON REPRODUCTIVE PERFORMANCE

| | *Study* | | | |
|---|---|---|---|---|
| | *Edwards and Pike (1997)* | | *Rooke et al. (2001c)* | |
| | *Control* | *Fishmeal* | *Control* | *Salmon oil* |
| Gestation length (d) | | | | |
| Gilt | 115.0 | 115.3- | - | |
| Multiparous | 115.3 | 115.7 $^{P=0.06}$ | 115.4 | 115.9*** |
| Total born / litter | 11.2 | 11.5 | 11.8 | 11.6 |
| Piglet birth-weight (kg) | 1.45 | 1.46 | 1.54 | 1.47* |
| Litter birth-weight (kg) | | | | |
| Gilt | 14.9 | 15.8 $^{P=0.08}$ | - | - |
| Multiparous | 17.0 | 17.3 | 18.0 | 17.7 $^{P<0.10}$ |
| Pre-weaning mortality (%) | | | | |
| Gilt | 20.2 | 13.8* | | - - |
| Multiparous | 13.1 | 11.9 | 11.7 | 10.2* |

Superscript after value indicates whether value is significantly different from control.

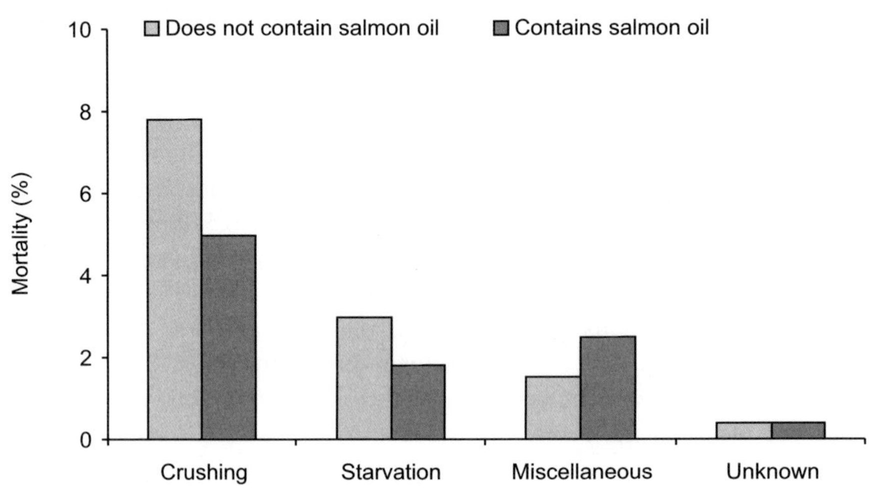


**Figure 6.5** Causes of pre-weaning mortality in piglets whose dams were fed diets not containing or containing salmon oil (17.5 g/kg) throughout pregnancy (Rooke *et al.*, 2001c).

mitochondrion independent of carnitine, have been reviewed recently by Odle (1998). Similarly, Bauman *et al.* (2001) reviewed conjugated linoleic acids and described their effects of growth and fat deposition. One intriguing and as yet unexplained observation is that of Bee (2000), who fed equivalent amounts of linoleic or conjugated linoleic acids to sows during pregnancy and lactation and followed the performance of their offspring. Unexpectedly and irrespective of the diet fed post-weaning, piglets whose dams were fed conjugated linoleic acids during pregnancy and lactation consumed more food and grew faster in the post-weaning period.

## Practical implications

The conclusions, from research at SAC and elsewhere, are that boar fertility and piglet survival may benefit from including a source of long chain PUFA in the diet of boar and sow. For the sow, it was suggested that inclusion of 10 g salmon oil /kg diet would provide an adequate supply of long chain PUFA (0.6% DE). There are several practical issues that may need to be addressed:

- Given concerns over sustainability of fish stocks, can 18:3 n-3 rich vegetable oils be substituted for fish oils? This matter has not been addressed in the boar and, although in the sow the efficiency of incorporation of dietary 18:3 n-3 into long chain n-3 PUFA was about 0.20 of pre-formed long chain PUFA when equal amounts were fed, whether feeding 5 times the amount of 18:3 n-3 would substitute for long chain PUFA has not been evaluated.
- The total amount of long chain n-3 PUFA, the relative amounts of 22:6 n-3 and 20:5 n-3 and cost of fish oils differ substantially between different oils. Nutritionally this may be important as the reduced infant growth, attributed by Carlsson *et al.* (1992; 1993) to feeding an excess of fish oil, was related to the relatively high 20:5 n-3 content of the oil.
- There may be differences between genotypes in utilisation of long chain n-3 PUFA by the sow as noted in growing pigs (e.g. muscle phospholipid fatty acids (Riette *et al.*, 1999) and sensitivity to short-term changes in nutrition (Cameron *et al.*, 2000).
- Inclusion of long chain PUFA in diets will increase their susceptibility to peroxidation. In the commercial scale trial (Rooke *et al.*, 2001c), no additional vitamin E was added to pregnancy diets but, in a batch of feed tested over 3 months, no decreases in PUFA content were detected. In more detailed studies, the vitamin E level of the diet was increased to 200 mg/kg as a precaution against peroxidation.
- In the sow, feeding a diet containing added long chain PUFA from day 60 of pregnancy is probably compatible with most feeding systems. In fact, convenience would usually dictate a longer period of feeding and there may be positive effects for this, given the observations of Perez-

Rigau *et al.* (1995) on piglet survival at 30 days of pregnancy. In the boar, changes in sperm composition were only observed after 30 – 40 days feeding, consistent with *de novo* spermatogenesis, and therefore continuous inclusion of long chain PUFA in the diet will be necessary to maintain sperm 22:6 n-3 concentrations. Finally, adding liquid oils may not be compatible with all feed mill practices, but this problem can be overcome by adding the oil as a blend containing 500g oil /kg diet (Rooke *et al.*, 2001c).

## References

Abayasekara, D.R.E. and Wathes, D.C. (1999) Effects of altering dietary fatty acid composition on prostaglandin synthesis and fertility. *Prostaglandins, Leukotrienes and Essential Fatty Acids,* **61**, 275-287.

Agricultural Research Council (1981) *The Nutrient Requirements of Pigs*. Commonwealth Agricultural Bureaux, Slough, UK.

Arbuckle, L.D., Rioux, F.M., Mackinnon, M.J., Hrboticky, N. and Innis, S.M. (1991) Response of (n-3) and (n-6) fatty acids in piglet brain, liver and plasma to increasing, but low, fish oil supplementation of formula. *Journal of Nutrition,* **121,** 1536-1547.

Arbuckle, L.D. and Innis, S.M. (1992) Docosahexaenoic acid in developing brain and retina of piglets fed high or low α-linolenoate formula with and without fish oil. *Lipids,* **27,** 89-93.

Azain, M.J. (1993) Effects of adding medium-chain triglycerides to sow diets during late gestation and early lactation on litter performance. *Journal of Animal Science*, **71**, 3011-3019.

Bauman, D.E., Corl, B.A., Baumgard, L.H. and Griinari, J.M. (2001) Conjugated linoleic acid (CLA) and the dairy cow. In *Recent Advances in Animal Nutrition 2001* pp 221-250 Edited by P.C. Garnsworthy and J. Wiseman. Nottingham University Press, Nottingham, UK.

Bee, G. (2000) Dietary conjugated linoleic acid consumption during pregnancy and lactation influences growth and tissue composition in weaned pigs. *Journal of Nutrition*, **130**, 2981-2989.

Bhathena, S., Berlin, E., McClure, D. and Peters, R.C. (2001) Effects of dietary fats on red blood cell membrane insulin receptor in normo- and hypercholesterolemic miniature swine. *Journal of Nutritional Biochemistry*, **12**, 529-535.

Calder, P.C. (2002) Dietary modification of inflammation with lipids. *Proceedings of the Nutrition Society*, **61**, 345-358.

Cameron, N.D., Wood, J.D., Enser, M., Whittington, F.M., Penman, J.C. and Robinson, A.M. (2000) Sensitivity of pig genotypes to short-term manipulation of plasma fatty acids by feeding linseed. *Meat Science*, **56**, 379-386.

Carlson, S.E., Cooke, R.J., Werkman, S.H. and Tolley, E.A. (1992) First year growth of preterm infants fed standard compared to marine oil *n-3* supplemented formula. *Lipids,* **27,** 901-907.

Carlson, S.E., Werkman, S.H., Peeples, J.M., Cooke, R.J. and Tolley, E.A. (1993) Arachidonic acid status correlates with first year growth in preterm infants. *Proceedings of the National Academy of Science,* **90,** 1073-1077.

Ding, S.-T. and Mersmann, H.J. (2001) Fatty acids modulate porcine adipocyte differentiation and transcripts for transcription factors and adipocyte-characteristic proteins. *Journal of Nutritional Biochemistry*, **12**, 101-108.

Edwards, S.A. and Pike, I. (1997) Effect of fishmeal on sow reproductive performance. *Proceedings of the British Society of Animal Science 1997*, p 55 (abstract).

Farnworth, E.R. and Kramer, J.K.G. (1988) Fetal pig development in sows fed diets containing different fats. *Canadian Journal of Animal Science*, **68**, 249-256.

Farnworth, E.R. and Kramer, J.K.G. (1989) Changes in the lipid composition of the internal organs of fetal pigs from sows fed different fats. *Canadian Journal of Animal Science*, **69**, 441-448.

Fritsche, K.L., Alexander, D.W., Cassity, N.A. and Huang, S.-C. (1993) Maternally-supplied fish oil alters piglet immune cell fatty acid profile and eicosanoid production. *Lipids*, **28**, 67-682.

Gerfault, V., Mourot, J., Etienne, M. and Mounier, A. (1999) Influence de la nature des lipides dans la regime de gestation de la truie sur ses performances et la composition corporelle des porcelaits a la naissance. *Journees Recherches Porcine en France*, **31**, 191-197.

Gerfault, V., Romao, M., Mourot, J., Etienne, M. and Mounier, A. (2000) Influence de la quantite et de la nature des lipides alimentaires pendant la gestation et la lactation des truies sur la developpement du tissu adipeux, les performances de croissance et la qualite de la viande des porcs charcutiers. *Journees Recherches Porcine en France*, **32**, 291-296.

Huang, M.-C. and Craig-Schimdt, M.C. (1996) Arachidonate and docosahexaenoate added to infant formula influence fatty acid composition and subsequent eicosanoid production in neonatal pigs. *Journal of Nutrition*, **126**, 2199-2208.

Innis, S.M. (2000a) The role of dietary n 6 and n-3 fatty acids in the developing brain. *Developmental Neuroscience*, **22**, 474-480.

Innis, S.M. (2000b) Essential fatty acids in infant nutrition: lessons and limitations from animal studies in relation to studies on infant fatty acid requirements. *American Journal of Clinical Nutrition*, **71** (supplement), 238S-244S.

Jump, D.B. (2002) Dietary polyunsaturated fatty acids and regulation of gene transcription. *Current Opinions in Lipidology*, **13**, 155-164.

Kojima, T., Zeniya, Y., Aoyama, Y., Kondo, A. and Yoshino, J. (1997) Dietary administration of fatty acids-enriched mold dried cell containing γ-linolenic acid to female pigs improves ovulation rate and embryo quality in summer. *Journal of Reproduction and Development,* **43**, 121-127.

Leskanitch, C.O. and Noble, R.C. (1999) The comparative roles of polyunsaturated fatty acids in pig neonatal development. *British Journal of Nutrition*, **81**, 87-106.

Li, Z., Kaplan, M.L. and Hachey, D.L. (2000) Hepatic microsomal and peroxisomal docosahexanoate biosynthesis during piglet development. *Lipids*, **35**, 1325-1333.

Malm, A., Pond, W.G., Walker, E.F.Jr., Homan, M., Aydin, A. and Kirtland, D. (1976). Effect of polyunsaturated fatty acids and vitamin E level of the sow gestation diet on reproductive performance and on level of alpha tocopherol in colostrum, milk and dam and progeny blood serum. *Journal of Animal Science*, **42**, 393-399.

Meat and Livestock Commission. (2001). *Pig Yearbook 2001.* Meat and Livestock Commission, Milton Keynes.

Nair, S.S.D., Leitch, J. and Garg, M.L. (2000) Suppression of inositol phosphate release by cardiac myocytes isolated from fish oil-fed pigs. *Molecular and Cellular Biochemistry*, **215**, 57-64.

Nair, S.S.D., Leitch, J. and Garg, M.L. (2001) N-3 polyunsaturated fatty acid supplementation alters inositol phosphate metabolism and protein kinase C activity in adult porcine cardiac myocytes. *Journal of Nutritional Biochemistry*, **12**, 7-13.

National Research Council (1998) *Nutrient Requirements of Swine, Tenth Revised Edition.* National Academy Press, Washington, D.C., USA.

Neuringer M., Connor W.E., Van Petten C. and Barstad, L. (1984) Dietary omega-3 fatty acid deficiency and visual loss in infant rhesus monkeys. *Journal of Clinical Investigation,* 7**3,** 272-276.

Odle J. (1998) Medium-chain triglycerides: a unique energy source for neonatal pigs. *Pig News and Information*, **20**, 25N-32N.

Paulenz, H., Taugbøl, O., Hofmo, P.O. and Saarem, K. (1995) A preliminary study on the effect of dietary supplementation with cod liver oil on the polyunsaturated fatty acid composition of boar semen. *Veterinary Research Communications*, **19**, 273-284.

Penny, P.C., Noble, R.C., Maldjian, A. and Cerolini, S. (2000) Potential role of lipids for the enhancement of boar fertility and fecundity. *Pig News and Information*, **21,** 119N-126N.

Père, M.-C. (2001) Effects of meal intake on materno-foetal exchanges of energetic substrates in the pig. *Reproduction, Nutrition, Developpement*, **41**, 285-296.

Perez-Rigau, A., Lindemann, M.D., Kornegay, E.T., Harper, A.F. and Watkins, B.A. (1995) Role of dietary lipids on fetal tissue fatty acid composition and fetal survival in swine at 42 days of gestation. *Journal of Animal Science*,**73**, 1372-1380.

Pettigrew, J.E. (1981) Supplemental dietary fat for peripartal sows: a review. *Journal of Animal Science*, **53**, 107-117.

Pope, W.F. (1994) Embryonic Mortality in Swine. In *Embryonic Mortality in Domestic Species,* pp 53-77. Edited by M.T. Zavy and R.D. Geisert. Boca Raton, Florida: CRC Press.

Raclot, T. and Oudart, H. (1999) Selectivity of fatty acids on lipid metabolism and gene expression. *Proceedings of the Nutrition Society,* **58**, 633-646.

Ramsay, T.G., Karousis, J., White, M.E. and Wolverton, C K. (1991) Fatty acid metabolism by the porcine placenta. *Journal of Animal Science,* **69**, 3645 - 3654.

Riette, L., van Laack, J.M. and Spencer, E. (1999) Influence of swine genotype on fatty acid composition of phospholipids in longissimus muscle. *Journal of Animal Science*, **77**, 1742-1745.

Rooke, J.A., Bland, I.M. and Edwards, S.A. (1998) Effect of feeding tuna oil or soyabean oil as supplements to sows in late pregnancy on piglet tissue composition and viability. *British Journal of Nutrition,* **80**, 273-280.

Rooke, J.A., Shanks, M. and Edwards S.A. (2000) Effect of feeding maize, linseed or tuna oils throughout pregnancy and lactation on sow and piglet tissue composition and piglet performance. *Animal Science,* **71,** 289-300.

Rooke, J.A., Shao, C.-C. and Speake, B.K. (2001a) The effect of feeding tuna oil upon porcine spermatozoa lipid and fatty acid composition and semen characteristics. *Reproduction* **121,** 315-322.

Rooke, J.A., Sinclair, A.G. and Edwards S.A. (2001b) Feeding tuna oil to the sow at different times during pregnancy has different effects on piglet long-chain polyunsaturated fatty acid composition at birth and subsequent growth. *British Journal of Nutrition,* **86,** 21-30.

Rooke, J.A., Sinclair, A.G., Edwards, S.A., Cordoba, R., Pkiyach, S., Penny, P.C., Penny, P., Finch, A.M. and Horgan, G.W. (2001c) The effect of feeding salmon oil throughout pregnancy on pre-weaning mortality of piglet. *Animal Science*, **73**, 489-500.

Rooke, J.A., Sinclair, A.G. and Ewen, M. (2001d) Changes in piglet tissue composition at birth in response to increasing maternal intake of long chain n-3 polyunsaturated fatty acids are non-linear. *British Journal of Nutrition,* **86,** 461-470.

Simopoulos, A.P., Leaf, A. and Salem, N.Jr. (2000) Workshop statement on the essentiality of and recommended dietary intakes for omega-6 and omega-3 fatty acids. *Prostaglandins, Leukotrienes and Essential Fatty Acids,* **63**, 119-121.

Speake, B.K., Surai, P.F. and Rooke, J.A. (2003) Regulation of avian and mammalian sperm production by dietary fatty acids. In press. In: *Lipid Metabolism and Male Fertility* Edited by S. De Vriese and A. Christophe. Champaign, Illinois: AOCS Press.

Sprecher, H. (2000) Metabolism of highly unsaturated n-3 and n-6 fatty acids. *Biochimica et Biophysica Acta*, **1486**, 219-231.

Thulin, A. J., Allee, G.L., Harmon, D.L. and Davis, D.L. (1989) Utero-placental transfer of octanoic, palmitic and linoleic acids during late gestation in gilts. *Journal of Animal Science,* **67**, 738 - 745.

Whelan, J. (1996) Antagonistic effect of dietary arachidonic acid and n-3 polyunsaturated fatty acids. *Journal of Nutrition*, **126,** 1086S-1091S.

Wood, J.D. and Enser, M. (1997) Factors influencing fatty acids in meat and the role of antioxidants in improving meat quality. *British Journal of Nutrition,* **78,** S49-S60.

Wuttke, W., Spiess, S., Knoke, I., Pitzel, L., Leonhardt, S. and Jarry, H. (1998) Synergistic effects of prostaglandin F-2 alpha and tumor necrosis factor to induce luteolysis in the pig. *Biology of Reproduction*, **58**, 1310-1315.

*This paper was first published in 2003*

7

# EARLY NUTRITION IN YOUNG POULTRY

J. DIBNER
*Novus International, Inc., St. Louis MO, USA*

## Introduction

Genetic selection has produced enormous increases in growth rate and feed efficiency of poultry. Selection also has been accompanied by changes in gastrointestinal structure and function. Studies suggest that changes in the gastrointestinal system associated with selection for efficiency are particularly notable in broiler chicks and turkey poults (Mitchell and Smith, 1991; Dunnington and Siegel, 1995). The importance of describing and understanding the growth of poultry during the first week of life has also increased because the first week has become a larger proportion of the whole life span, particularly for meat-type birds. Lilja (1983) has proposed that the ultimate growth of the bird is directly proportional to early development of those systems that supply substrate to the rest of the body, specifically the gastrointestinal and cardiovascular systems. It is also clear that achievement of growth potential is influenced by immune function (Coates *et al.*, 1954; Jukes *et al.*, 1956). A competent, but not overactive, immune capability is critical for steady provision of nutrients to demanding organs such as muscle.

The growth rate of broilers increases from day 0 to 10, reaching a maximum of about 20% per day (Nitsan *et al.*, 1991a). In order to achieve their genetic potential, birds must rapidly adapt to digestion of an exogenous diet in which nutrients are absorbed from the intestine and energy is supplied predominantly by carbohydrates. Factors that may influence early growth rate include amount of yolk sac residue, quality and intake of feed and water, pancreatic and intestinal enzyme levels, gastrointestinal tract surface area, nutrient transporters, and overall nutrient digestibility. Another process that must be considered is the fundamental change in energy metabolism from lipids to carbohydrates.

It has been demonstrated that the gastrointestinal system of young birds is not able to use certain ingredients, such as tallow, with the same efficiency as mature birds (Fredde *et al.,* 1960; Gomez and Polin, 1976; Polin *et al.,* 1980; Sell *et al.*, 1986). Ontogenic changes which accompany improved digestion include increased levels of pancreatic and intestinal enzymes (Krogdahl and Sell, 1989; Sell *et al.*, 1989; Noy and Sklan, 1995), increases in overall gut surface area for absorption (Nitsan *et al.,* 1991a; Nitsan *et al.*, 1991b; Sell *et al.*, 1991), and changes in nutrient transporters (Shehata *et al.*, 1981; Buddington and Diamond, 1989; Moreto *et al.*, 1991; Noy *et al.*, 1996). This chapter will consider these factors and their role in early growth of both chicks and poults.

## Residual yolk

Poultry chicks undergo a fundamental change in nutrient supply and metabolism upon emergence from the eggshell. During embryonic incubation, yolk lipid supplies the energy needs of the bird and is delivered from the yolk sac via the blood stream (Freeman and Vince, 1974). As hatch approaches, glycogen accumulates in the liver of the embryo and is used for energy during the hatching process. In addition, lipid is transferred to the liver and the yolk sac is internalized within the body wall (Romanoff, 1960). This lipid can be used to supply energy to the chick if required, but the composition of residual yolk lipid suggests that it is more efficient to use these lipids for cell membrane structure and central nervous system development (Noble and Ogunyemi, 1989; Anderson *et al.*, 1990). Thus, providing energy in the form of oral carbohydrate spares these unsaturated fatty acids for the phospholipid membranes of new cells.

The residual yolk is of very limited quantity (Phelps *et al.,* 1987a; Ding and Lilburn, 1996). In fact, the energy available from yolk lipids is barely sufficient to maintain the bird for 24 hours (Akiba and Murakami, 1995; Ding and Lilburn, 1996). During the first day after hatch, approximately 80% of residual yolk fat is transferred to the tissues and less than 10% remains after two days (Nitsan *et al.,* 1991a). Similarly, more than half of the protein contained in the yolk sac is transferred to the chick during the first two days of life, with virtually no protein remaining after 4 days (Nitsan *et al.,* 1991a). This protein, which contains substantial amounts of maternal antibodies, is better used to provide passive immune protection than to be broken down for use as amino acids. If the bird is in danger of starving, the maternal antibody may be used for nutrition, but this is clearly not the ideal situation as it leaves the chick unprotected against pathogens for the first two weeks of life.

## Ingestion of feed and water

Despite the presence of the lipid-rich residual yolk and reserves of lipid in the liver, delayed availability of feed and water is associated with a peak of early mortality, particularly in poults (Entenman *et al.,* 1940; Vanheel *et al.*, 1981; Phelps *et al.*, 1987b; Noble and Ogunyemi, 1989; Chamblee *et al.*, 1992). Although recent evidence indicates that some of the residual yolk makes its way into the intestine *via* the yolk stalk, the presence of the yolk sac has been found to be less important than oral intake of feed for gastrointestinal development (Uni *et al.*, 1998; Noy *et al.,* 1996; Sulaiman *et al.*, 1996). Thus, rapid availability and consumption of feed and water are crucial both to the immediate development of organ systems and to long term survival and performance (Fanguy *et al.*, 1980; Pinchasov and Noy, 1993).

From a performance standpoint, a delay in the initiation of feed and water intake can have long term consequences. The practice of holding birds in the brooder for up to 48 hours or until more than 90% of chicks have emerged from the shell is associated with higher mortality (Kingston, 1979; Fanguy *et al.,* 1980), lower placement weight (Fanguy *et al.,* 1980; Warriss *et al.*, 1991; Pinchasov and Noy, 1993; Casteel *et al.*, 1994), poorer four week (Hager and Beane, 1983) and long term (Vieira and Moran, 1999) performance, in comparison with birds removed immediately after hatching. There is also an indication that immune status may be compromised by delaying placement of chicks (Casteel *et al.,* 1994). Although three-day gut and liver weights are significantly reduced after removal of the yolk sac (Nitsan *et al.*, 1995), experiments in which such birds were either fed or fasted indicate that oral intake of nutrients is more important than residual yolk in the initiation of body-weight gain in the bird (Baranyiova, 1972b; Waldroup *et al.*, 1974; Twining, Nicholson and Thomas, 1978; Engku Azahan and Forbes, 1989).

## Digestive enzymes

Another aspect of the metabolic changes that occur with hatching is the change from blood-borne to oral nutrient intake. Oral nutrition requires the presence of digestive enzymes to break down macromolecules to a size that can be absorbed. Digestive enzymes first appear during incubation (Moran, 1985; Escribano *et al.*, 1988; Ikeno and Ikeno, 1991; Ikeno *et al.*, 1992; Pinchasov and Noy, 1994). Although levels appear to increase after hatch, their concentration per gram of feed intake does not change (Noy and Sklan, 1995; Uni *et al.*, 1995a). Despite never having ingested feed, the intestinal mucosa contains a high level of disaccharidase activity at hatch (Uni *et al.,* 1998).

In studies of digestive enzymes of lines selected for low and high eight-week body weight, Nitsan *et al.* (1991b) observed that chicks from the high-weight line have higher levels of trypsin and amylase at both 3 and 9 days of age than lines selected for low 8-week body weight. Similar data were reported by Dunnington and Siegel (1995) and by Uni *et al.* (1995b), who observed that such differences in digestive enzyme levels between light and heavy strains could be observed at 4 days after hatching but disappeared thereafter. Murakami *et al.* (1992) suggest that age-related changes in the amount of enzymes relative to digesta may cause variability or even limit growth over the first week of life.

The failure of chicks to respond to force-feeding with higher pancreatic enzyme secretion (Nitsan, 1974) can be contrasted with the older chick, which compensates for increased feed intake with higher pancreatic enzyme secretion (Nir *et al.*, 1978). Both lines of evidence suggest that, while digestive enzyme levels may not limit growth during the first week of life, levels and specific activities closely approximate requirements and that rapid increases in synthesis and secretion are required to keep up with increasing feed intake.

## Gastrointestinal surface area

Other research suggests that physical factors in the gastrointestinal system, such as gut length and surface area, are more likely to limit early growth than enzyme availability (Pinchasov and Noy, 1993; Nitsan *et al.,* 1991a; Sell *et al.,* 1991). For example, Ritz *et al.* (1995) concluded that increased early growth in birds fed diets supplemented with amylase was due to an increase in absorptive surface area in response to the presence of enzyme in the diet.

Research on lines selected for heavy weight indicates that the low body weight lines show lower relative intestine growth (Nitsan, *et al.,* 1991a), shorter villi and lower enterocyte density (Uni *et al.,* 1995a and b) than do heavy weight or fast growing lines (Lilja, 1983; Mitchell and Smith, 1991). Data reported by Nir *et al.* (1978) and by Barbato *et al.* (1984) suggest that surface area may limit growth even in older broilers that have been selected for rapid growth. These relationships may be age-dependent, in that Mitchell and Smith (1991) have reported that selection for heavier body weight may result in increased efficiency of absorption since relative total intestinal mucosa weight in 6-week old birds actually decreases with selection for higher body weight and feed efficiency.

In the chick, the effect of low surface area may be partly ameliorated by the slower feed passage rate (Golian and Polin, 1984; Noy and Sklan, 1995), although this may also be associated with relatively poor feed intake (Knoblock and Siegel, 1970). Poor feed intake is a particular problem in poults (Phelps *et al.,* 1987a). It should be noted that, although broilers generally show increasing feed consumption post hatch, even *ad libitum* availability of feed can be associated with a decline in weight over the first 24 hours after hatch (Pinchasov, 1991).

Increased absolute and relative mass of the gastrointestinal system, the nutrient supply system for animal growth, is observed during the first week of life (Nitsan *et al.,* 1991b). In fact, the absolute length of the small intestine increases over the first 5 days of life, even under fasting conditions (Baranyiova, 1972b). An increase in intestinal weight relative to body weight (Baranyiova, 1972b), and increases in villus length and intestinal diameter, however, require oral nutrient intake (Baranyiova and Holman, 1976).

## Nutrient transport systems

Amino acid and hexose transport systems in enterocyte cell membranes develop shortly before hatch and increase in density during the first week of life (Shehata *et al.,* 1981; Buddington, 1992; Noy *et al.,* 1996). Although it appears that transport systems do not limit early growth, transport capacities appear to be regulated to match or just slightly exceed nutrient inputs (Buddington and Diamond, 1989; Obst and Diamond, 1992). Recent evidence suggests that transport capacity of glucose may be limiting, particularly in birds selected for rapid growth (Fan, 1995; Croom *et al.*, 1999). In agreement with this is the report by Mitchell and Smith (1991) suggesting that increased absorption efficiency may accompany selection for improved performance. Indeed, any decrease in the relative mass of gut tissue with its high oxygen and metabolic requirements, high heat production and short epithelial cell life span could represent a significant improvement in overall maintenance requirements for the bird (Fan *et al.*, 1997).

## Nutrient digestibility

The combined efficiency of gastrointestinal processes is measured in digestibility experiments. For the chick, digestibility appears to vary for different nutrients, although increases in digestibility over the first week of life have been observed for carbohydrates (Phelps *et al.,* 1987a), proteins (Noy and Sklan, 1995) and fats (Senkoylu and Janssen, 1988; Noy and Sklan, 1995).

Saturated fats of long chain length appear to be among the most difficult of fats for the chick to digest (Wiseman and Salvador, 1991; Blanch *et al.*, 1995). Low lipid digestibility has been widely reported in chicks and in poults (Sell *et al.,* 1986) and appears to be associated with the ongoing maturation of the bile salt synthesis and reabsorption systems rather than deficiencies in lipase (Escribano *et al.,* 1988). This is supported by the observation that poor early digestibility of relatively saturated fats such as tallow can be improved with bile salt addition (Gomez and Polin, 1976) or soybean lecithin (Polin, 1980). Digestibility of relatively unsaturated fats, such as soyabean oil, is much better than tallow and not improved as much with age (Blanch *et al.,* 1995; Noy and Sklan, 1995). In a recent study of nutrient uptake, Noy and Sklan (1995) report no change in oleic acid uptake by the duodenum during the first 14 days after hatch. In that study, the fatty acid was supplied as micelles containing taurocholic acid, which would obscure poor digestibility associated with bile-salt deficiency in the chick.

## Energy metabolism

During the first five days of life, changes in serum lipid, lipoprotein and glucose levels indicate a fundamental shift from the lipid-based metabolism of the embryo to that dominated by carbohydrate in the neonate (Latour *et al.*, 1995). Even before hatch, concentration of blood sugar begins to increase with the onset of pulmonary respiration and then continues to rise until hatch (Freeman, 1965). At initiation of hatch there are moderate stores of liver glycogen, which are virtually depleted by the first day after hatch (Freeman, 1965).

The metabolic changes that occur during hatch are accompanied by an increase in serum cortisone, further suggesting a fundamental change in the energy metabolism of the chick (Latour *et al.* 1995). At the end of hatch in broilers, liver glycogen is depleted and blood ketone levels are high (Best, 1966), but following hatch, liver glycogen increases steadily as long as birds are eating a carbohydrate type of diet (Best, 1966; Baranyiova, 1972a). Fasted broilers, with or without yolk sacs, show no increase in liver glycogen (Baranyiova, 1972a) and also exhibit increased free fatty acids in the blood (Baranyiova and Standara, 1980). Latour *et al.* (1995) also suggest that the metabolic processes that regulate blood constituents have not been fully developed by day five, which results in non-homeostatic variations in serum levels of cortisone, triglycerides and glucose.

Chicks and poults show similarities in early carbohydrate metabolism, although the stress of a longer hatch time for poults (Moran and Reinhart, 1981) leads to more severe depletion of the glycogen stored during incubation (Rosebrough *et al.*, 1979). This necessitates a greater use of fat for energy in the poult (Entenman *et al.,* 1940; Best, 1966) resulting in ketosis. Two peaks of early mortality are observed in poults. High poult mortality at 4-5 days is related to a decline in intake associated with ketosis. Poor feed intake then leads to severe glycogen depletion, which is associated with a second mortality peak at 8 - 10 days (Phelps *et al.,* 1987a).

The importance of carbohydrate metabolism in day-old chicks has been examined through the administration of solutions of glucose or sucrose either orally or subcutaneously. Studies by Thaxton and Parkhurst (1976) and by Moran (1988) indicated an improvement in performance associated with administration of a water solution of glucose or sucrose to broiler chicks and poults. In subsequent studies, Moran (1989) and Pinchasov and Noy (1992) observed that the improvement in poult performance was maximized by the availability of other nutrients in addition to or immediately subsequent to glucose or sucrose administration. Thus, although the presence of residual yolk may be sufficient for good chick livability (Baranyiova, 1972a), early intake of carbohydrates is required for maturation of energy metabolism (Thaxton and Parkhurst, 1976; Moran, 1990) and a balance of amino acids and other nutrients is required to optimize subsequent performance (Moran, 1990; Pinchasov and Noy, 1992).

## Early nutrition and supply systems: gastrointestinal and cardiovascular function

Early nutrition and initiation of feeding seem to be essential for optimum performance. There are numerous reports in the literature that demonstrate the impact of delays in feeding on growth and livability (Fanguy *et al.,* 1980; Moran, 1990; Pinchasov and Noy, 1994). Delayed feeding has been shown to retard maturation of systems that begin developing in the chick only after ingestion of nutrients. This is particularly marked in the gastrointestinal system, including effects on liver and pancreas (Sell *et al.,* 1991). Gut development, not only villus growth but also enterocyte differentiation, depends in part on oral intake (Baranyiova, 1972b; Baranyiova and Holman, 1976). Intestinal motility, nutrient transport systems, pancreatic enzyme secretion and bile salt synthesis are all examples of systems that are partly developed at hatch, but whose development to adult levels requires oral intake (Nir *et al.*, 1988; Noy and Sklan, 1995; Palo *et al.*, 1995; Uni *et al.,* 1998).

Unless the gastrointestinal supply system can quickly mature and provide the necessary substrates, demanding organs, such as muscle, may never catch up. Studies of the benefits of early nutrition on the gastrointestinal system have shown that the absolute weight of the small intestine, pancreas and liver from fed birds remained significantly higher than those of birds fasted from days 0-4. Nutrients must be available quickly for optimal post-natal development of this supply system. Thus, early provision of nutrients affects not only immediate survival and disease resistance but also the ultimate attainment of genetic potential at organ, system and whole body levels.

Another supply system that must develop in order to achieve optimum animal growth is the cardio-pulmonary system. Rapidly growing poultry are susceptible to heart failure and ascites that originate as cardio-pulmonary insufficiency (Wideman *et al.*, 1996). Therefore, the development of the cardio-pulmonary system in the neonate needs to begin immediately after hatch and must be enough to support the other body systems.

Figure 7.1 shows the effect of early nutrition on gut weight and yolk sac weight over a four-day treatment period in turkey poults. These birds were fed a hydrated nutritional supplement (Oasis® chick supplement) formulated specifically for chick poultry or were fasted for the first four days of life. In terms of body weight, fasted poults lost 1.12 g and fed birds gained 1.0 g over the 4-day treatment period. Small intestine growth was significantly greater in the fed birds despite the presence of potential nutrients in the residual yolk of all birds (Figure 7.1). Interestingly, fasting did not change the rate of yolk utilization. Absolute yolk sac weights showed no accelerated use in fasted birds.

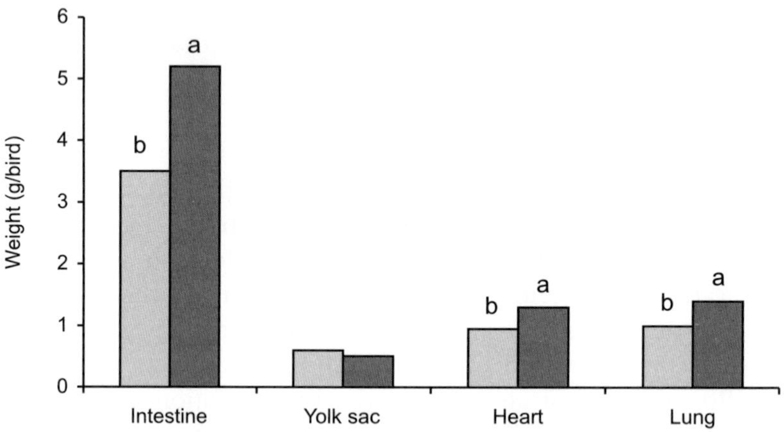


**Figure 7.1** Effect of early nutrition on the development of supply systems in the turkey poult. Birds were either fed or fasted from day of hatch to day 4 and then fed *ad libitum* a maize-soya starter diet. Organs were weighed on day 7. Significantly greater weights of intestine, heart and lung were observed in the fed birds (a,b P<.05). Residual yolk sac weights did not differ (▒ = fasted, ▓ = fed Oasis® chick supplement).

Figure 7.1 also shows the effect of early nutrition on heart and lung weights. Despite the fact that the fasted birds lost weight over the treatment period, relative heart and lung weights were higher in fed birds (data not shown). Figure 7.2 shows the relative heart weight as a function of time in birds that were fasted, fed Oasis® or fed a maize/soya bean meal starter diet. Relative heart weight in supplemented birds was fairly stable; while fasted birds showed a loss in relative heart weight during fasting followed by a tremendous compensatory growth upon feeding. The consequences of this burst of heart growth may well be negative, since early cardiac hypertrophy can be an indicator of the eventual development of cardiac insufficiency and ascites (Julian *et al.*, 1989; Wideman *et al.*, 1996) From these data it appears that the residual yolk is not able to provide enough substrate to achieve sustained cardio-pulmonary growth and that development of supply organs such as gut, heart and lungs is particularly responsive to early feeding.

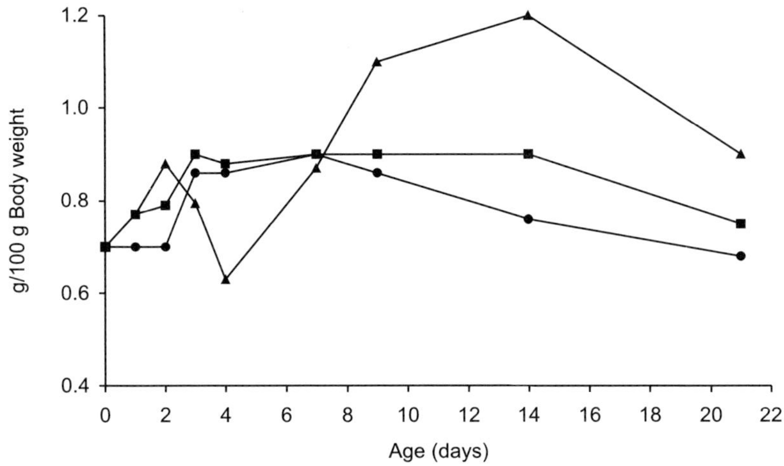


**Figure 7.2** Effect of early nutrition on the weight of the heart relative to body weight (g/100 g body weight). Relative heart weights of birds fasted (▲) or fed a corn soy diet (●) or Oasis® chick supplement (■) for days 0-4. Relative heart weight in the fed birds was very stable while fasted birds experienced wide fluctuations in heart weight with an initial loss in relative heart weight followed by compensatory over-growth upon feeding.

## Summary

In order to achieve their genetic potential for growth, chicks must undergo a shift in energy metabolism and nutrient supply dynamics immediately after emergence from the shell. The presence of residual yolk may be sufficient for survival, but not for optimum growth. Some of the residual yolk contents, such as maternal antibodies, cholesterol and polyunsaturated fatty acids have other functions than provision of nutrients to the chick. Prompt oral nutrition spares these compounds for passive immunity and cell membrane synthesis. Data indicate that a delay of even a day or two in the provision of food and water can result in substantial reductions in early growth of the gastrointestinal tract, liver and pancreas. Further studies of the role of various nutrients in the early nutrition of poults and broilers demonstrated that initiation of growth followed absorption of residual yolk but oral intake of carbohydrates was essential to the fulfillment of the growth potential of birds selected for rapid gain. Data suggest that the residual yolk may serve the critical functions of complementing nutrients ingested orally and facilitating efficient use of protein and energy during the first few days of life. A shift from blood-borne to oral nutrition, essential to provide substrates for the rapid growth of demanding organs, such as bone and skeletal muscle, requires rapid growth and maturation of the supply organs, including the gastrointestinal system. The cardio-vascular system must develop rapidly to meet the demands of rapid growth, as the final realization of genetic potential depends upon a prompt and steady supply of nutrients and oxygen above the levels required to maintain the bird.

## References

Akiba, Y. and Murakami, H. (1995) Partitioning of energy and protein during early growth of broiler chicks and contribution of vitteline residue. In *Proceedings of the 10th European Symposium on Poultry Nutrition*, pp 45-52. Antalya, Turkey.

Anderson, G. J., Connor, W. E. and Corliss, J. D. (1990) Docosahexanoic acid is the preferred dietary n-3 fatty acid for development of the brain and retina. *Pediatric Research*, **27**, 89-97.

Baranyiova, E. (1972a) Influence of deutectomy, food intake and fasting on liver glycogen content in chickens after hatching. *Acta Vet. Brno,* **41**, 149-159.

Baranyiova, E. (1972b) Influence of deutectomy, food intake and fasting on the digestive tract dimensions in chickens after hatching. *Acta Vet. Brno,* **41,** 373-384.

Baranyiova, E. and Holman, J. (1976) Morphological changes in the intestinal wall in fed and fasted chickens in the first week after hatching. *Acta Vet. Brno* **45**, 151-158.

Baranyiova, E. and Standara, S. (1980) Effect of deutectomy, fasting and environmental temperature on free fatty acid concentration in the blood plasma of chickens in the first week after hatching. *Acta Vet. Brno* **49**, 187-192.

Barbato, G. F., Siegel, P. B., Cherry, J. A. and Nir, I. (1984) Selection for body weight at eight weeks of age. 17. Overfeeding. *Poultry Science,* **63**, 11-18.

Best, E. E. (1966) The changes of some blood constituents during the initial post-hatching period in chickens. *British Poultry Science,* **7**, 23.

Blanch, A., Barroeta, A. C., Baucells, M. D. and Puchal, F. (1995) The nutritive value of dietary fats in relation to their chemical composition. Apparent fat availability and metabolizable energy in two-week-old chicks. *Poultry Science,* **74**, 1335-1340.

Buddington, R. K. and Diamond, J. M. (1989) Ontogenetic development of intestinal nutrient transporters. *Annual Review of Physiology,* **51**, 601-619.

Buddington, R. K. (1992) Intestinal nutrient transport during ontogeny of vertebrates. *American Journal of Physiology,* **32**, R503-509.

Casteel, E. T., Wilson, J. L., Buhr, R. J. and Sander, J. E. (1994) The influence of extended posthatch holding time and placement density on broiler performance. *Poultry Science,* **73**, 1679-1684.

Chamblee, T. N., Brake, J. D., Schultz, C. D. and Thaxton, J. P. (1992) Yolk sac absorption and initiation of growth in broilers. *Poultry Science,* **71**, 1811-1816.

Coates, M. E., Davies, M. K. and Kon, S. K. (1954) The effect of antibiotics on the intestine of the chick. *British Journal of Nutrition,* **9**, 110-119.

Croom, W. J., Brake, J., Coles, B. A., Havenstein, G. B., Christensen, V. L., McBride, B. W., Peebles, E. D. and Taylor, I. L. (1999) Is intestinal absorption capacity rate-limiting for performance in poultry? *Journal of Applied Poultry Research*, **8**, 242-252.

Ding, S. T. and Lilburn, M. S. (1996) Characterization of changes in yolk sac and liver lipids during embryonic and early posthatch development of turkey poults. *Poultry Science,* **75**, 478-483.

Dunnington, E. A. and Siegel, P. B. (1995) Enzyme activity and organ development in newly hatched chicks selected for high or low eight-week body weight. *Poultry Science,* **74**, 761-770.

Engku Azahan, E. A. and Forbes, J. M. (1989) Growth, food intake and energy balance of layer and broiler chickens offered glucose in the drinking water and the effect of dietary protein content. *British Poultry Science,* **30**, 907-917.

Entenman, C., Lorenz, F. W. and Chaikoff, I. L. (1940) The lipid content of blood, liver, and yolk sac of the newly hatched chick and the changes that occur in these tissues during the first month of life. *Journal of Biological Chemistry,* **133**, 231-241.

Escribano, F., Rahn, B. E. and Sell, J. L. (1988) Development of lipase activity in yolk membrane and pancreas of young turkeys. *Poultry Science,* **67**, 1089-1097.

Fan, Y. K. (1995) Effects of genetic selection on energetic efficiency of small intestinal glucose absorption. Ph. D. Dissertation, North Carolina State University.

Fan, Y. K., Croom, J., Christensen, V. L., Black, B. L., Bird, A. R., Daniel, L. R., McBride, B. W. and Eisen, E. J. (1997) Jejunal glucose uptake and oxygen consumption in turkey poults selected for rapid growth. *Poultry Science,* **76**, 1738-1745.

Fanguy, R. C., Misra, L. K., Vo, K. V., Blohowiak, C. C., and Krueger, W. F. (1980) Effect of delayed placement on mortality and growth performance of commercial broilers. *Poultry Science,* **59**, 1215-1220.

Fredde, M. R., Waible, P. E. and Burger, R. E. (1960) Factors affecting the absorbability of certain dietary fats in the chick. *Journal of Nutrition.* **70**, 447-452.

Freeman, B. M. (1965) The importance of glycogen at the termination of the embryonic existence of *Gallus domesticus. Comparative Biochemistry and Physiology,* **14**, 217-222.

Freeman, B. M. and Vince, R. L. (1974) *Development of the Avian Embryo*, London, Chapman and Hall.

Golian, A. and Polin, D. (1984) Passage rate of feed in very young chicks. *Poultry Science,* **63**, 1013-1019.

Gomez, M. X. and Polin, D. (1976) The use of bile salts to improve absorption of tallow in chicks, one to three weeks of age. *Poultry Science,* **55**, 2189-2195.

Hager, J. E., and Beane, W. L. (1983) Posthatch incubation time and early growth of broiler chickens. *Poultry Science,* **62**, 247-254.

Ikeno, T. and Ikeno, K. (1991) Amylase activity increases in the yolk of fertilized eggs during incubation in chickens. *Poultry Science,* **70**, 2176-2179.

Ikeno, T., Sakamoto, H., Ikeno, K. and Niwa, K. (1992) The embryo pancreas is a source of increased yolk amylase in the fertilized eggs of domestic fowls. *Experimental Animal,* **41**, 19-23.

Jukes, H. G., Hill, D. C. and Branion, H. D. (1956) Effect of feeding antibiotics on the intestinal tract of the chick. *Poultry Science*, **35**, 716-723.

Julian, R. J., Frazier, J. A. and Goryo, M. (1989) Right ventricular hypertrophy, right ventricular failure and ascites in broiler chickens caused by amiodarone-induced lung pathology. *Avian Pathology*, **18**, 161-174.

Kingston, D. J. (1979) Some hatchery factors involved in early chick mortality. *Australian Veterinary Journal* **55**, 418-421.

Knoblock, J. W. and Siegel, P. B. (1970) Ingestive behavior of day-old chicks. *Poultry Science,* **49**, 598-599.

Krogdahl, A. and Sell, J. L. (1989) Influence of age on lipase, amylase, and protease activities in pancreatic tissue and intestinal contents of young turkeys. *Poultry Science,* 68, 1561-1568.

Latour, M. A., Peebles, E. D., Boyle, C. R., Brake, J. D. and Kellogg, T. F. (1995) Changes in serum lipid, lipoprotein and corticosterone concentrations during neonatal chick development. *Biology of the Neonate* **67**, 381-386.

Lilja, C. (1983) A comparative study of postnatal growth and organ development in some species of birds. *Growth,* **47**, 317-339.

Mitchell, M. A. and Smith, M. W. (1991) The effects of genetic selection for increased growth rate on mucosal and muscle weights in the different regions of the small intestine of the domestic fowl (*Gallus domesticus*). *Poultry Science,* **99A**, 251-258.

Moran, Jr., E. T. (1985) Digestion and absorption of carbohydrates in fowl through perinatal development. *Journal of Nutrition,* **115**, 665-674.

Moran, Jr., E. T. (1988) Subcutaneous glucose is more advantageous in establishing the posthatch poult than oral administration. *Poultry Science,* **67**, 493-501.

Moran, Jr., E. T. (1989) Effects of posthatch glucose on poults fed and fasted during yolk sac depletion. *Poultry Science,* **68**, 1141-1147.

Moran, Jr., E. T. (1990) Effects of egg weight, glucose administration at hatch, and delayed access to feed and water on the poult at 2 weeks of age. *Poultry Science,* **69**, 1718-1723.

Moran, Jr., E. T. and Reinhart, L. (1981) Providing glucose to turkey hatching eggs via pressure differential antibiotic dipping: Effects on hatchability, poult quality and subsequent performance. *Poultry Science,* **60**, 1544-1548.

Moreto, M., Amat, C., Puchal, A., Buddington, R. K. and Planas, J. M. (1991) Transport of l-proline and a-methyl-d-glucoside by chicken proximal cecum during development. *American Journal of Physiology,* **260**, G457-G463.

Murakami, H., Akiba, Y. and Horiguchi, M. (1992) Growth and utilization of nutrients in newly-hatched chick with or without removal of residual yolk. *Growth, Development & Aging,* **56**, 75-84.

Nir, I., Nitsan, Z. and Ben-Avraham, G. (1988) Development of the intestine, digestive enzymes and internal organs of the newly hatched chick. Pp 861-864 In *Proceedings XVIII World's Poultry Congress*, Nagoya, Japan.

Nir, I., Nitsan, Z., Dror, Y. and Shapira, N. (1978) Influence of overfeeding on growth, obesity and intestinal tract in young chicks of light and heavy breeds. *British Journal of Nutrition,* **39**, 27-35.

Nitsan, Z. (1974) The effects of force-feeding on enzymes of the liver, kidney, pancreas and digestive tract of chicks. *British Journal of Nutrition,* **32**, 241-247.

Nitsan, Z., Ben-Avraham, G., Zoref, Z. and Nir, I. (1991a) Growth and development of the digestive organs and some enzymes in broiler chicks after hatching. *British Poultry Science,* **32**, 515-523.

Nitsan, Z., Dunnington, E. A. and Siegel, P. B. (1991b) Organ growth and digestive enzyme levels to fifteen days of age in lines of chickens differing in body weight. *Poultry Science,* **70**, 2040-2048.

Nitsan, Z., Turro-Vincent, I., Liu, G., Dunnington, E. A. and Siegel, P. B. (1995) Intubation of weight-selected chicks with soybean oil or residual yolk: effect on early growth and development. *Poultry Science,* **74**, 925-936.

Noble, R. C. and Ogunyemi, D. (1989) Lipid changes in the residual yolk and liver of the chick immediately after hatching. *Biology of the Neonate* **56**, 228-236.

Noy, Y. and Sklan, D. (1995) Digestion and absorption in the young chick. *Poultry Science,* **74**, 366-373.

Noy, Y., Uni, Z. and Sklan, D. (1996) Routes of yolk utilization in the newly hatched chick. *Poultry Science,* **75S**, 13. (Abstr.)

Obst, B. S. and Diamond, J. (1992) Ontogenesis of intestinal nutrient transport in domestic chickens (*Gallus gallus*) and its relation to growth. *The Auk,* **109**, 451-464.

Palo, P. E., Sell, J. L., Piquer, F. J., Vilaseca, L. and Soto-Salanova, M. F. (1995) Effect of early nutrient restriction on broiler chickens. 2. Performance and digestive enzyme activities. *Poultry Science,* **74**, 1470-1483.

Phelps, P. V, Edens, F. W. and Gildersleeve, R. P. (1987a) The posthatch physiology of the turkey poult - III. Yolk depletion and serum metabolites. *Comparative Biochemistry and Physiology,* **87A** 2, 409-415.

Phelps, P. V., Gildersleeve, R. P. and Edens, F. W. (1987b) Research Note: Effect of prefeeding on physiological parameters associated with turkey poult mortality. *Poultry Science,* **66**, 1882-1884.

Pinchasov, Y. (1991) Relationship between the weight of hatching eggs and subsequent early performance of broiler chicks. *Poultry Science,* **70**, 109-115.

Pinchasov, Y. and Noy, Y. (1992) A single post-hatch intubation of various nutrients improves subsequent early performance of young birds. *Proceeding 19th World Poultry Congress Amsterdam* **3**, 614-618.

Pinchasov, Y. and Noy, Y. (1993) Comparison of post-hatch holding time and subsequent early performance of broiler chicks and turkey poults. *British Poultry Science,* **34**, 111-120.

Pinchasov, Y. and Noy, Y. (1994) Early postnatal amylolysis in the gastrointestinal tract of turkey poults *Meleagris gallopavo. Comparative Biochemistry and Physiology,* **107A** 1, 221-226.

Polin, D. (1980) Increased absorption of tallow with lecithin. *Poultry Science,* **59**, 1652. (Abstr.)

Polin, D., Wing, T. L., Ki, P. and Pell, K. E. (1980) The effect of bile acids and lipase on absorption of tallow in young chicks. *Poultry Science,* **59**, 2738-2743.

Ritz, C. W., Hulet, R. M. Self, B. B. and Denbow, D. M. (1995) Growth and intestinal morphology of male turkeys as influenced by dietary supplementation of amylase and xylanase. *Poultry Science,* **74**, 1329-1334.

Romanoff, A. L. (1960) *The Avian Embryo, Structural and Functional Development.* The Macmillan Company, New York.

Rosebrough, R. W., Geis, E., Henderson, K. and Frobish, L. T. (1979) Control of glycogen metabolism in the developing turkey poult. *Growth,* **43**, 188-201.

Sell, J. L., Angel, C. R., Piquer, F. J., Mallarino, E.G. and Al-Batshan, H. A. (1991) Developmental patterns of selected characteristics of the gastrointestinal tract of young turkeys. *Poultry Science,* **70**, 1200-1205.

Sell, J. L., Kolodovsky, O. and Reid, B. L. (1989) Intestinal disaccharidases of young turkeys, temporal development and influence of diet composition. *Poultry Science,* **68**, 265-277.

Sell, J. L., Krogdahl, L. A. and Hanyu, N. (1986) Influence of age on utilization of supplemental fats by young turkeys. *Poultry Science,* **65**, 546-554.

Senkoylu, N. and Janssen, W. M. M. A. (1988) The influence of age, basic feed, fat type and inclusion levels upon apparent metabolizable energy values in chicken feeds. Pages 784-786 *in, Proceedings XVIII World's Poultry Congress*, Nagoya, Japan.

Shehata, A., Lerner, T. J. and Miller, D. S. (1981) Development of brush-border membrane hexose transport system in chick jejunum. *American Physiological Society,* **81**, G102-G108.

Sulaiman, A., Peebles, E. D., Pansky, T., Kellogg, T. F., Maslin, W. R. and Keirs, R. W. (1996) Histological evidence for a role of the yolk stalk in gut absorption of yolk in the post-hatch broiler chick. *Poultry Science,* **75S**, 48. (Abstr.)

Thaxton, J. P. and Parkhurst, C. R. (1976) Growth, efficiency, and livability of newly hatched broilers as influenced by hydration and intake of sucrose. *Poultry Science,* **55**, 2275-2279.

Twining Jr., P. V., Nicholson, J. L. and Thomas, O. P. (1978) Feed and water management of the broiler chick for the first 72 hours. *Poultry Science,* **57**, 1325-1328.

Uni, Z., Noy, Y. and Sklan, D. (1995a) Posthatch changes in morphology and function of the small intestines in heavy- and light-strain chicks. *Poultry Science,* **74**, 1622-1629.

Uni, Z., Noy, Y. and Sklan, D. (1995b) Development of the small intestine in heavy and light strain chicks before and after hatching. *British Poultry Science,* **36**, 63-71.

Uni, Z., Ganot, S. and Sklan, D. (1998) Posthatch development of mucosal function in the broiler small intestine. *Poultry Science* **77**, 75-82.

Vanheel, B., Vandeputte-Poma, J. and Desmeth, M. (1981) Resorption of yolk lipids by the pigeon embryo. *Comparative Biochemistry and Physiology,* **68A**, 641-646.

Vieira, S. L. and Moran, E. T., Jr. (1999) Effects of delayed placement and used litter on broiler yields. *Journal of Applied Poultry Research*, **8**, 75-81.

Waldroup, P. W., Hillard, C. M., Grigg, J. E. and Harris, Jr., C. J. (1974) The effectiveness of nutrient solutions given to young turkey poults in drinking water or by oral and parenteral dosage. *Poultry Science,* **53**, 1056-1060.

Warriss, P. D., Kestin, S.C. and Edwards, J. E. (1991) Responses of newly hatched chicks to inanition. *Veterinary Record,* **130**, 49-53.

Wideman, R. F., Jr., Kirby, Y. K., Tackett, C. D., Marson, N. E., McNew, R. W., (1996) Cardio-pulmonary function during acute unilateral occlusion of the pulmonary artery in broilers fed diets containing normal or high levels of

arginine-HCl. *Poultry Science,* **75(1)**, 1587-1602.
Wiseman, J. and Salvador, F. (1991) The influence of free fatty acid content and degree of saturation on the apparent metabolizable energy value of fats fed to broilers. *Poultry Science,* **70**, 573-582.

*This paper was first published in 2000*

8

# PHYTASE IN POULTRY NUTRITION

S.P. TOUCHBURN, S. SEBASTIAN and E.R. CHAVEZ
*Macdonald Campus of McGill University, Ste-Anne-de-Bellevue, Quebec, Canada H9X 3V9*

## Phosphorus

Phosphorus (P) is an important component in the animal body although it represents only 6 - 7.5 g/kg adult weight. 0.80 of body P is present in the skeletal structure. The remaining 0.20 is critical to homeostasis: in proteins such as enzymes, in lipids such as the phospholipids of membranes, in nucleic acids such as in DNA and adenosine triphosphate (ATP), the currency for energy exchange in the body. Because of its many interactions with calcium (Ca), the two elements are normally considered together. A dietary deficiency of P results in decreased growth and production or bone lesions. An early sign of deficiency is depressed appetite which, of course, leads to decreased growth but not necessarily lower efficiency of feed utilization. The digestibility of both Ca and P is depressed by an excess of either one but most commonly occurs because of an excess of Ca, the least expensive ingredient in feed.

## Sources of P

Sources of dietary P include the rock phosphates which are relatively unavailable to animals but the process of heating to eliminate fluorine alters their crystal structure and yields tricalcium-phosphate which is as digestible as animal product sources such as steamed bone meal (Scott, Nesheim and Young 1982). Along with the synthetic mono- and dicalcium phosphates, these products are generally considered to have an availability approaching 1.00. In contrast, plant sources of P are generally calculated to be only about 0.30 available to simple-stomached animals which normally consume mostly grains, oilseed meals and their by-products in which most of the P is in the form of phytic acid complexes.

Two recent developments have led to the expanding practice of adding phytase enzymes to the diets of pigs and poultry; first, the need to reduce P pollution of ground and surface waters from manure - a problem most critical in regions of high animal density and in some countries which are subject to strict regulation; second, the advent of genetically engineered micro-organisms capable of yielding acid phytase enzyme in sufficient concentration and at reasonable cost (Cantor, 1995). The high cost of P supplements of course, makes the use of these microbial phytase products even more attractive.

## Phytin

Phytin, phytic acid, phytate or myo-inositol hexaphosphate is the major storage form of phosphorus in plants, comprising 0.60 to 0.80 of the P in grains and their by-products (Ravindran *et al.*, 1995) and in oil seeds but only 0.15 to 0.30 in green plants (National Research Council, 1994). This storage form provides reactive anions capable of binding or chelating divalent or trivalent cations, forming insoluble salts. It also complexes with and binds proteins, rendering them resistant to proteolytic enzymes. It may also bind endogenous digestive enzymes, reducing their activity.

Phytate can be considered a unique compound since it bears six phosphate groups on one 6-carbon molecule of low molecular weight (Figure 8.1). At neutral pH, each of the phosphate groups has either one or two negatively charged oxygen atoms; hence various cations could strongly chelate between two phosphate groups or weakly with a single phosphate group (Figure 8.2). Thus phytate is considered a nutrient because it contains P but it can also be considered a toxin or anti-nutrient because it binds various essential mineral elements and reduces their availability for absorption from the diet (Reddy *et al.*, 1982). The concentration of phytate in feedstuffs depends on the part of the plant from which they are derived. Oilseed meals contain large amounts compared to cereal by-products and grain legumes (Ravindran *et al.*, 1995). Furthermore, the phytate is deposited in different parts of the seed as shown in Table 8.1 (Reddy *et al.*, 1982). In maize it is almost all in the germ; in wheat it is in the aleurone and the germ; in rice in the germ and the pericarp. In oilseeds the phytate is dispersed throughout the seed (Erdman, 1979).

## Phytase

### ENDOGENOUS PHYTASE IN POULTRY

Simple-stomached animals, like poultry and pigs, elaborate very little phytase, hence dietary phytates are largely undigested and end up in the manure.

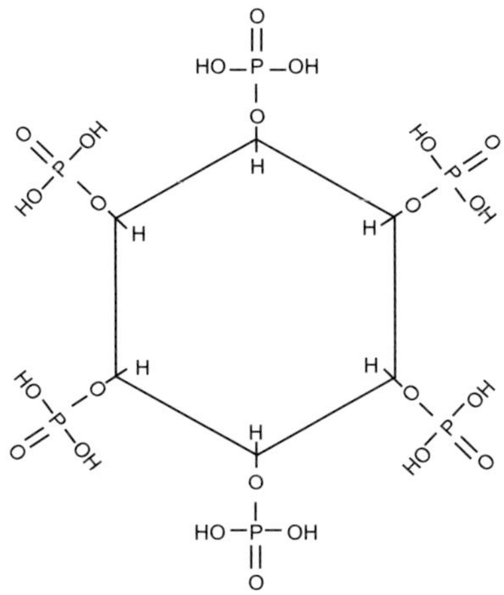


**Figure 8.1** Structure of phytic acid proposed by Anderson (1914). (After illustration by Reddy *et al.*, 1982).

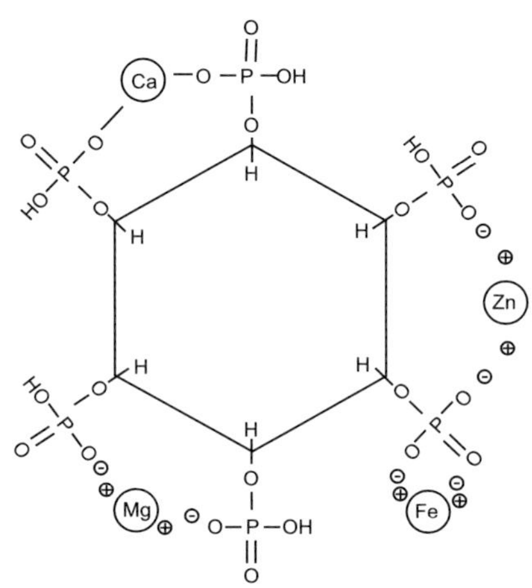


**Figure 8.2** Phytic acid chelate at neutral pH. (After Erdman, 1979)

However, on diets low in non-phytin P (nP), that is lacking in added mineral phosphates or animal products, chick intestinal phytase has been shown to increase more than three-fold over that in controls fed P-supplemented diets (Davies and Motzok 1972). Most recently, Maenz and Classen (1998) studied the kinetics of phytate hydrolysis by chicken small intestinal brush boarder membrane vesicles. Effective pH of the enzyme ranged from 5 to 6.5 with a maximum at 6, the pH of the intestinal unstirred water layer. Activity was highest in the duodenum and declined in the jejunum and still further in the ileum. Comparing 4-wk-old broilers and laying hens, they found the same specific activity in each category but the hens had 35% higher total activity.

**Table 8.1** PHYTIC ACID AND PHYTIC ACID P CONCENTRATION IN MORPHOLOGICAL COMPONENTS OF CEREALS

| *Cereal* | *Sample* | *Phytic acid (g/kg)* | *Phytic acid P (g/kg)* |
|---|---|---|---|
| Maize | Commercial hybrid | 8.9 | 2.5 |
| | Endosperm | 0.4 | 0.1 |
| | Germ | 63.9 | 18.0 |
| | Hull | 0.7 | 0.2 |
| Maize | High lysine | 9.6 | 2.7 |
| | Endosperm | 0.4 | 0.1 |
| | Germ | 57.2 | 16.1 |
| | Hull | 2.5 | 0.7 |
| Wheat | Soft | 11.4 | 3.2 |
| | Endosperm | 0.04 | 0.01 |
| | Germ | 39.1 | 11.0 |
| | Hull | 0.0 | 0.0 |
| | Aleurone | 41.2 | 11.6 |
| Rice | Brown | 8.9 | 2.5 |
| | Endosperm | 0.1 | 0.04 |
| | Germ | 34.8 | 9.8 |
| | Pericarp | 33.7 | 9.5 |

(After Reddy *et al.*, 1982)

They suggested that the expression of intestinal phytase activity is subject to regulatory mechanisms and is important in maintaining P status. This raises the possibility of selecting birds genetically for increased ability to secrete phytase or employing bioengineering successfully in introducing the phytase gene in poultry.

### *Genetic differences in poultry*

In early studies, Edwards (1983) reported that White Leghorn cockerels were able to utilise sub-optimal levels of P in a diet more efficiently than did commercial broilers as measured by growth, liveability and bone calcification. Differences were exaggerated by higher levels of Ca in the diet. The Athens-Canadian Randombred Control broiler population were intermediate in their response. Carlos and Edwards (1997) compared strains and crosses of young broiler chicks and found large individual differences in their ability to utilise phytate-P. Body weight, bone ash, toe ash, and plasma minerals were measured and it was concluded that, on a P-deficient diet, 21-day body weight might be a satisfactory criterion for selection studies. Zhang *et al.* (1998) compared broiler lines for their ability to utilise phytate-P. An unselected control line was compared with lines selected over eleven generations for a high- or low incidence of tibial dyschondroplasia and it was found the controls were superior in liveability, mortality and growth performance. However, variability was greater in the selected lines, which led to the conclusion that selection could be effective for improved utilization of phytate-P.

## ENDOGENOUS PHYTASE IN FEEDSTUFFS

Endogenous plant phytases may contribute to phytate hydrolysis. They are present in considerable amounts in the cereals, rye and wheat but their activity is highly variable. Maize, Sorghum and the oilseed meals are very low in phytase content (Eeckhout and de Paepe 1994). It is relevant to note that the optimum pH for plant phytase activity is in the range of 4.0-6.0 (Table 8.2) though some activity may be retained at pH 3.0. The activity will vary depending on cultivar, climate and handling conditions. Optimum temperatures range mostly from 40 to 55°C and activity of the phytase will be reduced if the diet or ingredients containing the enzyme are subjected to temperatures much above 60 to 65°C during processing.

**Table 8.2** OPTIMUM PH AND TEMPERATURE OF PHYTASE FROM CEREALS AND LEGUMES

| *Phytase source* | *Optimum pH* | *Temperature (°C)* | *Reference* |
|---|---|---|---|
| Triticale | 5.4 | 45 | Singh and Sedeh (19790 |
| Maize | 5.6 | 50 | Chang (1967) |
| Wheat flour | 5.15 | 55 | Peers (1953) |
| Wheat bran | 5.0 | - | Nagai and Funahashi (1962) |
| Rice aleurone particles | 4.0-5.0 | 45 | Yoshida *et al.* (1975) |
| Navy bean | 5.3 | 50 | Lolas and Markakis (1977) |
| Dwarf french bean | 5.2 | 40 | Gibbins and Norris (1963) |
| California small white bean | 5.2 | 60 | Chang (1975) |
| Mung bean (germinating) | 7.5 | 57 | Mandal and Biswas (1970) |

## Microbial phytase as poultry feed supplement

Rojas and Scott (1969) reported that phytase from the mould, *Aspergillus ficuum* improved the metabolizable energy value of cottonseed meal. It effectively rendered the P from phytate available to the birds and also freed some protein from the phytate complex. Nelson *et al.* (1971) also observed the improvement in phytin-P utilization from supplementation of the diet with this mould phytase. Subsequently, Simons *et al.* (1990) carefully prepared a batch of a crude phytase dry powder from *Aspergillus ficuum*. *In-vitro* studies showed the phytase to be active over a wide range in pH from 2.5 to 5.5. The microbial phytase supplement in the diets of broilers to 24 and 28 d of age overcame the poor growth performance of the birds fed the low-P basal diet. At a phytase dose level of 800 U/kg of diet, maximum apparent availability of P was obtained. The availability of the P rose to over 0.60 and the amount in the faeces decreased by 50%. It was also shown that the enzyme preparation had good stability at pelleting temperatures of 80°C with 0.46 activity remaining after pellet temperatures had reached 87°C (Table 8.3). Since that time, many studies have demonstrated the value of microbial phytase in broiler diets during the first 3 to 4 wk of life. More details are contained in the comprehensive review by Ravindran *et al.* (1995).

**Table 8.3** INFLUENCE OF MICROBIAL PHYTASE ON GROWTH PERFORMANCE AND RETENTION OF P IN BROILER CHICKENS FED MAIZE-SOYA BEAN MEAL DIETS

| *Source* | *Age (d)* | *Phytase units/kg* | *Non phytate-P in diet* | *% improvement* | | |
|---|---|---|---|---|---|---|
| | | | | *BW gain* | *FCR* | *P retention* |
| Simons *et al.* (1990) | 28 | 750 | 1.6 | 38 | 0.63 | 20 |
| Brox *et al.* (1994) | 22 | 500 | - | 13 | 3.4 | 15 |
| Aoyagi and Baker (1995) | 20 | 600 | - | 77 | 3.7 | - |
| Sebastian *et al.* (1996a) | 21 | 600 | 3 | 13.2 | 0.67 | 24 |
| Kornegay *et al.* (1996) | 21 | 600 | 2 | 36 | 2.6 | 5.3 |
| Yi *et al* (1996) | 20 | 600 | 4.5 | 11 | 3.53 | - |

With the advent of genetically engineered microorganisms capable of producing large amounts of phytase at much more reasonable cost, there has been a flurry of research in this area. Campbell and Bedford (1992), reviewing research on enzyme applications for non-ruminant feeds, commented that the renewed interest in dietary phytase comes with the realisation that phytase provides a cost-effective alternative to inorganic P supplementation and that it becomes of even greater importance where excessive P in animal waste is a national concern.

Table 8.3 lists a few of the many papers indicating that microbial phytase supplementation increases the availability of phytate P in young broiler chickens (Simons *et al.*, 1990; Mohammed *et al.* 1991; Broz *et al.*, 1994; Denbow *et al.*, 1995; Yi *et al.*, 1996; Kornegay *et al.*, 1996; Sebastian *et al.*, 1996a,b) and in young turkeys (Yi *et al.,* 1996a, Ravindran *et al.*, 1995; Qian *et al.,* 1996). The improvements in P retention by phytase supplementation ranged from 5.3% to 24% . Almost all of the trials involved chicks and turkey poults to 3- and some to 4-wk of age. Kornegay *et al.* (1997) concentrated on broilers in the 3- to 7-wk age period, supplementing a low-P maize-soyabean meal diet with 0, 200 or 400 U of phytase/kg of diet. It was observed that ileal digestibility and total retention of P (as a proportion of P intake) increased linearly with increasing phytase level. P excretion was reduced 35.4% by 200 U of phytase and 37.7% by 400 U of phytase per kg of diet. Calculated equivalency values averaged 290 U of phytase for 1 g of P based on improvements in toe- and tibia ash, and 231 U of phytase based on averages of body weight and gain. Thus, supplemental phytase proved to be very effective in broiler finisher diets.

The researchers at Virginia Polytechnic Institute and State University have also applied these equivalency calculations to young broilers and young turkeys. Yi *et al.* (1996) calculated an equivalency of 785 U of phytase for 1 g of P in young broilers fed a corn-soybean meal diet. Qian *et al.* (1996) determined these values for young male turkeys fed a maize-soyabean meal diet and found 963 U of phytase equivalency for 1 g of P when the nP level of the diet was 3.6 g/kg and 652 U of phytase with a dietary content of 2.7 g of nP/kg. In this trial it was observed that supplemental phytase yielded linear improvements in body weight gain, feed intake, feed-to-gain ratio, toe ash and apparent retention of Ca and P at each Ca:tP ratio and nP level. Widening the Ca:tP ratio had a detrimental effect at each phytase- and P level and was greatest at the lower levels of phytase and P. Many of these observations are in agreement with work in our laboratory with maize-soyabean meal broiler diets containing 3.5 g nP/kg (Sebastian 1996 a,b, Sebastian *et al.*, 1997). Supplemental microbial phytase yielded increases in feed intake, growth, bone mineralization and retention of P, Ca, Cu, Zn and N. In the first trial (Sebastian *et al.*, 1996a) the best results occurred with dietary Ca at 6.0 or 10 g/kg of diet versus 12.5 g/kg. In a subsequent similar trial (Sebastian *et al.*, 1996b), feed intake and gain were depressed when the diet contained 3.5 g nP and 10 g Ca/kg but performance was restored to normal when the Ca level was reduced to 6 g/kg, i.e., a lower nP:Ca ratio. This negative response to a widened nP:Ca ratio has been apparent in other studies (Qian *et al.*, 1996). Since microbial phytase is active over a wide range of pH, the optimum range being 2.5 to 5.5 (Simons *et al.*, 1990), it can be active in the crop (pH 5-6) and in the proventriculus and gizzard (pH 2-4). Excess Ca may raise the pH to the point of affecting phytase function. The low solubility of phytate chelates and complexes formed would then further inhibit absorption of Ca, P and other nutrients such as mineral cations and protein.

## Effect of microbial phytase on availability of cations

Theoretically, when phytic acid is hydrolysed by microbial phytase, all minerals bound to it will be released. There is ample evidence to indicate that microbial phytase supplementation improves the availability of Ca (Table 8.4) in broiler chickens (Schoner *et al.*, 1991; Broz *et al.*, 1994; Kornegay *et al.*, 1996; Sebastian *et al.*, 1996a) and turkeys (Qian *et al.*, 1996). In a broiler study designed to measure the effect of phytase on Ca availability, Schoner *et al.* (1994) reported that 500 U of microbial phytase were equivalent to 0.35 g Ca, as measured by body weight gain and 0.56 g Ca as measured by phalanx ash. Qian *et al.* (1996) reported that both P and Ca retention were sensitive to the addition of phytase at varying nP levels and Ca:total P ratios in turkeys. Calcium retention increased linearly as the amount of supplemented phytase increased, and decreased as the Ca:total P ratio became wider and as the level of nonphytate P increased (Qian *et al.*, 1996). In a study with turkeys, Kornegay *et al.* (1996) estimated the value of phytase based on body weight gain, gain:feed and digested Ca within a Ca range of 5.3 to 7.4 g/kg of diet and a phytase level up to 500 U /kg of diet. On this basis they suggested that 500 U of phytase are equivalent to approximately 0.87 g of Ca.

**Table 8.4** THE EFFECT OF SUPPLEMENTAL MICROBIAL PHYTASE ON AVAILABILITY OF MINERALS IN BROILER CHICKENS

| *Source* | *Age (d)* | *Phytase units/kg* | *Mineral* | *Improvement (% units)* |
|---|---|---|---|---|
| Yi *et al.* (1996) | 20 | 600 | ZN | 6.9 |
| Sebastion *et al.* (1996a) | 21 | 600 | Zn | 62.3 |
| Aoyagi and Baker (1995) | 20 | 600 | Cu | -21 |
| Sebastion *et al.* (1996a) | 21 | 600 | Cu | 19.2 |
| Simons *et al.* (1990) | 28 | 750 | Ca | 13.1 |
| Sebastian *et al.* (1996a) | 21 | 600 | Ca | 12.2 |

Zinc availability has been shown to be affected by phytate in chicks, pigs, rats and other species (Prasad, 1966). Zinc is the most vulnerable to phytate complexation based on *in vitro* studies. Thus, zinc deficiency is the most likely result from the feeding of a diet with phytate-containing plant seed protein. Oberleas and Harland (1996) reported that results clearly showed phytate was a significant factor in the genesis of zinc deficiency. Studies on the influence of phytase on other phytate-bound minerals are limited. Pallauf *et al.* (1992) found that phytase addition increased the apparent absorption of Mg, Zn, Cu and Fe by up to 13, 13, 7, and 9%, respectively, in pigs. The addition of 800 U of phytase /kg to a diet containing 27 mg of Zn/ kg increased the retention of Zn and decreased Zn excretion of chicks (Thiel and Weigand, 1992). Thiel *et al.* (1993) reported that the femoral Zn content of chicks fed a diet containing 30 mg Zn /kg plus 700 U of phytase /kg diet was equal to that of chicks fed a diet containing 39 mg of Zn/ kg of diet without phytase. Roberson and Edwards (1994) reported that phytase supplementation had no effect on Zn retention in broiler chicks, but improved its retention when given along with vitamin $D_3$. In a study conducted in our laboratory (Sebastian *et al.*, 1996a), it has been shown that microbial phytase supplementation increased the relative retention of Zn by 62.3% compared with control in broiler chickens fed a low P maize-soyabean meal diet (Table 8.4). Yi *et al.* (1996a) reported that Zn retention in broiler chickens was linearly increased by adding microbial phytase to a low-Zn basal diet. It was further indicated that 0.9 mg of Zn was released per 100 U of phytase over a range of 150 to 600 U of phytase. Based on Biehl *et al.*, (1995) estimates using tibia Zn, the Zn equivalency would be 0.63 mg Zn per 100 U of phytase when 600 U of phytase were added, but 0.46 mg Zn per 100 U of phytase when 1200 U of phytase were added.

Aoyagi and Baker (1995) studied the effect of microbial phytase supplementation on dietary Cu utilization in chickens; it was found that phytase supplementation to soyabean meal had no effect on Cu availability and in fact it reduced the Cu bioavailability by 21 % (Table 8.4). Sebastian *et al.* (1996a) showed that microbial phytase supplementation increased the relative retention of Cu by 19.3% in broiler chickens fed a low P maize-soyabean meal diet (Table 8.4). Studies on the influence of microbial phytase on other minerals are very limited.

## Effects of microbial phytase on availability of protein and amino acids

Theoretically, phytase supplementation must also be able to release the phytate-bound protein for utilization, but published data on this aspect are scanty. Officer and Batterham (1992) observed improvements of 7-12 % in the ileal digestibility of protein and essential amino acids in pigs fed a diet with a supplemental microbial phytase. Several studies have reported that phytase supplementation improved nitrogen digestibility in pigs (Mroz *et al.*, 1994; Yi *et al.*, 1994a) and nitrogen retention in broiler chickens (Farrell *et al.*, 1993) and in laying hens (Van der Klis *et al.*, 1997). Yi *et al.* (1996b) determined the effect of phytase on N and amino acid digestibility in female turkey poults; they found that, with a dietary level of 4.5 g of nonphytate P/kg, adding phytase to diets containing 225g crude protein (CP)/kg tended to improve the apparent and true ileal digestibility of N and amino acids with the exception of cystine and methionine (Table 8.5). In a recent study with male and female broiler chickens fed a maize-soyabean meal diet to 28-d, Sebastian *et al.* (1996b) showed that, in the males, phytase supplementation increased the apparent ileal digestibility (AID) of CP but had no influence on AID of any amino acid except methionine and phenylalanine. In contrast, in the females, adding phytase increased the AID of all amino acids except lysine, methionine, phenylalanine and proline (Table 8.5). The possible effect of phytase on protein and amino acid utilization is of immense practical interest and needs to be confirmed. The factors contributing to the variability of the response must also be identified.

## Supplemental phytase in diets for laying hens

Until recently, there has been very little interest in the effect of phytase in diets for laying hens. The reasons are obvious: first is the knowledge that young birds produce very low levels of the enzyme and have hence been shown to respond favourably to dietary supplementation. Secondly, the literature clearly documents the depressed response to supplemental phytase caused by elevated Ca levels in young broiler and turkey diets and it is known that higher Ca levels are usual for laying hen diets. Summers (1995) fed laying hens a diet in which the nP level was reduced from 4 to 3 g/kg and found no depression of egg production but a 20% reduction of the P content of the excreta. The 20% lower dietary P was achieved simply by reducing the amount of supplemental P from calcium phosphate and represented a considerable saving in feed cost. Van der Klis *et al. (*1997) fed White Leghorn hens practical diets providing Ca at 30 g/kg and nP at 2.7 g/kg with 250 or 500 U of phytase/kg of diet. Ileal absorption of Ca and P measured at 24 wk of age appeared to be near maximum with 250 U of phytase/kg and were not further improved by 500 U of phytase/kg of diet. Feeding a similar diet with 40 g Ca/kg of diet resulted in a drop of 12% in absorption of P. The 250 U of phytase/kg in the diet containing only 30 g Ca/kg released phytate-P equivalent to 1.3 g P from monocalcium phosphate (MCP). A second trial at 36 wk of age showed ileal hydrolysis of phytate-P such that 250 U released the equivalent of 0.89 g of P from MCP. This drop was attributed to the increased age of the latter hens (36 vs. 24 wk). In a long-term trial (18 to 68 wk age) a control diet providing 28 g of Ca- and 2.6 g of nP/kg of diet proved inadequate to support normal levels of egg production and egg weight. It also resulted in decreased tibia weight and bone ash content. Supplementation of the diet with either 100 U of phytase- or 0.33 g of MCP-P/kg was sufficient to maintain normal performance. Thus,

**Table 8.5** THE EFFECT OF MICROBIAL PHYTASE ON IMPROVING AVAILABILITY OF N AND AMINO ACIDS IN POULTRY[1]

| *Species* | *CP (g/kg)* | *Phytase (units/kg)* | *Improvement in the availability of N and amino acids (percentage units of control)* | | | | | | | | | | | *Source* |
|---|---|---|---|---|---|---|---|---|---|---|---|---|---|---|
| | | | *N* | *Essential amino acids* | | | | | | | | | | |
| | | | | *Met* | *Cys* | *Lys* | *Thr* | *Arg* | *His* | *Ile* | *Leu* | *Phe* | *Val* | |
| Turkey | 225 | 750 | 1.0 | 0.6 | 2.1 | 0.7 | 1.0 | 0.6 | 0.8 | 0.7 | 0.9 | 0.8 | 0.8 | Yi *et al.* (1996b) |
| | 280 | 750 | 1.5 | 0.5 | 3.1 | 1.3 | 1.2 | 1.1 | 1.3 | 1.9 | 1.5 | 1.6 | 1.8 | Yi *et al.* (1996b) |
| Broiler | 220 | 600 | 1.3 | 0.3 | - | 0.6 | 4.3 | 1.8 | 0.3 | 3.1 | 1.9 | 1.1 | 2.5 | Sebastian *et al* (1996b) |
| | | | | | *Non-essential amina acids* | | | | | | | | | |
| | | | | | *Pro* | *Asp* | *Ser* | *Glu* | *Gly* | *Ala* | *Try* | | | |
| Turkey | 225 | 750 | | | 0.8 | 0.9 | 1.2 | 0.8 | 1.1 | 0.8 | 1.3 | | | Yi *et al.* (1996b) |
| | 280 | 750 | | | 2.4 | 1.7 | 0.7 | 1.3 | 1.6 | 1.3 | 1.2 | | | Yi *et al.* (1996b) |
| Broiler | 220 | 600 | | | 0.2 | 3.7 | 4.1 | 2.1 | 0.8 | 1.9 | 2.8 | | | Sebastian *et al* (1996b) |

[1] Female

2.9 g of nP/kg proved adequate in a diet containing 28 g of Ca/kg. Similarly, Gordon and Roland (1997) fed laying hens a diet containing 40 g of Ca/kg with an nP level of 1 g/kg and found it to reduce the rate of egg production. Addition of 300 U of phytase/kg of diet restored the egg production to normal levels. In a subsequent study (Gordon and Roland, 1998), the same low level of nP, 1 g/kg of diet, was fed in a diet containing only 25 g of Ca/kg of diet. This low nP- low Ca diet resulted in poor performance (egg production, shell quality, feed consumption) all of which were normal in birds fed the same diet supplemented with 300 U of phytase/kg of diet. Nakashon *et al.* (1994) also observed inferior production performance and poor retention in a diet providing 2.5 g nP/kg and a Ca level of 35 g/kg of diet. Normal performance was recorded in birds fed this diet supplemented with a product of condensed cane molasses plus a lactobacillus fermentation probiotic. The lactobacillus product supplied active phytase but it also lowered the pH of the crop and gastro-intestinal tract which, the authors suggested, could increase the solubility of various chelates and thus explain the observed enhanced absorption of P and some cations.

In a trial with growing pullets to 18 weeks of age, Punna and Roland (1997) observed a depression in feed intake, body weight and bone quality on a diet containing only 1.3 g P/kg and Ca at 8.6 g/kg. Supplementation of this diet with 300 U of phytase/kg restored these values to levels matching those on diets containing P at 2.3, 3.3 and 4.3 g P/kg. These latter treatments showed no significant differences from each other.

## Supplemental phytase and 1,25-dihydroxycholecalciferol

Interests have recently converged concerning the relationships of supplemental phytase and vitamin $D_3$ in their effects on utilization of dietary Ca and P. Mitchell and Edwards (1996a,b) added microbial phytase, 600 U/kg of diet, or 1,25-dihydroxycholecalciferol (5 μg/kg of diet), or a combination of the two to a basal maize-soyabean meal diet already adequate in its content of vitamin $D_3$. Based on improvements in body weight, bone ash weight and phytate-P retention, it was calculated that either supplement alone could replace up to 1 g of inorganic P/kg of diet whereas the combination could replace up to 2 g of inorganic P/kg of diet. The authors stated that the interaction observed between these supplements suggests that they are involved in different mechanisms of action. Qian *et al.* (1997) fed young broiler chicks diets supplemented with phytase levels of 0, 300, 600 or 900 U/kg and 1,25-dihydroxycholecalciferol at 66 and 660 μg/kg alone or in combination. They observed linear improvements in weight gain, feed intake, toe ash and in P and Ca retention with increments of either supplement alone and a synergism of combined action. All of these parameters were positive at Ca:total P ratios of 1.1 to 1.4:1 but declined at the higher ratios of 1.7 and 2.0:1. Total P retention ranged from 0.509 to 0.680, which was similar to that reported by Simons et al. (1990). Baker *et al.* (1998) fed young broilers supplemental 1,25-dihychoxycholecalciferol levels from 0 to 37.5 µg/kg in a basal diet low in available P (1.0 g/kg) and Ca (6.3 g/kg). A linear, positive response to the added vitamin in weight gain and tibia ash content was observed. A supplemental level of 1,25-dihydroxy $D_3$ of 1250 µg/kg of diet yielded a further increase in bone ash without any apparent negative effects on performance. Carlos and Edwards (1998) explored the effect of supplementing the diets of laying hens during a 9-week trial period with either 5 µg of 1,25-dihydroxy $D_3$/kg or 600 U of microbial phytase /kg or a combination of the two. In young hens, either supplement alone increased the body weight, plasma dialyzable P and tibia ash. It also improved the P retention from the basal level of 0.43 to levels of 0.63 to 0.77. The effect was slightly greater in older hens. This level of improvement was similar to that reported by Van der Klis *et al.* (1997) in response to 250 and 500 U of phytase/kg of diet; the authors suggested that, based on bone ash values, the hens receiving the P-deficient diet would likely have developed P-deficiency cage layer fatigue whereas the others would probably not have.

Biehl *et al.* (1998) evaluated the efficacy of two new vitamin $D_3$ analogues in increasing the bioavailability of phytate-bound P from maize-soybean meal diets that were more than adequate in $D_3$ for young chicks. The analogues, one dihydroxy compound (20-epi-19-nor-1", 25-dihydroxycholecalciferol) and one monohydroxy compound (20-epi-19-nor-1" hydroxycholecalciferol) were compared to 1" hydroxycholecalciferol which at levels of 10 to 15 µg/kg of diet had been shown to optimise phytate-P utilization. The results showed the dihydroxy test compound to be equivalent to the 1"-hydroxy $D_3$ standard supplement whereas the monohydroxy test compound had only 0.45 as much phytate-P-releasing activity; it was suggested that conversion of these compounds to the fully active 1,25-dihydroxycholecalciferol occurs in the liver and that a portion is returned to the gut by biliary flow where it enhances the action of intestinal or microbial phytase.

## Recombinant phytase

The phytase supplement used until now has been predominantly from the mould *Aspergillus ficuum* var. niger, now called *A. niger*. Recent developments indicate an improvement to the potency and perhaps the convenience of using the phytase enzyme preparation. Sun *et al.* (1997) reported application of molecular biology to effect the transfer of the gene for the phytase, myo-inositol hexakisphosphate phosphohydrolase, EC 3.1.3.8, from *A. niger* to the yeast, *Saccharomyces cerevisiae*. By measuring the amount of inorganic P released from sodium phytate *in vitro* a 4-to-11-fold increase in the activity of the transformed yeast over that of the control yeast was estimated; it was suggested that about 20 g/kg of the recombinant yeast (dry matter basis) will be required to provide phytase supplementation in pig and poultry feeds.

Another transformed product was evaluated by Denbow *et al.* (1998), who tested a new product of raw, transformed soyabeans expressing recombinant phytase derived from *A. niger*, comparing it to Natuphos[1] phytase at levels of 0, 400, 800 or 1200 U/kg in diets fed to broiler chicks from 7 to 21d of age. The positive linear effect on body weight, feed efficiency, feed intake, toe ash and tibia sheer force of both phytase supplements paralleled those from incremental additions of nP with the exception that the phytase treatments reduced rather than increased P excretion.

## Conclusions

Phosphorus (P) is an important component of the animal body, both structurally and metabolically. In P deficiency the earliest sign is diminished appetite, which will be manifested in reduced growth rate, and later, reduced bone mineralization. Phosphorus is normally considered in conjunction with calcium (Ca) because these two elements are collectively involved in so many functions. The inorganic phosphates and animal products represent feed ingredients in which P availability approaches 1.00. In plant materials, particularly the grains, oilseeds and their by-products which represent the major portion of the diets of poultry and pigs, the P availability is only about 0.30. The plant storage form of P is phytic acid, myo-inositol hexaphosphate, a powerful chelating agent that binds di- and trivalent cations and protein, rendering the complex resistant to the digestive enzymes. It may even bind and inactivate these enzymes under certain circumstances.

Several phytases capable of hydrolysing phytates release the phosphates and the bound components making them available for absorption. Poultry intestinal mucosa secrete a phytase which is active at low concentrations of inorganic P. Its optimum pH of 2-5.5 is similar to that of microbial phytase. Genetic differences among breeds or strains of poultry suggest that the ability to elaborate this enzyme could be enhanced through selection but it is not, currently, a major factor affecting P availability.

Another phytase enzyme is present in some feedstuffs such as rye and wheat but the activity is extremely variable. Maize, sorghum and oilseeds have very little endogenous phytase. The optimum pH is considerably higher, pH 5-6, so its effectiveness for poultry would probably have to occur prior to consumption or primarily in the crop. Microbial phytases mainly from fungi and predominantly from *A. niger* were observed to exert an important benefit upon addition to poultry diets. They operate over a pH range of 2.5 to 5.5 and are considered to be active in the crop, proventriculus and gizzard. Furthermore, they resist feed processing temperatures up to 80°C.

Many studies with broiler chicks and some with turkey poults, mostly to 3 wk of age, have shown the increasing benefits of supplemental microbial phytase from 100 to over 1000 units of activity. Feed intake, growth rate, bone mineralization, increased absorption of P, Ca, Cu, Zn, protein and amino acids have been observed. In laying hens supplemental phytase has additionally enhanced egg production, egg size and egg shell quality. These responses have been enhanced by supplements of 1,25-dihydroxycholecalciferol, well above the established requirement level, with the action being apparently synergistic with that of phytase.

All of these responses are susceptible to the levels of Ca and nP or total P in the diet, being most effective at low levels and declining at higher levels. Reducing the dietary levels of Ca and P to match more closely the actual needs of the bird enhances the activity of the supplemental phytase and reduces the output of Ca and P in the faeces. The ultimate result is reduced cost and a more environmentally friendly operation. Finally, recombinant phytases in which the gene has been transferred to yeast or to soyabean will increase the enzyme potency and facilitate feed supplementation.

## References


Anderson, R.J. (1914) A contribution to the chemistry of phytin. *Journal of Biological Chemistry*, **17:** 171-190.

Aoyagi, S. and Baker, D.H.(1995) Effect of microbial phytase and 1,25-dihydroxycholecalciferol on dietary copper utilization in chicks. *Poultry Science*, **74**, 121-126.

Baker, D.H., Biehl, R.R. and Emmert, T.L. (1998) Vitamin $D_3$ requirements of young chicks receiving diets varying in calcium and available phosphorus. *British Poultry Science*, **39**, 413-417.

Biehl, R.R., Baker, D.H. and De Luca, H.F. (1995) Hydroxylated cholecalciferol compounds act additively with microbial phytase to improve phosphorus, zinc and manganese in chicks fed soy-based diets. *Journal of Nutrition*, **125**, 2407-2416.

Biehl, R.R., Baker, D.H. and De Luca, H.F. (1998) Activity of various hydroxylated vitamin $D_3$ analogues for improving phosphorus utilization in chicks receiving diets adequate in vitamin $D_3$. *British Poultry Science*, **39**, 408-412.

Broz, J., Oldale, P., Perrin-Voltz, A.H., Rychen, G., Schulze, J. and Simoes Nunes, C. (1994) Effects of supplemental phytase on performance and phosphorus utilization in broiler chickens fed a low phosphorus diet without addition of inorganic phosphates. *British Poultry Science*, **35**, 273-280.

Campbell, G.L. and Bedford, M.R. (1992) Enzyme applications for monogastric feeds: A review. *Canadian Journal of Animal Science*, **72**, 449-466.

Cantor, A.H. (1995) Using enzymes to increase phosphorus availability in poultry diets. Proceedings of Alltech's Eleventh Annual Symposium, Biotechnology in the Feed Industry. 349-353.

Carlos, A.B. and Edwards, H.M., Jr. (1997) Influence of genetics on the utilization of phytate phosphorus by broilers. *Poultry Science*, **76**, Supplement 1, 142 (S158).

Carlos, A.B. and Edwards, H.M., Jr. (1998) The effects of 1,25-dihydroxycholecalciferol and phytase on the natural phytate phosphorus utilization by laying hens. *Poultry Science*, **77**, 850-858.

Davies, M.I., and Motzok, I. (1972) Properties of chick intestinal phytase. *Poultry Science*, **51**, 494-501.

Denbow, D.M., Grabau, E.A., Lacy, G.H., Kornegay, E.T., Russell, D.R. and Umbeck, P.F. (1998) Soybeans transformed with a fungal phytase gene improve phosphorus availability for broilers. *Poultry Science*, **77**, 878-881.

Denbow, D.M., Ravindran, V., Kornegay, E.T., Yi, Z., and Hulet, R.M. (1995) Improving phosphorous availability in soybean meal for broilers by supplemental phytase. *Poultry Science*, **74**, 1831-1842.

Edwards, H.M., Jr. (1983) Phosphorus I. Effect of breed and strain on utilization of suboptimal levels of phosphorus in the ration. *Poultry Science*, **62**, 77-84.

Eeckhout, W. and de Paepe, M. (1994) Total phosphorus, phytate-phosphorus and phytase activity in plant feedstuffs. *Animal Feed Science and Technology*, **47**, 19-29.

Erdman, J.W., Jr. (1979) Oilseed phytates: Nutritional implications. *Journal of the American Oil Chemists Society*, **56**, 736-741.

Farrell, D.J., Martin, E., Preez, J.J., Bongarts, M., Sudeman, A., and Thomson, E. (1993) The beneficial effects of a microbial phytase in diets of broiler chickens and ducklings. *Journal of Animal Physiology and Animal Nutrition*, **69**, 278-286.

Gordon, R.W. and Roland, D.A., Sr. (1997) Performance of commercial laying hens fed various phosphorus levels, with and without supplemental phytase. *Poultry Science*, **76**, 1172-1177.

Gordon, R.W. and Roland, D.A., Sr. (1998) Influence of supplemental phytase on calcium and phosphorus utilization in laying hens. *Poultry Science*, **77**, 290-294.

Kornegay, E.T., Denbow, D.M., Yi, Z. and Ravindran, V. (1996) Response of broilers to graded levels of Natuphos phytase added to corn-soybean meal based diets containing three levels of nonphytate phosphorus. *British Journal of Nutrition*, **75**, 839-852.

Kornegay, E.T., Denbow, D.M. and Zhang, Z. (1997) Phytase supplementation of corn-soybean meal broiler diets from three to seven weeks of age. *Poultry Science* **76:** Supplement 1, p. 6 (Abstract).

Maenz, D.D. and Classen, H.L. (1998) Phytase activity in the small intestinal brush border membrane of the chicken. *Poultry Science*, **77**, 557-563.

Mitchell, R.D. and Edwards, H.M., Jr. (1996a) Effects of phytase and 1,25-dihydroxycholecalciferol on phytate utilization and the quantitative requirement for calcium and phosphorus in young broiler chickens. *Poultry Science*, **75**, 95-100.

Mitchell, R.D. and Edwards, H.M., Jr. (1996b) Additive effects of 1,25-Dihydroxycholecalciferol and phytase on phytate-P utilization and related parameters in broiler chickens. *Poultry Science*, **75**, 111-119.

Mohammed, A., Gibney, M.J. and Taylor, T.G. (1991) The effects of dietary levels of inorganic phosphorus, calcium and cholecalciferol on the digestibility of phytate-P by the chick. *British Journal of Nutrition*, **66**, 251-259.

Mroz, Z., Jongbloed, A.W. and Kemme, P.A. (1994) Apparent digestibility and retention of nutrients bound to phytate complexes as influenced by microbial phytase and feeding regimen in pigs. *Journal of Animal Science*, **72**, 126-132.

National Research Council (1994) Nutrient Requirements of Poultry, 9th revised edition, National Academy Press, Washington, D.C.

Nakashon, S.N., Nakau, H.S. and Mirosh, L.W. (1994) Phytase activity, phosphorus and calcium retention, and performance of Single Comb White Leghorn layers fed diets containing two levels of available phosphorus and supplemented with direct-fed microbials. *Poultry Science*, **73**, 1552-1562.

Nelson, T.S., Shieh, T.R., Wodzinski, R.J. and Ware, J.H. (1971) Effect of supplemental phytase on the utilization of phytate phosphorus by chicks. *Journal of Nutrition*, **101**, 1289-1294.

Oberleas, D. and Harland, B.F. (1996) Impact of phytate on nutrient availability. In *Phytase in Animal Nutrition and Waste Management*. Edited by M.B. Coelho and E.T. Kornegay. BASF Corporation, Mount Olive, New Jersey, U.S.A.

Officer, D.I. and Batterham, E.S. (1992) Enzyme supplementation of Linola TM meal for growing pigs. Proceedings of the Australian Society of Animal Production, **9**, 288-296.

Pallauf, V.J., Hohler, D. and Rimbach, G.(1992) Effect of microbial phytase supplementation to a maize-soya-diet on the apparent absorption of Mg,

Fe, Cu, Mn and Zn and parameters of Zn-status in piglets. *Journal of Animal Physiology and Animal Nutrition*, **68**, 1-8.

Prasad, A.S. (1996) Metabolism of zinc and its deficiency in human subjects. In *Zinc Metabolism* - 1996, pp 250-256. Edited by A.S. Prasad and C.C. Thomas. Springfield, Illinois, U.S.A.

Punna, S. and Roland, D.A., Sr. (1997) Effect of dietary supplementation of phytase on pullets fed varying levels of dietary phosphorus and calcium. *Poultry Science,* **76**, Supplement 1, page 6, No. 23.

Qian, H., Kornegay, E.T. and Denbow, D.M. (1996) Phosphorus equivalence of microbial phytase in turkey diets as influenced by calcium to phosphorus ratios and phosphorus levels. *Poultry Science*, **75**, 69-81.

Qian, H., Kornegay, E.T. and Denbow, D.M. (1997) Utilization of phytate phosphorus and calcium as influenced by microbial phytase, cholecalciferol, and the calcium : total phosphorus ratio in broiler diets. *Poultry Science*, **76**, 37-46.

Ravindran, V., Bryden, W.L. and Kornegay, E.T.(1995) Phytates: occurrences, bioavailability and implications in poultry nutrition. *Poultry and Avian Biology Reviews*, **6**, 125-143.

Ravindran, V., Kornegay, E.T., Denbow, D.M., Yi, Z. and Hulet, R.M. (1995) Response of turkey poults to tiered levels of Natuphos® phytase added to soybean meal-based semi-purified diets containing three levels of nonphytate phosphorus. *Poultry Science*, **74**, 1843-1854.

Reddy, N.R., Sathe, S.K. and Salunkhe, D.K. (1982) Phytates in legumes and cereals. *Advances in Food Research*, **28**, 1-91.

Roberson, K.D. and Edwards, H.M., Jr. (1994) Effects of 1,25-dihydroxycholecalciferol and phytase on zinc utilization in broiler chicks. *Poultry Science*, **73**, 1312-1326.

Rojas, S.W. and Scott, M.L. (1969) Factors affecting the nutritive value of cottonseed meal as a protein source in chick diets. *Poultry Science*, **48**, 819-835.

Schoner, F.J., Hoppe, P.P. and Schwartz, G. (1991) Comparative effects of microbial phytase and inorganic phosphorus on performance and retention of phosphorus, calcium and crude ash in broilers. *Journal of Animal Physiology and Animal Nutrition*, **66**, 248-255.

Schoner, F.J., Schwartz, G., Hoppe, P.P. and Wiesche, H. (1994) Effect of microbial phytase on Ca-availability in broilers. Third Conference of Pig and Poultry Nutrition in Halle, Germany, November 29-December 1.

Scott, M.L., Nesheim, M.C. and Young, R.J. (1982) Nutrition of the chicken, 3rd edition, M.L. Scott and Associates, Ithaca, New York, U.S.A.

Sebastian, S., Touchburn, S.P., Chavez, E.R. and Laguë, P.C. (1996a) The effects of supplemental microbial phytase on the performance and utilization of dietary calcium, phosphorus, copper and zinc in broiler chickens fed corn-soybean diets. *Poultry Science*, **75**, 729-736.

Sebastian, S., Touchburn, S.P., Chavez, E.R. and Laguë, P.C. (1996b) Efficacy of supplemental microbial phytase at different dietary calcium levels on growth performance and mineral utilization of broiler chickens. *Poultry Science*, **75**, 1516-1523.

Sebastian, S., Touchburn, S.P., Chavez, E.R. and Laguë, P.C.(1997) Apparent digestibility of protein and amino acids in broiler chickens fed a corn-soybean diet supplemented with microbial phytase. *Poultry Science*, **76**, 1760-1769.

Simons, P.C.M., Versteegh, H.A., Jongbloed, A.W., Kemme, P.A., Slump, P., Bos, K.D., Wolters, M.G.E., Buedeker, R.F. and Vershoor, G.J. (1990) Improvement of phosphorus availability by microbial phytase in broilers and pigs. *British Journal of Nutrition*, **64**, 525-540.

Summers, J.D. (1995) Reduced dietary phosphorus levels for layers. *Poultry Science*, **74**, 1977-1983.

Sun, W., Patterson, J.A., Woloshuk, C.P. and Muir, W.M. (1997) Expression of Aspergillus niger phytase in yeast Saccharomyces cerevisiae for poultry diet supplementation. *Poultry Science*, **76**, Supplement 1, No. 19, page 5.

Thiel, U. and Weigand, E. (1992) Influence of dietary zinc and microbial phytase supplementation on zinc retention and zinc excretion in broiler chickens. Proceedings of XIX World's Poultry Congress. World's Poultry Science Association, Amsterdam, The Netherlands.

Thiel, U., Weigand, E., Hoppe, P.P. and Schoner, F.J. (1993) Zinc retention of broiler chickens as affected by dietary supplements of zinc and microbial phytase. In *Trace Elements in Man and Animals* -1993, pp 658-660. Edited by M. Anke, D. Meissner and C.F. Mills.

Van der Klis, J.D., Versteegh, H.A.J., Simons, P.C. and Kies, A.K. (1997) The efficacy of phytase in corn-soybean meal-based diets for laying hens. *Poultry Science*, **76**, 1535-1542.

Yi, Z., Kornegay, E.T., Lindemann, M.D. and Ravindran, V. (1994) Effect of Natuphos phytase for improving the bioavailability of phosphorus and other nutrients on soybean meal-based semi-purified diets for young pigs. *Journal of Animal Science*, **72**, 7, Supplement 1.

Yi, Z., Kornegay, E.T. and Denbow, D.M. (1996a) Supplemental microbial phytase improves the zinc utilization in broilers. *Poultry Science*, **75**, 540-546.

Yi, Z., Kornegay, E.T. and Denbow, D.M. (1996b) Effect of microbial phytase on nitrogen and amino acid digestibility and nitrogen retention of turkey poults fed corn-soybean meal diets. *Poultry Science*, **75**, 979-990.

Yi, Z., Kornegay, E.T., Ravindran, V. and Denbow, D.M. (1996) Improving phytate phosphorus availability in corn and soybean meal for broilers using microbial phytase and calculation of phosphorus equivalency values for phytase. *Poultry Science*, **75**, 240-249.

Zhang, X., McDaniel, G.R. and Roland, D.A. (1998) Genetic variation of phytate phosphorus utilization from hatch to three weeks of age in broiler chicken lines selected for incidence of tibial dyschondroplasia. *Poultry Science*, **77**, 386-390.

*This paper was first published in 1999*

9

# EXOGENOUS ENZYMES AS PRO-NUTRIENTS IN BROILER DIETS

GORDON ROSEN
*66 Bathgate Road, Wimbledon, London SW19 5PH, England*

## Introduction

During the last ten years enzyme feed supplements have been widely adopted in broiler production. Their usage in broiler diets is targeted primarily at the enhancement of nutritive and economic values. Following an initial 60-year exploratory lag phase (1925-84), the commercial application of exogenous enzymes in broiler feeds expanded rapidly. The growth pattern in broiler developments is well reflected in the numbers of scientific and trade press publications collected for use herein. Excluding 21 undated, there were 126 in 1925-79, followed by 47, 120, 402 and 604 in subsequent half-decades to 1999, with a further 500+ in 1999-2001.

Exogenous enzymes are used to improve nutritive values measured as rates of live-weight gain, feed conversion efficiencies, and carcass qualities; to decrease body weight variation; and to reduce nutrient excretion into the environment, e.g. phytate phosphorus, by the use of microbial phytase. Rationalization of the choice of an enzyme and its optimal dosage, in its court of last resort, needs to be based on the results of controlled scientific tests under practical conditions. For reasons of economy in research and development, however, short-term metabolism and mode of action tests in starter birds have figured largely in programmes to underpin and promote the application of enzymes. Such tests on enzymes utilizing nutrient deficiency and/or impractical conditions have aided progress, but they are inevitably open to question concerning their quantitative reliability for posology in praxis [determining the correct dose in practice]. Accordingly, the primary objective of the Brozyme project presented herein is to quantify the influence of dosage and other important variables governing the nutritive and economic effectiveness of exogenous enzymes in broilers and thereby achieve more predictable and more consistent results.

## Brozyme. Scope, targets and nomenclature

Brozyme is the code name for the first in a series of comprehensive multifactorial assessments of the pro-nutrient effects of exogenous enzymes in the nutrition of farm animals (Rosen, 2000a). Pro-nutrients are substances, such as antimicrobials, anticoccidials, antihistomonials, enzymes, microorganisms, mineral earths, aromatics, botanicals, copper sulphate and organic acids, which improve the value of nutrients. The effects of pro-nutrients on nutritive value are positive, as diametric opposites of the negative effects of anti-nutrients.

Brozyme is a large-scale applied nutrition research project aimed at knowledge discovery in the mass of available literature data. It is devised to quantify the relative contributions and interactions of feed, genetic, environmental, managemental and enzymic independent variable factors in order to predict fair average values of net performance and profit improvement by exogenous enzymes. Its large resource of controlled test data, mined from the scientific and trade press, is used to generate optimal, statistically-significant algebraic models for the prediction of the effects of enzymes on key dependent variables, i.e., feed consumption, live-weight gain, feed conversion efficiency and mortality; and also, if and when data suffice, carcass, litter and environmental characteristics. In particular, Brozyme is aimed (i) to elaborate broadly-based dose-response relationships, more useful than individual dose-titration tests, in order to improve posology in praxis and (ii) to provide comprehensive, broadly-based enzyme product comparisons in place of inadequate single tests, which are unique in time, place and circumstances.

## PROBLEMS AND LOGISTICS

Inadequacies and errors in titles, key words and abstracts and untitled references create problems. Of 1,422 papers collected, 100 were irrelevant. Exclusion of replicated test reports is essential, but can be complicated, especially when replicate reports differ in detail. Experimental reports are also polymorphic in key details of feed processing, diet composition, stocking density, etc. Extensive international searches are required for sources of 10% or more of references in published bibliographies, when not easily available from major national libraries. Truncated definitions of enzyme preparations and the omission of enzyme dosage units require author contacts for details. Responses from authors fall well below 50%, though some may on occasions furnish missing details and results, not included in abstracts or short communications or which were not germane to their theme.

GENERIC ENZYME NOMENCLATURE

The Brozyme resource initially contained 252 different generic descriptors, 135 singles and 117 with 2-11 components. Some of the latter had more than one basic component e.g. two or three different beta-glucanases. Too few types accord with the 1992 recommendations on enzyme nomenclature of the Nomenclature Committee of the International Union of Biochemistry and Molecular Biology (Webb, 1992) or the listed alternatives within its divisions, sub-classes and sub-sub-classes. There is a need in Brozyme for a simple system to pinpoint and group those of primary importance and to distinguish declaration with and without enzyme units. A litero-numeric system has therefore been devised (Table 9.1).

At present Brozyme deals with nine basic generic types having sufficient tests for cardinal status. The remainder with fewer tests are placed together *pro tempore* in a holding group, 'miscellanase'. Table 9.1 also contains nine further descriptors used for preparations of 2-10 declared generic components, *viz*, diase, triase, up to decase. The notation scheme distinguishes components of known and unknown unit value by the use of upper and lower case identifiers respectively. Thus, TRI.AM.BE.XY contains declared concentrations of amylase, beta-glucanase and xylanase units and PH.be.xy denotes a phytase preparation of known potency with unmeasured beta-glucanase and xylanase side activities. In Brozyme modelling procedures the preparations, DI.BE.XY, DI.BE.XY.am and DI.BE.XY.pr are classified as diases with beta-glucanase and xylanase of known unit concentrations. Dummy variables are deployed for each three-component product to test for the significance of any differences due to declared, unquantified side activity.

The literature collection for Brozyme began on 01 April 1998. Its assembly, filing, data abstraction and computer filing was concluded for commencement of analysis on 01 February 2000. Studies to date are based on 1,322 publications from 1925-1999. Further collection during 1999-2001 for future research has so far increased the total to 1,888.

## Methodology

The main features and sequential steps in the modelling procedures employed in this study (Rosen, 1995) are summarized in Table 9.2.

The methodology consists of: (i) world-wide collection of controlled feeding test publications to provide a comprehensive data bank on broiler performance and allied numeric and descriptive variables; (ii) computer filing of data (Nie, Hadlai-Hull, Jenkins, Steinbrenner and Bent, 1975), eliminating repeats; (iii)

**Table 9.1** GENERIC ENZYME NOTATION SCHEME USED IN BROZYME

| *Enzyme* | *Code** | |
|---|---|---|
| | *u/g known* | *u/g unknown* |
| alpha-galactosidase | AL | al |
| amylase | AM | am |
| beta-glucanase | BE | be |
| lipase | LI | li |
| mannanase | MA | ma |
| phytase | PH | ph |
| polygalacturonase | PO | po |
| protease | PR | pr |
| xylanase | XY | xy |
| 'miscellanase' | M | m |
| diase | | DI |
| triase | | TRI |
| tetrase | | TET |
| pentase | | PEN |
| hexase | | HEX |
| septase | | SEP |
| octase | | OCT |
| nonase | | NON |
| decase | | DEC |

* A simple enzyme is defined as a preparation having a sole generic enzyme declared activity, specified by a letter code, in upper or lower case respectively, for known or unknown enzyme unit concentration. Mixtures of enzymes, having two or more declared generic enzyme activities, are specified, e.g., as DI.AL.AM; TRI.BE.LI.MA; TRI.PH.po.PR.XY, etc.

conventional multiple regression analysis (Draper and Smith, 1981), relating dependent to independent variables in statistically-significant regressions of minimum standard deviation (SD), maximum multiple correlation coefficient square ($R^2$) and significant partial regression coefficients, after excluding aberrant responses (residuals >3xSD). The models are then used to predict nutritional responses for requisite values of influential independent variables.

## Results

### DATA BANK CHARACTERISTICS

The data bank used for analysis, outlined in Table 9.3, was amassed from 1,322

**Table 9.2** TENETS AND PROCEDURES OF THE METHODOLOGY USED IN MULTIFACTORIAL ANALYSIS OF PRO-NUTRIENTS IN ANIMAL NUTRITION

- Collection of author-attributed published reports
- Scientifically-controlled feeding tests
- Abstraction of numeric and descriptive variables on record forms
- All available unselected data
- Computer filing of data bank
- Correction of errors; elimination of repeats
- Standard multiple regression analysis; relating dependent to independent variables; start to finish
- Best-fit algebraic models; highly statistically-significant regressions; minimum standard deviations; maximum multiple correlation coefficient squares; significant partial regression coefficients; exclusion of aberrant (>3 x SD) responses
- Models for statistically-significant sub-classes
- Calculation of nutritional responses and confidence limits for requisite variables
- Economic valuations to target live weight or duration.

publications dated 1925-1999. A large majority of 1,173 in this collection (89%) are of more recent vintage (1980-1999).

The collation of unique performance data sets is derived from only 575 papers (43%). In 98 reports the performance data were repeats (7.4%). Most of the balance were metabolic and mode of action research reports and reviews without performance data (34%), and allied subjects, e.g. analysis and stability (2.9%). Rejects (9.4%) lacked data on feed intake, or live weight, or duration (3.1%); had no negative control (3.0%); or reported responses as percentages (3.3%).

The 5,725 controlled-test data sets contain 2,106 negative controls and 3,619 enzyme-treated. Excluding 265 tests on pullets (7.3%), the 3,354 broiler tests comprise 2,573 from start to finish and 781 intermediates. The 2,573 is reduced, by lack of enzyme dosage units in 704 (27.4%), to 1,869 for comprehensive analysis of tests conducted on a total of approximately 410,000 broilers. Mortality data are reported in only 439 (23.5%) of the 1,869.

## INDEPENDENT VARIABLES

Many factors are known and many others are deemed likely to affect the magnitude of nutritional responses to exogenous enzymes in broiler diets. The potentially relevant independent variables for analysis in Brozyme are listed in Table 9.4, as broiler-, environment-, test conditions-, enzyme- and feed-related factors.

**Table 9.3** OUTLINE CHARACTERISTICS OF BROZYME DATA BANK

| | *n* |
|---|---|
| Publications | 1422 |
| Omitted | 100 |
| Utilized | 1322 |
| Performance data | 575 |
| Enzyme products | 432 |
| Generic types | 252 |
| Data sets (feed/gain/conversion) | 5725 |
| Negative controls | 2106 |
| Enzyme-treated | 3619 |
| Enzyme units known | 2670 |
| Negative controls (mortality) | 279 |
| Enzyme-treated | 534 |
| Enzyme units known | 439 |
| Dose-titration tests | 346 |
| Dose-titration tests (>5 doses) | 32 |
| Broiler tests | 3354 |
| Pullet tests | 265 |
| Intermediate phase broiler tests | 781 |
| Start to finish broiler tests | 2573 |
| Start to finish enzyme units known | 1869 |
| Start to finish enzyme units known (mortality) | 365 |

The total of 164 variables contains 12 countries, 8 antibacterials, 18 anticoccidials, 66 feed characteristics and 15 enzyme dosages, only a few of which are relevant in any given model. Nonetheless there are 50 or so variables for consideration in model development.

The main cereal grain substrate is known in 87% of the tests. They are barley (30.1%), wheat (28.4%), maize (25.7%), rye (5.8%), sorghum (3.1%), oats (2.9%), hulless barley (2.4%) and triticale (1.5%). The values for main vegetable protein source in the feeds reveal soya as very highly dominant (94%), with rape (1.5%) and lupin (1.3%) ahead of smaller proportions, in decreasing order, of sunflower, guar, bean, cottonseed, groundnut, pea and sesame. Animal protein sources are included in 54% of the feed formulations. Of the 39 types including admixtures, there are, as sole sources, fish (42.4%), herring (13.8%), meat and bone (6.2%), meat (4.2%) and casein (3.4%) and admixtures of fish with meat and bone (15.6%) and fish with meat (3.3%). Oil and/or fat feed supplements are used in 62% of the diets. Of the 56 types, the relative frequencies of usage are soya (21.3%), fat (16.6%), animal (12.9%), tallow (10.5%), vegetable (9.4%), animal plus vegetable (8.2%), maize (6.7%), poultry (3.8%), pig (2.3%) and others (2.1%).

**Table 9.4** BROZYME BROILER-, ENVIRONMENT-, TEST CONDITIONS-, FEED- AND ENZYME-RELATED INDEPENDENT VARIABLES

| *Variable* | *n* | *Variable* | *n* |
|---|---|---|---|
| negative control performance* | 4 | feed process (mash; processed) | 2 |
| duration | 1 | part-purified diet | 1 |
| year of test - 1900 | 1 | antibiotic | 8 |
| age at start | 1 | antibiotic dosage | 1 |
| sex (male; female; mixed; as-hatched) | 4 | anticoccidial | 12 |
| housing (cage; floor) | 2 | anticoccidial dosage | 1 |
| stocking density | 1 | sole cereal | 8 |
| not day-old birds | 1 | sole cereal content | 1 |
| selected sample birds | 1 | main cereal | 8 |
| diagnosed disease | 1 | main cereal content | 1 |
| mode of action/metabolism test | 1 | secondary cereal | 8 |
| factorial data | 1 | secondary cereal content | 1 |
| trade press | 1 | main/secondary cereal ratio | 1 |
| major country | 12 | animal protein | 11 |
| alpha-galactosidase dosage | 1 | animal protein content | 1 |
| amylase dosage | 1 | main vegetable protein | 10 |
| beta-glucanase dosage | 1 | main vegetable protein content | 1 |
| lipase dosage | 1 | added oil or fat | 11 |
| mannanase dosage | 1 | added oil or fat content | 1 |
| 'miscellanase' dosage | 1 | crude protein | 1 |
| phytase dosage | 1 | crude fat | 1 |
| polygalacturonase dosage | 1 | crude fibre | 1 |
| protease dosage | 1 | energy | 1 |
| xylanase dosage | 1 | lysine | 1 |
| diase dosage | 1 | methionine | 1 |
| triase dosage | 1 | methionine plus cystine | 1 |
| tetrase dosage | 1 | phosphorus | 1 |
| pentase dosage | 1 | available phosphorus | 1 |
| hexase dosage | 1 | calcium | 1 |
| phased enzyme dosage | 1 | | |
| enzyme source (major suppliers) | 8 | | |
| enzyme source (major brands) | 10 | | |

* FDIC feed intake; LWGC live-weight gain; FCRC feed conversion ratio; MORT mortality

Brozyme data are from 58 countries, of which the 12 largest contributors, furnishing 84.5% of the total, are USA (21.8%), Germany (11.3%), Canada (11%), UK (9.5%), Sweden (5.4%), Switzerland (5.3%), Australia (4.3%), Netherlands (3.9%), Poland (3.7%), Spain (2.8%), Czech/Slovak Republics (2.8%) and Denmark (2.7%).

## VARIATIONS IN RESPONSE

Overall variations in nutritional and mortality responses to exogenous enzymes in broilers are given in Table 9.5.

**Table 9.5** VARIATION IN FEED INTAKE, LIVE-WEIGHT GAIN, FEED CONVERSION RATIO AND MORTALITY EFFECTS OF EXOGENOUS ENZYMES IN BROILER NUTRITION

| *Variable* | *(n)* | *Effect* | | *Standard deviation* | *Coefficient of variation (%)* |
|---|---|---|---|---|---|
| All | | | | | |
| FDIeff | (2573) | +31.3g | (1.5)* | 139g | 444 |
| LWGeff | (2573) | +53.4g | (5.1) | 76.4g | 143 |
| FCReff | (2573) | -0.105 | (5.3) | 0.195 | 186 |
| MORTeff | (439) | -1.71% | (26) | 6.44% | 377 |
| Dosage units known | | | | | |
| FDIeff | (1869) | +31.9g | (1.4) | 146g | 458 |
| LWGeff | (1869) | +57.0g | (5.0) | 79.0g | 139 |
| FCReff | (1869) | -0.0999 | (5.1) | 0.194 | 194 |
| MORTeff | (365) | -1.80% | (26) | 6.93% | 385 |

* as percentage of negative control
FDIeff , feed intake effect; LWGeff, live-weight gain effect; FCReff, feed conversion ratio effect; MORTeff, mortality effect

For the 2,573 nutritional and 439 mortality effects, the coefficients of variation are 143% for live-weight gain, 186% for feed conversion ratio, 377% for mortality and 444% for feed intake. Their relative consistencies of response, measured by proportion of negative (adverse) plus zero responses, are 14% for live-weight gain, 17% for feed conversion ratio, 47% for mortality and 37% for feed intake. The corresponding coefficients of variation in the 1,869 data bank of tests with known dosage units are very similar with coefficients of variation of 139% for LWGeff, 194% for FCReff, 385% for MORTeff and 458% for FDIeff.

## PRELIMINARY MODELS

Initial investigations on generalized enzyme responses using the full 1,869 data resource were based on experience in modelling the effects of other pro-nutrients (Rosen, 1995). At the outset these showed that the feed, live-weight gain and feed conversion effects of enzymes are negatively (adversely) related to the control level of broiler performance, positively to the duration of feeding and favourably to the passage of time over the years. The same applies to smaller regressions for beta-glucanase, phytase, protease, xylanase, 'miscellanase', diases, triases and higher multi-component mixtures.

The triad of independent variables, control performance, duration and year of test, accounted for 7.6%, 9.9% and 47% respectively of the total variation in feed intake, live-weight gain and feed conversion ratio effects in the total of 1,869 broiler tests.

## 'BROILERASE'

Expansion of the preliminary models by testing a variety of additional variables to elaborate an overall generalised model, termed 'broilerase', produced feed, gain and conversion effect regressions with 8, 5 and 10 statistically-significant independent variables, respectively accounting for 14%, 11% and 54% of variation in response. The FCReff model, as detailed in Tables 9.6 and 9.7, is used hereafter in further investigations of factors determining broiler nutritional responses to enzymes. For comparison, Table 9.8 details broilerase FDIeff and LWGeff models.

The 10 significant terms in the FCReff model include 8 of the 9 in the FDIeff or LWGeff congeners. For FCReff, as would be expected, the FCRC and DUR terms are counteractive in beneficial and adverse contributions respectively as they increase with growth. Enzyme effectiveness has improved over the years, as seen in the negative XD term. Feed conversion improvement is better in malethan in as-hatched birds and in processed versus mash feed. The positive PPD, NDO and MMT terms quantify disadvantage in the evaluation of FCReff improvement using part-purified diets, older than day-old birds and metabolic and mode of action tests. Use of selected weight range birds instead of as-hatched markedly inflates the feed conversion improvement (-0.129). Broilerase improves FCReff logarithmically over the range 0.0014 – 979u/g feed. The only other significant independent variable indicates an inferior LWGeff in female cf. as-hatched, with a partial regression coefficient of -30.3g.

## ABERRANT RESPONSES

A detailed analysis of aberrant responses in the broilerase models revealed 103 in toto for FDIeff (32), LWGeff (31) and FCReff (33). Their aberrance is manifest in respective mean values of 516g (16.7%), 432g (42.4%) and -0.748 (-24.8%),

**Table 9.6** CODES AND DEFINITIONS OF VARIABLES IN BROILERASE FEED CONVERSION MODEL

| *Symbol* | *Definition* |
|---|---|
| n | number of tests |
| $R^2$ | multiple regression coefficient square |
| SD | standard deviation |
| FCReff | effect on feed conversion ratio |
| FDIeff | effect on feed intake (g) |
| LWGeff | effect on live-weight gain (g) |
| se | standard error |
| p | probability |
| FCRC | feed conversion ratio of control birds |
| FCR | feed conversion ratio of treated birds |
| FDIC | feed intake of control birds (g) |
| FDI | feed intake of treated birds (g) |
| LWGC | live-weight gain of control birds (g) |
| LWG | live-weight gain of treated birds (g) |
| DUR | duration of enzyme feeding (days) |
| XD | year of test – 1900 |
| TEUG | total enzyme units/g feed |
| log(TEUG+1) | logarithm to base 10 of TEUG+1 |
| PRO | processed feed = 1; mash = 0 |
| MAL | male = 1; as-hatched = 0 |
| PPD | part-purified diet = 1; practical diet = 0 |
| NDO | not day-old birds = 1; day-old = 0 |
| MMT | metabolic or mode of action test = 1; if not = 0 |
| SEL | weight band selected birds = 1; if not = 0 |

**Table 9.7** MULTIFACTORIAL GENERALISED MODEL FOR THE EFFECT OF BROILERASE ON FEED CONVERSION RATIO*

| FCReff = | 0.960 | - 0.400FCRC | + 0.00942DUR | - 0.00625XD | - 0.0334PRO | - 0.0289MAL |
|---|---|---|---|---|---|---|
| se | (0.061) | (0.010) | (0.000) | (0.001) | (0.007) | (0.007) |
| p | (<0.001) | (<0.001) | (<0.001) | (<0.001) | (<0.001) | (<0.001) |

n 1869

$R^2$ 0.537

SD 0.132

| | + 0.0685PPD | + 0.104NDO | + 0.0191MMT | - 0.129SEL | - 0.0257log(TEUG + 1) |
|---|---|---|---|---|---|
| se | (0.014) | (0.008) | (0.007) | (0.020) | (0.007) |
| p | (<0.001) | (<0.001) | (0.010) | (<0.001) | (<0.001) |

FCR = 0.960 + 0.600FCRC + 0.00942DUR - 0.00625XD - 0.0334PRO - 0.0289MAL + 0.0685PPD + 0.104NDO + 0.0191MMT - 0.129SEL - 0.0257log(TEUG+1)

$R^2$ 0.900

SD 0.132

* see Table 9.6 for codes and definitions of variables

**Table 9.8** MULTIFACTORIAL GENERALISED MODELS FOR THE EFFECTS OF BROILERASE ON FEED INTAKE AND LIVE-WEIGHT GAIN*

| | | | | | | |
|---|---|---|---|---|---|---|
| FDIeff= | | -223 | - 0.0827FDIC | + 9.99DUR | + 1.66XD | - 39.5log(TEUG+1) |
| n 1869 | se | (69.2) | (0.007) | (0.864) | (0.671) | (7.19) |
| $R^2$ 0.140 | p | (0.001) | (<0.001) | (<0.001) | (0.013) | (<0.001) |
| SD 136 | | | | | | |
| | | | - 31.2PRO | + 30.0PPD | + 33.9NDO | + 20.0MMT |
| | | | (7.32) | (14.2) | (9.20) | (7.55) |
| | | | (<0.001) | (0.035) | (<0.001) | (0.008) |
| | | | | | | |
| LWGeff = | | - 249 | - 0.0749LWGC | + 4.25DUR | + 2.97XD | - 13.5log(TEUG+1) |
| n 1869 | se | (35.5) | (0.005) | (0.297) | (0.368) | (3.88) |
| $R^2$ 0.111 | p | (<0.001) | (<0.001) | (<0.001) | (<0.001) | (0.001) |
| SD 74.6 | | | | | | |
| | | - 30.3FEM | | | | |
| | | (12.1) | | | | |
| | | (0.012) | | | | |

* see Table 9.6 for codes and definitions of variables

compared with norms of 23.5g (1.1%), 50.7g (4.5%) and -0.088 (-4.6%). Means for 7 aberrant MORTeffs are -14.9% (-59%), cf. -1.5% (-25%). Detailed inspection of aberrance test circumstances revealed high incidences of mash feeds, caged birds, not day-olds, part-purified diets and selected birds. Other dominant factors are phytase, deficiency diets, high mortality and diets based on barley, rye or oats. The role of cereal base was therefore investigated by the use of dummy variables for dietary main cereal bases, barley, hulless barley, maize, oats, rye, sorghum, triticale and wheat.

## INFLUENCE OF CEREAL BASE

Table 9.9 contains the broilerase models on the influence of cereal base, with significant effects for all grains except sorghum. Feed intake is increased by broilerase in diets based on oats, rye or barley, with respective partial regression coefficients of 77, 68 and 41g. It is decreased for wheat (-22g). Resultant effects on live-weight gain are 56, 47, 26 and -11g respectively and there are values of 36g for hulless barley and -15g for maize. Consequential significant improvements in FCReff pertain to oats (-0.114), rye (-0.123) or hulless barley (-0.108) and an adverse effect for triticale (+0.0696).

**Table 9.9** BROILERASE FDIEFF, LWGEFF AND FCREFF MODELS* CONTAINING MAIN CEREAL BASE DUMMY VARIABLES**

| | | | | |
|---|---|---|---|---|
| FCReff = 0.966 | - 0.373FCRC | + 0.00836DUR | - 0.0645XD | - 0.0334PRO - 0.0209MAL |
| | - 0.0275log(TEUG+1) | + 0.102NDO | - 0.110SEL + 0.0177CA | |
| | - 0.114OAT - 0.123 RYE | | - 0.108HUB | |
| | + 0.0696TRI | | | |
| FDIeff = - 379 | - 0.0835FDIC + 10.3DUR | + 3.17XD | - 22.4PRO | |
| | - 42.8log(TEUG+1) | + 35.6NDO | + 25.9MMT | |
| | + 76.7OAT + 68.2RYE | + 40.9BAR | - 22.2WHE | |
| LWGeff = - 339 | - 0.0685LWGC | + 4.38DUR | + 3.76XD | |
| | - 14.2log(TEUG+1) | | + 11.8MMT | |
| | + 56.3OAT + 46.8RYE | + 26.3BAR | + 36.0HUB - 11.3WHE | |
| | - 14.9MZ | | | |

* n 1869; $R^2$ 0.644/.172/.171; SD 0.129/133/72.1
** BAR = barley; HUB = hulless barley; MZ = maize; OAT = oats; RYE = rye; TRI = triticale; WHE = wheat

## CHRONOLOGICAL ASPECTS

The significance of year of test merited further study. The linear improvement of FCReff of -0.00625 per annum (Table 9.7) was re-examined in successive periods, 1964-79, 1980-89 and 1990-98. Highly-significant respective partial regression coefficients of XD were -0.0178, -0.00754 and -0.00423. Were this retrogression to continue on the same course, zero effect would be reached in 2004.

## ENZYME CONCENTRATION

Ongoing control performance improvements by the use of better breeds, feeds and management practices inevitably comports a reduced response over the years for any given enzyme dosage, analogous to changes actuating use of higher nutrient concentrations. This decline can be offset at least in part by higher enzyme dosage. As an example, the partial regression coefficients of FCRC and log(TEUG+1) (in Table 9.7) predict that a 2% improvement of FCRC 1.813 to 1.777, at 42 days for processed feed and MAL = PPD = NDO = MMT = SEL = 0, would require a near-quadruplication of dosage from 10 to 38 TEUGu/g feed to maintain FCReff = -0.042. N.B. Coincident changes in DUR and XD would also need to be taken into account in practice in any revision of TEUG.

## Discussion of results

In sketching future horizons for enzymes in farm animal nutrition, Marquardt and Bedford (2001) point to areas for additional research and development including "the use of models to predict responses to enzyme treatment and hence optimize economy and efficacy of usage". This coincides with the main objective of the Brozyme project presented herein. Moreover, Brozyme is aimed at the estimation of responses under practical conditions utilizing the existing pool of performance data in the elaboration of comprehensive dose-response relationships of exogenous enzyme preparations and of their overlapping limiting nutrients. The models produced, based solely on performance measurements, are congruous with, but not dependent upon, theories of modes of action. This empirical approach has greater potential in enzyme selection and dose optimization because it takes account of manifold variations in breeds, feeds and production conditions.

The collection and organization of the large volume of data for analysis in Brozyme research has revealed some interesting facets and vital statistics in the broad spectrum of independent variables which govern the effectiveness of exogenous enzymes. Test conditions and feed formulations are often angled away from praxis and test reports leave much to be desired even in refereed scientific journals. Apart from any complications due to the use of different assay procedures and standards, it is regrettable that more than a quarter of the performance data resource is virtually useless, in the absence of enzyme units. Furthermore, nomenclature is confused and imprecise. Hopefully the generic enzyme notation system developed for Brozyme might prove also to be useful in legislation and marketing or it might at least stimulate adaptations and/or improvements for general application.

The methodology used previously for other pro-nutrients, notably antibiotics and microorganisms, as adapted to enzyme studies, has functioned satisfactorily. It has manifested similar patterns of response and relativities of independent variables (Rosen, 2000b). After allowance for marked differences in duration, epoch, housing, sex, use of anticoccidials, etc. the efficacies of enzymes and antibiotics on average manifest equivalence (Rosen, 2001a). This finding, however, does not preclude potentially important differences between individual products used at optimal dosages.

The initial outputs in Brozyme research have uncovered or confirmed and illustrated some of the complexities of responses to enzymes in nutrition. Initial exploration of the significance and relative importance of independent variables determining the magnitude of enzyme responses in generalized 'broilerase' models using all 1,869 controlled tests has shown (i) that the magnitude of response is much more influenced by level of broiler performance and duration of feeding and date of test than by enzyme dosage; (ii) that the use of mash feed, unisex birds, not day-old and selected weight birds and part-purified diets cannot be relied upon for prediction of broiler responses in praxis; (iii) that in diets based on wheat and maize, feed intake is reduced, whereas it is increased with barleys, oats and rye; and (iv) that as broiler performance continues to improve over the years, higher enzyme dosages are required to maintain responses. The higher enzyme doses required are facilitated by the trend, due to improved production technology and increased competition, to the much lower prices seen in the approximate trisection of enzyme prices today, compared with introductory values in 1984-1991.

Brozyme then is a forerunner in a series of investigations planned on other species, Pigzyme, Layzyme, Turkzyme, Calfzyme and Rumzymes. Results of the first Brozyme enzyme-specific study are reported in Chapter 7 of this book on microbial phytase in broiler nutrition (Rosen, 2002). Currently a first study is in progress on the interactions of beta-glucanases and xylanases in the largest Brozyme diase collection, DI.BE.XY.

## Conclusions

The comprehensive collection of published data on the effects of exogenous enzymes in broiler nutrition and the elaboration of empirical multiple regression models have provided a summary perspective of the influence of several independent variable factors in the form of generalised broilerase models of effects on feed intake, live-weight gain and feed conversion ratio. It has also been demonstrated that the magnitude of nutritional responses is primarily dependent on the level of negative control broiler performance and duration of feeding and thereafter logarithmically by enzyme dosage. A move towards a higher proportion of efficacy tests in practical conditions would be a good future investment. These empirical models are used to predict nutritional responses to exogenous enzymes in praxis for the improvement of efficacy and net profit, while still taking account of the existing plentiful supply of data available from lower cost, short-term research screening tests. The divergent effects of broilerase in diets based on wheat and maize and those based on barleys, rye, maize and triticale will be followed up in models for individual enzyme types and will also be extended to study the effects of secondary cereals in commonly-used admixtures.

Key topics for discussion include the improvement of enzyme nomenclature and the format and detail of individual test reports; future test designs; methods of enzyme comparison; overlap of enzyme and limiting nutrient dose-response functions; biologically-relevant in vitro enzyme assays; enzymes plus or minus other pronutrients; and priorities for future research and development.

## References

Draper, N.R. and Smith, H. (1981) *Applied Regression Analysis, Second Edition.* John Wiley and Sons, Inc., New York.

Marquardt, R.R. and Bedford, M.R. (2001) Future horizons. pp. 389-398. In *Enzymes in Farm Animal Nutrition.* Edited by M.R. Bedford and G.G. Partridge, CABI Publishing, Wallingford, OX10 8DE.

Nie, N.H., Hadlai-Hull, C., Jenkins, J.G., Steinbrenner, K. and Bent, B.H. (1975) *Statistical Package for the Social Sciences. Second Edition.* McGraw Hill Book Company, New York.

Rosen, G.D. (1995) Antibacterials in poultry and pig nutrition. pp.143-172. In *Biotechnology in Animal Feeds and Animal Feeding*. Edited by R.J. Wallace and A. Chesson. VCH Verlagsgesellschaft mbH, D-69451 Weinheim.

Rosen, G.D. (2000a) Enzymes for broilers: a multi-factorial assessment. *Feed International*, **21(12)**, 14-18.

Rosen, G.D. (2000b) Multifactorial assessment of exogenous enzymes in broiler pronutrition: targets and problems. p11. In *Abstracts of Lectures and Posters of the 3rd European Symposium on Feed Enzymes*, Noordwijkerhout, 8-10 May 2000.

Rosen, G.D. (2001) Multi-factorial efficacy evaluation of alternatives to antimicrobials in pronutrition. pp. 24-25. In *Proceedings of the Spring Meeting, World's Poultry Science Association U.K. Branch.* University of York, 10-11th April, 2001.

Rosen, G.D. (2002) Microbial phytase in broiler nutrition. pp. 105-118. *Recent Advances in Animal Nutrition.* Edited by P.C. Garnsworthy and J. Wiseman. Nottingham University Press, Nottingham,

Webb, E.C. (1992) *Enzyme nomenclature 1992. Recommendations of the Nomenclature Committee of the International Union of Biochemistry and Molecular Biology on the Nomenclature and Classification of Enzymes.* Academic Press, Inc. New York.

*This paper was first published in 2002*

# 10

# MICROBIAL PHYTASE IN BROILER NUTRITION

G ROSEN
*66 Bathgate Road, Wimbledon, London SW19 5PH, England*

## Introduction

The effect of exogenous phytase from *Aspergillus ficuum* NRRL 3135 on dietary phosphorus (P) utilization by chicks was first reported by Nelson *et al.* (1971), evidenced as an increased percentage of bone ash in Single Comb White Leghorn cockerels. Commercial development of phytase in poultry nutrition was however delayed for two decades by the high cost of phytase and relatively little concern about phosphorus pollution of the environment. Research and development in fermentation technology reduced the cost of phytase and the growing concern by national and regional authorities about phosphorus water pollution initiated, in 1991, a rapid expansion of the commercial use of phytase to reduce phytate and inorganic P excretion. The scientific literature now contains many reports of studies confirming that phosphorus excretion can be reduced by 20-50% using dietary phytase. Local laws and financial penalties limiting the phosphorus content of litter and manure for land application have boosted the use of phytase in broiler, layer and pig feed formulations.

Research on the effects of phytase in phosphorus metabolism has been extended to studies on other nutrients, such as the improvement of the bioavailability of calcium and trace elements (Pallauf and Rimbach, 1999), the digestibility of proteins and amino acids and of energy utilization (Kies *et al.*, 2001). Integrated 'nutrient release economic benefit' ratings for protein plus lysine plus energy have been proposed, based on 'equivalence values' (BASF, 2000). The ratings are claimed in total to be worth four times the net financial value of the phosphorus application of phytase. Such economic benefits are calculated using 'nutrient matrix values' in least-cost feed formulation procedures incorporating safety margins on the amounts of nutrients released by phytase.

Measurement and application of the value of phytase in broiler nutrition is complicated by variations in response which are encountered in the use of enzymes as pro-nutrients. Effects on feed conversion are of primary interest, especially when feed represents 70% or more of the cost of production. Variation in the effects of enzymes on feed conversion ratio has been quantified in its coefficient of variation of 1.9 in a collection of 3,619 controlled tests (Rosen, 2000a). The evaluation of phytase as a pro-nutrient in broiler nutrition reported and discussed herein is part of a comprehensive Brozyme (exogenous enzymes in broilers) project (Rosen, 2000b). Its primary objective is to quantify in empirical models the significance and value of several feed-, breed- and management-related independent variables to facilitate the more precise application of phytase in broiler nutrition to improve nutritive values.

## Methodology

The main features and sequential steps in the modelling procedures (Rosen, 1995) employed in this study are summarised in Table 10.1. They comprise essentially: (i) world-wide collection of controlled feeding test publications to provide a comprehensive data bank on broiler performance and allied numeric and descriptive variables; (ii) computer filing of data (Nie, Hadlai-Hull, Jenkins, Steinbrenner and Bent, 1975), eliminating repeats; and (iii) conventional multiple regression analysis (Draper and Smith, 1981), relating dependent to independent variables in statistically-significant regressions of minimum standard deviation (SD), maximum multiple correlation coefficient square ($R^2$) and significant partial regression coefficients, after excluding aberrant responses (residuals >3xSD). The models are then used to predict nutritional responses to phytase for requisite values of influential independent variables.

**Table 10.1** TENETS AND PROCEDURES OF THE METHODOLOGY USED IN MULTIFACTORIAL ANALYSIS OF PRO-NUTRIENTS IN ANIMAL NUTRITION

- Collection of author-attributed published reports
- Scientifically-controlled feeding tests
- Abstraction of numeric and descriptive variables on record forms
- All available unselected data
- Computer filing of data bank
- Correction of errors; elimination of repeats
- Standard multiple regression analysis; relating dependent to independent variables; start to finish
- Best-fit algebraic models; highly statistically-significant regressions; minimum standard deviations; maximum multiple correlation coefficient squares; significant partial regression coefficients; exclusion of aberrant (>3 x SD) responses
- Models for statistically-significant sub-classes
- Calculation of nutritional responses and confidence limits for requisite variables
- Economic valuations to target live weight or duration.

## Results

The total phytase data resource on chicken growers contains the results of 420 feeding test measurements of phytase performance versus negative controls, of which 23 are layer stock. Of the 397 tests in broilers, 68 intermediate results, 18 without phytase units and 9 without diet composition were not relevant. After exclusion of 6 aberrants, the collation used for modelling numbered 296, including 33 with mortality data. The data bank characteristics of symbols used, with definitions, ranges and means of 31 numeric and descriptive variables, aberrant means and a set of variables used for a modern praxis example are summarised in Table 10.2. Table 10.3 compares the magnitude of the mean nutritional responses to phytase with those for other broiler enzymes. Table 10.4 details the best-fit multifactorial nutritional models of the effects of phytase in broilers on feed intake and live-weight gain with statistical details; response estimates therefrom are used for the computation of effects on feed conversion ratio.

Many of the independent variable means in Table 10.2 are remote from praxis values, e.g. 81% are tests on caged birds; 92% use mash diets; 18% are as-hatched (male, 77%; female, 5%). The negative control mean levels of performance for 24 days are feed consumption (1402g), live-weight gain (795g) and feed conversion ratio (1.664). The latter performance is inferior to current feed conversion standards, due to ongoing use of better breeds, feeds and management.

The mean nutritional responses to phytase are clearly different from those for other broiler enzymes (Table 10.3). They are shorter term at 24 compared with 32 days. Phytase increases feed intake much more than other enzymes and its effect is much more consistent. Their mean live-weight gain effects are closer in magnitude and coefficient of variation, so the effect of phytase on feed conversion is much smaller than that of other enzymes; and it is more variable. Phytase greatly reduces mortality compared with other enzymes, due to the use of a high proportion of severely-deficient diets.

The feed intake and live-weight gain effect models in Table 10.4 have in common seven highly-significant independent variable terms, namely, control performance, duration, year of test, phytase dosage, dietary phosphorus, cage housing and above average mortality. The live-weight gain effect is also influenced by maize as major grain, by the use of an anticoccidial and by dietary fat supplementation.

Broadly speaking, the triad of control performance, duration of enzyme feeding and year of experiment account for three times the amount of variation in response compared with that due to the phytase and phosphorus dosage pair. The counteractive logarithmic phytase and dietary phosphorus terms in the models clearly invite a caution in the use of 'equivalence values' for phytase

**Table 10.2** CODES AND DEFINITIONS, RANGES AND MEANS OF NUMERIC AND DESCRIPTIVE VARIABLES (N=296/33 RESPECTIVELY), ABERRANT TEST MEANS (N=6/3) AND VALUES USED IN A PRAXIS EXAMPLE

| *Symbol* | *Definition* | *Range* | *Mean* | *Praxis example* | *Aberrant mean* |
|---|---|---|---|---|---|
| FDIC | feed intake control (g) | 138 - 4851 | 1402 | 4133 | 2883 |
| FDI | feed intake phytase (g) | 144 - 4984 | 1483 | - | 3429 |
| FDIeff | FDI - FDIC (g) | -159 - 502 | 81.0 | - | 546 |
| LWGC | live-weight gain control (g) | 93 - 2222 | 795 | 2326 | 1310 |
| LWG | live-weight gain phytase (g) | 102 - 2226 | 853 | - | 1572 |
| LWGeff | LWG - LWGC (g) | -108 - 352 | 57.7 | - | 262 |
| FCRC | FDIC ÷ LWGC | 1.222 - 3.134 | 1.664 | 1.777 | 2.173 |
| FCR | FDI ÷ LWG | 1.233 - 2.97 | 1.641 | - | 2.132 |
| FCReff | FCR - FCRC | -0.330 - 0.189 | -0.023 | - | -0.042 |
| PHY | phytase in diet (u/kg) | 75 - 2500 | 634 | - | 45 |
| P | phosphorus in diet (g/kg) | 1.7 - 9.4 | 5.33 | 7 | 5.18 |
| DUR | duration (days) | 6 - 49 | 24.0 | 42 | 39.0 |
| XD | year of test - 1900 | 88 - 98 | 93.0 | 98 | 93.5 |
| DM5 | MORTC > 5% | 0 or 1 | 0.0338 | 0 | 1 |
| CA | cage birds | 0 or 1 | 0.811 | 0 | 0.667 |
| COC | anticoccidial fed | 0 or 1 | 0.203 | 1 | 0.5 |
| FAT | added fat diet | 0 or 1 | 0.932 | 1 | 0.5 |
| MZ | maize diet (>40%) | 0 or 1 | 0.632 | 0.632 | 0.833 |
| NMF | not mash feed | 0 or 1 | 0.084 | 1 | 0 |
| NDO | not day-old | 0 or 1 | 0.223 | 0 | 0 |
| MAL | male | 0 or 1 | 0.767 | 0 | 1 |
| FEM | female | 0 or 1 | 0.051 | 0 | 0 |
| AB | antibacterial fed | 0 or 1 | 0.277 | 1 | 0 |
| PPD | part-purified diet | 0 or 1 | 0.145 | 0 | 0 |
| MMT | metabolic/mode of action test | 0 or 1 | 0.493 | 0 | 0.5 |

| | | | | | |
|---|---|---|---|---|---|
| MORTC | mortality control (%) | 0 - 45 | 19.3 | 5 | 21.7 |
| MORT | mortality phytase (%) | 0 - 22.5 | 5.8 | - | 10.0 |
| MORTeff | MORT - MORTC (%) | -42.5 - 5.0 | -13.5 | - | -11.7 |
| PHY | phytase in diet (u/kg) | 200 - 1200 | 583 | - | 745 |
| P | phosphorus in diet (g/kg) | 3.8 - 8.0 | 5.23 | 7 | 5.18 |
| DUR | duration (days) | 21 - 49 | 31.0 | 42 | 39.0 |

**Table 10.3** COMPARISON OF MEAN NUTRITIONAL RESPONSES, COEFFICIENTS OF VARIATION (CV), CONTROL PERFORMANCES AND DURATIONS OF PHYTASE AND OTHER ENZYME TESTS IN BROILERS

| *Variable (units)* | *Phytase* | *CV* | *Other enzymes* | *CV* |
|---|---|---|---|---|
| n | 296 | | 1553 | |
| DUR (days) | 24.0 | | 31.6 | |
| FDIC (g) | 1402 | | 2374 | |
| FDIeff (g) | 81.0 (5.8*) | 1.4 | 12.3 (0.5) | 5.3 |
| LWGC (g) | 795 | | 1191 | |
| LWGeff (g) | 57.7 (7.3) | 1.3 | 49.1 (4.1) | 1.1 |
| FCRC | 1.664 | | 1.978 | |
| FCReff | -0.0226 (1.4) | 1.3 | -0.101 (5.1) | 2.9 |
| n | 33 | | 325 | |
| DUR (days) | 31.0 | | 41.2 | |
| MORTC (%) | 19.3 | | 5.1 | |
| MORTeff (%) | -13.5 (70) | 1.2 | 0.3 (5.9) | 4.4 |

* percentage of control

and phosphorus, if such values are measured in the lower deficiency (linear) segment for application in the upper near-sufficiency (curvilinear) region of the dose-response relationships.

Phytase nutritional research has been centred in short-term, nutrient-deficient, somewhat-impractical test conditions. For such test circumstances Table 10.5 has been constructed to illustrate the effects on feed conversion response of different phosphorus/phytase dosage pairs covering the range of test values. These Table 10.5 estimates show (a) that phytase fed at a substantially higher dosage (2500u/kg) approximately doubles the mean 2.5 to 5 points of feed conversion improvement in diets containing 5-9g/kg of phosphorus and (b) that the marginal FCReff improvement of 1 point at severely-limited phosphorus (1.7g/kg) content at currently-used phytase dosages (500-750 cf. 634u/kg in Table 10.2) is approximately trebled by 2500u/g. The larger FCReff improvements at adequate dietary phosphorus provision may indicate a response due to the alleviation of an insufficiency other than phosphorus.

These observations prompted the calculation of predicted phytase responses in modern birds performing at a good average standard, Type A, compared with a bird of 10% inferior FCRC performance, Type B. The standards set for 14-49 day-old Types A and B are given in Table 10.6.

**Table 10.4** MULTI-FACTORIAL NUTRITIONAL MODELS FOR THE FEED INTAKE AND LIVE-WEIGHT GAIN EFFECTS OF PHYTASE IN BROILERS*

| | | | | |
|---|---|---|---|---|
| FDIeff = | 1291 | -0.0825FDIC | + 11.0DUR | - 12.8XD |
| $R^2$ 0.353 se | (265) | (0.012) | (1.31) | (2.90) |
| SD 92.5 p | (<0.001) | (<0.001) | (<0.001) | (<0.001) |
| n 296 | | | | |
| | + 218log(PHY+1) | | - 208log(P+1) | |
| | (63.0) | | (62.4) | |
| | (0.001) | | (0.001) | |
| | + 124DM5 | | - 60.6CA | |
| | (30.5) | | (17.2) | |
| | (<0.001) | (<0.001) | | |
| LWGeff = | 836 | - 0.159LWGC | + 10.0DUR | - 9.38XD |
| $R^2$0.410 se | (172) | (0.018) | (1.00) | (1.89) |
| SD 58.0 p | (<0.001) | (<0.001) | (<0.001) | (<0.001) |
| n 296 | | | | |
| | + 164log(PHY+1) | | - 104log(P+1) | |
| | (40.5) | | (39.8) | |
| | (<0.001) | | (0.009) | |
| | + 38.8DM5 | | - 32.0CA | |
| | (19.7) | | (11.2) | |
| | (0.049) | | (0.005) | |
| | - 17.7MZ | + 28.8COC | + 63.0FAT | |
| | (7.89) | (9.39) | (15.8) | |
| | (0.026) | (0.002) | (<0.001) | |

FCR = (DFIC + DFIeff) ÷ (LWGC + LWGeff)
FCRC = DFIC ÷ LWGC
FCReff = FCR - FCRC

*(i) see Table 10.2 for codes and definition of variables;
(ii) PHY values are computed as u/g feed

Thence the valuations for Bird Types A and B presented in Table 10.7 relate to deficient (4gP/kg), marginally-deficient (5.5gP/kg) and adequate (7gP/kg) phosphorus dosages. The phytase dosage levels used are low (150u/kg), current (625u/kg) and high (2500u/kg), in line respectively with the European Union rejected minimum level (European Commission, 2000), the median of currently-recommended broiler dosages (500 and 750u/kg) and the maximum tested in published reports.

**Table 10.5** FEED CONVERSION EFFECTS IN PHYTASE RESEARCH CONDITIONS* FOR LOW, INTERMEDIATE AND HIGH PHOSPHORUS AND PHYTASE DOSAGE PAIRS

| *Dietary phosphorus (g/kg feed)* | *Phytase dosage (u/kg)* | *FCReff* |
|---|---|---|
| 1.7 | 75 | 0.006 |
| 5.3 | 75 | -0.006 |
| 9.4 | 75 | -0.013 |
| 1.7 | 634 | -0.009 |
| 5.3 | 634 | -0.021 |
| 9.4 | 634 | -0.028 |
| 1.7 | 2500 | -0.033 |
| 5.3 | 2500 | -0.046 |
| 9.4 | 2500 | -0.053 |

* FDIC = 1402g; LWGC = 795g; FCRC = 1.764; DUR = 24 days
CA = 0.811; DM5 = 0.0338; COC = 0.203; FAT = 0.932; MZ = 0.632; XD = 93

**Table 10.6** NEGATIVE CONTROL BROILER PERFORMANCE LEVELS* AT 14-49 DAYS-OLD FOR BIRD TYPE A, CURRENT GOOD PERFORMANCE, AND ITS 10% INFERIOR FCRC COUNTERPART, TYPE B

| | *Age (days)* | *FDIC (g)* | *LWGC (g)* | *FCRC* |
|---|---|---|---|---|
| A | 14 | 427 | 351 | 1.217 |
| | 21 | 1003 | 723 | 1.387 |
| | 28 | 1836 | 1217 | 1.509 |
| | 35 | 2906 | 1774 | 1.638 |
| | 42 | 4133 | 2326 | 1.777 |
| | 49 | 5444 | 2831 | 1.923 |
| B | 14 | 470 | 351 | 1.339 |
| | 21 | 1103 | 723 | 1.526 |
| | 28 | 2020 | 1217 | 1.660 |
| | 35 | 3197 | 1774 | 1.802 |
| | 42 | 4546 | 2326 | 1.954 |
| | 49 | 5988 | 2831 | 2.115 |

* used for Table 10.7 estimates

**Table 10.7** FEED CONVERSION EFFECTS OF NINE PHYTASE/PHOSPHORUS DOSAGE PAIRS FOR BIRD TYPES A* AND B* IN 14-49 DAY-OLD BROILERS UNDER PRACTICAL CONDITIONS**

| *Age* | *FCREFF* *phytase (u/kg)/phosphorus (g/kg) dosage pairs* | | | | | | | | |
|---|---|---|---|---|---|---|---|---|---|
| *(days)* | *125/4* | *125/5.5* | *125/7* | *625/4* | *625/5.5* | *625/7* | *2500/4* | *2500/5.5* | *2500/7* |
| A 14 | 0 | -0.026 | -0.048 | 0.007 | -0.016 | -0.036 | 0.021 | -0.001 | -0.017 |
| 21 | 0.015 | 0.006 | -0.002 | 0.013 | 0.004 | -0.004 | 0.009 | 0 | -0.007 |
| 28 | 0.024 | 0.019 | 0.016 | 0.020 | 0.015 | 0.011 | 0.011 | 0.007 | 0.003 |
| 35 | 0.026 | 0.024 | 0.022 | 0.021 | 0.019 | 0.017 | 0.011 | 0.009 | 0.007 |
| 42 | 0.023 | 0.022 | 0.021 | 0.018 | 0.017 | 0.016 | 0.007 | 0.006 | 0.005 |
| 49 | 0.016 | 0.016 | 0.015 | 0.010 | 0.010 | 0.010 | -0.001 | -0.002 | -0.002 |
| B 14 | -0.015 | -0.037 | -0.056 | -0.015 | -0.036 | -0.053 | -0.014 | -0.032 | -0.048 |
| 21 | -0.001 | -0.009 | -0.015 | -0.007 | -0.015 | -0.021 | -0.020 | -0.027 | -0.033 |
| 28 | 0.009 | 0.006 | 0.003 | 0.002 | -0.011 | -0.004 | -0.012 | -0.015 | -0.018 |
| 35 | 0.012 | 0.011 | 0.010 | 0.005 | 0.004 | 0.003 | -0.009 | -0.010 | -0.011 |
| 42 | 0.010 | 0.009 | 0.009 | 0.002 | 0.002 | 0.002 | -0.012 | -0.012 | -0.012 |
| 49 | 0.002 | 0.002 | 0.003 | -0.006 | -0.005 | -0.005 | -0.020 | -0.020 | -0.020 |

* defined in Table 10.6
** CA = 0; DM5 = 0; COC = 1; FAT = 1; MZ =0.632

The mean feed conversion responses are +0.007 for Bird A and -0.010 for Bird B as would be expected. Age has an interesting influence on the response pattern at 14 through 49 days. Early mean response in young birds falls to no response at 17 and 32 days for Birds A and B respectively. Thereafter there is an indication of feed conversion improvement in both types beyond 42 days. This may also be held to indicate different mechanisms of response to phytase in starter birds and in birds produced to heavy slaughter weights.

The Table 10.4 models can also be used to calculate FCReff responses for maize versus other cereal-based rations and for feed with and without an anticoccidial. For the performance levels tested in Tables 10.5 and 10.7, maize base is inferior by 2-3 points and the presence of an anticoccidial in the diet improves FCR by 3-6 points.

In the average phytase test condition scenario, the mean FCReff for birds in cages and on the floor differs by less than 1 point. For older birds of 35-49 days there is no difference between cage and floor responses for 625-2500u/kg. But for tests on day-olds for short durations to 14 and 21 days the use of caged versus floor-reared birds is predicted to enhance FCReff by 6 and 2 points respectively.

The mean effect of phytase on broiler mortality in 33 test reports is a sizeable reduction from MORTC = 19.3% to MORT = 5.8%, mainly in those tests on low dietary phosphorus (3.8-5.2g/kg).

## Discussion of results

The opinion expressed by Yan (2001) in a recent comprehensive literature review of nutritional strategies to reduce phosphorus excretion 'that it remains a controversial subject whether phytase can improve feed conversion ratio of broilers' is reflected in the results of the current study of 296 controlled feeding tests. Microbial phytase has improved feed conversion ratio by an average of only 1.4% as against a mean value of 5.0% in 1,553 tests on other exogenous enzymes in broilers, consequent on the disparate effects on feed intake of 5.8 and 0.5% respectively. The coefficient of variation of phytase feed conversion ratio effects of 2.9 is more than double that of 1.3 for the other enzymes group.

Current phytase recommended dosages of 500-750u/kg are geared towards the reduction of phosphorus excretion. In contrast it is quite evident herein that the improvement of nutritive value by phytase would be markedly enhanced by the use of substantially higher dosages, up to at least 2500u/kg.

The phytase models in Table 10.4 can be used to quantify the increase in dosage required to offset a reduction in response at a given dosage, resulting from the improvement of broiler performance over the years. There is a need too to re-appraise dosages relating to the cereal base composition of broiler diets, illustrated herein by the mean 2-3 point inferior feed conversion effect of phytase in maize-soy diets. In a direct comparison, Wu, Ravindran, Morel, Thomas, Camden and Hendriks (2001) found a 1.5 point better feed conversion response in wheat- versus maize-diets in males to 21 days post-hatching. Another aspect worthy of more detailed study is the influence of individual anticoccidials on the efficacy of phytase in broilers.

The biphasic pattern in starter and slaughter birds of feed conversion response to phytase revealed herein requires more detailed investigation, including dose-titrations to ascertain optimal dosages. At constant dosages the initial improvement in starter birds fades rapidly to little or no response at ages of 35-42 days, beyond which response returns in heavier-weight birds. This course of events was seen in practical feeding tests by Scheideler and Ferket (2000) from day-old to market ages of 49 and 63 days. In females the feed conversion response to 500u/kg changed from -0.02 at 21 days to +0.01 and 0 at 35 and 49 days respectively. In males fed normal, moderate and low phosphorus diets the mean feed conversion improvements at 21, 42 and 63 days averaged -0.019, -0.007 and -0.071, while phytase also improved liveability and decreased tibial dyschondroplasia. A second example is found in the studies of Yan *et al.* (2000) using both normal and reduced dietary phosphorus. Mean responses to 1000u/kg of phytase were -0.013 at 21 days, +0.035 at 42 days and -0.095 at 56 days with respective mortality effects of +0.1, -3.3 and -9.9%. It will be of considerable interest to determine whether the early and late responses reside in phosphorus insufficiency or in that of other limiting nutrients. It is noteworthy in this connection that at present the rationale for protein-associated responses to added phytase remains largely speculative, according to Selle *et al.* (2000).

The feed intake and live-weight gain effect models (Table 10.4) have counteractive logarithmic dosage terms in phytase and phosphorus. Bearing in mind the wide range of P equivalency phytase values of 500-1100 (Yan, 2001), these highly-significant logarithmic terms in the regressions confirm that P equivalences determined in the linear or near-linear segment of the P dose-response function are not quantitatively suitable for use in other situations closer to nutritional practice. This strengthens the observation of Yan (2001) that P equivalency values are not suitable as at present propounded and operated. Yan (2001) also advocates the need for expansion of research under more practical conditions so that animal performance will not be sacrificed when P equivalences are used in diet formulation. This need is strongly supported by the comparisons herein of the efficacy of phytase in research and practical situations. The partial regression coefficients in these phytase models could provide first-aid for the adjustment of equivalences, until the large scientific literature resource of P equivalence measurements has been comprehensively re-analysed to provide significant best-fit regressions of phytase equivalence on dietary P content for live-weight gain, feed conversion ratio, bone characteristics and of course P excretion.

Improved efficiency in the use of phytase in broiler nutrition would be facilitated by the separation of the distinctive requirements and economic values of the two different endpoints of lower phosphorus excretion and enhanced nutritive value. Closely-related topics for future research are inherent in recent trends advocating admixture in practice of phytase with NSP enzymes plus the debate about the role of NSP enzyme side-activities in phytase preparations. Routine 2 x 2 or larger factorial feeding tests on phytase are required on the importance and possible overlap of admixture and of side-activities, in which trials to slaughter weight would be definitive. Such studies would also contribute to a better definition of broiler phosphorus requirements. In summary, two questions may be posed. Do 'nutrient release', ileal digestibility, or other partial metabolic indicators accurately predict net results, reflecting nutritive values? Can one expect coincident nutritional responses to phosphorus, lysine, protein and energy in a given diet or should this tetrad be accorded successive attention in step-wise elimination of individual limiting nutrient insufficiencies?

For the future, the next phase of multifactorial analyses of phytase in broilers will encompass the investigation of further independent variables, e.g. dietary calcium, lysine, sulphur amino acids, energy, nitrogen, etc.; tests for interactions of independent variables; comparisons of the bioefficacy of different phytase sources; and expansion of the data base to include material from 175 more recent publications (1999-2001). A brief survey of the latter's areas of investigation, test objectives, methodology and nutritional responses reveals similarities with the existent data base. Nonetheless, revision and updating of the partial regression coefficients to represent a larger resource and the search for further significant independent variables could well be advantageous.

Finally, there is a need to investigate why, in the multi-factorial analysis of phytase to date, so-called available (non-phytate) P has proved to be less often significant than total P. The need to clarify available phosphorus terminology has recently been emphasised by Angel and Applegate (2001). The emergence of an agreed unified definition for available phosphorus would be invaluable. Alternatively, net phosphorus utilisation may have to be deployed in order to facilitate the revision of phosphorus requirements in broilers with and without exogenous phytase.

## Conclusion

The user of phytase in broiler feed formulation is faced with a perplexing set of uncertainties in the overlap of pro-nutrient and pollution abatement objectives, with their bifocal endpoints exacerbated as they are by sizeable variations in response. Comprehensive multifactorial analysis of 296 phytase feeding tests has provided nutritional models to facilitate the optimisation of dosage for enhanced nutritive value in practice; to assist in feeding test design; and to suggest promising avenues for future research. Much remains to be discovered about phytase products in order to balance its practical application with phosphorus ingredient qualities, with genetic advances and with new sources of vitamin D and therewith to specify appropriate phosphorus and phytase dosage pairs to meet, as yet to be defined, optimal phosphorus requirements for broiler production.

Key topics for discussion include: the use of dosage partial regression coefficients to adjust P equivalences for praxis; individual versus simultaneous use of nutrient matrix values; the bioefficacies of different phytases; phytase side-activities; phytase admixtures with NSP and/or other enzyme products; future research requirements and interactions of (a) plant, animal and mineral sources of P, (b) phytase posology, (c) genetically-modified improved raw materials, (d) vitamin D and (e) revised broiler P requirements.

## References

Angel, R. and Applegate, T. (2001) Phytase use - what do we know? In *Proceedings of the 62nd Minnesota Nutrition Conference*, September 11-12, 2001. pp. 250-263. Bloomington MN.

BASF (2000) Nutrients released, economic benefits and ration formulation with phytase. In *BASF Technical Symposium 2000 Series DC0001: Natuphos phytase: validation of phosphorus, amino acids and energy matrix values in poultry and swine*. pp. 121-155. BASF Corporation, Mount Olive, NJ.

Draper, N.R. and Smith, H. (1981) *Applied Regression Analysis, Second Edition*. John Wiley and Sons, Inc., New York.

European Commission. (2000) Opinion of the SCAN on the use of enzymatic product Natuphos[R] 5000 (3-phytase; EC 3.1.3.8) as feed additive (adopted on 27 April 2000).

Kies, A.K., Van Hemert, K.H.F. and Sauer, W.S. (2001) Effect of phytase on protein and amino acid digestibility and energy utilisation. *World's Poultry Science Journal*, **57**, 109-126.

Nelson, T.S., Shieh, T.R., Wodzinski, R.J. and Ware, J.H. (1971) Effect of supplemental phytase on the utilization of phytate phosphorus by chicks. *Journal of Nutrition*, **101**, 1289-1294.

Nie, N.H., Hadlai-Hull, C., Jenkins, J.G., Steinbrenner, K. and Bent, B.H. (1975) *Statistical Package for the Social Sciences. Second Edition*. McGraw Hill Book Company, New York.

Pallauf, J. and Rimbach, P. (1999) Effect of supplemental phytase on mineral and trace element bioavailability and heavy metal accumulation in pigs with different type of diets. In *Phytase in Animal Nutrition and Waste Management*, BASF Reference Manual DC9601. Second Revised Edition, 1999. Edited by M.B. Coelho and E.T. Kornegay, BASF, Mount Olive, NJ.

Rosen, G.D. (1995) Antibacterials in Poultry and Pig Nutrition. In *Biotechnology in Animal Feeds and Animal Feeding*. pp.143-172. Edited by R.J. Wallace and A. Chesson. VCH Verlagsgesellschaft mbH, D-69451 Weinheim.

Rosen, G.D. (2000a) Multifactorial assessment of exogenous enzymes in broiler pronutrition: targets and problems. p11. In *Abstracts of Lectures and Posters of the 3rd European Symposium on Feed Enzymes*, Noordwijkerhout, 8-10 May 2000.

Rosen, G.D. (2000b) Enzymes for broilers: a multi-factorial assessment. *Feed International*, **21(12)**, 14-18.

Scheideler, S.E. and Ferket, P.R. (2000) Phytase in broiler rations - effects on carcass yields and incidence of tibial dischondroplasia. *Journal of Applied Poultry Research*, **9**, 468-475.

Selle, P.H., Ravindran, V., Caldwell, R.A. and Bryden, W.L. (2000) Phytate and phytase: consequences for protein utilisation. *Nutrition Research Reviews*, **13(2)**, 255-278.

Wu, Y.B., Ravindran, V., Morel, P.C.H., Thomas, D.V., Camden, B.J. and Hendriks, W.H. (2001) Evaluation of microbial phytase in broiler diets. pp. 54-60. In *Advancing Poultry Production,* Massey Technical Update Seminar, Palmerston North, July 2001. Edited by V. Ravindran. Massey University, New Zealand.

Yan, F. (2001) Nutritional strategies to reduce phosphorus excretion by broilers. PhD dissertation, University of Arkansas, Fayetteville, AR.

Yan, F., Kersey, J.H., Fritz, C.A., Waldroup, P.W., Stilborn, H.L., Crumb Jr., R.C., Rice, D.W. and Raboy, V. (2000) Evaluation of normal yellow dent corn and high available phosphorus corn in combination with reduced dietary phosphorus and phytase supplementation for broilers grown to market weights in litter pens. *Poultry Science*, **79(9)**, 1282-1289.

*This paper was first published in 2002*

11

# HIGH-ENERGY DIETS FOR POULTRY - EFFECTS OF DIET COMPOSITION ON PERFORMANCE AND CARCASS QUALITY

JULIAN WISEMAN
*University of Nottingham, Sutton Bonington Campus, Loughborough, Leics LE12 5RD*

## Introduction

It is widely recognised that performance and carcass quality of broilers is influenced considerably by variations in energy and nutrient inputs during growth. However, addition of fats to diets to achieve required levels of apparent metabolisable energy (AME), together with high dietary levels of AME *per se*, may promote excess lipid accretion in fast-growing broiler chickens fed under *ad libitum* conditions. The consequences of such high levels of body fat relate both to evisceration losses and to the fat content of saleable meat. These have been the subject of many previous investigations examining the effects of nutrition, in particular manipulation of the energy:protein ratio (E:P), on carcass quality (e.g. Bartov *et al.* 1974a). It is generally considered that AME cannot be regarded in isolation from E:P. This chapter will discuss, initially, the consequences of changing E:P (under a variety of circumstances) for performance and carcass characteristics, although a consideration of protein quality is outside the scope of this discussion. Similarly, discussion of actual AME values of high-energy ingredients may be found elsewhere (e.g. Wiseman, 2001 for fats; Short *et a*l 1999; Wiseman 2000; Wiseman *et al* 2000, for wheat, which is the major energy-yielding commodity for poultry diets in much of Europe and other regions of the World).

Maintaining fat deposition at acceptable levels, whilst producing chicken meat economically from current commercial strains of broiler chickens, will be a compromise between achieving a satisfactory carcass and realising the potential of the bird for maximum live-weight gain. However, fat deposition is an integral part of broiler growth and its extent and distribution throughout the carcass is an important aspect of meat quality. Hakansson *et al.* (1978*a,b*) examined the distribution of lipid in tissues within broiler carcasses, as influenced by dietary nutrient concentration and age, but no data for individual fat depots were reported.

A subsequent area that will be considered is 'catch-up' growth. It has been suggested that feed (and dietary energy) restriction early in the life of the broiler, followed by a refeeding period, may improve efficiency of feed utilization and reduce fat content of the carcass (Kubena *et al.,* 1974; Plavnik & Hurwitz 1985; Jones & Farrell 1992*a*), although it is likely that this response might be accompanied by a smaller finisher body weight (Jones and Wiseman 1985). Such early feed restriction has been considered in the context of prevention of metabolic diseases (e.g. ascites) associated with growth rates that are too rapid. Other studies have failed to confirm this catch-up following early feed restriction (Deaton *et al.,* 1973; Griffiths *et al.,* 1977). Susbilla *et al.* (1994) demonstrated that early feed restriction did improve subsequent growth rate, although no differences were observed for feed conversion ratio and carcass fat content; Jones and Farrell (1992*b*) examined body fat growth. However, the majority of these studies have tended to consider the consequences of diet changes at one point in time (slaughter) rather than over time up to slaughter, although Susbilla *et al.* (1994) examined the growth pattern of internal organs.

There has been considerable interest recently in the manipulation of fatty acid profiles of broiler meat (e.g. see review by Leskanich and Noble, 1997). Notwithstanding the current trend (at least in the UK) for dietary fat levels to be reduced (in favour of increasing cereal starch so as to maintain overall AME), change in carcass fatty acids, in response to dietary changes, is an important area for study. It allows accurate dietary regimes to be developed to produce carcasses with a specific fatty acid profile.

Developments in carcass quality are generally assuming greater importance as broiler meat markets in many regions move from a volume-dominated to a quality- controlled position.

## Effect of E:P on performance and carcass quality

Maximisation of lean-tissue growth rate is one of the fundamental objectives of any meat-producing animal enterprise. Lean-tissue (muscle) accretion is an energy-demanding process, which suggests that dietary protein (P - assumed to be of optimum quality) inputs can only result in lean tissue gain if there is adequate dietary energy (E) intake. E:P may be altered by varying E at constant P, maintaining E and varying P or by altering both simultaneously.

Narrowing E:P by reducing AME whilst maintaining P (quantitatively and qualitatively) was studied (Trial 1 - Jones and Wiseman, 1985; Trial 2 - University of Nottingham unpublished data) as the literature appeared to offer conflicting evidence on the effect of this variable during starter (0 to 23 days of age) and finisher (24 to 49 days of age) time periods. For example, Griffiths *et al.* (1977) concluded that the starter regime imposed had no effect on abdominal fat pad (AFP) weight at eight weeks of age, in contrast to the observations of Kubena *et al.* (1974) and March and Hansen (1977). The AFP is commonly employed as an indicator of total carcass fat content; correlations between the two are usually high.

Trial 1 was based on constant P at varying E and the second (Trial 2) employed varying P at constant E. Dietary regimes are presented in Tables 11.1A and 11.1B respectively. The transfer between starter and finisher diets was at 23 days of age. Performance, together with basic carcass responses from Trial 1 are presented in Table 11.2A. The data indicate that a low-energy starter diet was associated with less carcass fat at 24 days of age and that this effect persisted until slaughter at 49 days of age. However, this was associated with a smaller bird and a poorer feed conversion ratio. Consequently, an economic appraisal of such a regime would not favour any approach that compromised the two major performance indicators, which are rate and efficiency of live-weight gain. Nevertheless, if financial incentives for carcass quality were introduced, as in other livestock production systems, then modifying carcass fat content may be an attractive proposition.

**Table 11.1A** DIETARY REGIMES EMPLOYED IN TRIAL 1 (JONES AND WISEMAN, 1985)

| | *AME levels (CP constant)* | | | | | |
|---|---|---|---|---|---|---|
| *Diet* | *L* | | *M* | | *H* | |
| | *AME (MJ/kg)* | *CP (g/kg)* | *AME (MJ/kg)* | *CP (g/kg)* | *AME (MJ/kg)* | *CP (g/kg)* |
| 0 - 23 d | | | | | | |
| Starter | 10.78 | 230 | 12.78 | 230 | 14.78 | 230 |
| E:P (kJ AME/g CP) | 46.9 | | 55.6 | | 64.3 | |
| 24 - 49d | | | | | | |
| Finisher | 10.78 | 200 | 12.78 | 200 | 14.78 | 200 |
| E:P (kJ AME/g CP) | 53.9 | | 63.9 | | 73.9 | |

**Table 11.1B** DIETARY REGIMES EMPLOYED IN TRIAL 2 (UNIVERSITY OF NOTTINGHAM, UNPUBLISHED DATA)

| *Diet* | *CP levels (AME constant)* L | | M | | H | |
|---|---|---|---|---|---|---|
| | *AME (MJ/kg)* | *CP (g/kg)* | *AME (MJ/kg)* | *CP (g/kg)* | *AME (MJ/kg)* | *CP (g/kg)* |
| 0 - 23 d | | | | | | |
| Starter | 12.75 | 190 | 12.75 | 230 | 12.75 | 270 |
| E:P (kJ AME/g CP) | 67.1 | | 55.4 | | 47.2 | |
| 24 - 49d | | | | | | |
| Finisher | 12.75 | 170 | 12.75 | 203 | 12.75 | 235 |
| E:P (kJ AME/g CP) | 75.0 | | 62.8 | | 54.3 | |

**Table 11.2A** SELECTED PERFORMANCE AND CARCASS DATA FROM TRIAL 1 - L, M AND H REFER RESPECTIVELY TO DIETARY LEVELS OF AME (FROM JONES AND WISEMAN, 1985)

| *Starter* | | *FI (kg/b)* | *LWG (kg/b)* | | | *FCR Period* | *Overall* | |
|---|---|---|---|---|---|---|---|---|
| L | | 1.09 | 0.50 | | | 2.180 | | |
| M | | 1.11 | 0.63 | | | 1.762 | | |
| H | | 1.09 | 0.73 | | | 1.493 | | |
| | *Finisher* | *FI (kg/b) Period* | *LWG (kg/b) Period* | *LWG (kg/b) 0 - 49d* | *FI (kg/b) 0 - 49d* | | | *Carcass Fat (g/kg DM)* |
| | L | 4.17 | 1.48 | 1.98 | 5.26 | 2.818 | 2.657 | 326 |
| L | M | 3.52 | 1.58 | 2.08 | 4.61 | 2.228 | 2.216 | 362 |
| | H | 3.29 | 1.68 | 2.18 | 4.38 | 1.958 | 2.009 | 399 |
| | L | 4.11 | 1.62 | 2.25 | 5.22 | 2.537 | 2.320 | 364 |
| M | M | 4.16 | 1.68 | 2.31 | 5.27 | 2.476 | 2.281 | 387 |
| | H | 3.49 | 1.72 | 2.35 | 4.6 | 2.029 | 1.957 | 412 |
| | L | 4.08 | 1.51 | 2.24 | 5.17 | 2.702 | 2.308 | 379 |
| H | M | 4.27 | 1.52 | 2.25 | 5.36 | 2.809 | 2.382 | 403 |
| | H | 3.73 | 1.65 | 2.38 | 4.82 | 2.261 | 2.025 | 438 |

**TABLE 11.2B** SELECTED PERFORMANCE AND CARCASS DATA FROM TRIAL 2 - L, M AND H REFER RESPECTIVELY TO DIETARY LEVELS OF CP (UNIVERSITY OF NOTTINGHAM, UNPUBLISHED DATA)

| *Starter* | | *FI (kg/b)* | *LWG (kg/b)* | | | *FCR Period* | *FCR Overall* | |
|---|---|---|---|---|---|---|---|---|
| L | | 1.30 | 0.64 | | | | 2.031 | |
| M | | 1.28 | 0.74 | | | | 1.730 | |
| H | | 1.29 | 0.82 | | | | 1.573 | |
| | *Finisher* | *FI (kg/b) Period* | *LWG (kg/b) Period* | *LWG (kg/b) 0 - 49d* | *FI (kg/b) 0 - 49d* | | | *Carcass Fat (g/kg DM)* |
| | L | 3.24 | 1.32 | 1.96 | 4.54 | 2.455 | 2.316 | 362 |
| L | M | 3.03 | 1.26 | 1.90 | 4.33 | 2.405 | 2.279 | 346 |
| | H | 3.53 | 1.31 | 1.95 | 4.83 | 2.695 | 2.477 | 346 |
| | L | 3.47 | 1.27 | 2.01 | 4.75 | 2.732 | 2.363 | 384 |
| M | M | 3.45 | 1.34 | 2.08 | 4.73 | 2.575 | 2.274 | 303 |
| | H | 3.63 | 1.46 | 2.20 | 4.91 | 2.486 | 2.232 | 320 |
| | L | 3.7 | 1.25 | 2.07 | 4.99 | 2.960 | 2.411 | 368 |
| H | M | 3.78 | 1.36 | 2.18 | 5.07 | 2.779 | 2.326 | 335 |
| | H | 3.29 | 1.25 | 2.07 | 4.58 | 2.632 | 2.213 | 281 |

Differences between treatments in Trial 2 were also important. Although dietary protein affected performance, in terms of live-weight gain and food conversion ratio, there was a suggestion that the very high protein diet was used less efficiently. This implies that the excess protein was catabolized rather than contributing to increased lean-tissue deposition. Interestingly, this response was associated with a reduction in carcass fat, suggesting that dietary energy was used in catabolism of excess protein rather than being deposited as fat. This therefore represents a further means of altering carcass quality, although feeding high (supra-optimal) protein diets would be associated with increased nitrogen excretion (which would have serious environmental consequences) and may be metabolically challenging to the bird as it attempts to accommodate excessive protein degradation.

The consequences of changing nutrient regimes can also be viewed over time following modelling of data. Table 11.3 presents data from a programme in which three starter diets were fed from 0 to21days of age, all with E:P of 57.2 (achieved by varying both E, MJ/kg, and P, g/kg; 11.39/199, 12.77/224, 14.15/248 for H, C and L respectively) and three finisher diets were fed from 22 to 70 days of age, with E:P of 64.8 (11.85/183, 13.07/202, 14.29/220 for

**Table 11.3** ESTIMATES OF TIME (d) TO REACH SPECIFIC LIVE WEIGHT (g) AND WEIGHT OF CARCASS COMPONENTS (g) AT THIS LIVE WEIGHT

| *Diet* | *Live weight (g)* | | | | | | | | |
|---|---|---|---|---|---|---|---|---|---|
| | *1000* | *1250* | *1500* | *1750* | *2000* | *2250* | *2500* | *2750* | *3000* |
| Time to reach Live weight (d) | | | | | | | | | |
| HH* | 24 | 29 | 32 | 35 | 39 | 42 | 46 | 50 | 55 |
| HL | 27 | 32 | 36 | 40 | 44 | 47 | 52 | 56 | 61 |
| CC | 27 | 31 | 35 | 38 | 42 | 46 | 49 | 53 | 58 |
| LH | 30 | 33 | 36 | 39 | 43 | 46 | 49 | 53 | 57 |
| LL | 32 | 36 | 40 | 44 | 48 | 53 | 57 | 61 | 66 |
| Carcass Component | | | | | | | | | |
| Carcass Protein (g) | | | | | | | | | |
| HH | 166 | 214 | 264 | 314 | 365 | 417 | 469 | 521 | 573 |
| HL | 170 | 226 | 284 | 342 | 400 | 456 | 510 | 563 | 612 |
| CC | 178 | 230 | 282 | 334 | 385 | 436 | 484 | 532 | 577 |
| LH | 171 | 225 | 279 | 333 | 386 | 438 | 488 | 536 | 581 |
| LL | 181 | 239 | 296 | 350 | 402 | 451 | 497 | 538 | 577 |
| Carcass Fat (g) | | | | | | | | | |
| HH | 93 | 124 | 159 | 198 | 240 | 286 | 337 | 394 | 456 |
| HL | 82 | 113 | 147 | 181 | 217 | 252 | 288 | 322 | 355 |
| CC | 88 | 121 | 158 | 196 | 238 | 277 | 317 | 358 | 399 |
| LH | 97 | 134 | 174 | 217 | 262 | 309 | 359 | 410 | 463 |
| LL | 82 | 106 | 131 | 159 | 189 | 222 | 258 | 299 | 345 |

H, C and L respectively. This gave five treatment combinations - HH, HL, CC, LH and LL. Representative birds were slaughtered at regular intervals, allowing assessment of responses through use of the Gompertz equation (Wiseman and Lewis 1999). Performance (in terms of time taken to reach a specific live weight) was influenced considerably by diet, as was carcass composition (in terms of fat and protein content)

## CONTROL OF FEED INTAKE

In the studies of Leeson *et al* (1996a and b) conflicting evidence was presented on the ability of the broiler to compensate feed intake for differing dietary AME concentrations. Whilst feed intake increased with decreasing AME concentration, intake of AME (MJ over the experimental period studied; 35-49d ) was reduced (from 35.3 to 28.0 MJ and from 34.7 to 28.8MJ) irrespective of E:P (Leeson *et al* 1996a). Intake of AME actually increased when the experimental period was 0-49d (Leeson *et al* 1996b). Bartov (1998) subsequently observed that increasing dietary AME had no effect on feed intake but, consequently, was associated with an increase in AME intake (54.4 to 58MJ) over the experimental period (from 7-49d). The hypothesis that the bird is able to control its energy intake is therefore not tenable.

General observations (see Table 11.4) tend to support the principle of a modest control of feed intake (to an extent determined by many factors, including E:P), but this 'compensatory mechanism' is insufficient, so increasing dietary AME concentration is associated with increasing AME intake.

**TABLE 11.4** INFLUENCE OF DIETARY AME (MJ/KG) ON FEED INTAKE (FI, KG/BIRD) AND AME INTAKE (MJ/BIRD)

Data are from:

T1 Jones and Wiseman, 1985; T2 University of Nottingham, unpublished data; T3 Wiseman and Lewis, 1999

| | *FI (kg.bird)* | *AME (MJ/kg)* | *AME consumed (MJ/bird)* |
|---|---|---|---|
| T1 | 4.17 | 10.78 | 45.0 |
| | 3.52 | 12.78 | 45.0 |
| | 3.29 | 14.78 | 48.6 |
| | 4.11 | 10.78 | 44.3 |
| | 4.16 | 12.78 | 53.2 |
| | 3.49 | 14.78 | 51.6 |
| | 4.08 | 10.78 | 44.0 |
| | 4.27 | 12.78 | 54.6 |
| | 3.73 | 14.78 | 55.1 |
| T2 | 3.24 | 12.75 | 41.3 |
| | 3.03 | 12.75 | 38.6 |
| | 3.53 | 12.75 | 45.0 |
| | 3.47 | 12.75 | 44.2 |
| | 3.45 | 12.75 | 44.0 |
| | 3.63 | 12.75 | 46.3 |
| | 3.70 | 12.75 | 47.8 |
| | 3.78 | 12.75 | 48.2 |
| | 3.29 | 12.75 | 41.9 |
| T3 | 3.74 | 14.29 | 53.4 |
| | 3.76 | 11.85 | 44.5 |
| | 3.49 | 13.07 | 45.7 |
| | 3.59 | 14.29 | 51.2 |
| | 3.69 | 11.85 | 43.7 |

## COMPENSATORY GROWTH RATE

Data from HH and LH (Wiseman and Lewis, 1999) were used to examine the effects of early feeding of diets with low nutrient and energy concentration, followed by a return to a more adequate diet, on the ability of birds thus treated to achieve rates of performance comparable with those fed adequately throughout. Gompertz values for 'M' (the age in days at which growth is maximum) were 33.3 and 38.0 for HH and LH respectively, indicating that maximum growth rate was achieved earlier on the HH treatment. Similarly, A + C (asymptote) values (which represent mature weight) were higher for HH (4.40 kg) than for LH (4.15 kg), suggesting a more persistent growth rate. Whilst these data and analyses suggest that HH birds were always heavier than LH, these differences became progressively smaller with increasing age. Rogers *et al.* (1987), with a more acute restriction of early feed, also observed that Gompertz asymptote values were always below those of the control group. These observations on the influence of dietary treatment support conclusions on time taken to reach specific live weights (as presented in Table 11.3).

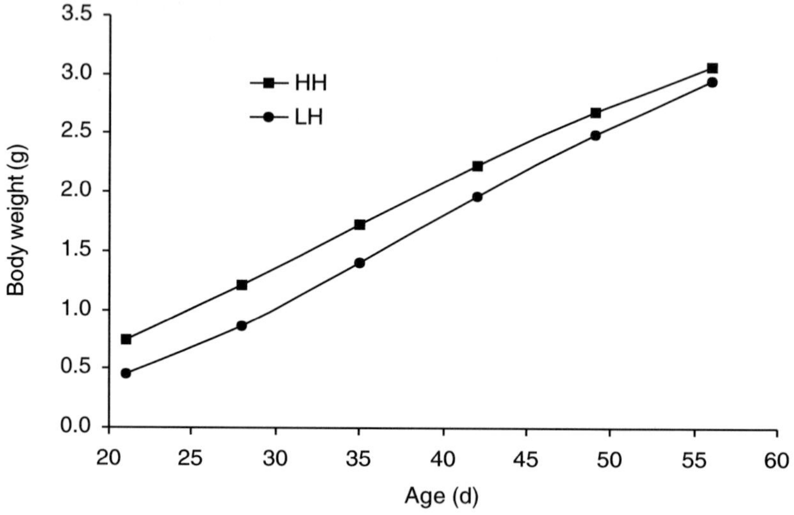


**Figure 11.1** Comparison between fully fed (HH) and early-feed restriction followed by re-alimentation (LH) on broiler growth (from Wiseman and Lewis, 1999)

Early feed restriction in broilers has been investigated because of the possible reductions in body fat, but not overall body weight, that might result. There was the suggestion (Wiseman and Lewis, 1999) that LH birds gradually approached the live weight of HH (see Figure 11.1), a response that was associated with increasing feed intake by LH (but which did not reach that of HH). Comparisons between treatments for carcass protein and fat content require separation on the basis of whether time or live weight is the independent variable. LH birds had slightly higher carcass protein and fat contents when comparisons were at the same live weight (Figure 11.2); on the basis of time (Figure 11.3) carcass fat and protein contents for LH approached, but did not reach, those for HH.

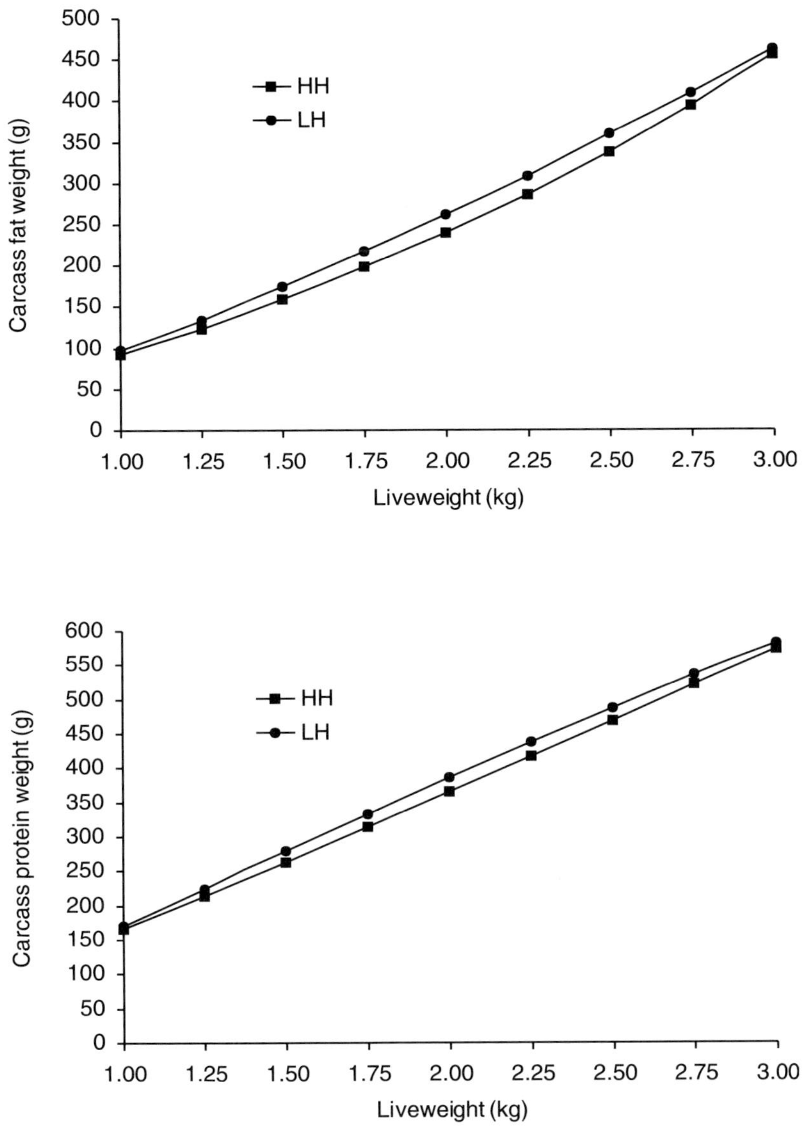


**Figure 11.2.** Comparison between fully fed (HH) and early-feed restriction followed by re-alimentation (LH) on composition of live weight in broilers based on live weight (from Wiseman and Lewis, 1999)

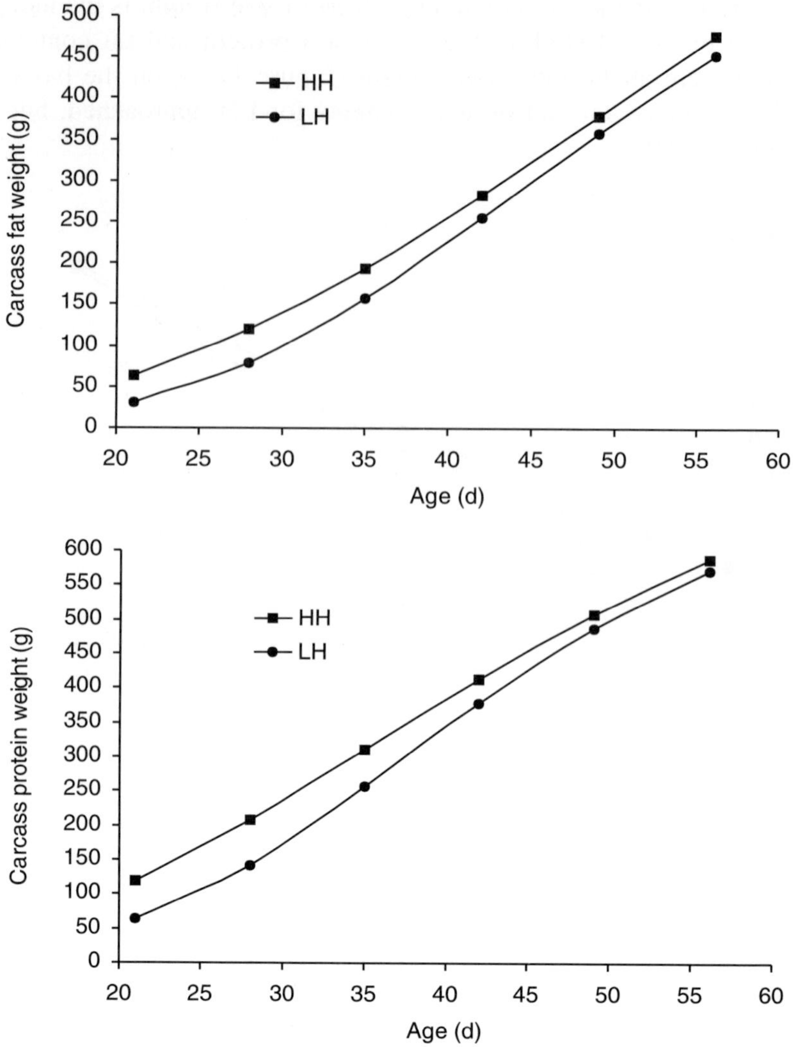


**Figure 11.3.** Comparison between fully fed (HH) and early-feed restriction followed by re-alimentation (LH) on composition of live weight in broilers based on time (from Wiseman and Lewis, 1999)

Plavnik & Hurwitz (1985) observed that there was a lower proportion of abdominal fat (the depot most often employed to characterize overall fatness of broilers) following early feed restriction, which may also have contributed to the better feed efficiency of these birds. It was further argued that reduced fatness was attributable to impaired hyperplasia of adipocytes (as observed by March & Hensen, 1976). Jones & Farrell (1992b) concluded that the success of early feed restriction in reducing carcass fat (but no other component) was attributable to a temporary delay in fat deposition. However, the older the birds, the greater the likelihood that this advantage would disappear. The results of the study of Wiseman and Lewis (1999) support this latter observation, although LH birds were always fatter at a given weight than HH when total fat content was considered. However there was variation with individual fat depots where LH birds were less fat. This suggests differential responsiveness of individual fat depots to nutrient and energy intake. Hargis and Creger (1980) reduced nutrient and energy intake for the first 7 days of life whereas Arafa *et al.* (1983) reduced energy intake during the last 10 days of the growth period following a commercial starter. Both studies reported a reduction in carcass fat at 49 days of age.

The ability of birds to compensate for early nutrient and energy restriction in terms of lean tissue weights is, according to Jones & Farrell (1992b) dependent upon the severity of this restriction. Susbilla *et al.* (1994) observed that the weight of breast and thighs at 40d of age was not influenced by feed restriction. It is likely that the study of Wiseman and Lewis (1999) was more severe in this context as the content of white (i.e. breast) muscles from birds fed HH was always, albeit marginally, greater at the same live weight than birds fed on LH. The effect of feeding diets of low energy and nutrient content early in life was different when considering dark meat, where the small differences recorded were in favour of LH, particularly at higher weights.

## LIPID:PROTEIN RATIOS

The composition of lipids is considerably more variable than that of other components in broilers. Whilst there may be a genetic maximum body lipid composition, the level of this component is subject to a number of variables; those associated with diet are essentially the provision of dietary energy relative to the bird's energy and nutrient (specifically protein / amino acid) requirements. Thus, if protein accretion is at a genetic maximum, additional dietary energy supplied beyond the requirement to support such accretion will result in increased lipid deposition. Conversely, energy intake below requirement will risk lipid catabolism and a consequent reduction in lipid content (a further complication is the dietary E:P as considered earlier). Lipid:protein ratios have been employed to separate genotypes (e.g. Hancock *et al* 1995) which would, accordingly, require different energy and nutrient regimes in order for them to grow optimally. In the study of Wiseman and Lewis (1999), lipid:protein ratios ranged from 1.27, 0.62, 0.78, 1.02 to 1.65 respectively for HH, HL, C, LH and LL diet combinations which is further demonstration of the significant influence of diet on carcass composition. Changes in lipid:protein ratios, as influenced by diet within the same genotype, are presented in Table 11.5 (on the basis of either live weight or time).

**Table 11.5** CARCASS LIPID:PROTEIN RATIOS (WISEMAN AND LEWIS, 1999)

a. At specific live weight

| *Live weight (g)* | *Diet Combinations* | | | | |
|---|---|---|---|---|---|
| | *HH* | *HL* | *C* | *LH* | *LL* |
| 1000 | 0.56 | 0.48 | 0.49 | 0.57 | 0.45 |
| 1250 | 0.58 | 0.50 | 0.53 | 0.60 | 0.44 |
| 1500 | 0.60 | 0.52 | 0.56 | 0.62 | 0.44 |
| 1750 | 0.63 | 0.53 | 0.59 | 0.65 | 0.45 |
| 2000 | 0.66 | 0.54 | 0.61 | 0.68 | 0.47 |
| 2250 | 0.69 | 0.55 | 0.64 | 0.71 | 0.49 |
| 2500 | 0.72 | 0.56 | 0.66 | 0.73 | 0.52 |
| 2750 | 0.76 | 0.57 | 0.67 | 0.77 | 0.55 |
| 3000 | 0.80 | 0.58 | 0.69 | 0.80 | 0.60 |

b. At specific time

| *Time (d)* | *Diet Combinations* | | | | |
|---|---|---|---|---|---|
| | *HH* | *HL* | *C* | *LH* | *LL* |
| 21 | 0.54 | 0.46 | 0.44 | 0.48 | 0.54 |
| 28 | 0.58 | 0.49 | 0.50 | 0.55 | 0.47 |
| 35 | 0.63 | 0.51 | 0.56 | 0.61 | 0.45 |
| 42 | 0.68 | 0.54 | 0.61 | 0.67 | 0.45 |
| 49 | 0.75 | 0.56 | 0.65 | 0.73 | 0.47 |
| 56 | 0.81 | 0.57 | 0.68 | 0.79 | 0.51 |

## EFFICIENCY OF USE OF AME FOR GAIN

It is evident from the three Nottingham trials reported that there are major differences between diets in terms of both growth performance and carcass quality. However, although food conversion ratios were also influenced by diet, it remains to be established whether the efficiency of utilisation of AME varied between treatments.

Accordingly, data were analysed further by regressing AME intake on weight gain to derive the efficiency of utilisation of dietary energy (e.g. g weight gain / MJ AME consumed) and results are presented in Table 11.6A, 11.6B and 11.6C respectively for Trials 1, 2 and 3.

**Table 11.6A** FEED INTAKE AND EFFICIENCY OF UTILISATION OF AME FOR GROWTH (TRIAL 1, FROM JONES AND WISEMAN, 1985)

| *Starter* | *Diet* | *Food Intake kg/bird* | *Calculated AME MJ/kg as fed* | *AME intake* | *Efficiency of AME utilisation - lwt gain (g) / AME intake (MJ)** |
|---|---|---|---|---|---|
| | L | 1.09 | 10.78 | 11.75 | 42.6 |
| | M | 1.11 | 12.78 | 14.19 | 44.4 |
| | H | 1.09 | 14.78 | 16.11 | 45.3 |
| Finisher | | | | | |
| L | L | 4.17 | 10.78 | 44.95 | 32.9 |
| | M | 3.52 | 12.78 | 44.99 | 35.1 |
| | H | 3.29 | 14.78 | 48.63 | 34.5 |
| M | L | 4.11 | 10.78 | 44.31 | 36.6 |
| | M | 4.16 | 12.78 | 53.16 | 31.6 |
| | H | 3.49 | 14.78 | 51.58 | 33.3 |
| H | L | 4.08 | 10.78 | 43.98 | 34.3 |
| | M | 4.27 | 12.78 | 54.57 | 27.9 |
| | H | 3.73 | 14.78 | 55.13 | 30.0 |

* Live-weight gain presented in Table 11.2A

**Table 11.6B** FEED INTAKE AND EFFICIENCY OF UTILISATION OF AME FOR GROWTH (TRIAL 2; UNIVERSITY OF NOTTINGHAM, UNPUBLISHED DATA)

| *Starter* | *Diet* | *Food Intake kg/bird* | *Calculated AME MJ/kg as fed* | *AME intake* | *AME utilisation - lwt gain (g) / AME intake (MJ)** |
|---|---|---|---|---|---|
| | L | 1.30 | 12.75 | 16.58 | 38.6 |
| | M | 1.28 | 12.75 | 16.32 | 45.3 |
| | H | 1.29 | 12.75 | 16.48 | 50.0 |
| Finisher | | | | | |
| | L | 3.24 | 12.75 | 41.31 | 32.0 |
| L | M | 3.03 | 12.75 | 38.63 | 32.6 |
| | H | 3.53 | 12.75 | 45.08 | 29.1 |
| | L | 3.47 | 12.75 | 44.24 | 28.7 |
| M | M | 3.45 | 12.75 | 43.98 | 30.5 |
| | H | 3.63 | 12.75 | 46.28 | 31.5 |
| | L | 3.7 | 12.75 | 47.18 | 26.5 |
| H | M | 3.78 | 12.75 | 48.20 | 28.2 |
| | H | 3.29 | 12.75 | 41.95 | 29.8 |

* Live-weight gain presented in Table 11.2B

**Table 11.6C.** FEED INTAKE AND EFFICIENCY OF UTILISATION OF AME FOR GROWTH (TRIAL 3; FROM WISEMAN AND LEWIS, 1999)

| | *Cumulative:* AME intake MJ | Weight gain g | *Weekly:* AME intake MJ | Weight gain g | *Efficiency of AME utilisation for weight gain* g gain/MJ intake | Week |
|---|---|---|---|---|---|---|
| HH | 10.12 | 470 | 10.12 | 470 | 46.5 | 4 |
| | 22.78 | 983 | 12.67 | 513 | 40.5 | 5 |
| | 37.45 | 1486 | 14.66 | 503 | 34.3 | 6 |
| | 53.37 | 1940 | 15.93 | 454 | 28.5 | 7 |
| | 69.79 | 2327 | 16.42 | 387 | 23.6 | 8 |
| | 86.00 | 2643 | 16.21 | 316 | 19.5 | 9 |
| | 101.47 | 2893 | 15.46 | 250 | 16.2 | 10 |
| HL | 8.01 | 371 | 8.01 | 371 | 46.3 | 4 |
| | 18.31 | 789 | 10.30 | 418 | 40.6 | 5 |
| | 30.63 | 1227 | 12.32 | 438 | 35.5 | 6 |
| | 44.49 | 1659 | 13.86 | 432 | 31.2 | 7 |
| | 59.32 | 2066 | 14.83 | 407 | 27.4 | 8 |
| | 74.53 | 2436 | 15.21 | 369 | 24.3 | 9 |
| | 89.59 | 2762 | 15.06 | 326 | 21.6 | 10 |
| CC | 9.09 | 398 | 9.09 | 398 | 43.8 | 4 |
| | 20.19 | 851 | 11.09 | 453 | 40.8 | 5 |
| | 33.21 | 1327 | 13.02 | 475 | 36.5 | 6 |
| | 47.98 | 1793 | 14.78 | 467 | 31.6 | 7 |
| | 64.25 | 2230 | 16.27 | 436 | 26.8 | 8 |
| | 81.70 | 2622 | 17.44 | 392 | 22.5 | 9 |
| | 99.97 | 2964 | 18.27 | 342 | 18.7 | 10 |
| LH | 9.18 | 413 | 9.18 | 412 | 44.9 | 4 |
| | 21.06 | 944 | 11.88 | 531 | 44.7 | 5 |
| | 35.28 | 1511 | 14.23 | 567 | 39.9 | 6 |
| | 51.26 | 2042 | 15.98 | 531 | 33.2 | 7 |
| | 68.29 | 2496 | 17.03 | 454 | 26.7 | 8 |
| | 85.66 | 2860 | 17.37 | 364 | 21.0 | 9 |
| | 102.73 | 3139 | 17.08 | 279 | 16.3 | 10 |
| LL | 7.64 | 316 | 7.64 | 316 | 41.4 | 4 |
| | 17.61 | 704 | 9.97 | 387 | 38.9 | 5 |
| | 29.79 | 1131 | 12.19 | 427 | 35.1 | 6 |
| | 43.89 | 1566 | 14.10 | 435 | 30.9 | 7 |
| | 59.46 | 1982 | 15.57 | 416 | 26.7 | 8 |
| | 75.97 | 2361 | 16.51 | 379 | 23.0 | 9 |
| | 92.91 | 2694.0 | 16.94 | 333 | 19.6 | 10 |

Although there is the suggestion that starter diets with higher nutrient and energy concentrations might be associated with greater efficiencies, no such trend was apparent for the finisher diets introduced from 24 days of age.

A similar conclusion could be drawn from Trial 3. Mean efficiencies of utilisation of AME for weight gain were 36.9, 37.9, 37.1, 39.0 and 35.5 g/MJ respectively for HH, HL, CC, LH and LL over all time periods; these efficiencies are somewhat lower than in Trials 1 and 2 because Trial 3 extended to 10 weeks - a point when efficiencies are declining rapidly. The reduction in efficiency is probably associated with changing composition of live-weight gain with time where the more efficient muscle growth is progressively replaced by the less efficient fat growth. Differences between these means were not significant (P=0.827) confirming that the influence of diet on growth performance is based substantially on energy intake and not on efficiency of utilisation of energy and nutrients *per se*; with the qualification that nutrients are provided in adequate amounts.

## Altering fatty acid profiles of broiler meat

This is an increasingly topical area as advice to the human consumer continues to advocate an increase in the intake of polyunsaturated fatty acids (specifically the n-3 or omega 3 families, e.g. COMA, 1984; DHSS 1994). Numerous studies have demonstrated how closely carcass fatty acids of poultry reflect those of the diet. Time over which changes take place has received some attention. Bartov *et al.* (1974b) recommended a withdrawal of polyunsaturated fat source between 3 and 4 weeks prior to slaughter and Lopez-Ferrer *et al.* (1999), together with Gonzalez-Esquerra and Leeson (2000), confirmed that the response of carcass to dietary fatty acids was greater with longer feeding periods. However, the rate at which carcasses respond to dietary changes has not been studied in detail.

Information on the rate of change would be valuable to those who wish to increase the degree of unsaturation of fatty acids in broiler meat. Such information might also be used to reduce the risks of lowering the melting point of adipose tissue, which has been associated with excessive degrees of fatty acid unsaturation. Finally, because of the well-established effect of age on the AME values of fats (e.g. Wiseman *et al.*, 1999) it is common to feed relatively unsaturated fats early in life (when the differential between AME of unsaturated and saturated fats is greatest) to be replaced subsequently by relatively saturated sources. It is important to point out that degree of saturation of carcass lipid is generally not thought to be associated with the 'oily bird' syndrome. Although Hammershoj (1997) observed that birds fed on diets containing soya bean oil had a greater skin tearing frequency and reduced skin elasticity, most other studies have implicated impaired collagen structure and cross-linking (e.g. Ramshaw *et al* 1986; Granot *et al*, 1991).

In a programme of work conducted at the University of Nottingham (unpublished data), broilers were fed iso-energetic and iso-nitrogenous diets based on fats and oils of varying unsaturation before being transferred (at 21 days of age) to a diet based on the considerably more saturated tallow. A serial-slaughter approach allowed modelling of the rate of change of carcass fatty acids based on the function (Salmon and O'Neil, 1973):

$y = A + BR^X$, where y is an increase or decrease in fatty acid concentration at a given value of X,

R = exp(-k), an estimate of the rate at which fatty acid levels change in the asymptotic region of the response,

A = an estimate of the fatty acid concentration towards which each response tends to approach (the asymptote),

B = an estimate of the rate of change of fatty acid in the initial portion of the curve,

X = number of days between the baseline and slaughter weights.

The data (Figure 11.4) indicate that the pattern of change in carcass fatty acids is substantially complete within approximately 20 days of dietary change (although it is not possible to determine categorically whether these changes are simple dilution of the existing fatty profile or actual replacement of one fatty acid by another). Intriguingly, the data also suggest that different carcass components respond differently. Thus, the abdominal fat pad (one of the major storage sites of adipose tissue in the broiler) is much more responsive than the thigh meat. Breast meat is very unresponsive to dietary changes; as fat extracted from this region will be predominantly functional lipid, as opposed to storage lipid, the lack of response is presumably due to homeostatic mechanisms.

## Conclusions

It is evident that alteration of carcass composition of broilers is achievable through a number of dietary routes, including changes to dietary energy: protein ratios (by changing one or both). There can be no optimum diets recommended as these will depend on the circumstances under which they are fed and the desired product. What is intriguing, however, is that analysis of responses can be reduced substantially to a consideration of feed intake. Finally, for those markets wishing to identify a specific fatty acid profile, diet is a means whereby this may be achieved although, similarly, definitions of what is optimum are not possible.

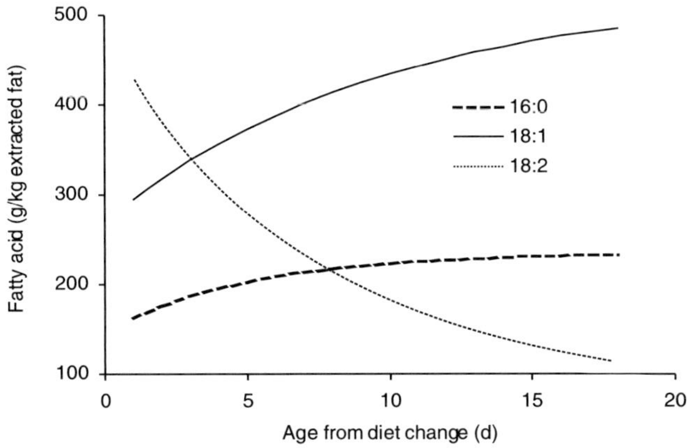


(a) Fatty acid profile of abdominal fat pad (AFP); 16:0, 18:1 and 18:2 are, respectively, palmitic, oleic and linoleic acids.

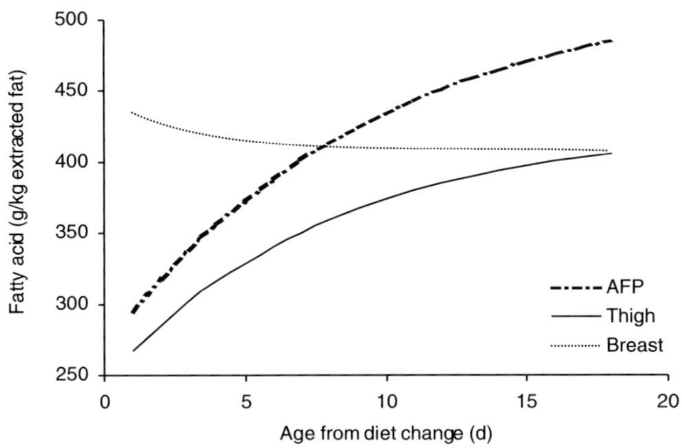


(b) Pattern of change of 18:1 in specific carcass components.

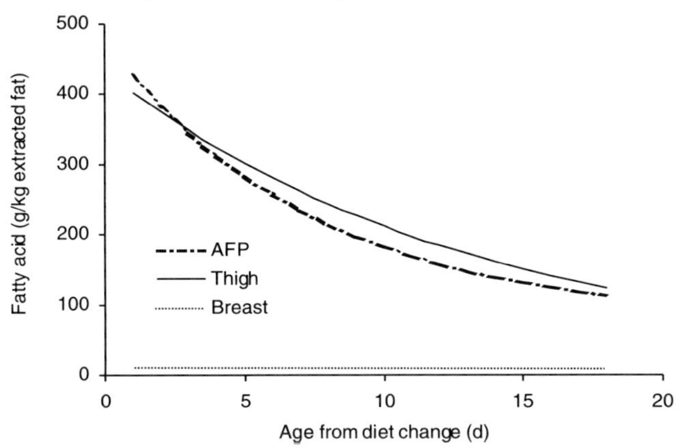


(c) Pattern of change of 18:2 in specific carcass components.

**Figure 11.4.** Rate of change of carcass fatty acids in response to a dietary change (from safflower oil to tallow) at 21 days of age (day zero in responses; University of Nottingham unpublished data).

## References


Arafa, A.S., Boone, M.A., Janky, D.M., Wilson, M.R., Miles, R.D. and Harms, R.M. (1983) Energy restriction as a means of reducing fat pads in broilers. *Poultry Science,* **62,** 314-320.

Bartov, I. (1998) Lack of interrelationship between the effects of dietary factors on food withdrawal on carcase quality of broiler chicks. *British Poultry Science,* **39**, 426-433.

Bartov, I, Bornstein S. and Lipstein, B. (1974a) Effect of calorie to protein ratio on the degree of fatness in broilers fed on practical diets. *British Poultry Science*, **15,** 107-117.

Bartov, I., Lipstein, B. and Bornstein, S., (1974b) Differential effects of dietary acidulated soybean oil soapstock, cottonseed oil soapstock and tallow on broiler carcass fat characteristics. *Poultry Science,* **53,** 115-124.

COMA (1984) Department of Health and Social Security, Diet and cardiovascular disease. Report on Health and Social Aspects No. 28. London HMSO.

Department of Heath and Social Security (1994) Report of Health and Social Subjects No. 46. Nutritional aspects of cardiovascular disease. London HMSO

Deaton, J.W., Reece, F.N., Kubena, L.F., Lott, B.D. and May, J.D. (1973) The ability of the broiler chicken to compensate for early growth depression. *Poultry Science,* **52,** 262-265

Gonzalez-Esquerra, R. and Leeson, S. (2000) Effects of menhaden oil and flaxseed in broiler diets on sensory quality and lipid composition of poultry meat. *British Poultry Science,* **41,** 481-488.

Granot I., Pines, M., Plavnik, I., Wax, E., Hurwitz, S. and Bartov, I. (1991) Skin tearing in broilers in relation to skin collagen - effect of sex, strain, and diet. *Poultry Science,* **70,** 1928-1935

Griffiths, L. Leeson, S. and Summers, J.F. (1977) Fat deposition in broilers: effect of dietary energy to protein balance and early life restriction on productive performance and abdominal fat pad size. *Poultry Science,* **56,** 638-646.

Hakansson, J., Eriksson, S. and Svensson, S.A. (1978*a*) The influence of feed energy level on chemical composition, growth and development of different organs of chicks. Report No.57. Swedish University of Agricultural Science, Department of Animal Husbandry.

Hakansson, J., Eriksson, S. and Svensson, S.A. (1978*b*) The influence of feed energy level on chemical composition of tissues and on the energy and protein utilisation of broiler chicks. Report No. 59. Swedish University of Agricultural Science, Department of Animal Husbandry.

Hammershoj, M. (1997) *Acta Agriculturae Sscandinavica,* **47,** 197-205

Hancock, C.E., Bradford, G.D., Emmans, G.C. and Gous, R.M. (1995) The evaluation of the growth parameters of six strains of commercial broiler chickens. *British Poultry Science,* **36,** 247-264.

Hargis, P.H. and Creger, C.R. (1980) Effects of varying dietary protein and energy levels on growth rate and body fat of broilers. *Poultry Science,* **59,** 1499-1504.

Jones, G.P.D. and Farrell, D.J. (1992*a*) Early-life restriction of broiler chickens. II. Methods of application, amino acid supplementation and the age at which restriction should commence. *British Poultry Science,* **33,** 579-587.

Jones, G.P.D. and Farrell, D.J. (1992*b*) Early-life restriction of broiler chickens. II. Effects of food restrictions on the development of fat tissue. *British Poultry Science,* **33,** 589-601.

Jones, R.L. and Wiseman, J. (1985) Effect of nutrition on broiler carcase composition: influence of dietary energy content in the starter and finisher phases. *British Poultry Science,* **26,** 381-388.

Kubena, L.F., Chen, T.C., Deaton, J.W. and Reece, F.N. (1974) Factors influencing the quantity of abdominal fat in broilers. 3. Dietary energy levels. *Poultry Science,* **53,** 974-978.

Leeson, S., Caston, L. and Summers, J.D. (1996a) Broiler response to energy or protein dilution in the finisher diet. *Poultry Science,***75,** 522-528.

Leeson, S., Caston, L. and Summers, J.D. (1996b) Broiler response to diet energy. *Poultry Science,* **75,** 529-535.

Leskanich, C.O and Noble, R.C (1997) Manipulation of the n3 polyunsaturated fatty acid composition of avian eggs and meat. W*orlds Poultry Science Journal,* **53,** 155-183.

Lopez-Ferrer, S., Baucells, M.D., Barroeta, A.C. and Grashorn, M.A. (1990) N-3 enrichment of chicken meat using fish oil: alternative substitution with rapeseed and linseed oils. *Poultry Science,* **78,** 356-365.

March, B.E. and Hansen, G. (1976) Lipid accumulation and cell multiplication in adipose bodies in White Leghorn and broiler-type chicks. *Poultry Science,* **56,** 886-894.

Plavnik, I. and Hurwitz, S. (1985) The performance of broiler chicks during and following a severe feed restriction at an early age. *Poultry Science,* **64,** 348-355.

Ramshaw, J.A.M., Rigby, B.J., Mitchell, T.W.and Nieass, A. (1986)Changes in the physical and chemical properties of skin collagen from broiler-chickens exhibiting oily bird syndrome. *Poultry Science,* **65,** 43-50.

Rogers, S.R., Pesti, G.M. and Marks, H.L. (1987) Comparison of three nonlinear regression models for describing broiler growth curves. *Growth,* **51,** 229-239.

Salmon, R.E. and O'Neil, J.B., 1973. The effect of dietary fat and storage temperature on the storage stability of turkey meat. *Poultry Science,* **52,** 314-317.

Short, F.J., Wiseman, J. and Boorman, K.N. (2000) The effect of the 1B/1R translocation and endosperm texture on amino acid digestibility in near-isogenic lines of wheat for broilers. *Journal of Agricultural Science,* **134,** 69-76.

Susbilla, J.P., Fraankel T.L., Parkinson, G. and Gow, C.B. (1994) Weight of internal organs and carcase yield of early food restricted broilers. *British Poultry Science,* **35,** 677-685.

Wiseman, J. (2000) Correlation between physical measurements and dietary energy values of wheat for poultry and pigs. *Animal Feed Science and Technology,* **84,** 1-11.

Wiseman, J. (2001) The quantitative contribution of fat to metabolisable energy. In "26th Poultry Science Symposium", edited by J.M. McNab, CAB International, Wallingford. p 137-150.

Wiseman, J. and Lewis, C.E. (1999) Influence of dietary energy and nutrient concentration on the growth of body weight and of carcass components of broiler chickens. *Journal of Agricultural Science,* **131,** 361-371.

Wiseman, J., Nicol, N.T. and Norton, G. (2000) Relationship between apparent metabolisable (AME) values and *in vivo / in vitro* starch digestibility of wheat for broilers. *Worlds Poultry Science Journal,* **56,** 1-14.

Wiseman, J. Powles, J. and Salvador, F. (1998) Comparison between pigs and poultry in the prediction of the dietary energy value of fats. *Animal Feed Science and Technology,* **71,** 1-9.

*This paper was first published in 2001*

12

# THE PRACTICAL RELEVANCE OF THE KINETICS OF STARCH DIGESTION IN BROILERS

P.J. VAN DER AAR, R. E. WEURDING, H. ENTING AND B. VELDMAN
*Institute of Animal Nutrition " De Schothorst", Meerkoetenweg 26, 8218 NA, Lelystad, The Netherlands*

## Introduction

Starch is the main component of poultry diets (where it supplies more than 50% of the apparent metabolisable energy AME). Often, the coefficient of starch digestibility is considered to be almost 1.0. However, incomplete starch digestion in broiler chickens was observed for wheat (Rogel *et al.*, 1987), barley (Hesselman and Åman, 1986), peas (Longstaff and McNab, 1987) and isolated starch of different origins from several feedstuffs (Yutste *et al.*, 1991).

The AME of wheat is positively correlated with starch digestibility (Rogel *et al.*, 1987, Wiseman *et al.*, 2000) and inversely correlated with non-starch polysaccharide (NSP) content (Choct *et al.*, 1999). In many feed evaluation systems, starch content is not a specific component in energy calculation but is part of the nitrogen-free extract (NFE). This has consequences for the energy value of the raw material, especially for raw materials that vary in starch content.

The physical and chemical properties of starch depend on the starch source and the technological treatments to which it has been subjected. This variation may not only affect the extent but also the rate by which it is digested in the gastrointestinal tract. Rate of digestion may be of importance particularly in poultry since the rate of passage through the intestinal tract is high relative to other species. A high rate of digestion in the small intestine ensures an almost complete digestion in the small intestine, whereas a slow rate of digestion may result in a larger amount of the starch being fermented in the cecae or more indigestible starch.

In this chapter the effect of rate of starch digestion on performance of broilers is discussed.

## Differences in starch characteristics between feedstuffs

In modern feed formulations different starch sources with varying starch characteristics are used. These differences can refer to the composition and structure of the starch granules and / or of the feedstuff itself. The starch granules may be very susceptible to enzymatic breakdown, but if the granules are embedded in a protective layer, then the granules are less accessible to the digestive enzymes, particularly amylases. Starch degradability is a function of granule surface area, starch structure and degree of crystallinity (Moran, 1982).

## Granule size

Franco *et al.* (1992) investigated the effect of granule size on *in vitro* starch hydrolysis rate in cassava and maize starch. Granule size classes were: small (< 10 μm), intermediate (between 10 and 15 μm) and large (> 16 μm). It was found that small granules were hydrolysed more rapidly than large granules (especially in the cassava starches). Microscopic observations indicated different modes of enzyme action in small and large granules. It was suggested that starch structure might be different in granules of different size. Small granules also showed higher initial gelatinisation temperatures and lower amylose contents for both starch sources. Small granules from cassava possessed less crystalline regions than large granules, which may explain the higher rate of starch hydrolysis in these granules. In the literature a wide range for granule sizes are reported for different starch sources (Table 12.1). Starch granules from rice, tapioca, sorghum, maize and oats are small to intermediate, whereas starch granules from peas, faba beans and potatoes are relatively large (Cone and Wolters, 1991).

## Amylose content

Starch in conventional starch sources contains 17 to 33% amylose. Amylose content is related to the growth stage of the plant. The amylose proportion in the granule as well as the molecular size of amylose and amylopectin increases during growth of the granule (Swinkels, 1985). This might explain some of the results found by Franco *et al.* (1992). Plant breeding in barley, maize, rice and sorghum has produced both waxy starch types and high-amylose starch types varieties. Waxy starch contains only amylopectin and hardly any amylose. Amylose content in starch granules of high amylose maize varieties may be as high as 50 to 70%. The conventional starch sources can roughly be divided in three classes with high, intermediate and low amylose contents. Legume starches contain on average 33% amylose, cereal starches 25 % and tubers are relatively low in amylose (potato 20% and tapioca 17%). Rice is a cereal grain that is different from the other cereals with respect to amylose content of starch (17%).

**Table 12.1** GRANULE SIZE AND SHAPE OF DIFFERENT STARCH SOURCES

| *Starch source* | *Type* | *Granule size range (diameter, μm)* | *Average* | *Shape* | *Source* |
|---|---|---|---|---|---|
| Maize | cereal | 3-26 | 15 | round, polygonal | 1 |
| Potato | tuber | 5-100 | 33 | oval, spherical | 1 |
| Wheat | cereal | 2-10 | 15 | lenticular | 1,3 |
| | | 20-35 | | round | 3 |
| Tapioca | tuber | 4-35 | 20 | oval, truncated | 1 |
| Sorghum | cereal | 3-26 | 15 | round, polygonal | 1 |
| Rice | cereal | 3-8 | 5 | polygonal, angular | 1 |
| Barley | cereal | 20-25 | | round | 3 |
| | | 2-6 | | lenticular | 3 |
| Triticale | cereal | 19 | 15 | round | 3 |
| Rye | cereal | 28 | 12 | round, lenticular | 3 |
| Oats | cereal | 3-10 | | polyhedral | 3 |
| Waxy maize | cereal | 3-26 | | round, polygonal | 1 |
| Amylomaize | cereal | 3-24 | | round, deformed | 1 |
| Mung bean | legume | 10-32 | | oval, irregelar | 2 |
| Faba bean | legume | 20-48 | | round | 2 |
| Smooth pea | legume | 20-40 | | oval, spherical | 2 |
| Wrinkled pea | legume | 6-80 | | oval, round | 2 |
| | | | | round | 2 |

1)Swinkels, 1985; 2) Hoover and Sosulski, 1991; 3) Hoseney, 1986.

High amylose starches are often considered less digestible. Amylopectin is a much larger molecule than amylose and therefore the surface area per molecule is substantially larger. Additionally the hydrogen bonds linking the glucose chains in amylose starch make the amylose molecules less susceptible to hydrolysis by amylase, compared to the amylopectin molecules. If starch is subjected to heat treatments, the amount of resistant starch formed is linearly correlated with the the formation of starch that is resistant to *in vitro* digestion (Sievert and Pomeranz,1989).

The effect of amylose on crystallinity remains unclear. Zobel (1988) reported degrees of crystallinity for several starch sources. No clear relation between amylose content and crystallinity was found, although the starch sources extremely high in amylose seem to indicate that a low amylose content can result in a higher degree of crystallinity. Since the crystallinity in the starch granules comes from amylopectin, it is logical that higher amylose contents result in less crystallinity. In their review on the physico-chemical and functional aspects of starch, Eliasson and Gudmundsson (1996) confirmed this relationship. The fact that starch sources with different amylose contents in starch can have a similar degree of crystallinity suggests differences in amylopectin structure (chain length, branching pattern).

## Technology

An important property of starches in animal feed is their behaviour during processing. Feeds are exposed to heat, pressure, moisture or a combination of these processes all of which influence the gelationasation of the starch. In general, the more intensive the technological treatment the higher the degree of gelatinisation resulting in a faster digestion. The temperature range over in which starches gelatinise vary between raw materials and the amount of water present during processing. The gelatinisation range of barley, oats and triticale is relatively low compared to those of amylo maize, rice and sorghum. Therefore the effect of processing on the digestibility characteristics of starches vary between starch sources (Swinkels,1985). Furthermore other physico-chemical properties of starches are altered by treatment. Heat and pressure treatment alter the viscosity of the staches. Starch from potato results in a high viscosity while starch from wheat, maize and sorghum have a low viscosity after heat treatment. These properties will influence the digestion kinetics.

Other properties including water holding capacity, solubilty and swelling power vary among starch sources. These properties all may exert an effect on the rate rate of digestion of starch.

## Starch source and digestibility

The digestibility of starch varies between different origins of the starch. Yutste *et al*, (1991) studied the digestibility of isolated starches of different origin. The differences observed in these experiments were mainly associated with differences in structure of the starches. In addition, within a raw material, the digestibility of starch can vary. Rogel *et al*, (1987), obtained differences in starch digestibility between wheat varieties from 0.82 to 1.00. However, if the starch from poorly digestible sources was isolated and incorporated in diets, the starch was as digestible as the starch from well-digested wheats. This indicates the starch fraction from low energy wheats is less accessible to digestive enzymes.

Not only the extent of digestibility but also the rate in which the starch is digested depends on the source. The extent to which the starch is digested in the various regions of the small intestine depends on the origin of the starch. The differences are not only absolute but also relative. The smaller the proportion of the ileal digestible starch digested in the proximal region, the slower the starch digestibility is. Weurding *et al.* (2001) observed that starch sources with a similar faecal digestibility had different digestibilities in the posterior jejunum (Table 12.2.) Tapioca starch had a digestibility at the level of the posterior ileum of 0.97 whereas sorghum starch had a digestibility in that region of the intestine of of 0.83. The starch from legumes not only had a lower total tract digestibility but also a smaller fraction was digested in the first part of the intestine.

**Table 12.2** COEFFICIENTS OF DIGESTIBILITY OF STARCH IN DIFFERENT SEGMENTS OF THE SMALL INTESTINE FOR BROILER CHICKENS FED DIETS CONTAINING DIFFERENT STARCH SOURCES[1,2]

| *Starch source* | *Posterior jejunum* | *Anterior ileum* | *Posterior ileum* | *Total tract* |
|---|---|---|---|---|
| Wheat | 0.882[ef] | 0.929[d] | 0.944[d] | 0.938[d] |
| Maize, hammer-milled | 0.888[fg] | 0.953[e] | 0.969[ef] | 0.974f[g] |
| Maize, roller-milled | 0.913[g] | 0.966[f] | 0.974[f] | 0.977[g] |
| Maize, waxy | 0.839[d] | 0.943[de] | 0.966[e] | 0.972[f] |
| Common beans, heat-treated | 0.361[b] | 0.629[b] | 0.723[b] | 0.745[b] |
| Barley | 0.898f[g] | 0.973[g] | 0.981[g] | 0.983[h] |
| Sorghum | 0.837[d] | 0.930[d] | 0.953[d] | 0.954[e] |
| Peas | 0.574[c] | 0.730[c] | 0.804[c] | 0.810[c] |
| Horse beans | 0.570[c] | 0.748[c] | 0.815[c] | 0.815[c] |
| Tapioca pellets | 0.977[h] | 0.987[h] | 0.989[h] | 0.989[i] |
| Raw potato starch | 0.198[a] | 0.253[a] | 0.329[a] | 0.317[a] |
| Brown rice, not polished | 0.851[de] | 0.948[e] | 0.968[e] | 0.973[f] |

Weurding *et al.*, 2001

The determining factor of the observed differences is probably the accessibility to enzymes. An *in vitro* method developed by Weurding *et al.* (2001) has a high predictive value of the amount of starch digested in the various regions of the intestine. By this method not only the effect of starch source but also the effect of different technological treatments on the rate of starch digestion can easily be determined

## Relevance of the rate of starch digestion.

A series of experiments was designed to determine the effect of rate of starch digestion on the performance of broilers. The first experimental diets were formulated with the same ileal digestible starch content. The digestible ileal starch was determined in an earlier experiment. (Weurding *et al.*, 2000). The rapidly digestible starch originated from cassava and maize whereas the starch from the relatively slow digesible starch sources was from peas and sorghum. The results are presented in Table 12.3.

**Table 12.3** BODY WEIGHT, WEIGHT GAIN, FEED INTAKE AND FEED CONVERSION RATIO OF FEMALE BROILER CHICKENS RECEIVING EITHER HIGH (H) OR LOW (L) AMOUNTS OF SLOWLY DIGESTIBLE STARCH (SDS) (*N*=6).

| *Period* *SDS (g/kg)* | *Parameter* | *H* *52* | *L* *7* | *SEM* | *Starch effect P-value* |
|---|---|---|---|---|---|
| 0 - 15 days | Body weight (g) | 434 | 406 | 6 | < 0.01 |
| | Feed intake (g) | 577 | 568 | 12 | 0.62 |
| | FCR | 1.464 | 1.555 | 0.023 | 0.02 |
| 15 - 31 days | Weight gain (g) | 926 | 862 | 6 | < 0.01 |
| | Feed intake (g) | 1578 | 1528 | 15 | 0.04 |
| | FCR | 1.703 | 1.772 | 0.011 | < 0.01 |
| 31 - 38 days | Weight gain (g) | 463 | 461 | 7 | 0.86 |
| | Feed intake (g) | 939 | 911 | 13 | 0.17 |
| | FCR | 2.030 | 1.976 | 0.016 | 0.04 |
| 0 - 38 days | Body weight (g) | 1823 | 1729 | 13 | < 0.01 |
| | Feed intake (g) | 3093 | 3002 | 32 | 0.07 |
| | FCR | 1.734 | 1.777 | 0.009 | 0.01 |

From day 1–31 the diets formulated with slower digestible starch resulted in somewhat higher feed intake and significantly improved weight gain and feed conversions. During the last week of the experiment (day 31-38) weight gain and intake did not significantly differ, but the feed conversion was better for the slower starch. From this experiment it was concluded that, during the first weeks, broilers may benefir from slower digestible starch sources.

In the next experiment the effect of rate of starch digestion was studied. Two diets were formulated based on a different rate of starch digestion. The diet formulated with the slowly digestible starch contained peas and maize as starch sources, whereas the rapidly disgestible starch originated from wheat and cassave. Variation in rate of starch digestibility was also created by technological treatment of the starch sources. Before incorporation into the diets the starch-rich raw materials were not treatedor either cold pelletized or expanded.

*In vitro* starch digestibility data showed that the technological treatments hardly affected the rate of digestion of the rapidly digestible starch sources.

However, the rate of digestion of the slowly digestible starch sources was increased by the technological treatments with the effect of expanding being greater than the effect of pelleting. The increase of the rate of digestion of the starch by selecting specific raw materals resulted again in a better FCR for the diets containing the slow digestible starch. The technological treatments did not exert an influence on the FCR through difeerences in feed intake. However, expanding the slow digestible starch resulted in faster hydrolyzable starch and also in a less efficient use of the AME in the diet. (Table 12.4.)

**Table 12.4** EFFECT OF STARCH SOURCE (SS) AND PROCESSING ON BROILER PERFORMANCE

| | *SS* | | *PM* | | | *TW* | | |
|---|---|---|---|---|---|---|---|---|
| | *PROCESS* | *0* | *SP* | *EP* | *O* | *SP* | *EP* | *SED* |
| 0-39 days | Body weight, g | 2087[bc] | 2143[ab] | 2092[abc] | 2039[c] | 2151[a] | 2098[abc] | 29 |
| | Feed intake, g | 3613[c] | 3640[c] | 3611[c] | 3627[c] | 3846[a] | 3743[b] | 50 |
| | FCR, g/g | 1.765[b] | 1.731[c] | 1.760[b] | 1.815[a] | 1.822[a] | 1.819[a] | 0.014 |
| | AMECR, kJ/g | 20.82[b] | 20.73[b] | 21.74[a] | 21.42[a] | 21.67[a] | 21.56[a] | 0.17 |

[1] PM = peas and maize based diet; TW = tapioca and wheat based diet; 0 = starch sources untreated; SP = starch sources steam pelleted; EP = starch sources expander pelleted.
Means in a row without a common superscript differ, $P< 0.05$.

The physiological mechanism(s) responsible for the different responses of broiler chickens to slowly and rapidly digestible starch need to be elucidated. A few possible mechanisms can be suggested. Firstly, rapid glucose absorption results in different metabolic responses than those associated with slow glucose absorption. Rapid glucose absorption results in substantial conversions to lactate in the gut wall. This way, the peak glucose supply to the blood is buffered (Riesenfeld *et al.*, 1982). In the liver, lactate is converted back to glucose. When starch digestion is slow, less glucose will be converted to lactate, thus saving energy. Secondly, rate of glucose absorption affects the post prandial insulin response (Björck *et al.*, 2000) and the insulin sensitivity (Wolever, 2000). Insulin plays a key role in protein deposition during growth (Fox, 1996). A high starch digestion rate results in a rapid, short term increase in the blood insulin level. A slow starch digestion, on the other hand, results in a lower, but longer lasting insulin response which may result in a more efficient protein deposition and thus a better feed conversion ratio for broiler chickens. Thirdly, the level of synchronisation of energy (starch) and protein digestion may affect feed efficiency. These three possible mechanisms are all directly related to starch digestion rate. A fourth possible mechanism is indirectly related to starch digestion rate, but directly related to site of starch digestion. The energy demands of the mucosae and muscle tissues along the small intestine must be met by the diet (McBride and Kelly, 1990). Glucose and amino acids may be oxidised for this purpose (Fleming *et al.*, 1997). A more gradual starch digestion, resulting in a higher glucose supply to the lower part of the small intestine, may spare amino acids at that site. Thus, more amino acids may be available for protein deposition (muscle growth) when broiler chickens are fed a diet containing sufficient slowly digestible starch.

## Protein sparing effect

In a pilot experiment, it was observed that additional amino acid supply in the diets compensated for the negative effects of technological treatment on feed conversion (Weurding *et al.*, 2001) Therefore, it was postulated that the protein sparing effect of slow digestible starch sources seems to be the most likely hypothesis. Weurding (2002) showed that the optimal digestible amino acid levels in broiler diets depend on the rate of starch digestion. In diets with rapidly digestible starch sources the effect of additional amino acid supply is larger than in the diets with slow digestible amino acids. The effect of additional amino acids in 2 different diets on growth and feed conversion in the growing period from day 9 to day 30 are presented in Figure 12.1. The amino acid supply is expressed as digestible lysine. However, all essential amino acids were increased in proportion. The effect of additional amino acids was larger for the diet with rapidly degradable starch than for the slowly digestible starch. The effect of additional amino acids was also still relevant at higher levels. Based on these data it can be calculated that for diets in which the starch is rapidly digested the amino acid requirement in the diets might be approximately 7 % higher to obtain maximal performance results.

## Effect on microflora

The rate of starch digestion may not only exert an effect on the amino acid utilization in the small intestine but it may also affect the composition of the microflora. Diets with more slowly digestible starch contain more resistant starch. This starch entering the hind gut will be a substrate for the microflora in the caeca. Due to its relatively fast fermentability, resistant starch may lead to shifts in the composition of the flora. In 2 experiments the effect on *C. perfringens* and Lacobacilli were measured. In one experiment more resistant starch resulted in lower *C. perfringens* counts, whereas the Lactobacilli counts were not affected. In another experiment (Weurding *et al.*, 2002) the effect on the counts of these bacteria were not significantly different. However, especially

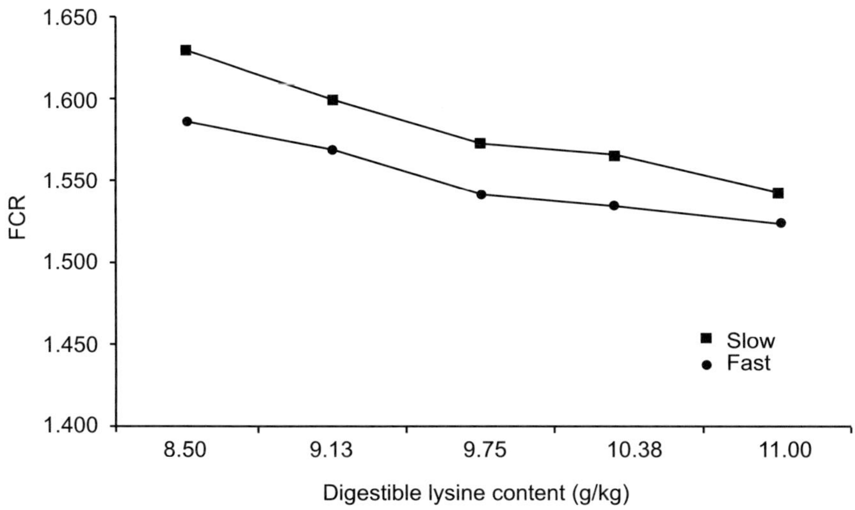


**Figure 12.1** The effect of digestible lysine on feed conversion in diets with slow and fast digestible starch over day 9 to 31 of the growing period.

the effect on *C.perfringens* may be of potential importance since necrotic enteritis seems to become a larger problem in feeding strategies without antibiotics.

## Practical relevance

The practical relevance of including the rate of starch digestibility in the formulation of feeds depends on the common practice of feed formulation. From the reported experiments it can be concluded that in feed production systems were the feed is hardly exposed to technologies in which heat is involved (mash or mild pelleting), differences in starch degradation rate between feedstuffs is a factor to take into account. In these diets the protein-sparing effect might be an important economic factor. However, if the processing involves high temperatures, for microbial decontamination, the effect is of less or no relevance.

## References

Björck, I., H. Liljeberg, and E. Östman, 2000. Low glycaemic-index foods. *British Journal of Nutrit British Poultry Science* **37**: 609-621.83 (Suppl. 1): S149-S155.

Choct, M., Hughes, R.J., Wang, J., Bedford, M.R., Morgan, A.J. and Annison, G.,

1996. Increased small intestinal fermentation is partly responsible for the anti-nutritive activity of non-starch polysaccharides in chickens.

Cone, J.W. and Wolters, M.G.E., 1991. Fysisch-chemische eigenschappen van zetmeel in relatie tot de afbreekbaarheid met pensvocht en enzymen. Rapport. *C.V.B. tabel 1996*.

Fleming, S. E., K. L. Zambell, and M. D. Fitch, 1997. Glucose and glutamine provide similar proportions of energy to mucosal cells of rat small intestine. *American Journal of Physiology* **273**: G968-978.

Fox, S. I., 1996. *Human Physiology*, pp 588, Wm. C. Brown.

Franco, C.M.L., Preto, S.J. R. and Ciacco, C.F., 1992. Factors that affect the enzymatic degradation of natural starch granules - effect of the size of the granules. *Starch* **44** (11): 422-426.

Hesselman, K. AND Åman, P., 1986. The effect of ß-glucanase on the utilization of starch and nitrogen by broiler chickens fed on barley of low- or high-viscosity. *Animal Feed Science and Technology* **15**: 83-93.

Hoover, R., 1995. Starch retrogradation. *Food Reviews International* **11** (2): 331-346.

Hoseney, R.C., 1986. Chapter 2: Cereal starch. In: *Principles of cereal science and technology* pp 33-68.

Longstaff, M. and McNab, J.M., 1987. Digestion of starch and fibre carbohydrates in peas by adult cockerels. *British Poultry Science* **28**: 261-285.

McBride, B.W., Kelly, J.M., 1990. Energy cost of absorption and metabolism in the ruminant gastrointestinal tract and liver: A review. *Journal of Animal Science* **68**, 2997-3010.

Moran, E.T., 1982. Starch digestion in fowl. *Poultry Science* **61**: 1257-1267.

Riesenfeld, G., A. Geva, and S. Hurwitz, 1982. Glucose homeostasis in the chicken. *Journal of Nutrition* **112**: 2261-2266.

Rogel, A.M., Annison, E.F., Bryden, W.L. and Balnave, D., 1987. The digestion of wheat starch in broiler chickens. *Australian Journal of Agricultural Research* **38**: 639-649.

Swinkels, J.J.M., 1985. Sources of starch, its chemistry and physics. In: *Starch Conversion Technology*. Ed: Beynum van G.M.A. and Roels, J.A.. pp 15-46.

Weurding, R.E., A. Veldman, WA.G. Veen, P.J. van der Aar, and M.W.A. Verstegen, 2001*a*. Starch digestion rate in the small intestine of broiler chickens differs between feedstuffs. *Journal of Nutrition* **131**: 2329-2335.

Weurding, R.E., Veldman, A., Veen, W.A.G., Van der Aar, P.J. & Verstegen, M.W.A., 2001*b*. *In vitro* starch digestion correlates well with rate and extent of starch digestion in broiler chickens. *Journal of Nutrition* **131**: 2336-2342.

Wiseman, J., Nicol, N.T. and Norton, G., 2000. Relationship between apparent metabolisable (AME) values and *in vivo* / *in vitro* starch digestibility of wheat for broilers. *World's Poultry Science Journal* **56**: 305-318.

Wolever, T.M.S., 2000. Dietary carbohydrates and insulin action in humans. *British Journal of Nutrition* **83**, Suppl. 1, S97-S102.
Yutste, P., Longstaff, M.A., McNab, J.M. and McCorquodale, C., 1991. The digestibility od semipurified starches from what, cassava. pea, bean and potato by adult cockerels and young chicks. *Animal Feed Science and Technology* **35**: 289-300.

*This paper was first published in 2003*

13

# PUTTING POULTRY NUTRITION INTO PRACTICE: EXPERIENCE FROM THE FIELD

D FILMER
*FLOCKMAN™, Brent Knoll, Somerset, TA9 4DT*

## Introduction

Feed contributes over 75% of the costs of poultry meat production in the UK and has a major effect on bird performance, welfare and health. Proper management of nutrition is therefore vital if the correct balance between production, profit, bird health and welfare, and environment considerations are to be achieved.

Traditionally, broilers are fed a series of feeds of decreasing protein content from day old to slaughter. Thus the first starter feed may be fed for the first 10 days and the next grower feed for the following 14 days etc. Because the birds' needs change gradually with age, each feed can only be correctly balanced for a particular day. Assuming that the nutritionist who designed the feeds was competent, this day will be at approximately the mid point of the age range over which the feed is used. In the above case, this will be day 5 for the starter and day 17 for the grower. At the end of the starter phase, the feed will be too high in protein and will lead to excessive nitrogen excretion; at the beginning of the grower phase, the feed will be too low in protein and will be inadequate to support optimal growth. Figure 13.1 shows the feeding of four feeds, of descending protein content, for various time intervals and superimposes an "Ideal protein" curve where the protein content is a function of age and changes gradually over the life span of the broiler. This is in contrast to the "step feeding" of protein typical of most current broiler feeding systems.

One answer to this inadequacy is to use a greater number of feeds over the life cycle, with the ultimate logical solution of one feed for each day of life. However, even a few more feeds causes manufacturing, delivery and control problems and is not practical. A commercial solution is to provide a high and a low protein feed in two separate silos at the poultry production house. Augers convey each feed to a common weigher/mixer, which, under computer control, can make the optimal mixed diet according to the age and needs of the birds.

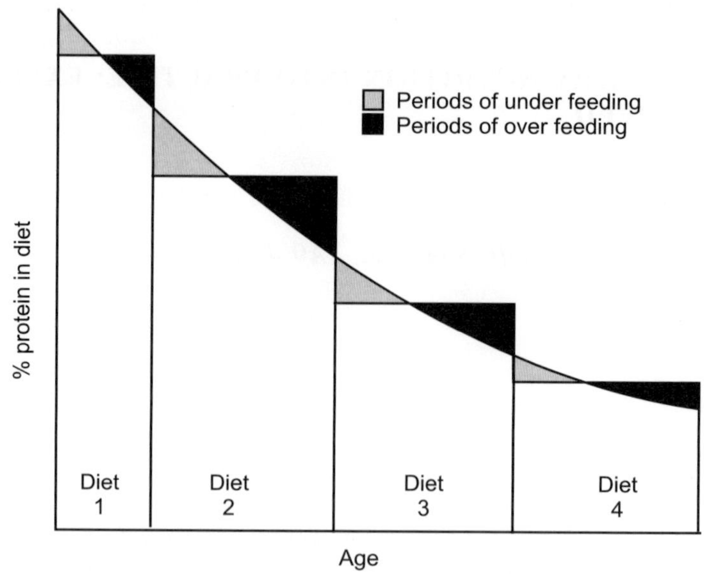


**Figure 13.1** Typical 'step feeding' of protein to broilers from day-old to slaughter

## Concept 1 - Daily nutrient intake versus feed composition

Traditionally, the nutritional requirements of growing birds have been stated in terms of feed composition for an age range, as illustrated in Figure 13.1. However, birds need the correct daily intakes of the critical nutrients to enable them to perform at a given level. These nutrients need to be defined for a given strain and sex of growing bird for each day of life.

The factors that contribute to these daily intakes are :-

1) Feed composition - e.g. Lysine expressed as 1g/100g of feed or 10g/kg of feed
2) Daily Feed Intake - e.g. 100g of feed / day

From these two factors the resultant daily nutrient intake can be calculated

e.g. 100 g of feed x 1g lysine / 100g feed = 1g lysine intake / day

The requirement therefore is 1g (or 1000mg) lysine for the given day. Table 13.1 shows the daily digestible lysine intake requirements to enable a defined strain and sex of bird to grow along a defined growth curve.

**Table 13.1** DAILY DIGESTIBLE LYSINE INTAKE TARGETS FOR BROILERS

| *Day* | *mg/bird/day* | *Day* | *mg/bird/day* | *Day* | *mg/bird/day* | *Day* | *mg/bird/day* |
|---|---|---|---|---|---|---|---|
| 0 | 64 | 16 | 718 | 32 | 1144 | 48 | 1316 |
| 1 | 100 | 17 | 754 | 33 | 1161 | 49 | 1321 |
| 2 | 138 | 18 | 789 | 34 | 1176 | 50 | 1326 |
| 3 | 178 | 19 | 823 | 35 | 1191 | 51 | 1331 |
| 4 | 220 | 20 | 855 | 36 | 1205 | 52 | 1336 |
| 5 | 262 | 21 | 887 | 37 | 1218 | 53 | 1340 |
| 6 | 305 | 22 | 916 | 38 | 1230 | 54 | 1343 |
| 7 | 348 | 23 | 945 | 39 | 1241 | 55 | 1346 |
| 8 | 391 | 24 | 972 | 40 | 1252 | 56 | 1349 |
| 9 | 434 | 25 | 998 | 41 | 1262 | 57 | 1351 |
| 10 | 477 | 26 | 1022 | 42 | 1271 | 58 | 1353 |
| 11 | 519 | 27 | 1046 | 43 | 1280 | 59 | 1355 |
| 12 | 561 | 28 | 1068 | 44 | 1288 | 60 | 1355 |
| 13 | 601 | 29 | 1089 | 45 | 1296 | 61 | 1356 |
| 14 | 641 | 30 | 1108 | 46 | 1303 | 62 | 1356 |
| 15 | 680 | 31 | 1127 | 47 | 1309 | 63 | 1356 |

Figure 13.2 shows this in graphical form as a digestible lysine intake profile. This simple concept is difficult for many to understand and even more difficult to comprehend in terms of the implications for the correct feeding of birds that the concept implies. For example, given that on a specific day a bird needs 1g lysine, how does the bird obtain that quantity? From the above illustration, if the bird eats 100g feed/d, then that feed should contain 1g lysine / 100g (or 10g/kg). However, if the bird is eating only 90g/d, then the feed will need to contain 1g lysine / 90g (or 11.1g/kg). The consequence of this nutrient intake concept is that there must be a logical sequence in deciding on the ideal diet composition for each day of the growing bird's life.

Step 1 Define the daily nutrient intake required
e.g. 1000mg (1g) of digestible lysine on day 25 (A)

Step 2 Estimate feed intake
e.g. 100g / day (B)

Step 3 Calculate diet
A/B = 1000mg lysine / 100g = 10mg lysine / g, equivalent to 10g lysine /kg diet.

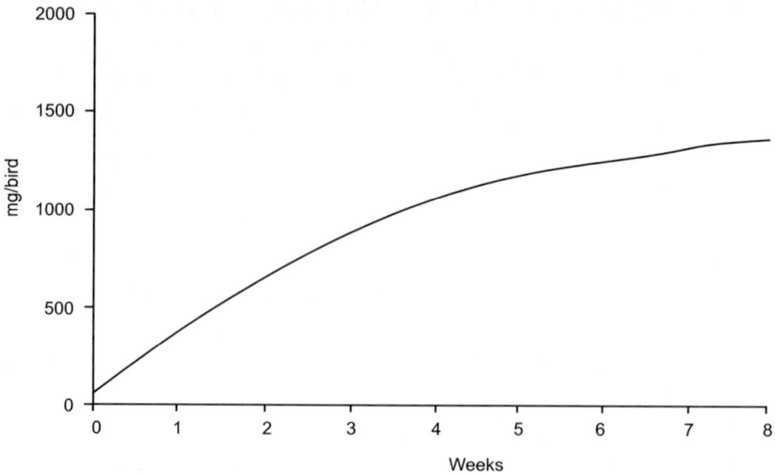


**Figure 13.2** Daily digestible lysine intake requirements of broilers (mg/bird/day)

However, there is a major practical problem with this approach, even assuming that correct nutrient intake profiles can be constructed, which is the estimation of feed intake in advance of preparing the feed formulation. It is known that many factors affect feed intake from day to day and from house to house. The major factors are age, sex and strain of the birds, but these are modified by bird weight and health status. Environmental factors, such as temperature, humidity and airflow, have known effects as they affect the rate at which heat loss occurs. Birds need to lose heat in order to maintain appetite, so depressions in appetite and performance occur in hot humid conditions with inadequate airflow. Similarly, appetite increases in cool conditions due to greater heat loss, leading to higher intakes of protein, as well as the energy-yielding components of the feed. This effect often leads to higher growth rates on diets inadequate in protein as this is the only way the birds can get an adequate daily intake of protein and amino acids necessary to support their genetic potential for live-weight gain. This effect is often seen in turkey pole barns with inadequate insulation. The growth response under cold conditions is thus a measure of the inadequacy of the diet.

Factors affecting the ability of the birds to lose heat, such as feather cover, the thermal insulation of the house, the type of floor and litter including its thickness and thermal conductivity, all affect feed intake. High stocking densities, where birds crowd together, prevent their body heat from escaping. If birds settle in groups and huddle together, they effectively insulate each other and this is a natural mechanism for keeping warm in cold conditions. This activity should be prevented in hot conditions by disturbing birds that are sitting down together; this releases heat that has been retained beneath the birds by the collective carpet of feathers that such behaviour produces. Misting systems, which introduce coarse droplets onto the birds, can have a major effect on heat loss. When water droplets hit the birds, their first reaction is to stand up. This has the same effect as walking amongst the birds. The second effect is to stimulate preening. This is self-grooming by birds of their own feathers. By this action, the birds distribute the water droplets round their bodies, including onto their skin. Birds have no sweat glands, so evaporation of water from the skin is a natural mechanism for heat loss. A study of the Jungle Fowl shows that this is a major mechanism for keeping cool in hot conditions. Simulation of natural mechanisms for keeping cool can be exploited by such sophisticated systems. However, the introduction of very fine water particles or fogging, can have the opposite effects. The birds' main mechanism for heat loss is by evaporative cooling from their lungs. The rate of loss of heat from the lungs depends on the difference in Relative Humidity (RH) of the inhaled air and the exhaled air. If dry air is inhaled, it can absorb more moisture at the lung surface, so more evaporation and heat loss can occur. The cooler blood supply is then distributed round the body. However, if the humidity of the inhaled air is already high, there is little opportunity for evaporation to take place at the lung surface, and heat loss can be severely reduced. The use of fogging systems or cooling pads, through which warm air enters the building, may well cool the air entering the building, but it does so by increasing the humidity of the air. This cooler air may appear beneficial to a human, and it will affect temperature sensors in the air of the house, but it can have negative effects on the birds. It is well known that introducing fogging into houses in hot, very humid conditions is counterproductive. The other mechanism to increase heat loss is panting. The more air of a given RH that can pass over the lung surface per unit time, the greater the heat loss.

A major factor affecting feed intake is the energy concentration of the feed. Birds eat less high-energy feeds than low energy feeds. Some breed companies, such as BUT (British United Turkeys) provide two guides to daily feed intakes. The first (Table 13.2, column 'A') is for high energy American type feeds based on maize, whilst the second (Table 13.3, column 'B') shows daily feed intakes for age for UK-type feeds based on wheat. There is a known relationship between dietary energy concentration and feed intake for various breeds and strains; nutritionists take this into account when designing feeds for optimal economic performance. However there may be considerable differences between the theoretical energy concentration in the feed and that in the feed actually delivered to the poultry unit. Firstly, there is normal variation in the energy concentration of the raw materials making up the feed. This can show a coefficient of variation of 5% to 10%. Secondly, there can be errors in feed manufacture. The most likely cause of variation will be the

**Table 13.2** EXTRACT FROM TABLE B10, BIG 6 - COMMERCIAL MALE DATA, (BUT 2002)

| *Age (Weeks)* | *Liveweight (kg)* | *Weekly feed intake (kg)* | | *Weekly cumulative FCR* | |
|---|---|---|---|---|---|
| | | *Feed "A" ** | *Feed "B" ** | *Feed "A" ** | *Feed "B" ** |
| 1 | 0.16 | 0.15 | 0.16 | 0.96 | 0.99 |
| 2 | 0.39 | 0.32 | 0.34 | 1.23 | 1.28 |
| 3 | 0.75 | 0.54 | 0.57 | 1.37 | 1.42 |
| 4 | 1.26 | 0.82 | 0.85 | 1.47 | 1.53 |
| 5 | 1.92 | 1.08 | 1.16 | 1.52 | 1.61 |
| 6 | 2.74 | 1.41 | 1.51 | 1.58 | 1.68 |
| 7 | 3.68 | 1.73 | 1.86 | 1.65 | 1.76 |
| 8 | 4.73 | 2.03 | 2.19 | 1.72 | 1.83 |
| 9 | 5.86 | 2.21 | 2.24 | 1.77 | 1.90 |
| 10 | 7.05 | 2.46 | 2.74 | 1.82 | 1.97 |
| 11 | 8.28 | 2.69 | 2.99 | 1.88 | 2.03 |
| 12 | 9.54 | 2.90 | 3.22 | 1.94 | 2.12 |

Note * See Table 13.3 for ME of Feeds"A" and "B"

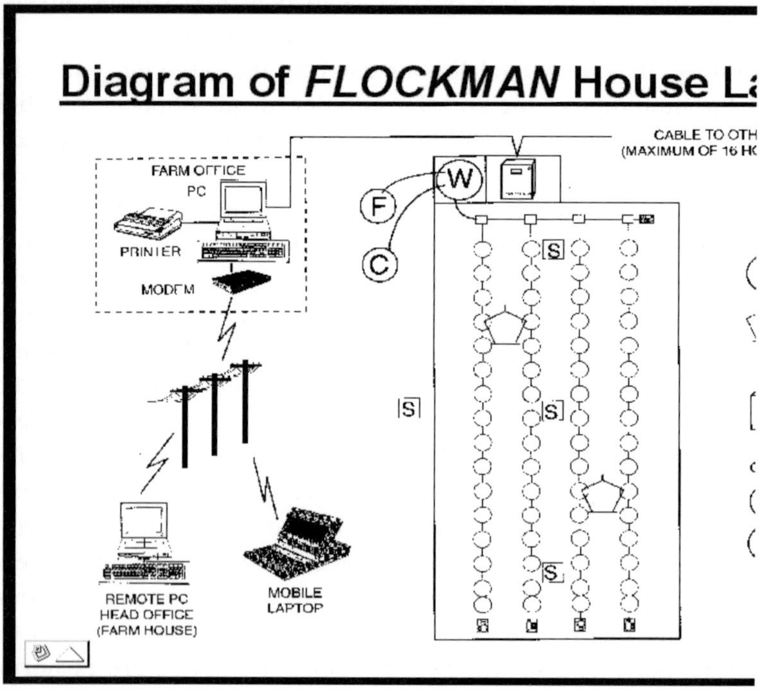


**Figure 13.3** Diagram of a ***FLOCKMAN***™ house layout for broilers

**Table 13.3** ME OF FEED"A" (MAIZE BASED) AND FEED "B" (WHEAT BASED) MJ/kg

| *Weeks fed from and to* *Males* | *Females* | *Maize based Feed "A"* | *Wheat based Feed "B"* |
|---|---|---|---|
| 0 - 4 | 0 - 4 | 12.2 | 11.8 |
| 4 - 8 | 4 - 8 | 12.8 | 12.0 |
| 8 - 12 | 8 - 11.5 | 13.4 | 12.2 |
| 12 - 16 | 11.5 - 15 | 13.6 | 12.2 |
| 16 - 20 | 15 - 18 | 14.0 | 12.4 |
| 20 - 24 | N/A | 14.0 | 12.6 |

level of fat incorporated into the feed. For these two reasons, it is impossible for a nutritionist to know precisely the actual energy concentration in each delivery of feed to the poultry unit.

## METHODS OF ESTIMATING AD-LIBITUM FEED INTAKE

The most common method used in commercial practice is to use published tables of feed intakes issued by the breed companies. These can form a good basis for initial estimations, but can and should be modified by the operator or integrator in the light of experience, using feed back from commercial sites.

Additionally, mathematical modelling techniques can be employed. These use some of the known factors affecting appetite, such as age and weight of the bird, expected growth rate, temperature, humidity, insulation of the house, theoretical energy concentration of the feed. However, they cannot take all of the factors into account, as these will vary from house to house in unpredictable ways. Furthermore, the main growth modelling systems attempt to predict intake for each day of a bird's life, even before the birds are placed. Such forecasts into the future are bound to be inaccurate, as is seen when predicted intakes by such methods are compared to actual intakes. Unfortunately, most animal growth models rely on predictions of feed intake in order to predict performance on various diets and dietary regimes. Although such predictions have some value, they are clearly not accurate enough to enable diet calculations to be made in real time, so as to deliver specific daily nutrients to the birds.

The third method is not to predict feed intake at all, but to measure it in real-time at each poultry house. Here there is no estimate involved. This is the approach that is incorporated into the ***FLOCKMAN***™ system to ensure that the daily intakes of nutrients are as close to those set up in the nutrient profiles as possible.

CONCLUSIONS FROM THE DAILY NUTRIENT INTAKE APPROACH

Firstly, a different feed formulation is required each day. Secondly, this formulation cannot be predicted accurately in advance, because feed intake is not predictable accurately in advance. A solution is to weigh the total daily feed intakes accurately in real-time, to extrapolate forward one day, look up the table for the nutrient intakes required for that day and then to calculate the composition of a feed which, at the extrapolated feed intake, will deliver the required nutrient intakes. From the analysis of the two component feeds stored at the poultry house, the mix ratio required to produce the calculated diet can be determined. Finally, the feeds are mixed in batches of 20-25kg and delivered to the birds via the normal feeding system in the house (Filmer, 1991). A diagram of a ***FLOCKMAN***™ house layout is shown in Figure 13.3. Accuracy is enhanced by feed control (see Concept 3 p. 235).

## Concept 2 - Use of whole cereal as the low protein feed

The feeding of unground cereals to birds is not a new concept as it was common practice before intensive poultry meat production started, at which time feed manufacturers marketed and sold complete feeds with all the components finely ground. Although originally these were sold as meals or mash feeds, they were soon superseded by steam pelleted or crumbed feed, as these were associated with higher daily feed intakes and better performance. Ideas of each pellet containing all the nutrients needed by the birds, balanced in ideal proportions, were effectively marketed. The concept of a "balanced beakful" proved popular. The use of extruded products for broilers, containing fully ground components, has been the norm for the last 50 years.

Ideas of the importance of texture in the feed did not re-emerge until 20-25 years ago. Firstly, observations were made that coarse layers meals were popular with some farmers, who claimed that they gave better performance than the same formula in ground mash form. Secondly, some Dutch farmers were using a proportion of whole wheat mixed with standard broiler pellets – apparently successfully. Thirdly, work by Emmans (1977) and Cowan and Michie (1978), showed that offering broilers and turkeys a choice between a compound feed and whole cereal produced satisfactory results. The proportion of cereal selected depended on the individual bird's performance potential, with birds of lower performance choosing a higher proportion of cereal than those of higher performance. In addition, work in Australia by Cumming (1992) showed that choice feeding of whole wheat to broilers led to a reduction in excreted coccidial oocysts. Two treatments were examined, one of which was standard broiler feed; the other was the same feed together with free-choice access to whole wheat. Both treatments were reared in coccidial-free conditions and both were subsequently infected with equal quantities of coccidial oocysts. Excreted oocysts were subsequently measured (Table 13.4).

**Table 13.4** OOCYST COUNTS IN BROILERS OFFERED A COMPLETE DIET OR THE SAME DIET PLUS FREE-CHOICE ACCESS TO WHOLE WHEAT

| *Replicate* | *Complete diet* *Oocyst output '000* | *Free choice* *Oocyst output '000* |
|---|---|---|
| 1 | 180 | <10 |
| 2 | 170 | <10 |
| 3 | 150 | 10 |
| 4 | 140 | <10 |
| 5 | 150 | 20 |
| 6 | 140 | <10 |
| 7 | 170 | <10 |
| 8 | 150 | 10 |
| 9 | 150 | 10 |
| 10 | 100 | <10 |
| Mean | 150 | <10 |

Cumming (1992) concluded that the stronger, more muscular gizzards that were developed in the free-choice groups, had effectively damaged or destroyed a high proportion of the introduced oocysts by their grinding action. This was independent of whether or not non-soluble grit was fed.

## ROLE OF THE GIZZARD IN DIGESTION BY POULTRY

Apart from the powerful grinding action disrupting coccidial oocysts, the gizzard has an important role in avian digestion. It is a remarkable organ, unique to avians and dinosaurs, which contains a hard, ridged keratinised inner lining surrounded by powerful musculature. When presented with large hard particles, such as whole grains, the inability of these to pass through the sphincter muscle exit from the gizzard, stimulates the grinding action. This continues, so reducing the gizzard contents to smaller particulate sizes that eventually can pass out into the small intestine. The evolutionary process has clearly equipped birds to deal with the wide array of berries, grains, insects and vegetation that are their normal dietary constituents. The absence of large particles in standard fully ground and pelleted broiler feed does not trigger the grinding motion and the gizzard is effectively removed from its important role in digestion. When whole cereal is present, the action not only grinds the cereal grains, but also reduces the particle size of the protein components in the compound feed, so presenting a greater surface area for subsequent attack by digestive enzymes. The physical size and movement of the gizzard, and the fact that is attached to other parts of the digestive system, influences the function of the other digestive components. For example the proventiculus, which produces hydrochloric acid, is stimulated to produce greater quantities leading to a reduction in pH of the digesta. This is probably due to the physical removal of the secreted HCl from the sites of secretion. The effect on digesta pH is well documented but the potential effects on the production of higher quantities of digestive enzymes are worthy of research investigation.

Lower pH changes the gut microflora, as bacteria are sensitive to pH. Gut bacteria adversely affected by lower pH include salmonella and *E. coli*, so the change in pH due to whole cereal feeding is likely to be beneficial. The pH change also changes the viscosity of the gut contents making the digesta more liquid. This eases the penetration of digestive enzymes and enables better physical contact between enzyme and substrate, resulting in higher digestibility. More liquid digesta also assists the movement of the end products of digestion to the microvilli of the small intestine leading to better absorption. The effect of this is an increase in protein digestion and a reduction in nitrogen excretion. In turn this reduces ammonia production in the litter and the incidence of sticky litter. It is an observation that whole wheat feeding also leads to dryer, more friable litter. This may be due to the better digestibility and absorption of limiting amino acids leading to less need to de-aminate and excrete non-essential amino acids, which are normally in excess supply. Such de-amination, conversion to uric acid and excretion needs a liquid medium. Less excretion needs less water intake and lowers the observed water to feed ratio.

## INDUSTRY CHANGES AT THE TIME OF FEEDSTUFFS DE-CONTROL IN THE LATE 1950S

The plentiful supply of feedstuffs, following the rationing of animal feeds, which had been imposed during the 1940s and early 1950s, enabled the broiler industry to develop rapidly. Many innovations took place, with new strains of chicken from America specifically developed for fast growth and good meat production becoming available. Larger housing was developed, with birds confined indoors with no access to pasture, seeds, grain, vegetation, insects, grit, etc. Mechanisation of feeding systems was developed, including chain feeders, cable and flight delivery systems and feed pans. The latter were supplied via interconnecting pipes with centre-less augers operated automatically by auger motors when sensors detected that feed levels in the pans were low. Feed delivery from compound feed mills changed from 112 lb (50 kg) jute or hessian sacks to bulk delivery in new types of feed lorries.

Bags were still required for tube feeders, but these bags were made of paper and weights were reduced to 25kg. Most feeding practice changed to *ad libitum*, which seemed to be necessary for the new types of feeding systems being introduced.

Birds in these new situations faced many changes: -

a) *Ad-libitum* feeding instead of twice daily
b) Fully ground feed instead of partly whole grains
c) No access to vegetation, seeds, insects and grit
d) No access to sunlight with its Vitamin D activity benefits
e) 23-24 hours of artificial light in many cases
f) Higher stocking densities.

To offset this, housing provided sheltered accommodation, where the environment could be controlled to achieve optimum conditions and which was free from predation.

Some of the first problems that hit the industry were severe outbreaks of coccidiosis. This was thought to be due mainly to the higher stocking density. The lack of an active gizzard did not appear, at that time, to be implicated. In retrospect, it should have been realised that hosts and parasites/diseases evolve together so that the host tolerates the invader and can control attacks on its system. The gizzard appears to be a major mechanism for controlling coccidia to manageable and tolerable proportions. The work of Cumming (1992) showed over a 15-fold reduction in control in the absence of an active gizzard, implying that the lack of whole grain feeding was probably the major item in the severe outbreaks of coccidiosis that the industry suffered at that time.

However, the pharmaceutical industry was not slow to develop ever more effective coccidiostats, which provided the defence that the birds originally provided for themselves. Elaborate dose-response trials established the optimal dose rate for each coccidiostat for effective control and those levels were enshrined in law and policed actively by government officials. The argument that different, lower, levels would be required by birds with active gizzards, compared to those with inactive ones, appears to have been ignored.

## Concept 3 - Meal time feeding

A study of the Red Jungle Fowl (*Gallus gallus*), which is the ancestor of the domestic fowl, should be of considerable interest and relevance to the industry today. The bird is used to a hot climate with high humidity levels. It forages rapidly as soon as dawn breaks, before temperatures rise rapidly, and fills its crop with seeds, grains, berries, insects and vegetation. During the heat of the day, it shelters in the undergrowth away from direct sunlight and seeks wet patches where it preens to assist cooling by evaporation. During this time, it lives on the feed stored in its crop. When the sun goes down, it again forages rapidly in the cooler evening and fills its crop again for the second time in 24 hours. It then seeks a roost for the night, safe from predators where it sleeps for 6+ hours, living again on the stored food until it awakes gradually at dawn, ready to forage again as before.

## MEAL-TIME FEEDING IN THE UK DURING THE 1930S

The husbandry system during the 1930s had more similarities to the Jungle Fowl scenario than current intensive systems and is described below.

Birds were kept in night arks or small sheds at night, up to a maximum of 50 – 100 birds. Early in the morning, the stockman put a given quantity of mash feed (usually soaked in water, hot in the winter), into individual troughs close to or within each unit. When all houses had their allocated feed put in their respective troughs, all pop-holes to the houses were opened quickly, the birds rushed out and started active feeding. The stockman observed the birds whilst they were feeding and noted, among other things, how quickly or slowly they ate the allocated feed. If they left the troughs before all the feed was consumed, a note was made, and less was offered the next day. If the birds cleared up the feed too quickly and then visited troughs at other houses to find more, another note was made and more feed was allocated the next day.

There was thus a feedback mechanism whereby the stockman adjusted the birds' daily feed intake by observing their behaviour. The birds ranged on grassland during the day. Houses were moved regularly to fresh pasture as soon as the existing location became bare. During the late afternoon, a scratch feed, usually of mixed whole grains (wheat, barley, sorghum, maize, etc.), was scattered directly onto the grass. Birds would scratch around until the last grains were found and consumed. Examination of birds at both feeding times showed that the rapid eating led to the development of full crops. At dusk most birds would return to their respective houses. Pop-holes were then closed for the night as protection from predators.

## KNOWLEDGE OF FEED INTAKE ON AD LIBITUM FEEDING SYSTEMS

Control of intake by the stockman was not possible when the industry adopted *ad libitum* feeding. With feed available in troughs, tube feeders, feed pans, etc., which were mechanically replenished 24 hours a day, knowledge of how much the birds were actually eating each day was lost. Until the advent of feed weighing systems, nutritionists had to make assumptions concerning daily feed intakes. It is true to say that, even today, most commercial nutritionists know a lot more about feed formulations than they do about daily feed intakes.

The first automatic feed weighers were tipper weighers, where feed was augured in until a change in the centre of gravity of the containing hopper reached a threshold point. The hopper would then tip and the contents would be discharged. Tipping was continuous in both directions and a mechanical counter recorded the number of tips. Unfortunately the weight of feed dispensed at each tip depended on the flow characteristics and bulk density of the feed being weighed, so was not constant. Errors of 5% or more were common. Modern batch weighers based on accurate load cells and linked to computers can now provide excellent data. The quantity of feed weighed out per day can be accurately recorded, stored on disk and reproduced numerically and graphically. Comparisons of actual versus expected daily intakes can be made.

For those interested in bird behaviour, and how feed intake is distributed throughout a given day, records can be taken in subsets of the day. For example the proportion weighed out in eight equal periods of three hours can be recorded and automatically presented to the stockman and nutritionist etc. The current ***FLOCKMAN***™ system can record the quantity of feed weighed out in each 6-minute period of the day, so 10 records are taken each hour and 240 in each 24-hour period. At the same times, the quantity of water consumed is recorded, as is the ON/OFF status of the house lights and the enabled/disabled status of the lane augers. Such data can be quite revealing and can initiate ideas of ideal patterns of feed distribution during the day in relation to various lighting programmes.

Breed companies provide most commercial data on expected feed intakes as well as expected daily bodyweights. Such tables can be presented as daily feed intake profiles, daily liveweight profiles (growth curves), daily liveweight gain profiles, etc.

## DETAILED STUDY OF AD LIBITUM FEEDING RESULTS

Houses equipped with accurate automatic feed and bird weighers can reveal critical information from which improvements in management techniques can be revealed. Such a study was carried out in 1995 on a commercial broiler farm. Figure 13.4 shows typical results of actual performance of mixed sex commercial broilers fed *ad libitum* throughout life. Birds were below the breed targets for the first 2 weeks, exceeded them between 3 and 4½ weeks of age, but subsequently declined progressively to finish below target. A more revealing way of presenting the same data is to show the deviation from the

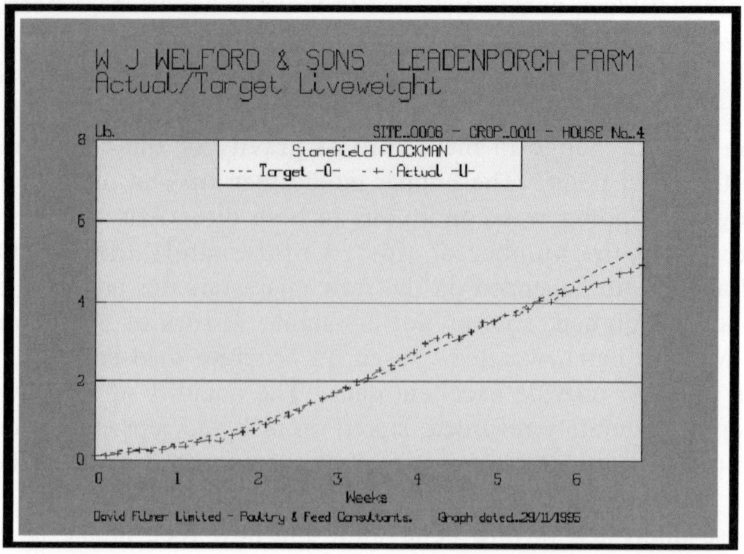


**Figure 13.4** Live weight of broilers fed *ad libitum* compared with breed target live weight

breed target as in Figure 13.5. This shows that birds on average exceeded target by 8-9% at about 4 weeks, but ended up 8-9% below the breed target at slaughter.

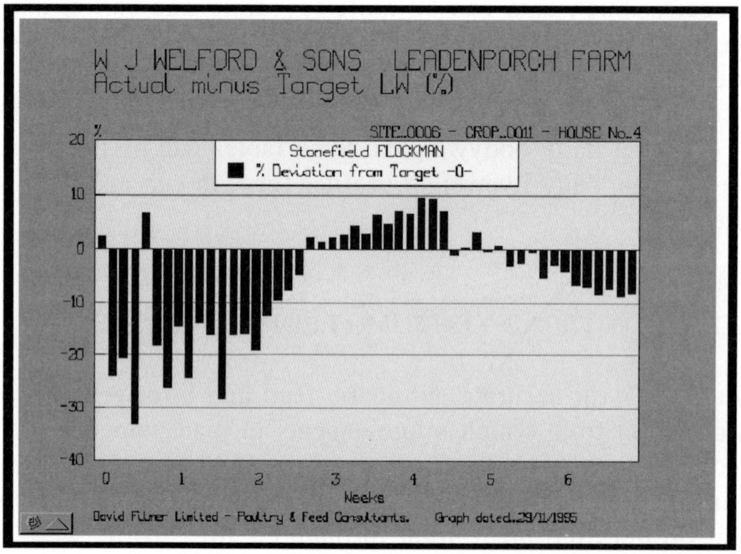


**Figure 13.5** Deviation from breed target live weight of broilers fed ***ad libitum***

More revealing still, is to plot the daily live-weight gain (Figure 13.6). This was quite erratic, with several days actually showing losses.

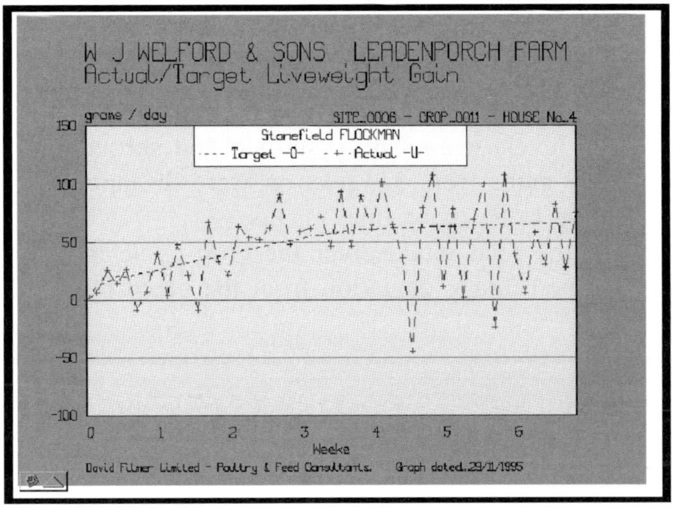


**Figure 13.6** Live-weight gain in broilers fed ***ad libitum*** as a proportion of breed target live-weight gain

In order to smooth out these irregularities, to enable the trends in daily live-weight gain to be seen more clearly, the 3-day running average for live-weight gain can be plotted (Figure 13.7).

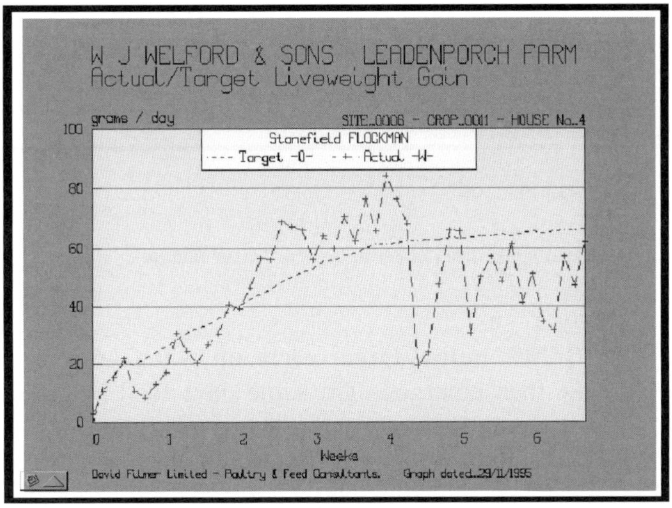


**Figure 13.7** Three-day running average live-weight gain as a proportion of breed target live-weight gain in broilers fed ***ad libitum***

The value for each day is the average of the recorded gain for that day plus the day before and the day after. Trends are now obvious, with gains exceeding target from 2 weeks of age until just after 4 weeks. At that time the 3-day average for the mixed sex flock exceeded 80 g/d. A collapse in subsequent daily gain then occurred, which has often been seen on *ad libitum* feeding systems. It would appear that birds can grow excessively fast for short periods, but that these high levels cannot be sustained and subsequently a recovery stage follows. Daily gains from 5 weeks on were disappointingly below the breed targets, leading to the poor final results.

Examination of the feed intake over the crop cycle is revealing. Figure 13.8 shows this as percentage deviation from the breed target.

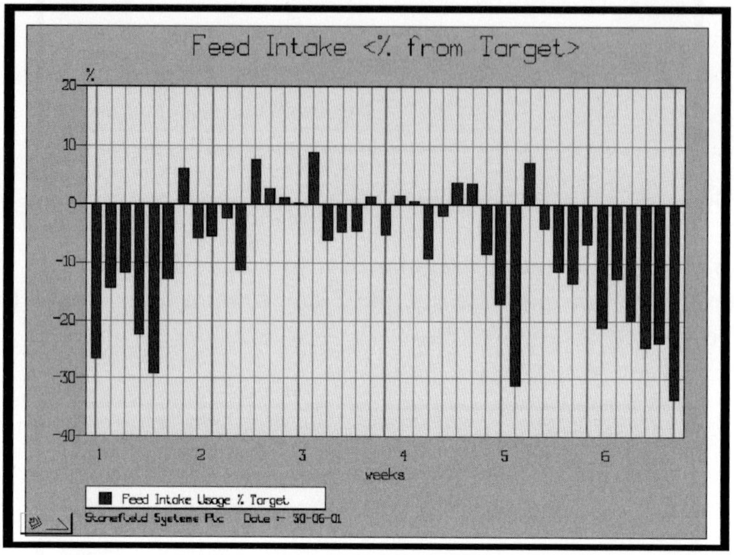


**Figure 13.8** Deviation of feed intake from target in broilers fed ***ad libitum***

Feed intake was 10-20% below target early on when growth was poor. A pattern of feed intake then emerges. On some days feed intake exceeds breed target by 5-8%. Subsequently feed intake drops as though the birds, having been satiated on the high feed intake, have lost their appetite. A cyclical pattern emerges with peaks and troughs of appetite. Several days of low feed intake occurred at 5 weeks followed by another peak. From that time on feed intake declined, which was associated with the poor growth rates seen at that time.

## CONCLUSIONS FROM AD LIBITUM FEEDING DATA

1) Feed intake and LWG on *ad libitum* feeding is erratic from day to day
2) Birds often grow early on at rates that they cannot sustain
3) Typically liveweight gain then falls off
4) Birds often finish well below the target weight at slaughter, although they were 5-10% above breed target at 4 weeks of age

From these conclusions, a theory was developed that if daily feed intake could be better controlled, daily live-weight gain would be more consistent.

## FIRST ATTEMPT AT CONTROLLED FEEDING

This was based on disabling the feed system during parts of the day. It was common practice at the time to disable the feed system for several hours during the day with the purpose of allowing the feed pans to become empty so that there was no build-up of stale feed at the bottom of the feed pans.

Various timetables for enabling and disabling the feeders were tried, such as: -

| | | |
|---|---|---|
| 2 hours enabled, | 4 hours disabled | i.e. 4 feeds a day |
| 4 hours enabled, | 4 hours disabled | i.e. 3 feeds a day |

These systems were not successful, as the birds soon learnt the times that the feeders did not run and ate more in the times they did to compensate. Total feed intakes and variation were not reduced.

## SECOND ATTEMPT AT CONTROLLED FEEDING

This was based on the 1930s' system of feed control described earlier. A given quantity of feed is fed per bird per day, based on breed intake tables for the strain and sex involved. Since it was necessary to feed the flock as a group, it was important to know the number of birds in the house each day. This can be estimated from the numbers housed at the start of the crop and the daily mortality. Thus, the quantity of feed to be weighed out per day will equal the number of birds in the house multiplied by the daily feed / bird taken from the feed intake profile for that particular day, with the scale factor set to 100%. This quantity is now divided by the number of feeds to be fed during the day, to arrive at the quantity to be weighed out per feed. The method is to weigh out this quantity at each mealtime and stop the augers supplying the feed pans as soon as this quantity is reached. The time that elapsed since the feed augers started at the beginning of that feed period was then recorded. This was designated the "Reached Time". These reached times were then tabulated for each period for each day and also displayed as graphs where variation in reached times for each period could be examined.

The same principle was adopted as used by the stockman in the 1930s. This was to offer more feed the next day if the reached times were getting shorter, or to offer less feed the next day if they were getting longer. This was done by changing the feed intake scale factor. Experience showed that once the birds' appetites were controlled, the scale factor could be increased or decreased by 1-2% upward or 2-3% downward per day without losing control. If the scale factor was increased too much, too quickly, the birds would eat the higher quantity, but would become satiated and lose appetite the next day. The skill was to keep an edge on the birds' appetites by feeding them just below what they would have eaten given free access to feed.

As well as watching the reached times before deciding to change the scale factor for the next day, the manager would also compare the actual daily live-weight gains with the targets. If the 3-day live-weight gain exceeded 80g/day for mixed sex flocks, 90g/day for males or 70g/day for females, the scale factor would be reduced to slow them down to avoid the inevitable subsequent fall off in daily live-weight gain described earlier. In addition, if the daily live-weight gain began to exceed the target growth curve, (as in Figure 13.7 at about 4 weeks of age), intake was again cut back. The idea was to control growth to as near the target live-weight gain curve as possible throughout the crop. The nutritional argument for this is that if birds exceed the target weights before the final age, they have a heavier body mass to maintain and therefore higher maintenance requirements for energy and protein turnover are required. This contributes to inefficiency. In addition, if birds put on too much weight from surplus energy that they consume, this is laid down as fat. Fat contains more energy, gram for gram, than does lean tissue, again leading to energy inefficiency. Both these sources of inefficiency lead to deterioration in the final overall feed efficiency of flocks fed *ad libitum*.

This system of controlled feeding was first put into practice in 1995, with a skilled broiler grower who had previously won the BP Nutrition/NFU Broiler Efficiency Award at the UK Poultry Fair in 1991 and 1993. Figure 13.9 shows actual daily body weight compared to targets, whilst Figure 13.10 shows the deviation per day from the targets. These deviations were within 2-3% of targets from 2 weeks of age onwards. Significantly, Figure 13.11 shows that daily live weight gains were much less erratic than on *ad libitum* feeding, particularly up to 5 weeks of age. Figure 13.12 shows the 3-day average daily gains and it will be seen that these daily gains did exceed 80g/day and, although an attempt was made to arrest the normally observed subsequent fall away, this was only partially successful. However, a good recovery over the last few crop days brought the crop in at 1-2% above target.

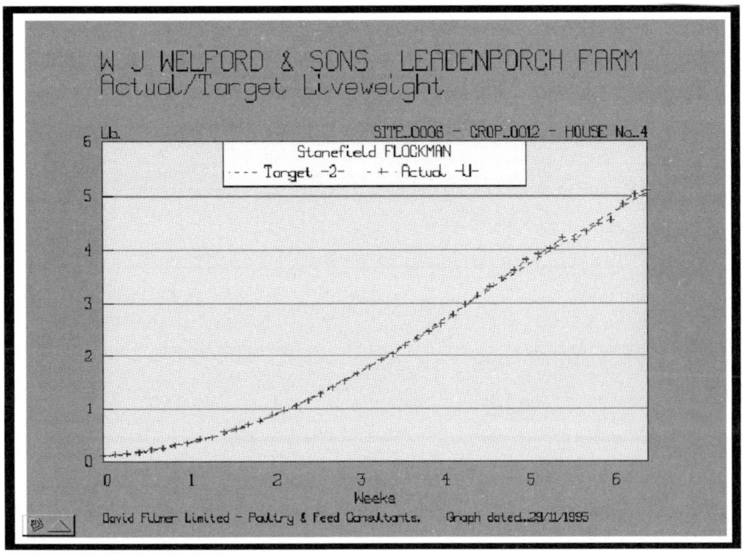


**Figure 13.9** Live weight compared with target in broilers under ***controlled*** feeding

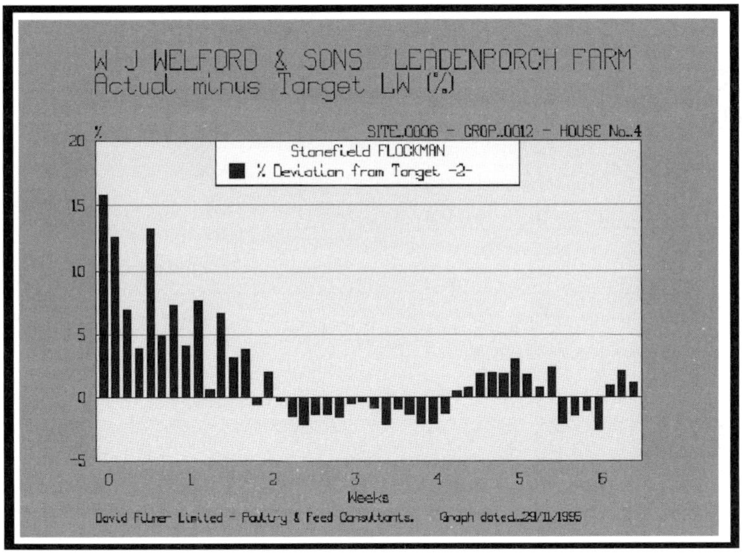


**Figure 13.10** Deviation from target live weight in broilers under ***controlled*** feeding

Feed intakes per day as a deviation from target are shown in Figure 13.13. The Y-axis of this graph is from -40% to + 20%, as on the equivalent *ad libitum* feed intake graph (Figure 13.8). Only on one occasion did feed intake fall below 88% of the daily target, whereas the *ad libitum* graph shows 12 occasions.

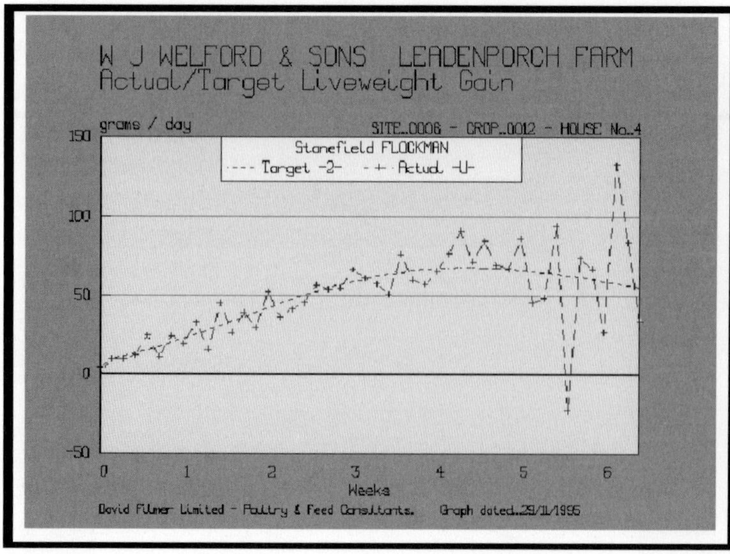


**Figure 13.11** Daily live-weight gain compared with target in broilers under ***controlled*** feeding

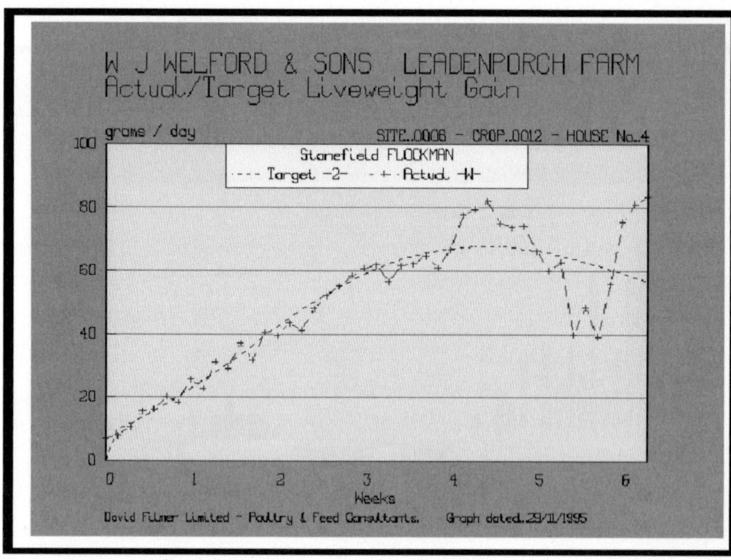


**Figure 13.12** Three-day rolling average live-weight gain compared with target in broilers under ***controlled*** feeding

This single occasion was associated with the single daily live-weight gain below 10 grams over the whole crop, compared with 8 occasions on *ad libitum* feeding.

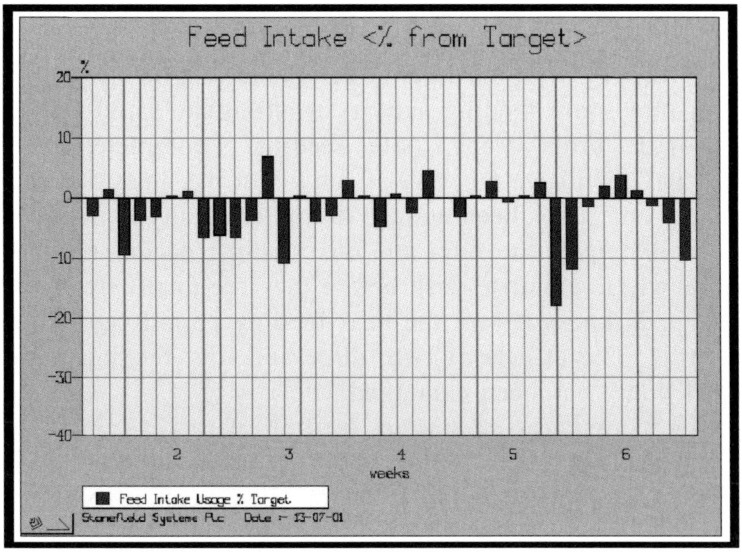


**Figure 13.13** Deviation of feed intake from targey in broilers under ***controlled*** feeding

It would appear that a reduction in variability of feed intake really is associated with a reduction in variability of live-weight gain/day.

## ADVANTAGES OF THE SECOND ATTEMPT AT CONTROLLED FEEDING

1) Problems are associated with over rapid growth rates which affect the largest, fastest growing males in the flock. Controlled feeding reduced late mortality of the bigger birds specifically from heart attacks, ascites and SDS (sudden death syndrome). Solving these problems had a substantial beneficial effect on overall feed conversion and profit.
2) Birds were less fat because feed control on average was beneath the levels of *ad libitum* feeding intakes.
3) Observations showed that leg quality was improved, with fewer lame birds. This was probably associated with the improved behavioural activity of the birds, leading to better health and fitness. Compared with *ad libitum* feeding, the day is divided into several feeding cycles instead of the uneventful day on *ad libitum* feeding. There is considerable bird activity at feeding times, followed by rest periods when all the birds in the house have full crops. This is much better for the birds' health and welfare. The lighting programme was also synchronised with the feeding cycle, so that lights are off for a time before the feeders are run and

remain off until all the pans are filled. Lights then ramp up slowly to simulate dawn, which reduces stress on the birds, and leads towards orderly feeding without undue excitement. Lights are on fully at the time of maximum feeding activity to stimulate rapid feed intake and filling of the birds' crops. After feeding is complete, and birds have rested, they then have a period of activity at the times that the feed pans are empty and it has been noticed that litter quality is improved and that more scratching in the litter and dust bathing occurs. Lights then dim down slowly to simulate dusk before they are totally extinguished. The period of darkness before the next feeding period can be adjusted for each cycle. The effects of two, three and four feeding periods within each 24 hours has been examined.

4) Table 13.5 compares *ad libitum* feeding of turkeys on standard feeds (A) with using a proportion of whole wheat in the diet and control fed (B). There was less variation in factory live weights with (B)

**Table 13.5** COMPARISON OF TURKEYS REARED CONVENTIONALLY WITH TURKEYS OFFERED SOME WHOLE WHEAT UNDER CONTROLLED FEEDING CONDITIONS.

| | *Ad libitum* *No whole wheat (A)* | *Control fed +* *whole wheat (B)* | *Difference* *(B-A) as % (A)* |
|---|---|---|---|
| Age of birds (days) | 56 | 56 | 0 |
| Mean weight (g) | 4242 | 4337 | 2.2 |
| Weight gain (g/day) | 154 | 154 | 0 |
| Growth curve weight (g) | 4557 | 4557 | 0 |
| Diff. from curve (g) | -315 | -220 | 30 |
| No. of birds weighed | 861 | 808 | -6 |
| Standard Deviation (g) | 391 | 371 | -5 |
| Coefficient of Variation | 9.2% | 8.5% | -7.5 |
| Uniformity | 67.3% | 71.5% | +6.4 |
| % outside 10% of mean | 32.7% | 28.5% | -12.8 |

The proportion of birds falling outside 10% of the mean weight was reduced from 32.7% to 28.5%; a reduction of 12.8%.

From observations, the explanation for improved uniformity of the flock is as follows: -

a) Larger birds on *ad libitum* feeding eat large quantities of feed and probably are larger because they eat more. Under controlled feeding systems they can only eat at meal times because the feed pans run out of feed and are completely empty for several hours between meals.

Although they fill their crops at meal times, their total daily feed intakes are reduced, and they therefore grow less quickly, are less fat and are more active and healthy. Because of this, mortality is much less (Filmer, 2001).

b) Smaller birds are at the lower end of the dominance hierarchy or "peck order". Under *ad libitum* conditions, when a small bird tries to eat, there is usually a more dominant bird at the feed pan, which prevents the small bird from feeding adequately. However, with controlled feeding, the dominant birds feed first at the start of the meal time event. They eat rapidly and are soon satiated and give way to the second dominance group. They too feed rapidly and in turn give way to subsequent groups. Finally, the birds at the bottom of the dominance hierarchy get their turn, and can also get full crops without disturbance, because all the more dominant birds are already satisfied and are resting. Thus the smaller birds eat more under controlled feeding and grow faster than under *ad libitum* conditions.

1) All birds develop their crop capacity, which under *ad libitum* feeding remain undeveloped and non-functional. The mass of feed stored in the crop remains present for some hours, before passing fully into the gizzard and digestion system proper. During this time, the feed is soaked in a warm, liquid medium and undergoes softening, expansion and disruption of some of the cells of feedstuffs of vegetable origin. This probably assists the release of cell contents for more thorough attack by digestive enzymes during the digestive process. Yalda and Forbes (1995) offered replicate groups of broilers the same daily quantities of commercial broiler feed dry matter. One group was fed the normal form of dry pellets and the other was fed the same feed, but as a wet mash after soaking in water for several hours. They observed that the group fed the soaked feed out-performed the dry-fed group in both live weight and feed efficiency. It is likely that the crop is an important part of the digestive system for avians and enables them to derive the maximum benefit from their feed. This has implications for reductions in excreted nitrogen, phosphorus and other pollutants in the faeces, litter and exhaust emissions from intensive poultry houses.

## DISADVANTAGES OF THE SECOND METHOD OF CONTROLLED FEEDING

The method works well in the hands of skilled stockmen, especially those having experience of feeding dairy and beef cattle, which are fed in a similar way. Results were poor, however, with less skilled or disinterested farm managers; often not as good as *ad libitum* feeding, where such people can have little influence on feed intake. The method also needed regular examination of the reached times and the graphs showing live weights and particularly daily live-weight gains. Skilled interpretation and experience was needed to convert these observations into changes in the feed intake scale factor for the next day. All this proved to be excessively time consuming, particularly on large sites where 8-10 houses were managed by one farm manager. The general conclusion reached by large integrators was that, although the system could work well, in practice it was too complicated for large-scale commercial use. It was considered essential to develop a simple system, requiring minimal input from farm managers, if there was to be large-scale commercial success.

## THIRD ATTEMPT AT CONTROLLED FEEDING

This was based on observations in poultry houses where the second system was in use. It could be seen that as soon as individual birds in the house were satiated and had full crops they lost interest in feed and went off to rest. It seemed logical to continue feeding the birds until all the birds, including the least dominant, had full crops. The challenge was to produce a sensor that would determine when this occurred, so as to send a signal back to the computer to stop the feed system. Fortunately, a method to achieve this objective was found and the intellectual property rights (IPRs) registered. The system is called "Automated Controlled Feeding" as it is totally automatic and needs no intervention by the site manager. The method still retains the ability to disable the feed system if the 24 hour feed consumption reaches a pre-set proportion of the normal daily feed intake (set by the daily feed intake scale factor).

## BENEFITS OF "AUTOMATED CONTROLLED FEEDING"

The main benefit is that there is a direct and instant feedback from the birds, which controls their immediate feed intake, instead of waiting for the manager to interpret eating times, and then to set the feed intake scale factor for the next day. This is particularly apparent in turkey pole barns, which are largely un-insulated, and where house temperatures are affected greatly by external temperatures. Should a sudden drop in external temperature occur, the birds will immediately respond by wanting to eat more before they reach satiation. The automatic system responds immediately to the demand for greater energy intake. The previous system had to wait until the manager noted the change in reached times. Even in this situation, the intelligent manager, who has noted the temperature fall, may anticipate the increased demand for energy and make an ad-hoc upward change in the scale factor. However, there are many variables that affect the birds' energy needs, as listed earlier, so the stockman's estimate can be no more than an intelligent guess. The birds however, can integrate all these factors, and are the best judges of their energy needs. The automated system is also independent of the number of birds in the house, so errors in the records of birds placed or daily mortality are irrelevant, nor does it depend on the breed feed intake targets being accurate.

A major practical and commercially important benefit is that no time commitment is required from the site manager for the system to operate. Finally, field results show that results are better with "Automated Controlled Feeding" than even skilled stockmen can produce. Table 13.6 compares 2 crop results (Crops 17 & 18) on the old manual system, with a further two (Crops 19 & 20) on the automated system. Each crop consisted of 2 houses each of 40,000 birds. The target for the major integrator involved was 2.75kg at 49 days. These results are posted on the Internet at *www.flockman.com*.

**Table 13.6** RESULTS FROM CROPS OF BROILERS FED ON A MANUAL SYSTEM AND THE "AUTOMATED CONTROLLED FEEDING" SYSTEM

| | *Crops 17 & 18 (manual system)* | *Crops 19 & 20 (automated feeding system)* | *Benefit to automated feeding* | *Benefit (% )* |
|---|---|---|---|---|
| Age (days) | 48.25 | 48.0 | 0.25 | 0.5 |
| Weight (kg) | 2.60 | 2.72 | 0.12 | 4.5 |
| FCR | 1.99 | 1.91 | 0.08 | 4.0 |
| Mortality (%) | 5.8 | 2.23 | 3.57 | 60 |
| EPEF[1] | 253 | 292 | 39 | 15 |
| Whole wheat (g/kg) | 155 | 160 | 5 | 3 |

[1] European Production Efficiency Ratio = $\left[\dfrac{Liveweight(kg)\times Liveability(\%)}{Age(days)\times FCR}\right]\times 10{,}000$

where Liveability = 100-mortality (%); FCR = Food Conversion Ratio

## 4th Concept - Integrated management system

Figure 13.14 shows age-related automatic linking between the pre-set lighting programme, the feeding schedule, the automated controlled feeding and the control of daily nutrient intakes. Simulated dawn and dusk, over a period,

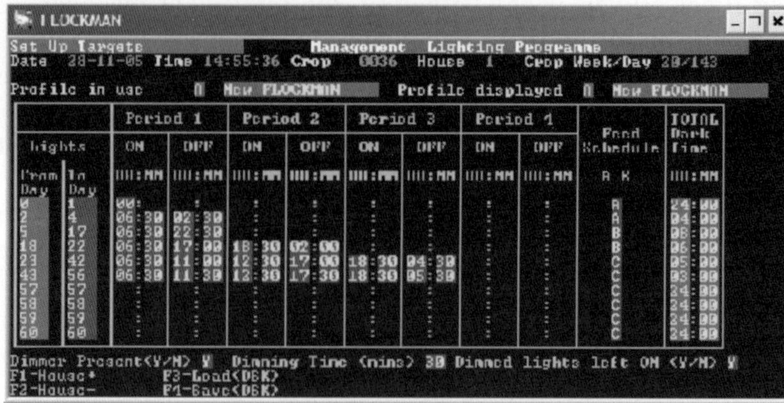


**Figure 13.14** Integrated lighting and feeding schedule for broilers

separates dark from light and light from dark periods respectively. Meal times are synchronised with the lighting programme for the appropriate day and the frequency of meals per day is automatically changed on the due crop days. In the example illustrated, feeding is changed from *ad libitum* to twice a day on day 5 and from 2 to 3 times a day on day 23. Temperature, humidity and daily lysine intake targets are all scheduled in on the due crop days.

All the various profiles are pre-set at the start of the crop by skilled supervisors, so that daily entries by farm staff can be zero. Even feed deliveries and daily mortality do not have to be entered. However, farm manager or supervisor intervention is still possible, with adjustments to environment profiles, such as temperature, target weights and scale factors for rate of change of daily wheat levels, lysine intake and feed intake being capable of manual adjustment daily. Of course, skill and experience are required to change these powerful control mechanisms effectively. Nevertheless, the system is designed to run automatically unless overridden for very good reasons. It should be noted that the feed intake and lysine intake scale factors operate independently from each other. Thus, for example, feed intake can be increased whilst maintaining daily lysine intakes (the ratio of whole wheat to feed increases automatically to ensure this). Similarly, lysine intakes can be increased whilst maintaining daily feed intakes (in this case by automatically decreasing the proportion of whole wheat). This is not possible with ordinary single feed systems as both feed and lysine intake change simultaneously in the same proportions. The ability to manipulate each independently presents a powerful tool for nutritional control of carcass composition, such as breast meat yield.

In summary, the new simple system minimises or eliminates daily entries on farm, is easy to set up and easy to use. It also incorporates feed and water spillage alarms. Farm managers like it as it helps them get good results without undue effort. Supervisors like it as it enables them to standardise lighting, feeding, temperature and other profiles together with performance targets and achieve greater uniformity across the various sites for which they are responsible. It does not need constant attention, as did the previous system, because the birds themselves actually decide when they have satisfied their energy needs.

The benefits are: -

a) less feed wastage, because the feed pans are regularly fully eaten out
b) better digestion because of crop activity, leading to improved litter conditions
c) more active, cleaner and healthier birds with improved behavioural patterns
d) less heavy bird mortality and better overall feed conversion efficiency
e) less variation in weight of birds into the factory
f) more control over average factory weights, dressing percentage and breast meat yields
g) improved profitability, resulting in payback of investment costs in approximately 12 months or less

## 5th Concept - Automatic changes to nutrient intakes if birds begin to deviate from targets

Current systems of deciding diets or daily nutrient intakes are prescriptive. In other words, assumptions are made that if a series of feeds are fed, or if a daily nutrient intake profile is followed, all crops of birds will perform as predicted. In reality, whilst this may be true on average, this does not happen consistently. Some flocks perform better or worse than expected for a whole variety of reasons. What is really needed is a system that detects if the flock is deviating from the desired growth curve, and then automatically makes appropriate adjustments in real-time to bring birds back on target. A continuous feedback system compares daily live weight and live-weight gain with daily targets. Deviations can be corrected by changing daily intakes either of energy or balanced protein or both to bring birds back on target.

This concept was accepted in 1997 by MAFF as suitable for funding under their LINK scheme for sustainable livestock production. A 3-year project was set up entitled "Integrated Management Systems for Poultry", which started in 1998. Industrial partners were Premier Poultry, Stonefield Systems and David Filmer Limited. The academic partner was the Silsoe Research Institute. Existing ***FLOCKMAN***™ equipment was installed in 8 modern, 23,000-bird broiler houses, at a site owned by Premier Poultry. Planning of the trial work was a group exercise, assisted by Dr Colin Fisher who acted as a consultant to the group on broiler modelling. Model construction and statistical analyses were undertaken by the mathematics department at Silsoe.

A new type of mathematical growth model was required. Normal growth models attempt to predict the outcome of various feeding regimes and feed compositions over the whole life cycle using predictions of feed intake. The new model did not have to predict feed intake as this was continuously measured. The real-time model is designed to make predictions of the next few day's growth, using all the live weight, feed intake and nutrient intake data it has collected up to date. Thus, it has an advantage over old models, which are based on predicted nutrient intakes, in that it can work on actual feed and nutrient intakes to date. The model recalculates every 24 hours, using the last 24 hours performance data to refine its predictions. A major difference is that the new model calculates any changes to feed intake and/or balanced protein intake that are necessary in order to bring the flock performance back on target. In order to do this, the model needed new data on the responses of commercial flocks of broilers to changes in energy and/or balanced protein intakes when birds had deviated from planned targets. A series of nutrition experiments were therefore set up on the 8-house commercial site, where birds were first fed inadequately, and then given various combinations of energy and/or protein intakes. Responses were recorded and built into the new model.

The model is now complete and the link between it and the ***FLOCKMAN***™ program established. This takes the next day's settings for energy and balanced lysine intakes from the model and makes the necessary adjustments to the two scale factors. The project has demonstrated that a feeding system in which broilers are weighed continuously and their diet and feed intake adjusted on a daily basis, is a more effective way of controlling the growth of broilers, than is the conventional method of feeding a prescribed nutrition program and hoping that it has the desired results. The model now fits the data extremely well, as can be seen from Figure 13.15 for House 7, Crop 23 before fitting the growth model, compared to Figure 13.16 for the same birds after fitting the growth model. The project ended in December 2001 and has been followed by a series of evaluation trials to establish performance on various commercial sites before widespread introduction of the system to the market place.

## Future developments

This is the first real-time growth model for broiler production and severalextensions flow logically from it. Firstly, the objective function could be modified to include achieving target weights at least cost; minimising cost

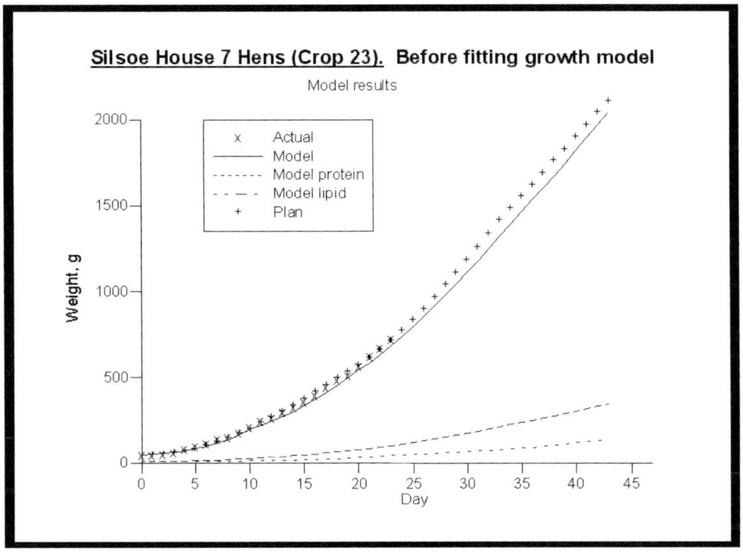


**Figure 13.15** Live weight of broilers under integrated management before fitting growth model

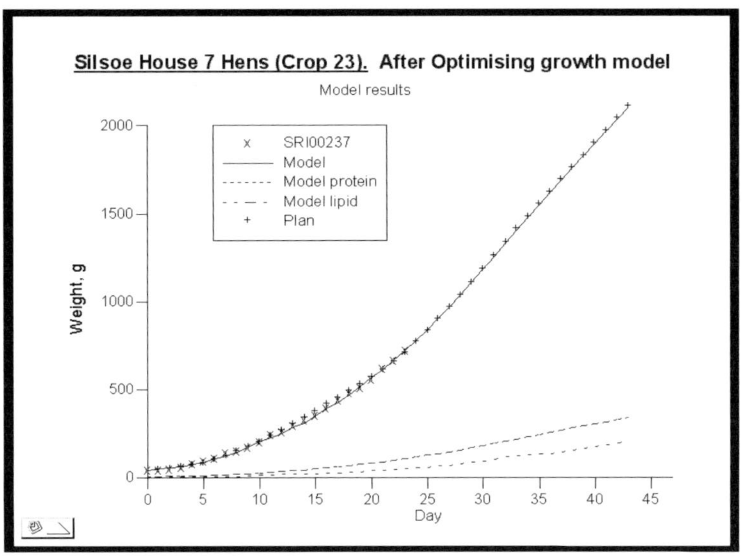


**Figure 13.16** Live weigth of broilers under integrated management after optimising growth model

per kg body weight or breast meat; or maximising margin per bird placed or per square metre per year. Further integration, incorporating costs and effects of maintaining temperature / humidity and/or cutting pollution would be possible. An exciting development is that the model can now "learn" from a "feedback loop", comparing its own predictions to what actually happened. Internal adjustments to the model are then made automatically so that the model can effectively fit itself into the circumstances found within a given integrator's operation. Stacey *et al.* (2004) describes this development and also gives field results. This automatically takes into account differences in nutrient levels ascribed to feed ingredients and/or differences in growth curves and their related nutrient intake profiles that do, no doubt, exist between various integrators. Commercial adaptation to other species, such as turkeys, is a priority. Developments of ***FLOCKMAN***™ systems for underdeveloped operations without the need for a farm PC may be achievable.

It is considered that the development of the first real-time growth model for broilers will be the first of a new generation of systems that will enable manipulation of nutritional inputs to be automated to the benefit of the integrator, the bird and the consumer.

## References

Cumming, R. B. (1992). Mechanisms of biological control of coccidiosis in chickens. in *Proceedings of Australian Poultry Science Symposium.* February 1992. University of Sydney, Sydney, NSW. Vol. 4. Pages 46 - 51

Cowan, P.J. and Michie, W. (1978). The use of barley in choice feeding of the turkey. *British Poultry Science* **19**, 1-6.

Emmans, G.C. (1977). The nutrient intake of laying hens given a choice of diets in relation to their production requirements. *British Poultry Science* **18**, 227-236.

Filmer, D. (1991). A new system for livestock feeding. in *Feeds & Feeding* July / August 1991. Pages 30-33.

Filmer, D. (2001). Nutrition and managing growth. in *Managing Broiler Lameness*, University of Bristol, School of Veterinary Science, 10 October 2001. Pages 24-38.

Stacey, K.F., Parsons, D.J., Frost, A.R., Fisher, C., Filmer, D. and Fothergill, A. (2004) An automatic growth and nutrition control system for broiler production. *Biosystems Engineering* **89**, 363-371.

Yalda, A.Y. and Forbes, J.M. (1995). Food intake and growth in chickens given food in the wet form with and without access to drinking water, *British Poultry Science* **36**, 357-369.

*This paper was first published in 2002*

14

# NATURAL PIGMENTS: PRACTICAL EXPERIENCES

MARÍA F. SOTO SALANOVA
*Villaviciosa de Odón, Madrid, Spain*

## Introduction

It is clear that yolk colour plays a key role in consumer decisions when evaluating the quality of an egg. It is also obvious that the colour target to be achieved will depend greatly on the specific preferences of a given country, or area within a country. From the clear yellow demanded by countries like Holland or the United Kingdom, to the intense oranges preferred by Germany or certain areas of Spain, there is a broad range of possibilities.

The aim of this chapter is to show results of practical trials carried out at the Nutreco Poultry research Centre on the subject.

## Market demand for yolk colour

The colour of the egg yolk is one of the most important attributes of egg quality throughout the world. Within the European market, more than 60% of people have a specific opinion about egg yolk colour, whatever that may be. Consumer preferences vary widely from country to country and, in may cases, from region to region. For example, a deep orange colour (RYCF 13-14) is preferred by the German market, whereas fairly pale egg yolks (RYCF 7-8) are favoured by countries like Sweden (or the USA).

In Spain, for example, egg yolk colour is considered as an important egg quality attribute, closely following albumen consistency and eggshell hardness (3.95, from 1=less important to 6=very important) (Roche, 1997). Spanish consumers prefer deep orange colours (Roche, 1999): 62% prefer RYCF 14, 22% RYCF 12, and only 16% prefer paler colours. In the UK, the situation is slightly different, with more people favouring colours between RYCF 10 and

12 (Wakeman, 2000). However, that preference varies according to region: i.e., in the Birmingham area, the preferences for RYCF 10, 12, or 14 are similar (24 to 29%), whereas in the Sheffield area, almost 40% of the people prefer eggs with RYCF 14. In all cases, and irrespective of the area where the study was carried out, 50% of people indicated that a uniform colour was an important attribute in an egg.

In summary, achieving a specific yolk colour is clearly a demand of the market. Whatever their preference, people have specific ideas about what the colour of the egg yolk should be.

## Carotenoids: colour and health

Poultry cannot synthesize pigments, which are fat-soluble compounds that are deposited in the yolk, giving it a specific colour. The pigments found in nature are carotenoids, which are hydrocarbonated compounds derived from beta-carotene. More than 600 have been identified in nature, and they are present naturally in plants, algae and bacteria. Carotenoids are usually symmetrical and bicyclical molecules, possessing a long carbonated chain with double bonds responsible for the colour, as they absorb light in the visible region. As stated above, birds cannot synthesize carotenoids, so they have to rely upon a daily supply to produce the typical yellow-golden egg yolks expected by the consumer. Birds have the ability to deposit dietary carotenoids in the egg yolk. Carotenoids are digested, absorbed and metabolized in a similar way to fats. Once inside the body, and depending on specific needs, they may have physiological as well as pigmenting functions.

Some of the known physiological functions of carotenoids are as follows:

- like beta-carotene, some of them have pro-vitamin A activity, and are active in the prevention of cancer and cardiovascular diseases
- others, like canthaxanthin, have been shown to have a role protecting the embryo against the oxidative processes that take place in the egg during incubation
- they are strong metabolic antioxidants, and are also used for communication through signs and colours (courting, warning, camouflage, etc)
- they are involved in immune response, cell and tissue oxygenation and maintaining water balance.

## Yellow carotenoids in feed: sources

Not all the carotenoids found in nature have pigmenting ability. Among those that do, only a few are efficiently deposited in the egg yolk. These are mainly lutein, zeaxanthin, and apo-ester. Lutein and zeaxanthin are commonly found in maize, alfalfa, and marigold extracts. Carotenoids such as beta-carotene, cryptoxanthin, or violaxanthin are metabolised by the hen and have no practical pigmenting properties. The difference between the total xanthophylls and the pigmenting xanthophylls in raw materials may explain the colour variability found in the final product. For example, beta-carotene and other non-pigmenting carotenoids may account for 10-15% of the total xanthophylls in marigold extracts.

The visual yolk colour that it is perceived is produced by the pigmenting carotenoids deposited in the yolk, and it is a combination of the deposition and colouring capacity of those carotenoids. For example, around 40-50% of the apo-ester consumed by layers is deposited in the egg yolk, whereas only 10-15% of lutein or zeaxanthin is deposited. Zeaxanthin absorbs at a higher wavelength than apo-ester, and this, in turn, higher than lutein. Therefore, their colouring capacity varies in the same direction: lutein is pale yellow, and zeaxanthin gives a more orange colour to the egg yolks, the apo-ester falling in-between.

The raw materials most used in feed for pigmenting purposes: maize (plata, and yellow), maize gluten meal, alfalfa meal, grass meals, or tagetes, contain variable amounts of zeaxanthin and lutein. For example, plata maize has a high zeaxanthin content (700-800 g/kg), responsible for the deep colour in eggs of hens fed this raw material. On the other hand, yellow maize has 400-500 g zeaxanthin/kg; this difference, if overlooked when formulating, will cause losses and variability in colour. Marigold extracts, containing around 900 g lutein/kg, and only a little zeaxanthin, confer a softer colour to eggs when added to the feed. Another factor to take into account is the inherent variability, even when using a single raw material: factors such as season, weather, harvesting year, storage, etc., will highly influence the xanthophyll content of these raw materials, and thus may be a source of colour variation in the final product.

Stability in storage may also influence the effectiveness of these raw materials. Marigold extracts, for example, may differ little in composition, but might vary in pigmentation, due to differences in stability caused by origin and processing conditions.

## Red pigments in feed: achieving the desired colour

By using high levels of one (or a combination) of the yellow sources, we can reach around 10 on the RYCF scale. However, yellow reaches a saturation point (desirable to avoid off-colours), but, if a more intense orange is desired, a source of red xanthophylls should be used. As the yellow xanthophylls, only a few of those found in nature are deposited in the egg yolk. These are, mainly: capsanthin (and capsorubin), citranaxanthin, and canthaxanthin. Capsanthin/capsorubin are commonly found in red peppers, whereas cantaxanthin was originally identified in the mushroom *Chanterellus cinnabarinus*. Again, the visual yolk colour perceived is produced by the pigmenting carotenoids deposited in the yolk, and it is a combination of the deposition and colouring capacity of that carotenoid. For example, in the case of the reds, around 40-50% of the canthaxanthin consumed is deposited in the egg yolk, whereas it is only 10-20% in the case of citranaxanthin, or 10% in the case of capsanthin/capsorubin. Instead, capsanthin/capsorubin absorbs at a higher wavelength than citranaxanthin, and this, in turn, higher than canthaxanthin, and therefore, their colouring capacity will also vary in the same direction: canthaxanthin will be mostly orange, whereas capsanthin/capsorubin will give a deep red colour to the egg yolks.

Thus, a given yolk colour can be obtained by combining different levels of yellow and red xanthophylls, although an adequate yellow base must be always present, and then, the red xanthophylls are used to obtain the orange, more or less intense, demanded by the market.

In summary, it is sometimes difficult (or even impossible) to reach the yolk colour required by the market using only raw materials. Relying on natural feed ingredients (maize gluten, maize, and alfalfa) is risky due to their variability. Adding pigments will allow the desired colour in final products to be reached without relying, at least completely, on raw materials. Also, it will allow the range of raw materials used in poultry feed formulations to be increased.

## The pigments market

The source of carotenoids for poultry makes no difference, either from the scientific or the legal point of view. The European Union additive legislation regulates only molecules, irrespective of origin. In practice, all pigments can be considered as natural colours, as they have been identified and isolated from Nature, and the process of yolk coloration also proceeds naturally in the laying hen. It should be remembered that carotenoids, in addition to their colour characteristics, have many biological functions ensuring healthy growth and reproduction.

The quality of marigold and paprika extracts depends on:

- The level of trans isomers (the higher the better)
- The level of saponification (should be as high as possible)

- The stability against oxidation (they often need vacuum-sealed packaging and antioxidants)
- Nowadays, some extracts are further chemically isomerized to obtain higher concentrations of some carotenoids, e.g. zeaxanthin.

The market for marigold and paprika extracts is often dependent on international supply and demand, determined by the annual harvest and the Euro/USD exchange rate. There are many products on the market and manufacturing losses range from 10 to 70% of the original product, arising during harvest, drying, extraction, saponification, production, storage, and, when performed, chemical isomerization.

## Practical experience at the Nutreco Poultry Research Centre

A series of trials was carried out at the Nutreco Poultry Research Centre to obtain in-house information on the pigmenting ability of a series of products available in the market. In all trials, the husbandry conditions were the same, and can be summarized as follows:

- Laying hens were housed individually.
- Hens were fed a white (barley-wheat) diet, with no added colour, for three weeks to eliminate all potential colour from previous feed.
- The hens then received a wheat-barley-based diet supplemented with different carotenoid sources for a further three weeks.
- Three eggs per hen were collected at the end of the 3-week period to monitor egg yolk pigmentation in both fresh and boiled eggs.
- Production parameters (feed intake, lay percentage, feed conversion, broken eggs) were monitored weekly to ensure no differences were observed and that variation in pigmenting would only be due to the treatments applied.
- Egg yolk colour was evaluated using two different methods:

    1. Roche Colour Fan: a subjective method, in which the colour of the yolk is compared with a colour scale from 1 to 15, assigning a number of that scale to each yolk. The value obtained was the average from three individual measurements.
    2. Minolta colorimeter: an objective method, measuring the amount of light reflected by the yolk when a light beam is shone on the yolk. The colour is measured by three parameters in the CIElab system:

        L : Luminosity
        a*: Red tones
        b*: Yellow tones

In the first trial, combinations of yellow (tagetes) and red (paprika) carotenoids were tested. The yellow source was a marigold extract in powder form, previously dehydrated, stabilized, homogenized and saponified (*Tagetes erecta*). This yellow source contained 20 g total xanthophylls/kg, 80% of which was lutein, 6% zeaxanthin, and approximately 14% was non-pigmenting carotenoids. The red source was a paprika extract in powder form, previously dehydrated, stabilized, homogenized and saponified (*Capsicuum annum).* This red source contained 5 g total xanthophylls/kg, 54% of which was capasnthin, 5% capsorubin, and variable amounts of lutein, cryptoxanthin, and non-pigmenting carotenoids. The following dosage combinations of yellow and red carotenoids were used:

- 150 ppm yellow, 600 or 900 ppm red
- 300 ppm yellow, 0, 300, 600, 900, or 1200 ppm red
- 450 ppm yellow, 0, 300, 600, 900, or 1200 ppm red

For this trial, a "negative" control with 6.1 ppm apo-ester, and 1.7ppm canthaxanthin was used.

**Table 14.1** YOLK COLOUR PRODUCED WITH COMBINATIONS OF YELLOW (TAGETES) AND RED (PAPRIKA) CAROTENOIDS

| *Treatments* | *RYCF* | *Minolta* | |
|---|---|---|---|
| | | *a** | *b** |
| Control | 12.7 | 6.1 | 46.6 |
| 6.1ppm apo-ester | | | |
| 1.7ppm canthaxanthin | | | |
| Yellow: 150ppm | | | |
| 600ppm red | 7.6 | -1.9 | 37.4 |
| 900ppm red | 10.7 | 0.5 | 38.7 |
| Yellow: 300ppm | | | |
| 0ppm red | 4.9 | -8.0 | 40.7 |
| 300ppm red | 7.3 | -4.8 | 41.3 |
| 600ppm red | 8.9 | -2.4 | 39.9 |
| 900ppm red | 10.0 | -0.5 | 39.6 |
| 1200ppm red | 11.8 | 2.5 | 41.8 |
| Yellow: 450ppm | | | |
| 0ppm red | 5.8 | -7.1 | 44.5 |
| 300ppm red | 7.9 | -4.1 | 41.9 |
| 600pmm red | 9.7 | -1.1 | 38.9 |
| 900ppm red | 11.0 | 1.8 | 44.6 |
| 1200ppm red | 11.9 | 3.1 | 41.9 |

As expected, the RYCF, and the a* and b* values (measured with the Minolta) increased with increasing dietary levels of yellow and red extracts (Table 14.1). However, values of RYCF of 10 or more could be achieved only at the highest levels of red extract (900 or 1200ppm). The a* values (red) obtained were low overall, suggesting that only the higher levels of red extract would be suitable for most markets (Generally demanding a good orange coloration of the egg yolk, obtained with a saturated yellow and increasing levels of red according to the specific demands of each market). The b* values, indicating the yellowness of the egg yolk, were less variable than those of a*, and did not change in a linear manner as observed with the a* values.

In another trial, an unknown source of concentrated carotenoids was tested against a "negative" control with 6.1ppm apoester, and 1.7ppm canthaxhanthin. The only available information on the product was that the concentrate contained 15 g total xanthophylls/kg, and that a dosage of 1500ppm was needed to reach above 8-9 on the RYCF scale. A fairly pale yellow egg yolk was produced that only reached 5.1 on the RYCF scale. The a* (red) value was -5.0, and the b* (yellow) value was 32.9.

Another trial was conducted with a marigold-derived product containing 15g total xanthophylls/kg and 60% zeaxanthin (Marigold 60). The typical composition of marigold (80% lutein and 6% zeaxanthin) was changed through an isomerization process using high temperature, time, and an alkali, to contain 25% lutein, and 60% zeaxanthin. Since zeaxanthin absorbs light at a higher wavelength than lutein, a higher concentration of this molecule should give a more orange colour. The levels tested against a "negative" control, containing 5.9ppm apo-ester and 2.04ppm cantaxanthin, were 200, 400, 600, 800, and 1000 ppm.

**Table 14.2** PIGMENTATION OF FRESH (AND BOILED) EGGS FROM HENS FED INCREASING DIETARY LEVELS OF MARIGOLD 60

| *Treatments* | *RYCF* | *Minolta* | |
|---|---|---|---|
| | | *a** | *b** |
| Control | 12.6 (5.7) | 7.9 (6.6) | 37.8 (50.8) |
| 5.9ppm apo-ester | | | |
| 2.04ppm canthaxanthin | | | |
| Marigold 60 | 5.5 (0.1) | -3.9 (-4.9) | 33.2 (37.1) |
| 200ppm | 6.1 (0.3) | -3.4 (-4.7) | 36.1 (39.8) |
| 400ppm | 7.2 (0.9) | -2.1 (-3.3) | 37.6 (45.0) |
| 600pmm | 8.2 (1.7) | -0.2 (-1.9) | 41.1 (47.9) |
| 800ppm | 8.5 (2.7) | 0.2 (-0.9) | 41.0 (50.9) |

The colour of the egg yolk increased from 5.5 (at 200ppm marigold 60) to 8.5 (at 1000ppm marigold 60) in the RYCF scale (Table 14.2). None of the marigold 60 treatments reached RYCF 10, despite the high zeaxanthin level in the marigold extract. In fact, a linear plus quadratic response was found between dose of marigold 60 and the RYCF values measured in the fresh eggs, described by the equation RYCF= $4.2951+9.2136(1\text{-}e^{-0.5227dose})$, which seemed to plateau around RCYF 9. The Minolta values a* (redness) and b* (yellowness) followed a similar pattern. The levels of redness were low, irrespective of dose; in contrast, high levels of yellowness were achieved by adding 800 or 1000 ppm marigold 60.

The results obtained for boiled eggs (Table 14.2; in brackets) corroborate those obtained for fresh eggs. Almost no colour was measurable with the RYCF, and the level of redness was very low, irrespective of dietary treatment. However, the yellowness values (b*) indicate a good saturation that increased with dose.

Two trials were run with four paprika extracts to determine their pigmentation ability, as well as their storage stability, either in the premix, or in the final feed.

**Table 14.3** CAROTENOID CONTENT OF FOUR PAPRIKA EXTRACTS

| | *ppk1* *ppm (%)* | *ppk2* *ppm (%)* | *ppk3* *ppm (%)* | *ppk4* *ppm (%)* |
|---|---|---|---|---|
| Pigmenting | (68) | (78) | (71) | (81) |
| Capsanthin | 2818 (55) | 2540 (60) | 2263 (50) | 2502(57) |
| Capsorubin | 92 (2) | 63 (1) | 89 (2) | 82 (2) |
| Zeaxanthin | 517 (10) | 563 (13) | 478 (10) | 461 (11) |
| Lutein | 49 (1) | 153 (4) | 432 (9) | 504 (11) |
| Non-pigmenting | (32) | (22) | (29) | (19) |
| ß-carotene | 633 (12) | 271 (6) | 446 (10) | 238 (5) |
| Cryptoxanthin | 389 (8) | 291 (7) | 321 (7) | 225 (5) |
| Violaxanthin | 589 (12) | 384 (9) | 540 (12) | 372 (8) |
| Total carotenoids | 5087 (100) | 4265 (100) | 4569 (100) | 4384 (100) |

All four paprika products were supposed to contain 5 g total carotenoids/kg. However, the variation observed was quite high (Table 14.3). Also, the concentration of pigmenting (and therefore, no-pigmenting) carotenoids varied widely among the four products. Thus, for example, ppk1 contained the highest amount of total carotenoids (5087mg). However, it had the lowest concentration of pigmenting carotenoids (68%).

The pigmentation ability of the four paprika extracts was tested in a trial in which diets were formulated to reach RYCF 11 or 14. A fifth treatment, in which the carotenoid used was canthaxanthin, was also tested. The amounts of product added to reach those levels varied greatly among the four paprika extracts, ranging from 700 to 1820g to reach RCYF 11, and from 1800 to 4900g to reach RYCF 14. The a* (redness) values varied greatly among the products, making it very difficult to draw clear conclusions.

The storage stability of these red pigments was also studied (Soto-Salanova and Hernández, 2001). All products were stored under the same conditions (25 °C, 60% humidity) for up to 3 months, and they were stored either as received, mixed in a vitamin-mineral premix, or in a final feed (layer hen mash). Samples were analyzed monthly, and compared with the values at Day 0. The stability of the pigments varied greatly among the products and the variability in stability increased from the product "as received", to the final feed, the most unstable of all the forms being the total premix.

## Conclusions

In summary, special attention must be paid to source of pigments, in terms of colour, carotenoid composition, efficacy, stability, etc. In practice, experience gives the best answer. Whenever possible, products should be tested under production conditions to suit particular final needs.

## References

Soto-Salanova, M.F., and J.M. Hernández, 2001. Effect of storage time on the stability of several carotenoid sources (paprika xanthophylls vs. Canthaxanthin) in premix and layer mash feed: Difference between yolk-pigmenting carotenoids and total xanthophylls. 13th European Symposium on Poultry Nutrition, Blakenberge, Belgium, Sep 30, 2001.

Wakeman, W., 2000. Dark yolk colour is a key attribute. *Poultry World* **5**,14.

15

# NUTRIENT REQUIREMENTS FOR GRAZING HORSES: DEVELOPMENT OF AN OPTIMAL PASTURE SUPPLEMENT

RHONDA M. HOFFMAN[1] AND DAVID S. KRONFELD[2]
[1]*Department of Animal Science, The University of Connecticut, Storrs, CT, USA*
[2]*Department of Animal and Poultry Sciences, Virginia Polytechnic Institute and State University, Blacksburg, VA, USA*

## Introduction

Most commercial horse feeds are supplements for use with forages – pastures or hays. Most supplements are based on cereal grains containing abundant starch, which is alien to the nutritional heritage of the horse. Common experience has been supported by epidemiological and experimental studies that associate grain concentrates with several digestive and metabolic disorders – colic, laminitis, gastric ulcers and, perhaps, developmental orthopedic disease and some forms of exertional rhabdomyolysis (Sprouse *et al.*, 1987; Clarke *et al.*, 1990; Valberg, 1995). The key etiologic factors may be overloads of hydrolyzable and rapidly fermentable carbohydrates (Figure 15.1). To circumvent these problems and promote performance, a series of studies at the Middleburg Agricultural Research and Extension Center have been developing a pasture supplement that features fibre and fat in lieu of starch and sugar (Hoffman *et al.*, 1996). The biological studies have been complemented by statistical investigation of optimal ranges of nutrients and the application of sensitivity analysis to ration evaluation and supplement formulation (Kronfeld *et al.*, 1994; Kronfeld, 1998b). This paper will summarize major findings and address certain dilemmas, starting with interpretation of nutrient requirements.

## Requirements, Allowances and Optimal Ranges

Current nutrient requirements of horses (NRC, 1989) are conceptually like those of the dog and cat – best regarded as mean minimums intended to avoid undesired effects (Figure 15.2). In contrast, the nutrient requirements of

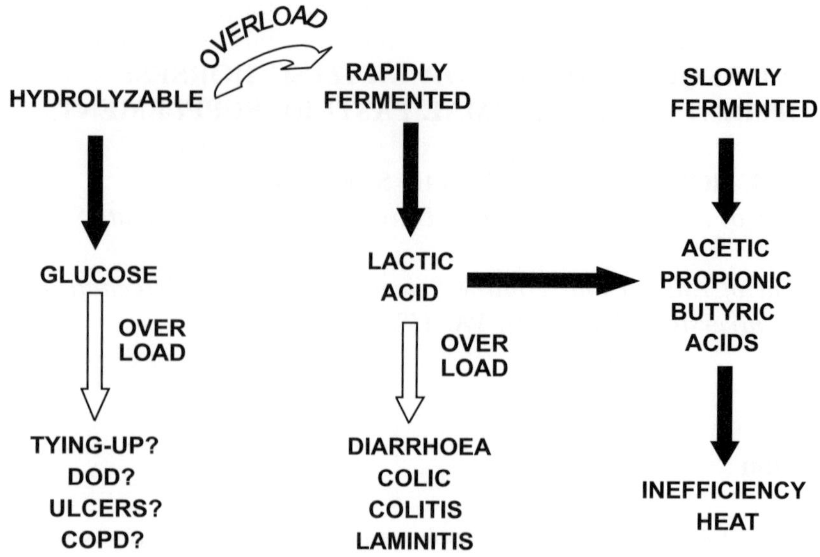


**Figure 15.1** Overloads of sugars (molasses and rapidly growing pastures), hydrolyzable starches (grains), and rapidly fermentable carbohydrates (soluble fibres) are commonly thought to precipitate certain digestive and metabolic disorders in the horse. Slow fermentation of insoluble fibres (mainly cellulose) sustains healthy function of the large bowel. (Modified from Kronfeld, 1998a).

production animals are mean values for desired effects. Recommended dietary allowances (RDAs) for humans are aimed at the mean plus two standard deviations, statistically sufficient for 0.98 of the population (Food and Nutrition Board, 1991). Noting that the nutrient requirements of dogs and cats, as proposed by the National Research Council, had little practical value for formulating pet foods, the Association of American Feed Control Officials (an alliance of government and industry, to which American regulatory agencies usually defer) developed nutrient profiles for dogs and cats. These canine and feline allowances emphasized practical experience and, unlike the human RDAs, lacked any systematic statistical basis.

The nutrient requirements of production animals and the allowances for humans, dogs and cats aim to reach the lower ends of optimal ranges of nutrient intakes (Figure 15.2). No such allowances have been offered by national committees for the horse. Following the plan of the human RDAs, equine allowances for essential nutrients should be at least 1.3-times the minimum requirements (NRC, 1989). Experimental and epidemiological studies suggest, however, that at least double the current minimums are needed for vitamin A (Donoghue *et al.*, 1981; Greiwe-Crandell *et al.*, 1997), zinc (Bridges and Moffitt, 1990), and copper (Knight *et al.*, 1988; Hurtig *et al.*, 1990). Given the numerous interactions among micronutrients, perhaps the minimums for all, rather than only three, should be doubled to yield useful allowances.

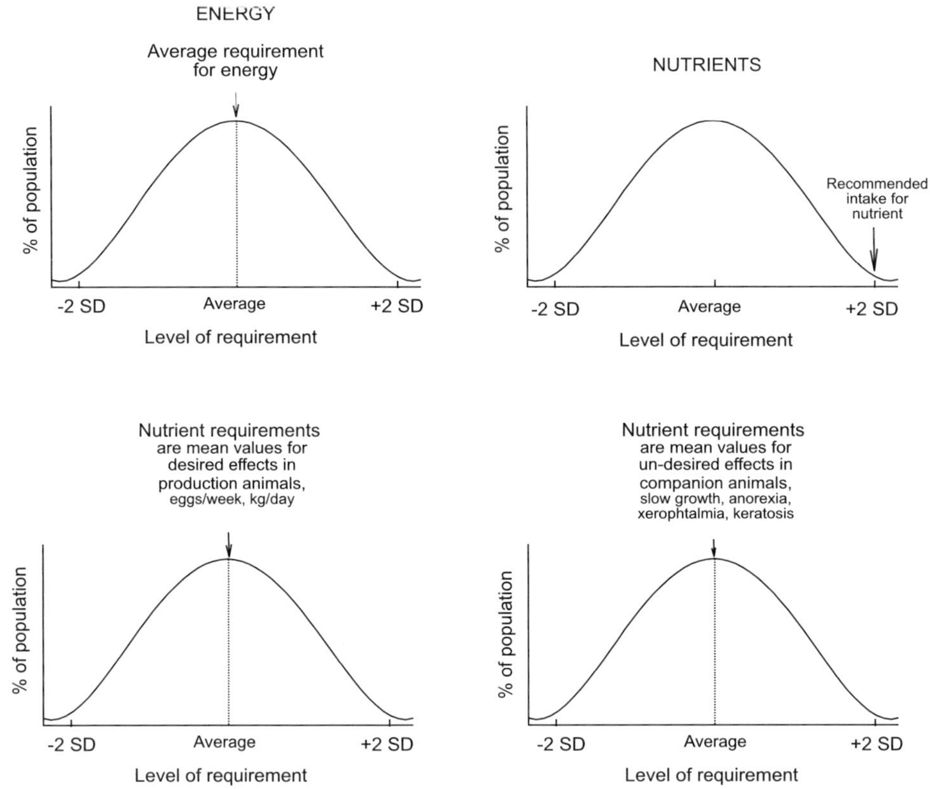


**Figure 15.2** The human recommended dietary allowances (RDAs) are means for specified populations (upper left), but the RDAs for nutrients are two standard deviations above mean requirements, so are adequate for 98% of the population (upper right, modified from Food and Nutrition Board, 1989). The nutrient requirements for livestock are mean values for specified production levels (lower left). In contrast, the nutrient requirements of companion animals are mean minimums to avoid undesired effects (lower right), hence are adequate for only half of the population.

Current digestible energy (DE) requirements for maintenance are mean estimates calculated from body weight (NRC 1989). The data were from four horses confined in metabolism stalls and multiplied by 1.43 for activity. Variation was negligible and failed to reflect the large variation in dry matter (DM) intake found in practice (Table 5-4 in NRC, 1989). If these ranges represent 90% confidence intervals, then the coefficient of variation ranges from 8% for maintenance to 12% for lactation and intense work, and 16% for growth. These coefficients of variation for DM and presumably DE intakes could be applied to nutrients for which corresponding coefficients are unknown, following the

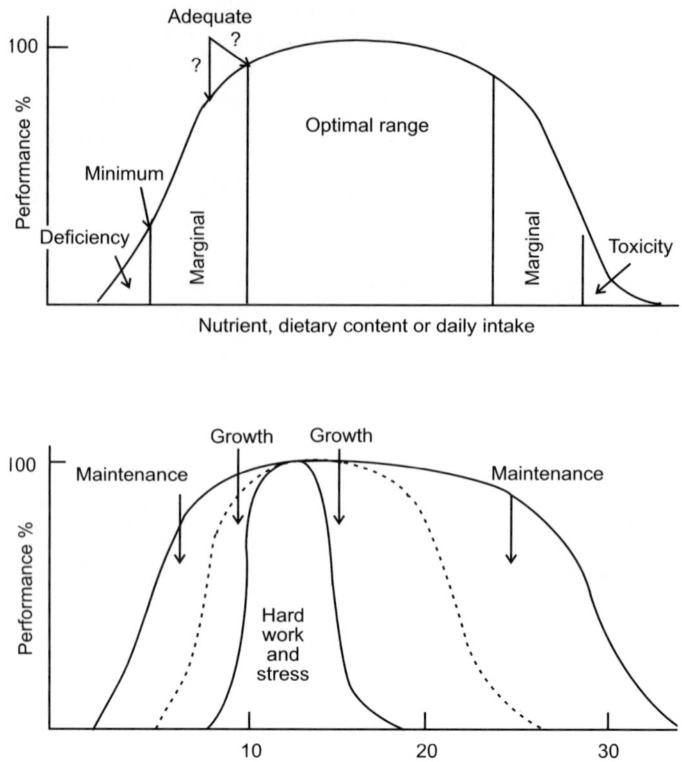


**Figure 15.3** The beneficial influence of dietary content or nutrient intake rises to a plateau, the optimal range, then declines. The plateau is broad for undemanding situations, but narrows as demands increase, for example, for growth, lactation, hard work and stress. (Modified from Kronfeld *et al*., 1994).

precedent of the human RDAs. Also, these coefficients of variation need to be kept in mind when estimating pasture consumption of grazing animals for the purposes of ration evaluation or supplement formulation (Kronfeld, 1998a). A palatable and presumably completely consumed supplement throws all of the variation into the estimate of pasture intake (Figure 15.4).

Reconciling American with European recommendations for horses involves multiple interconversions and numerous assumptions. The USA uses DE in MCal (NRC, 1989), the Germans use DE in MJ (Meyer, 1992), and the French use net energy (NE) in MCal (Martin-Rosset, 1990). The USA uses crude protein (CP) per kg DM, the Germans digestible protein (DP) per MJ DE, the French DP per MCal NE.

The NE systems are preferable because of large differences in efficiency of utilization of nutrients that follow one of five paths: glucose and other simple sugars; lactate and pyruvate (metabolized largely via glucose); acetate and butyrate; long-chain fatty acids; and amino acids (Vemorel and Martin-Rosset, 1993; Kronfeld, 1996). In formulating feeds, however, expressing nutrients

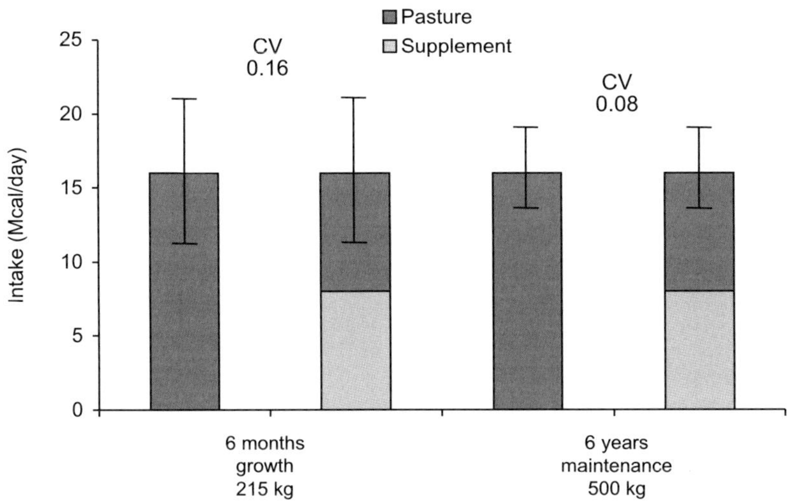


**Figure 15.4** Huge variation in estimates of daily intakes of pasture by grazing horses is exacerbated by the provision of a palatable supplement that is completely consumed. It requires the application of sensitivity analysis (Kronfeld, 1998b) in ration evaluation and supplement formulation. (Modified from Kronfeld, 1998a).

on a DM basis is usually better than any energy basis, because as energy concentration declines, so do bioavailabilities of many nutrients, and the opposing effects of these two variables tend to cancel out.

## Sensitivity analysis

For practical purposes, variation in intake, ranges of nutrient concentrations and known systematic errors can be handled by sensitivity analysis (Kronfeld, 1998b). A survey of pasture composition in central and north-central Virginia determined ranges (90% confidence intervals) of nutrient concentrations in initially 20, then 30 and later, 130 samples. Another set of ranges represented target zones for energy density and nutrient concentrations. A third set of ranges suggested DM intakes (NRC, 1989), hence approximate variation in DE intakes The range of supplement:pasture intakes of DM was 25:75 to 50:50. These ranges were used to calculate most of the nutrient contents of a supplement (Kronfeld, 1998b). The procedures are illustrated with the Pearson Square in Appendix A, and may be facilitated by ration formulation software.

Sensitivity analysis was used to formulate a trace element premix (Kronfeld *et al.*, 1996). Target ranges for the microminerals in whole ration were 1.5- to 3-times current recommendations for growth (NRC, 1989). Endogenous trace mineral concentrations were estimated using published values for the ingredients in the supplement, and the variation in intake and the composition of the 130 forage samples was considered. Sensitivity analysis was applied to test the soundness and flexibility of the formulation. These principles could be applied in any other locale, where ranges of microminerals have been determined in the forages.

The vitamin premix was less innovative. It was assumed endogenous vitamins were zero and the supplement was fortified to provide 2-times the current recommendations for vitamins A, D, E and thiamine (NRC, 1989), assuming that the supplement provided 0.25 of the DM intake. In addition, riboflavin, niacin, biotin, folic acid, $B_{12}$ and ascorbic acid were included on the basis of studies in other species and consultation with Dr. Ted Frye (Hoffman LaRoche, Nutley, NJ).

## Pasture intake

The huge variation in estimates of pasture intake (Figure 15.4) has prompted development of more precise methods, especially using markers. In ruminants, chromic oxide and ytterbium have been perhaps the most common external markers used to estimate fecal output (Blaser *et al.*, 1986). Lignin and acid insoluble ash have been used extensively as internal markers to estimate digestibility (Sunvold and Cochran, 1991). More recently, chromic oxide has been used to develop a model of faecal kinetics in the horse (Holland *et al.*, 1998b). Markers currently being evaluated for their ability to estimate digestibility in the horse include alkanes (Ordakowski, 1998), ytterbium and yttrium (Holland, 1998).

## Pasture composition

The energy and nutrient contents of pasture change with season and stage of growth. Relatively high sugar, protein and water contents are present in the spring and early summer (Blaser *et al.*, 1986). Fibre content increases with stem elongation, and energy, protein, phosphorus, and ß-carotene contents decrease as seeds are shed through late summer, autumn and winter. In a survey of twelve farms in northern Virginia (Kronfeld *et al.*, 1996), pastures were found marginal or deficient, compared with current recommendations (NRC, 1989), in zinc, copper and selenium throughout the year, and in phosphorus and vitamin A in the winter. The variation in nutrient composition and resultant inadequacies affect grazing animals with pasture as their primary habitat. Thus, these nutrients became the subject of field studies.

## Mineral supplementation

### PHOSPHORUS

Blood serum analysis indicated phosphorus depletion in weanlings but not in mares fed an all-forage diet of pasture and hay, that was marginal or deficient in phosphorus (Greiwe-Crandell *et al.*, 1992). Supplementation of pasture with phosphorus via a pelleted concentrate in another group of weanlings led to adequate serum phosphorus concentrations. Unsupplemented pregnant mares had hyperphosphatemia and hyperphosphaturia, which were regarded as paradoxical to the low phosphorus in the diet. The hyperphosphaturia was accompanied by calciuria, suggesting mobilization of calcium and phosphorus from bone in pregnant mares that would ensure a sufficient supply for the foetus (Greiwe-Crandell *et al.*, 1992).

### SELENIUM

Mares and weanlings fed only pasture and hay showed no clinical signs of selenium deficiency, but blood serum analysis reflected the low concentrations of selenium found in the pasture and hay (Greiwe-Crandell *et al.*, 1992). Selenium supplementation, via a pelleted concentrate, of another group maintained on pasture and hay, effectively maintained serum selenium concentration. Compared with supplemented weanlings, those fed only pasture and hay had more clinically-severe cases of an equine herpes virus type 4 infection, perhaps exacerbated by inadequate selenium intake.

### ZINC AND WEANING STRESS

The social dislocative stress of weaning may affect appetite, metabolism and immune competance. Foals raised on pasture and supplemented with a concentrate coped better with weaning stress, as assessed by behavior and adrenocorticotropic hormone response tests, than foals raised on pasture and hay only (Hoffman *et al.*, 1995). The pastures and hays were marginal or deficient in phosphorus, zinc and copper. The supplement provided two times more phosphorus, seven times more zinc and five times more copper than the forages. The advantage of feeding the concentrate may have been due to its mineral content. Serum zinc was lower during weaning in foals that had access to only pasture and hay, compared with those that were supplemented (Hoffman *et al.*, 1995). Zinc interferes with copper absorption; thus, copper deficiency may be caused by excess dietary zinc. Foals fed zinc in concentrations of 1000 or 2000 mg/kg, as compared to those fed 40 or 250 mg/kg, were severely lame after less than 10 weeks and had fractures of growth plate and articular cartilage (Bridges and Moffitt, 1990). A tentative target range for zinc may be 2- to 4- times the NRC minimum.

### COPPER

Copper is an essential cofactor for the metalloenzyme lysyl oxidase, which is essential for the cross-linking of collagen. Copper concentrations in pasture of farms surveyed in northern Virginia only marginally met the NRC minimum recommendation (Kronfeld *et al.*, 1996). A negative correlation between copper concentration in foal diets and degree of osteochondrosis was reported by Knight *et al.* (1985). In a subsequent study (Knight *et al.*, 1988), mares were fed normal and high levels of copper in late gestation and early lactation, and their foals were fed correspondingly normal and high levels of copper. The data were considered inconclusive (NRC, 1989), but were confirmed by epidemiological and experimental studies (Bridges and Harris, 1988; Williams *et al.*, 1989; Hurtig *et al.*, 1990). Recent research has demonstrated that copper supplementation of pregnant mares may reduce the risk of skeletal abnormalities in foals (Pearce *et al.*, 1998). Tentative target ranges may be 2- to 3-times the current mean minimum requirements of copper for pregnancy and growth.

## Vitamin supplementation

### VITAMIN A

Seasonal differences in vitamin A status of grazing mares was demonstrated using serum retinol concentrations and a relative dose response test (Greiwe-Crandell *et al.*, 1995a). Serum retinol concentrations and the relative dose response in newborn foals were linearly correlated with corresponding data from their dams (Greiwe-Crandell *et al.*, 1996). Supplementation with vitamin A at twice the NRC (1989) recommendation marginally compensated for seasonal differences (Greiwe-Crandell *et al.*, 1995b). Supplementation of depleted mares with retinol acetate reduced the incidence of retained placenta and flexor deformities and increased birth weights of foals (Greiwe-Crandell, 1995b). Considering these studies and previous reports (Donoghue *et al.*, 1981; Maenpaa *et al.*, 1988), the optimal range for vitamin A intake may be between 2- and 5- times the minimum NRC recommendation.

SYNTHETICS

A water-dispersible form of ß-carotene appeared to be ineffective in improving the vitamin A status of horses (Watson *et al.*, 1995; Greiwe-Crandell *et al.*, 1997). Moreover, the common synthetic, oxidized form of folic acid may interfere with absorption of the naturally occurring, active, reduced forms in rats, pigs and, perhaps, horses (Toribio *et al.*, 1998).

## Protein supplementation

Optimal dietary protein ranges for growth or hard work may be the most debated topic in horse nutrition. A quadratic curve applied to data from growth studies in the literature indicated maximum weight gain at a crude protein (CP) concentration of 160 g/kg DM, with 1.0 SE below the peak at 130 and 190 g/kg DM (Graham-Thiers and Kronfeld, unpublished data). Reports in the literature have indicated lysine as the first (Ott, Asquith and Feaster, 1981), and threonine as the second (Graham *et al.*, 1994), limiting amino acids for proper growth of young horses. Equine athletes may benefit from minimizing protein quantity and maximizing quality, which would minimize production of acid, heat and urea without compromising needs for stress and repair. In addition, dietary protein restriction would reduce ammonia in stables and nitrogen contamination of pasture.

A current pasture study on mares and foals is being conducted to compare a low protein supplement fortified with lysine and threonine with a typical (150 g CP/kg DM) supplement level (Staniar, W. B., personal communication). A similar comparison in exercising horses indicated that horses fed restricted protein fortified with lysine and threonine had a slight but significant moderation of the acidogenic effect of repeated sprints (Graham-Thiers *et al.*, 1998).

## Carbohydrate supplementation

Proximate analysis of carbohydrates relates to plant anatomy (Henneberg and Stohmann, 1864; Van Soest, 1963). The botanical fractions fit reasonably well with the digestive physiology of ruminants, but not hind-gut fermenters such as the horse. A proximate analysis to suit the digestion and metabolism of hind-gut fermenters would determine three groups of carbohydrates (Blaxter, 1989; Gray, 1992; Kronfeld, 1996):

- Hydrolyzable carbohydrates that yield glucose and other simple sugars.

- Rapidly fermented carbohydrates that yield mainly propionate and lactate, which are metabolized via glucose and pyruvate.
- Slowly fermented carbohydrates that yield mainly acetate and butyrate, which are metabolized via acetyl-CoA.

Instead, the common American system for livestock (Van Soest, 1963) measures acid-detergent fibre (ADF, lignin and cellulose), neutral detergent fibre (NDF), which is ADF plus hemicellulose in cell walls, and non-structural carbohydrates (NSC). Ruminant nutritionists estimate NSC, as calculated by difference, and thus include fermentable components such as some hemicellulose, pectins, gums, mucilages, oligosaccharides and resistant starches, as well as hydolyzable starches and sugars (Van Soest *et al.*, 1991). The NSC fraction may be calculated differently by subtraction of total dietary fibre (TDF; Hall, 1989). However, TDF does not include fermentable, non-hydrolyzable oligosaccharides and resistant starches, so this calculation of NSC also fails to delineate the hydrolyzable carbohydrates.

A common system used in human nutrition measures non-starch polysaccharides (NSP) and separates rapidly and slowly hydrolyzable carbohydrates (Englyst *et al.*, 1982; Englyst *et al.*, 1996). It has not been accepted widely in livestock nutrition because it makes no provision for lignin and the influence of lignification on the rate of fermentation, which affects the proportions of propionate and lactate versus acetate and butyrate.

Hydrolyzable carbohydrate has been measured in 107 forage samples and 25 concentrates (Hoffman and Kronfeld, unpublished data), using amylose and amylopectinase (Davis, 1976; Smith, 1981). The traditional method of estimating NSC by difference overestimated the fraction of the hydrolyzable carbohydrate present. Hydrolyzable carbohydrate correlated with NSC and accounted for about one-third of the NSC in forages and about two-thirds of the NSC in concentrates. Hydrolyzable carbohydrate fluctuated from month to month in pasture, but not relatively more than fermentable carbohydrate fractions (Wilson *et al.*, 1997). These partially seasonal, but also unpredictable, changes reinforced the need to provide a broad spectrum of carbohydrates in our pasture supplement.

The key feature of the pasture supplement developed is an array of fibre sources, perhaps ironically because forage is usually regarded as the main source of fibre in the equine diet. At times, however, the fibre content of pasture is low, and a supplement of slowly fermentable fibre is needed to sustain digestive health; this has been recognized for many years. The key development is the need for a full spectrum of carbohydrates, which is intended to promote a diverse microbial population. This symbiotic system should adapt readily to any abrupt change in pasture carbohydrates and sustain an adequate slow fermentation, yielding mainly acetate and butyrate, at times when overloads of hydrolyzable and rapidly fermentable carbohydrates may be exaggerating production of lactate (Figure 15.1).

## Fat supplementation

Given the emphasis on fibres, the energy concentration of the supplement developed needed to be sustained by additional fat. This design is the reverse of our complete ergogenic feed for the equine athlete, which features fat first, then slowly fermentable carbohydrate in sufficient amounts to preserve the equilibrium in the lower bowel.

The substitution of fat and fibre for hydrolyzable carbohydrates has various advantages, including reduced risk of digestive disorders and improved performance (Potter *et al.*, 1992; Kronfeld, 1996). Preference tests demonstrated higher acceptability of maize oil than other vegetable oils or animal fats (Holland *et al.*, 1998a). Spontaneous activity and reactivity were reduced (i.e. improved tractability) by dietary supplementation with maize oil and mixtures of soya lecithin and maize oil (Holland *et al.*, 1996). Fat supplementation may also be effective in controlling certain forms of exertional rhabdomyolysis (Kronfeld, 1998; Valberg, 1995). Rice bran, which contains 0.18-0.25 g/kg fat, has become a common fat supplement for horses in the last few years.

## Supplementation for growth

Our fat-and-fibre supplement (FF) has been tested against a sugar-and-starch supplement (SS), which is a copy of a typical, best-selling concentrate (Omalene-200™, Purina Mills, St Louis, MO). This is important, because control diets have been sub-standard in some equine studies. Results are also compared with industry standards for reproduction and growth.

The main advantage of FF over SS was noted in growth curves of yearlings (Hoffman *et al.*, 1996). Yearlings fed SS exhibited a spring slump, evident as a decreased rate of gain in body weight and condition. Similar growth slumps were noted in Ontario and Kentucky foals, around 360 to 400 days of age (Hintz *et al.*, 1979; Thompson, 1995). The slump in growth rate may be due to a metabolic change, or a result of seasonal differences in nutrient composition of pasture, easily attributed to the high sugar, starch and water content of spring pasture. This spring slump in body weight and condition was eliminated in yearlings fed FF (Hoffman *et al.*, 1996). Furthermore, compensatory growth was noted in yearlings raised on SS but not those fed FF. Compensatory growth has been associated with developmental skeletal problems, including flexural deformities (Hintz *et al.*, 1976).

## Supplementation and bone

Bone mineral content of the equine third metacarpal was estimated from radiographs standardized with aluminum wedges (Hoffman *et al.*, 1997). Bone mineral content (BMC) of the third metacarpal increased with body weight and age. Two plateaus were noted: the first coincided with a change in diet from mainly milk to mainly pasture and supplement, and the second with a decrease in activity on ice and packed snow. These plateaus appeared more evident in the SS group than the FF group. Thus, the FF supplement may reduce fluctuations in the rate of increase in bone density as well as body weight and body condition during growth.

However, BMC was lower from September to May, about 5 to 13 months of age, in growing horses fed the FF supplement. Perhaps the availability of calcium may have been compromised by the formation of calcium soaps with fat (Palmquist, Jenkins and Joyner, 1986), or through cation exchange and the water holding capacity of fibre (Allen *et al.*, 1985) in the intestine. Perhaps additional calcium provided in the FF supplement will compensate for this effect (Wilson and Hoffman, unpublished data).

## Supplementation and milk

Another advantage of the provision of a pasture supplement rich in fat and fibre was noted in milk and colostrum composition of mares (Hoffman *et al.*, 1998). The fatty acid profile indicated consistently higher linoleic [18:*2(n-6)*] acid in milk from mares supplemented with the fat and fibre concentrate over the first six months of lactation. Research in human nutrition has indicated a role for linoleic acid in the prevention of gastric ulcers (Kearney *et al.*, 1989). Linoleic acid is a precursor of prostaglandin E, and stimulation by linoleic acid increased gastroduodenal prostaglandin formation (Grant *et al.*, 1988). Prostaglandins are involved in the prevention of gastric ulcers by enhancing mucosal protective factors. Foals typically have a high incidence of gastric ulcers (Murray *et al.*, 1990), and prevention is important from both clinical and production standpoints.

Mares fed maize oil and fibre had increased protein ($P = 0.015$) and a 4.2 fold increase in immunoglobulin G ($P = 0.028$) concentration in colostrum sampled at 6 to 12 hours after foaling (Hoffman *et al.*, 1998). It was hypothesized that the maize oil contributed additional vitamin E activity that enhanced immunoglobulin synthesis in the mares. A subsequent study indicated that dietary vitamin E, supplemented during late gestation at twice the NRC minimum, increased concentrations of IgG, IgA and IgM in equine colostrum, with a resultant increase in passive transfer of IgG and IgA, but not IgM, to foals (Hoffman, unpublished data).

## Conclusions

These studies have shown that mixed grass-legume pastures used for horses need supplementation with phosphorus, selenium, copper, zinc and vitamin A. Providing a fat-and-fibre supplement designed to complement the pasture avoided the spring slump in growth of yearlings and increased immunoglobulin-G and linoleic acid in mares' milk. Improvement is needed in determining optimal ranges of nutrients, in measuring pasture intake, and in differentiating physiologically oriented carbohydrate fractions. Meanwhile, the application of sensitivity analysis should enhance the flexibility, effectiveness and safety of forage supplements.

## References

Allen, M. S., McBurney, M. I. and Van Soest, P. J. (1985) Cation-exchange capacity of plant cell walls at neutral pH. *Journal of Scientific Food Agriculture*, **36**, 1065–1072.

Blaser, R. E., Hammes R. C. Jr., Fontenot, J. P., Bryant, H. T., Polan, C. E., Wolf, D. D., McClaugherty, F. S., Kline, R. G. and J. S. Moore. (1986) *Forage-Animal Management Systems.* Bulletin 86-7. Virginia Agricultural Experiment Station, Virginia Tech, Blacksburg.

Blaxter, K. (1989) *Energy Metabolism in Animals and Man.* Cambridge University Press, New York.

Bridges, C. H. and Harris, E. D. (1988) Experimentally induced cartilaginous fractures (osteochondritis dissecans) in foals fed low-copper diets. *Journal of the American Veterinary Medical Association*, **193**, 215–221.

Bridges, C. H. and Moffitt, P. G. (1990) Influence of variable content of dietary zinc on copper metabolism of weanling foals. *American Journal of Veterinary Research*, **51**, 275–280.

Clarke, L. L., Roberts, M. C. and Argenzio, R. A.. (1990) Feeding and digestive problems in horses. *Veterinary Clinics of North America, Equine Practice*, **6**, 433–451.

Davis, R. E. (1976) A combined automated procedure for the determination of reducing sugars and nicotine alkaloids in tobacco products using a new reducing sugar method. *Tobacco Science,* **20**, 39–144.

Donoghue, S., Kronfeld, D. S., Berkowitz, S. J. and Copp, R. L.. (1981) Vitamin A nutrition of the equine: growth serum biochemistry and hematology.

*Journal of Nutrition*, **111**, 365–374.

Englyst, H. N., Veenstra, J. and Hudson, G. J. (1996) Measurement of rapidly available glucose (RAG) in plant foods: a potenital *in vitro* predictor of the glycaemic response. *British Journal of Nutrition*, **75**, 327–337.

Englyst, H. N., Wiggins, H. S. and Cummings, J. H. (1982) Determination of the non-starch polysaccharides in plant foods by gas-liquid chromatography of constituent sugars as alditol acetates. *Analyst*, **107,** 307–318.

Food and Nutrition Board (1989) *Recommended Dietary Allowances*, National Academy Press, Washington, DC.

Graham, P. M., Ott, E. A. , Brendemuhl, J. H. and TenBroeck, S. H. (1994) The effect of supplemental lysine and threonine on growth and development of yearling horses. *Journal of Animal Science*, **72**, 380–386.

Graham-Thiers, P. M., Kronfeld, D. S., Kline, K. A. and Harris, P. A. (1998) Dietary protein influences acid-base responses to repeated sprints. *Proceedings 5th International Conference on Equine Exercise Physiology*, p 115. Japan.

Grant, H. W., Palmer, K. R., Kelly, R. W., Wilson, N. H. and Misiewicz, J. J. (1988) Dietary linoleic acid, gastric acid, and prostaglandin secretion. *Gastroenterology*, **94**, 955–959.

Gray, G. M. (1992) Starch digestion and absorption in nonruminants. *Journal of Nutrition*, **122**, 172–177.

Greiwe-Crandell, K. M., Kronfeld, D. S., Gay, L. S. and Skan, D. (1995a) Seasonal vitamin A depletion in grazing horses is assessed better by the relative dose response test than by serum retinol concentration. *Journal of Nutrition*, **125**, 2711–2716.

Greiwe-Crandell, K. M., Kronfeld, D. S., Gay, L. S., Sklan, D. and Harris, P. A. (1996) Vitamin A status of neonatal foals assessed by serum retinol concentration and a relative dose response test. *Pferdeheilkunde*, **12**, 181–183.

Greiwe-Crandell, K. M., Kronfeld, D. S., Gay, L. S., Sklan, D., Tiegs, W., and Harris, P. A. (1997) Vitamin A repletion in Thoroughbred mares with retinyl palimate or b-carotene. *Journal of Animal Science*, **75**, 2684–2690.

Greiwe-Crandell, K. M., Kronfeld, D. S. and Sklan, D. (1995b) Vitamin A and beta-carotene supplementation in horses on different forage systems. *Annales de Zootechie*, **44 (Suppl. 1)**, 308.

Greiwe-Crandell, K. M., Morrow, G. A. and Kronfeld, D. S. (1992) Phosphorus and selenium depletion in Thoroughbred mares and weanlings. *Pferdeheilkunde*,**1**, 96–98.

Hall, J. M. (1989) A review of total dietary fibre methodology. *Cereal Foods World* **34**, 526–528.

Henneberg, W. and Stohmann, F. (1864) Beitrage zur Begrundung einer rationellen Futterung der Wiederkauer II. *Braunschweig*, **29**, 48.

Hintz, H. F., Hintz, R. L., and Van Vleck, R. L. (1979) Growth rate of Thoroughbreds. Effect of age of dam, year and month of birth, and sex of foal. *Journal of Animal Science*, **48**, 480–487.

Hintz, H. F., Schryver, H. F., and Lowe, J. E. (1976) Delayed growth response and limb conformation in young horses. *Proceedings, Cornell Nutrition Conference*, Ithaca.

Hoffman, R. M., Kronfeld, D. S., Herbein, J. H., Swecker, W. S., Cooper, W. L. and Harris, P. A. (1998) Dietary carbohydrates and fat influence milk composition and fatty acid profile of mare's milk. *Journal of Nutrition*, **128**, 2708S-2711S.

Hoffman, R. M., Kronfeld, D. S., Holland, J. L. and Greiwe-Crandell, K. M. (1995) Preweaning diet and stall weaning method influences on stress response in foals. *Journal of Animal Science*, **73**, 2922–2930.

Hoffman, R. M., Kronfeld, D. S., Lawrence, L. A., Cooper, W. L., Dascanio, J. J. and Harris, P. A. (1996) Dietary starch and sugar versus fat and fibre: growth and development of foals. *Pferdeheilkunde*, **12**, 312–316.

Hoffman, R. M., Lawrence, L. A., Kronfeld, D. S., Dascanio, J. J., Cooper, W. L. and Harris, P. A. (1997) Dietary carbohydrates and fat influence radiographic bone mineral content of growing foals. *Proceedings of the 15th Equine Nutrition and Physiology Society*, pp 191–192. Ft. Worth, TX.

Holland, J. L. (1998) *Pasture intake, digestibility and fecal kinetics in grazing horses*. Ph.D. Dissertation, Virginia Tech, Blacksburg.

Holland, J. L., Kronfeld, D. S. and Meachem, T. N. (1996) Behavior of horses is affected by soy lecithin and corn oil in the diet. *Journal of Animal Science*, **74**, 1252–1255.

Holland, J. L., Kronfeld, D. S., Rich, G. A., Kline, K. A., Fontenot, J. P. and Meachem, T. N. (1998a) Acceptance of fat and lecithin containing diets by horses. *Applied Animal Behavioral Science*, **56**, 91–96.

Holland, J. L., Kronfeld, D. S., Sklan, D. J. and Harris, P. A. (1998b) Fecal kinetics estimated by a chromium marker in the horse. *Journal of Animal Science*, **76**, 1937–1944.

Hurtig, M. B., Green, S. L., Dobson, H. and Burton, J. (1990) Defective bone and cartilage in foals fed a low-copper diet. *Proceedings of the American Association of Equine Practitioners*, **36**, 637–643.

Kearney, J., Kennedy, N. P., Keeling, P. W. N., Keating, J. J., Grubb, L., Kennedy, M. and Gibney, M. J. (1989) Dietary intakes and adipose tissue levels of linoleic acid in peptic ulcer disease. *British Journal of Nutrition*, **62**, 699–706.

Knight, D. A., Gabel, A. A., Reed, S. M., Embertson, R. M., Tyznik, W. J. and Bramblage, L. R. (1985) Correlation of dietary mineral to incidence and severity of metabolic bone disease in Ohio and Kentucky. *Proceedings of the American Association of Equine Practitioners*, **31**, 445–461.

Knight, D. A., Weisbrade, S. E., Schmall, L. M. and Gabel, A. A. (1988) Copper supplementation and cartilage lesions in foals. *Proceedings of the American Association of Equine Practitioners*, **33**, 191.

Kronfeld, D. S. (1998a) Clinical assessment of nutritional status of the horse. In *Metabolic and Endocrine Problems of the Horse*, pp 185–217. Edited by T. D. G. Watson. Saunders, London.

Kronfeld, D. S. (1998b) A practical method for ration evaluation and diet formulation: an introduction to sensitivity analysis. In: *Advances in Equine Nutrition*, pp 77–88.Proceedings of the 1998 Equine Nutrition Conference for Feed Manufacturers, Kentucky Equine Research, Inc., Versailles.

Kronfeld, D. S. (1996) Dietary fat affects heat production and other variables of equine performance, especially under hot and humid conditions. *Equine Veterinary Journal (Supplement)*, **22**, 24–34.

Kronfeld, D. S., Cooper, W. L., Crandell, K. M., Gay, L. S., Hoffman, R. M., Holland, J. L., Wilson, J. A., Sklan, D. and Harris, P. A. (1996) Supplementation of pasture for growth. *Pferdeheilkunde*, **12**, 317–319.

Kronfeld, D. S., Ferrante, P. L. and Grandjean, D. (1994) Optimal nutrition for athletic performance, with emphasis on fat adaptation in dogs and horses. *Journal of Nutrition (Supplement)*, **124**, 2745S–2753S.

Maenpaa, P. H., Pirhonen, A. and Koskinene, E. (1988) Serum profiles of vitamins A, D and E in mares and foals during different seasons. *Journal of Animal Science*, **66**, 1418–1423.

Martin-Rosset, W. (1990) *L'alimentation des Chevaux*, INRA, Paris.

Meyer, H. (1992) *Pferdefutterung*, Verlag Paul Parcy, Hamburg.

Murray, M.L., Murray, C.M., Sweeney, H.J., Weld, J., Wingfield Digby, N.J. and Stoneham, S.J. (1990) Prevalence of gastric lesions in foals without signs of gastric disease: an endoscopic survey. *Equine Veterinary Journal*, **22**, 6-8.

NRC. (1989) *Nutrient Requirements of Horses (5th Edition)*, National Academy Press, Washington, DC.

Ordakowski, A. L. (1998) *Alkanes are potentially useful internal markers of digestive functions in the horse*, M.S. Thesis. Virginia Tech, Blacksburg.

Ott, E. A., Asquith, R. L. and Feaster J. P. (1981) Lysine supplementation of diets for yearling horses. *Journal of Animal Science*, **53**, 1496–1503.

Palmquist, D. L., Jenkins, T. C. and Joyner, A. E. (1986) Effect of dietary fat and calcium sources on insoluble soap formation in the rumen. *Journal of Dairy Science*, **69**, 1020–1025.

Pearce, S. G., Grace, N. D., Firth, E. C. and Fennesey, P. F. (1998) Effect of copper supplementation on the evidence of developmental orthopaedic disease in pasture-fed New Zealand Thoroughbreds. *Equine Veterinary Journal*, **30**, 211–219.

Potter, G. D., Hughes, S. L., Julen, T. R. and Swinney, D. L. (1992) A review of research on digestion and utilization of fat by the equine. *Pferdeheilkunde*, **1**, 119–123.

Smith, D. (1981) Removing and analyzing total nonstructural carbohydrates from plant tissue. In: *University of Wisconsin-Madison Research Report R2107*, Agricultural Bulletin Building, Madison.

Sprouse, R. F., Garner, H. E. and Green, E. M. (1987) Plasma endotoxin levels in horses subjected to carbohydrate induced laminitis. *Equine Veterinary Journal*, **9**, 25–28.

Sunvold, G. D. and R. C. Cochran. (1991) Technical note: evaluation of acid detergent lignin, alkaline peroxide lignin, acid insoluble ash, and indigestible acid detergent fibre as internal markers for prediction of alfalfa, bromegrass and prairie hay digestibility by beef steers. *Journal of Animal Science*, **69**, 4951–4955.

Thompson, K. (1995) Skeletal growth rates of weanling and yearling thoroughbred horses. *Journal of Animal Science*, **73**, 2513–2517.

Toribio, T., Bain, F. T., Mrad, D. R., Messer, N. T., Sellars, R. S. and Hinchcliff, K. (1998) Congenital defects in new-born foals of mares treated for equine protozoal myeloencephalitis during pregnancy. *Journal of the American Veterinary Medical Association*, **212**, 697–701.

Valberg, S. J. (1995) Exertional rhabdomyolysis and polysaccharide storage myopathy in Quarter Horses. *Proceedings of the American Association of Equine Practitioners*, **41**, 228–230.

Van Soest, P. J. (1963) Use of detergents in the analysis of fibrous feeds. *Association of Official Analytical Chemists*, **46**, 829.

Van Soest, P. J., Robertson, J. B. and Lewis, B. A. (1991) Methods for dietary fibre, neutral detergent fibre and nonstarch polysaccharides in relation to animal nutrition. *Journal of Dairy Science*, **74**, 3583–3597.

Vermorel, M. and Martin-Rosset, W. (1993) The French horse net energy system (UFC): concepts, scientific bases and structure. *Proceedings 44th Annual Meeting of the European Association for Animal Production*, pp 1–25. Aarhus, Denmark.

Watson, E. D., Cuddeford, D. and Burger, I. (1996) Failure of b-carotene absorption negates any potential effect on ovarian function in mares. *Equine Veterinary Journal*, **28**, 233–236.

Williams, M., Stowe, H. and Stickle, R. (1989) Relationships of nutrition and management factors to incidence of equine developmental orthopedic disease: a field survey. *Proceedings of the 7th International Conference on Production Disease in Farm Animals*, p 32. Ithaca, NY.

Wilson, J. A., Kronfeld, D. S., Cooper, W. L. and Sklan, D. (1997) Seasonal variation in the nutrient composition of northern Virginia forages. *Proceedings of the 15th Equine Nutrition and Physiology Society*, pp 336–331. Ft. Worth, TX.

*This paper was first published in 1999*

## APPENDIX – SENSITIVITY ANALYSIS IN RATION FORMULATION

GIVEN: Forage Cu concentration average of 9 mg/kg, with a range of 6–12 mg/kg Cu.

The concentrate:forage ratio will be between 25:75 and 50:50, with an average of 33:67.

TARGET: Total intake of 20 mg/kg Cu, with lower and upper intakes between 15 and 30 mg/kg Cu.

TASK: Determine an appropriate Cu concentration in a supplement to complement the forage.

1. Calculate using the average values and a modified Pearson's square.
   9 mg/kg Cu in Forage.
   Concentrate:Forage ratio of 33:67.
   20 mg/kg Cu TARGET.

Forage 9 — $z$ — 0.67 forage

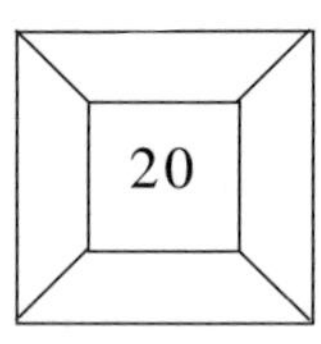


Concentrate $x$ — $y$ — 0.33 concentrate

*a)* $y = 20 - 9 = 11$:

Forage 9 — $z$ — 0.67 forage

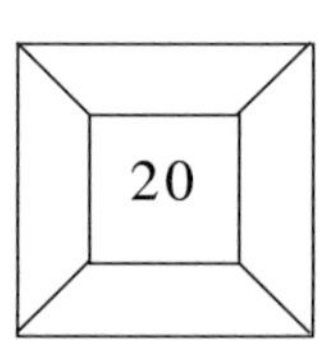


Concentrate $x$ — **11** — 0.33 concentrate

b) $\frac{z}{67} = \frac{11}{33} \qquad z = 22$

| | | | | |
|---|---|---|---|---|
| Forage | 9 | 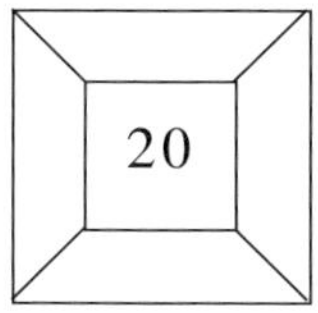 | **22** | 0.67 forage |
| Concentrate | ***x*** | | 11 | 0.33 concentrate |

c) ***x*** = 22+20 = 42, appropriate concentration of Cu in the concentrate.

| | | | | |
|---|---|---|---|---|
| Forage | 9 | 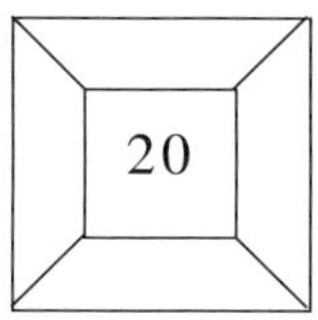 | 22 | 0.67 forage |
| Concentrate | ***42*** | | 11 | 0.33 concentrate |

2. Complete sensitivity analysis for the ranges of intakes, given 42 mg/kg Cu in the concentrate, forage ranges of 6–12 mg/kg Cu, and concentrate:forage ratios of 25:75, 33:67, and 50:50.

| | *Forage* | *Concentrate:Forage Ratios* | | |
|---|---|---|---|---|
| | *Cu, mg/kg* | *25:75* | *33:67* | *50:50* |
| lower | 6 | 15 | 18 | 24 |
| middle | 9 | 17 | 20 | 26 |
| upper | 12 | 20 | 22 | 27 |

(e.g. Forage Cu = 6; Concentrate:Forage = 25:75, then [42*0.25 + 6*0.75] = 15)

In this case, all total intake concentrations of Cu fit within the target range (15–30 mg/kg); therefore, no further iterations are needed for the concentrate's Cu content.

16

# SPECIALITY DIETS FOR HORSES

Anne Rodiek
*California State University, Fresno, California, USA*

## Introduction

Many products are marketed in, for example, both the United Kingdom and the United States for horses with different dietary needs or in different physiological states. This trend appears to have followed the companion-animal food industry, with foods specially designed to meet the nutrient needs of growing, mature and older animals. Diets for growing horses, mature horses, and "senior" horses have been available for several years. More recently, diets to meet more specific dietary needs have become available, including various speciality diets for performance horses and diets for horses with respiratory ailments or with hyperkalemic periodic paralysis. Some of the claims made regarding the attributes of these "designer diets" appear to be well supported by scientific research, some appear to be logical extensions of scientific research, and some appear not to be related to science at all.

The scientific knowledge of horse nutrition is not as advanced as for other farm species, or even many companion animals. This is due partly to lack of funding for equine research, but is also due to the lack of easily measurable parameters of success. Horse rations that promote maximal rate of growth are easier to formulate (and their efficacy proven) than rations that promote "optimum or paced" growth rate, that provide "calm energy", or that improve athletic performance, because all of these desirable outcomes are difficult to assess quantitatively. Because of the difficulty in scientifically evaluating the effects of rations on somewhat nebulous characteristics, it is tempting to accept testimonials as evidence of efficacy in place of scientific evidence. Scientifically, this is a dangerous practice. However, it is probably not wrong to extrapolate, in at least some cases, from research in other species, or to broaden the application of specific research in the formulation of rations that attempt to meet real needs in the horse industry. In all cases, both the feed manufacturer and the customer would be well advised to understand how nutrients/feed/rations promote their claimed effects and to separate the science-founded claims from the non-science claims. It is the objective of this chapter to summarise some of the generally accepted, science-based, nutritional concepts that can be used to formulate or assess some of the speciality diets popular today, with particular emphasis on energy requirements.

## Feeding older horses

Little research has been conducted on "old" horses. Even the age at which horses should be considered old is highly variable from horse to horse. In general, old horses that have trouble maintaining their weight have problems with improper worming, poor dentition or debilitating disease. Older horses also frequently have decreased ability to digest fibre, protein and phosphorus compared with young horses. Malabsorption of nutrients may be caused by chronic parasite damage or other alterations in the digestion processes in the small or the large intestine. Older horses may benefit from diets that are highly digestible and more concentrated in nutrients than young horses. Diets formulated for weanlings or yearlings have higher levels of nutrients and may better meet the needs of older horses with decreased digestion or absorption capabilities. Recommended nutrient concentrations/ kg of diet include: 120-140 g crude protein, 6 – 8 g calcium and 3 – 4 g phosphorus (Ralston, 1997). Feeds should be highly digestible and protein should be high quality. Raw materials such as soyabean meal, sugar beet pulp, processed grains and vegetable oil are more easily digested than others. Complete feeds that are pelleted and extruded and contain forage as well as concentrate (complete feeds) may increase intake. Coarse or poor quality hays should be avoided or minimised. Forage intake should not be discouraged, as gut fill is important. From a management perspective, the body condition of old horses should be carefully managed so that horses do not become too fat or too thin. Obesity will probably exaggerate arthritic conditions. Thin horses have little body reserves in case of illness and will probably suffer more in the cold. Adequate water intake is important.

Specific disease conditions may require specific dietary changes. Horses with pituitary dysfunction are frequently glucose intolerant and should not be given diets high in soluble carbohydrate (grains). They also often have low blood levels of vitamin C and therefore may benefit from vitamin C supplementation.

Horses with renal failure should receive diets low in protein (less than 120 g/kg), calcium (less than 6 g/kg) and phosphorus (less than 3 g/kg).

Microbial supplements, excess vitamins and herbs are frequently added to rations for older horses, but their scientific merit is largely unsubstantiated.

## Feeding athletic horses

Unlike the older horse, a large amount of research has been devoted to optimising nutrition for the athletic horse. However, because horses compete in such a wide variety of athletic activities, the research has been broad and sometimes difficult to compare, and the goals of various diets are different and sometimes even conflicting.

It is well accepted that equine athletes require rations of high energy concentration. The sources of the energy are generally either carbohydrates (cereal grains) or fats (vegetable oils or animal fat). The digestion, absorption and metabolism of these components are quite different, and the timing and form of the absorbed energy-yielding components may be factors that affect energy availability for different athletic endeavours.

High-fat diets (up to 150 g/kg or more) provide concentrated energy, not only to fuel athletic performance, but also to maintain body weight during training. Fats, both from dietary or adipose tissue sources, can only be metabolised aerobically and cannot supply energy directly during anaerobic work. However, some research indicates that dietary fat not only enhances the efficiency and amount of fat utilised during work, but also promotes preferential selection of fat as a metabolic fuel over glycogen during aerobic work. This fat preference may reduce glycogen utilisation until very high levels of work are required, and thus enhance glycogen availability during high intensity, anaerobic work. Several studies on fat supplementation to horses in training and performing high intensity work have been inconclusive. One study showed that fat supplementation (70 g added fat/kg diet) to a cereal-grain/forage diet increased both pre-exercise muscle glycogen levels (20.31 vs. 24.06 mg muscle glycogen/g wet tissue, for unsupplemented and fat-supplemented horses, respectively, 21 days into a feeding regime) and total muscle glycogen utilisation (8.05 vs. 11.30 mg muscle glycogen/g wet tissue in unsupplemented and fat-supplemented horses, respectively) during anaerobic work (Hughes *et al.*, 1995). Another study reported no difference in either parameter in fat-supplemented horses (Eaton, Hodgson, Evans, Bryden and Rose, 1995). Similarly, inconclusive results have been shown in studies designed to examine the effects of fat supplementation on lactic acid production during anaerobic work, although there is some tendency to believe generally that, when fat utilisation is increased, lactic acid accumulation is diminished.

Horses performing low intensity, prolonged work appear to be most likely to benefit from high fat supplementation. Endurance horses are frequently fed diets high in fat, low in soluble carbohydrate, low in protein and high in fibre. Vegetable oil, sugar beet pulp and high quality grass hays are popular, supplemented with electrolytes to balance the losses in sweat, particularly in hot climates or during competition.

Horses involved with high intensity work (racehorses in particular) may be fed fat, but generally are also fed liberal amounts of cereal grains. There are two schools of thought about how race horses should best be "fuelled". Some believe that high-fat diets are best because of their overall higher energy concentration and because of their "glycogen-sparing" effect. Others believe that fat is not a suitable energy substrate for horses as fat cannot be catabolised anaerobically. These latter individuals believe that carbohydrate is the better source, particularly during sprint work, because glucose can be metabolised anaerobically, making it available for the very intense, short-duration work of racing. Much of the difference in opinion about optimum metabolic fuel is caused by different opinions or findings on the limiting factors in various types of work. In very short duration, high intensity work, depletion of muscle glycogen stores, or even depletion of glycogen in fast twitch muscle fibres, may be the limiting factor in racing performance. In somewhat longer duration, but still quite intense work, accumulation of lactic acid and the feeling of pain and fatigue associated with its accumulation may be the first factor that causes work intensity to be diminished. Of course, all of these factors depend not only on diet, but also on fitness, muscle fibre type distribution and stride attributes of the horse, as well as numerous other factors, some which remain to be identified.

In the future, there may be enough nutritional information to warrant the production of diets specially formulated for horses competing in high intensity, short duration (primarily anaerobic) work and for horses competing in low intensity, long duration (primarily aerobic) work. There are already some supplements marketed that allegedly contain complex, concentrated carbohydrates for quick boosts in energy or for improved recovery after strenuous exercise. These supplements may provide readily available energy for some types of exercise. They should be used conservatively, however, to determine their most useful application, and also to guard against potentially harmful carbohydrate-overload.

In all diets for athletic horses, the supply of adequate levels of forage is necessary to maintain gut health and to maintain adequate water and electrolytes in the large intestine.

It is generally agreed that high protein levels do not enhance athletic performance. However, legume hays should not be discounted entirely as they are higher in energy and some minerals, and often more palatable than grass hays, so may make a greater contribution to the energy and nutrient requirements of horses.

Not only ration content, but also timing of a meal prior to exercise may affect a particular athletic performance, or at least affect the availability of energy substrates during work performance. Different feeds produce different blood concentrations of glucose and free fatty acids over different time courses after consumption. Several studies have shown that blood glucose (and insulin) levels peak approximately 2 to 3 hours after eating (Stull and Rodiek, 1988; Hintz, Argenzio and Schryver, 1971; and Glade, Gupta and Reimers, 1984) and that different feeds produce different glycaemic (blood glucose) responses. Maize, and a combination of maize and alfalfa, produced greater peak concentrations of glucose than iso-energetic amounts of alfalfa hay or a combination of maize and maize oil in resting horses (Stull and Rodiek, 1988). If exercise starts when glucose levels are high, glucose is used to a greater extent to fuel the exercise. If exercise starts when glucose levels are low, fatty acids are mobilised to a greater extent. Stull and Rodiek (1995) reported that exercising horses showed greater declines in blood glucose concentrations when exercised 1 or 4 hours after a meal (supplying approximately 17.2 MJ of digestible energy) of maize than after a meal of alfalfa hay or when fasted. During exercise, glucose concentrations in maize-fed horses fell below pre-feeding concentrations, while glucose in alfalfa-fed and fasted horses gradually rose through exercise. Blood insulin concentrations mirrored the glucose responses, being higher in the maize-fed horses. Lactic acid concentrations tended to be higher in horses given maize than fasted horses or horses fed alfalfa hay. Free fatty acid levels responded approximately inversely to the glucose levels, showing highest levels during exercise in the fasted horses and lowest levels in the maize-fed horses (Figures 16.1 and 16.2).

When exercise is of short duration and intense, the goal may be to provide quickly-available, high blood glucose levels. When exercise is of long duration, however, having large amounts of glucose being catabolised and causing a drop in blood glucose levels early in work may not be ideal. This is a relatively new area of nutritional research but, in the future, feed labels may contain information not only about amounts of feed to be offered, but also about the timing of meals before exercise (soon before or long before) to enhance further the ability of the diet to optimise athletic performance.

## Feeding laminitis-prone horses (feeding "natives")

In contrast to the equine athletes, where maximising energy intake is often the goal, there are other types and breeds of horses and ponies that are the "air ferns" of the equine world. They are the ultimate "good doers," seemingly able to maintain themselves on nothing and get fat on anything, no matter how meagrely they are fed. The metabolic differences in these animals have not been established conclusively, but many animals that maintain weight very easily also seem to be more sensitive to laminitis when overfed even relatively minimally. Some evidence points to pituitary or thyroid dysfunction, associated with detrimental alterations in glucose metabolism, as predisposing factors for laminitis.

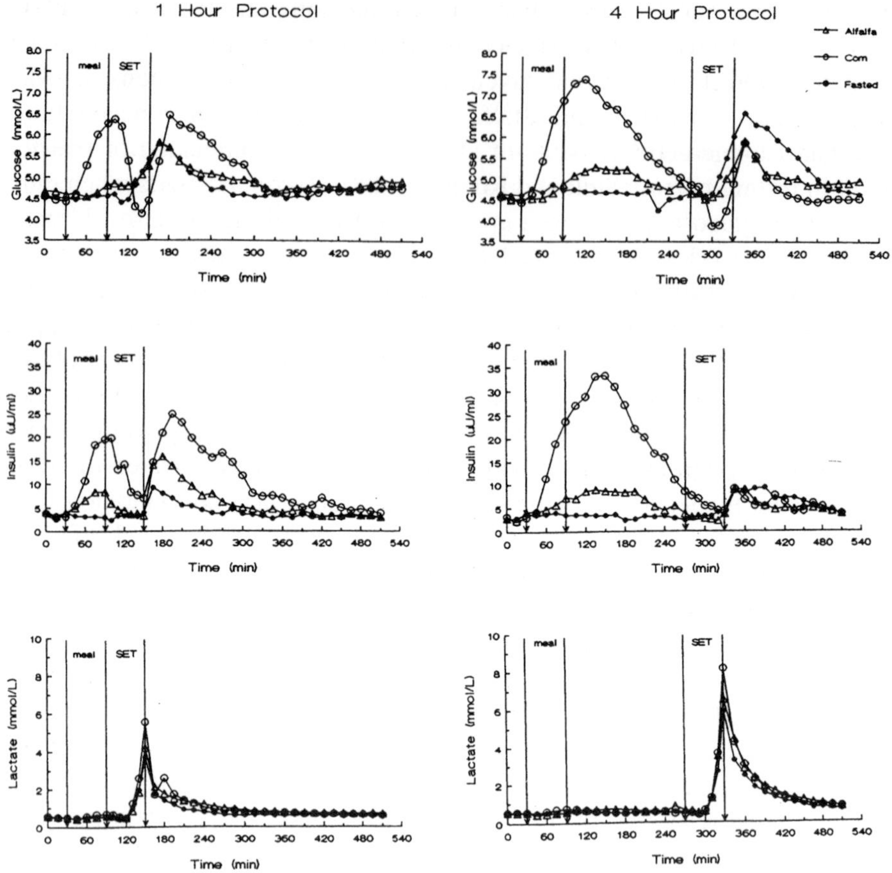


**Figure 16.1** Mean plasma glucose, serum insulin and plasma lactate concentrations of fasted, maize-fed, or alfalfa-fed horses exercised (SET) 1 or 4 hours after eating.

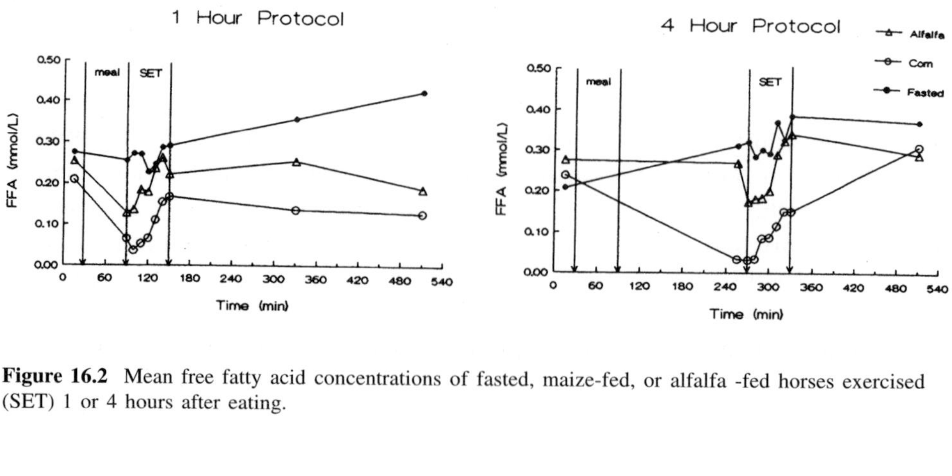


**Figure 16.2** Mean free fatty acid concentrations of fasted, maize-fed, or alfalfa -fed horses exercised (SET) 1 or 4 hours after eating.

Soluble carbohydrates are strongly associated with laminitis, particularly if they pass to the large intestine and are fermented by the microbes therein. Microbial fermentation of soluble carbohydrates results in acid production (primarily lactic acid), damage to the mucosa of the large intestine, and escape of toxins from the digestive system into the circulation. More than one theory has been proposed regarding how blood-borne toxins from the digestive system cause laminitis in the hooves, but the concept of an ultimate cause being carbohydrate-overload in the large intestine is generally accepted. Grain is not the only feed material that supplies soluble carbohydrates; pasture grasses can also cause problems because of their high concentration of fructans (polysaccharides of fructose) that largely by-pass the small intestine and are fermented by microbes in the large intestine. Longland *et al.* (1999) showed that fructan concentration varied greatly in a common species of United Kingdom pasture grass (*Lolium perenne*), due to variety as well as seasonal and diurnal variation. Fructan content of *Lolium perenne* varied throughout the year, with lowest levels (100 to 140 g/kg dry matter) in April and highest levels (300 to 420 g/kg dry matter) in July. Time of day and environmental conditions were also shown to influence fructan concentration. Fructan levels were lowest during the evening and morning hours (0 to 140 g/kg dry matter) and highest about midday (140 to 300 g/kg dry matter). Warm, sunny weather produced higher fructan concentrations than cool, rainy weather.

Formulating low energy, high fibre and palatable feeds is both the key and the challenge. Horses should not be given rations where the feed allocation is less than 15 g/kg body weight, since a minimum of dietary bulk is required for optimum health of the digestive tract. Rations must also meet needs for vitamins and minerals, which may mean supplementation is needed if the ration is based on grass hay (particularly for trace minerals and vitamin E and possibly also for protein). Long hay, coarse mixes or cubes are preferred over pelleted diets as the latter are usually consumed more readily, and pass through the digestive tract faster, than diets comprised of forages with larger particle size. Newer methods of manufacturing cubes compress the hay pieces along the long axis of the cube instead of the short axis of the cube, further increasing the size of the hay pieces incorporated into each cube. "Softer" cubes are preferred to "hard, glassy" cubes as they are easier to chew. Slow rates of eating pacify the horse for longer periods of time and are also more natural, considering the "nibbler" vs. "meal eater" evolution of the horse. A slower rate of passage increases the amount of time that feed is retained in the digestive tract. This enhances microbial digestion and also increases the feeling of satiety.

Palatability of grass hays can sometimes be increased by the addition of molasses (sparingly) or other feed flavourings; horses generally like apple or aniseed flavouring. On the one hand, it is not economical to pay for processing and bagging of hay when long-stem, baled hay can be fed (and is a superior source of long fibre) but, on the other hand, a specially blended feed for at-risk animals is more likely to contain the proper amounts and distribution of supplemental vitamins and minerals throughout the mix. If long-stem hay is preferred, a supplement of vitamins and minerals of low dietary energy concentration can be mixed with alfalfa hay or wheat bran as a relatively low energy, low soluble-carbohydrate, palatable carrier.

From a management perspective, overweight horses, ponies of almost all descriptions, and previously-foundered horses/ponies should be fed as continuously as possible. This means that several small meals should be offered daily instead of only two "bolus" feedings. Clarke *et al.* (1990) summarised the physiological changes that occur in the digestive tract and the circulatory system when ponies were fed a single large meal. It was reported that, when ponies ingested a large single meal (as opposed to several smaller meals), blood volume decreased by approximately 15% (approximately 1 litre in a 160 kg pony) within one hour of feeding. The post-feeding reduction in blood volume was regained within two hours of eating; however, a second, smaller decrease was detected six hours after eating, attributable to colonic secretion during microbial fermentation in the caecum and colon. Meal feeding also promoted a faster rate of passage, allowing a greater proportion of the ration, particularly a greater proportion of soluble carbohydrates, to reach the large intestine. This resulted in intense fermentation, as demonstrated by decreased luminal pH and increased organic acid production, similar to what is observed during carbohydrate overload that results in laminitis. These cyclic changes in blood volume and rate of microbial fermentation may not be harmful *per se* but, when these stresses are compounded by other stressors, they may push a horse or pony over the "brink" into colic or laminitis.

Another management consideration is housing of overweight or laminitis-prone animals. Like should be housed with like, and group-feeding of horses with widely different nutritional needs should be minimised. An older or larger horse or pony can easily bully younger or smaller pasture-mates and over-consume dangerous amounts of feed. Free exercise is generally considered to be beneficial to burn excess energy consumed and to enhance circulation in the lower legs.

## Palatability of feeds

Rations formulated for horses require not only that feed ingredients meet the nutrient and energy requirements of the horses for which they are formulated, but also that diets are millable and palatable. Horses generally prefer maize oil to other plant and animal fat sources. One study ranked palatability of common horse feeds in order, based on time of consumption (D'Ambrosi, 2000). Table 16.1 shows the relative palatability ranking of 16 different common equine feeds, categorised by feed type, with oats as a standard in each category.

**Table 16.1** RELATIVE PALATABILITY RANKING OF COMMON HORSE FEEDS*

| *Ranking of feeds* | *Cereal grains* | *Hays* | *Other feeds* |
|---|---|---|---|
| 1 | Maize, steam-rolled | Oats, whole | Oats, whole |
| 2 | Oats with molasses (100 g/kg) | Alfalfa, baled | Wheat bran, loose |
| 3 | Barley, steam-rolled | Alfalfa, cubed (large) | Alfalfa with molasses (100 g/kg) |
| 4 | Wheat, whole | Timothy, baled | Sugar beet pulp, loose |
| 5 | Oats, whole | Winter forage (various cereals, primarily oats) | Carrots, fresh, sliced |
| 6 | Oats with vegetable oil (100 g/kg) | Bermuda grass, baled | Rice bran, pelleted |

(D'Ambrosi, 2000)

* Maize: *Zea mays*
Oats: *Avena sativa*
Barley: *Hordeum aestivum*
Wheat: *Tricium aestivum*
Alfalfa: *Medicago sativa*
Timothy: *Phleum pratense*
Winter forage, primarily oats: *Avena sativa*
Bermuda grass: *Cynodon dactylon*
Wheat bran: *Triticum aestivum*
Sugar beet pulp: *Beta saccharifera*
Carrots: *Daucus ssp*
Rice bran: *Oryza sativa*

## Feeding the 'hot' horse

This is an area in which science-based nutrition appears to be left behind. No studies, to date, have been published that show the effects of specific feeds or diets on measurable behaviours. The concept of "grain high", while popular, is without scientific substantiation. It makes sense that a horse with excess energy intake may display more exuberant behaviour than a horse that is deficient in energy, but the idea that grain makes horses behave badly, or that fat supplementation promotes better behaviour, is based on testimonial evidence only. The same must be said about herbal supplements, although the knowledge of the author on this subject is limited.

## Summary

The demand for speciality diets for horses exceeds the scientific knowledge of the special nutritional, physiological and management needs of these horses. While it is tempting to formulate rations that "might" improve various conditions, it is probably better to educate horse owners about which nutritional formulations are science-based and which are not. It makes owners better able to care for their horses and helps them to understand the potential and the limitation of nutrition to influence the health and well being of their horses.

## References

Clarke, L.L., Roberts, M.C. and Argenzio, R.A. (1990) Feeding and digestive problems in horses: Physiologic responses to a concentrated meal. In *The Veterinary Clinics of North America. Equine Practice – 1990*, pp 433- 450. Guest edited by H.F. Hintz. W.B. Saunders Co. Philadelphia, PA, USA

D'Ambrosi, R.D. (2000) Personal communication.

Eaton, M.D., Hodgson, D.R., Evans, E.L., Bryden, W.L. and Rose, R. J. (1995) Effect of a diet containing supplementary fat on the capacity for high intensity exercise. In *Equine Exercise Physiology 4 – 1995 (Proceedings of the Fourth International Conference on Equine Exercise Physiology)*, pp 353 –356. Edited by N.E. Robinson. Equine Veterinary Journal Limited, Newmarket, Suffolk, UK.

Glade, M.J., Gupta, S. and Reimers, T.J. (1984) Hormonal responses to high and low planes of nutrition in weanling thoroughbreds. *J. Animal Sci.*, 59: 658-665.

Hintz, H.F., Argenzio, R.A. and Schryver, H.F. (1971) Digestion coefficients, blood glucose levels and molar percentage of volatile acids in intestinal fluid of ponies fed varying forage-grain ratios. *J. Animal Sci.*, 33: 992-995.

Hughes, S. J., Potter, G.D., Greene, L.S., Odom, T.W. and Murray-Gerzik, M. (1995) Adaptation of thoroughbred horses in training to a fat supplemented diet. In *Equine Exercise Physiology 4 – 1995 (Proceedings of the Fourth International Conference on Equine Exercise Physiology)*, pp 349 - 352. Edited by N.E. Robinson. Equine Veterinary Journal Limited, Newmarket, Suffolk, UK.

Longland, A.C., Cairns, A.J. and Humphreys, M.O. (1999) Seasonal and diurnal changes in fructan concentration in *Lolium perenne*: implications for the grazing management of equines pre-disposed to laminitis. *Proceedings of the 16th Equine Nutrition and Physiology Symposium*, Raleigh, North Carolina. pp 258-259.

Ralston, S.L. (1997) Geriatric Horse Nutrition. In *The Veterinarian's Practical Reference to Equine Nutrition – 1997*, pp 27 – 31. Edited by Kent N. Thompson. Published jointly by The American Association of Equine Practitioners and Purina Mills, Inc., St. Louis, MO, USA.

Stull, C. and Rodiek, A. (1988) Responses of blood glucose, insulin and cortisol concentrations to common equine diets. *J. Nutrition,* 118: 206-213

Stull, C. and Rodiek, A. (1995) Effects of post prandial interval and feed type on substrate availability during exercise. In *Equine Exercise Physiology 4 – 1995 (Proceedings of the Fourth International Conference on Equine Exercise Physiology)*, pp 362 - 366. Edited by N.E. Robinson. Equine Veterinary Journal Limited, Newmarket, Suffolk, UK.

*This paper was first published in 2001*

17

# EQUINE NUTRITION: SOME UNIQUE FEATURES, FUNCTIONS AND FRAILTIES OF THE DIGESTIVE SYSTEM OF THE HORSE

D CUDDEFORD
*Royal (Dick) School of Veterinary Studies, Roslin, EH25 9RE, UK*

## General introduction

The horse has evolved as a "trickle feeder", ingesting small amounts of herbage over extended periods of time. Fresh herbage in the United Kingdom has a low dry matter (DM) content, ranging between 150 and 250 g/kg, in contrast to that say growing on the Russian Steppe or on rangeland, where DM may be as high as 900 g/kg. Consequently, the horse may naturally consume a low or high DM diet. However, this feed material is acquired slowly over an extended period of time so that the gastrointestinal tract (GIT) has evolved to cope with a fairly continuous, but low rate of food intake. Thus, the apparently complicated and convoluted large intestine is able to regulate the flow of digesta through this organ to enable a satisfactory fermentation to occur. Grass-fed horses rarely experience gut-related problems, other than those occurring as a result of parasitism. The functionality of the horse's GIT is seriously challenged by "modern" horse feeding practices that almost always involve the feeding of dry (>800 g DM/kg), high nutrient-concentration diets as large, distinct meals, rather than there being food of low nutrient concentration available *ad libitum.* Episodic feeding of horses has been shown (Argenzio *et al.*, 1974) to institute major physiological changes within the animal; these changes have not been recorded in the grass-fed horse. Some of the hormonal shifts that occur have been linked to the onset of Developmental Orthopaedic Disease (a syndrome encompassing a number of bone diseases) in growing, meal-fed weanling foals (Glade and Reimers, 1985). The horse's GIT did not evolve to handle a large bulk of dry food that, together with added secretions, places a large, sudden volumetric load on a relatively small stomach. The need for digestive secretions causes massive fluid shifts between compartments to enable this to happen and, at the same time, creates a physiological situation analogous to that of a major haemorrhage. The extent of any long-term effects of these hormonal changes on durability of joints, bone formation and structure during the lifetime of a horse has yet to be ascertained.

Lignified, dry and fairly rigid fibrous material will not "flow" easily through the horse's GIT unless it is effectively comminuted. Otherwise, it would have great difficulty in negotiating the folds, bends, valves and strictures that characterise the large intestine of the horse (Figure 17.1). Impactions of food in the horse's large intestine are common (0.31 of colic cases; Mair and Hillyer, 1997), often at the site of the pelvic flexure. This in itself creates a major problem for the horse, but it is exacerbated by the accumulation of gas, resulting from the ongoing fermentation, that will cause colic and, at the worst, rupture of the bowel, usually followed by death. The anatomical features of the horse's gut, together with a post-gastric fermentation, make the horse vulnerable to dietary mismanagement in a way not seen in ruminants. Thus, effective nutrition of horses presents challenges beyond those of just establishing animal requirements and designing appropriate diets to meet nutrient needs. This chapter attempts to describe some of the features particular to the nutrition of the horse and to provide some insight into the conundrums that they present.

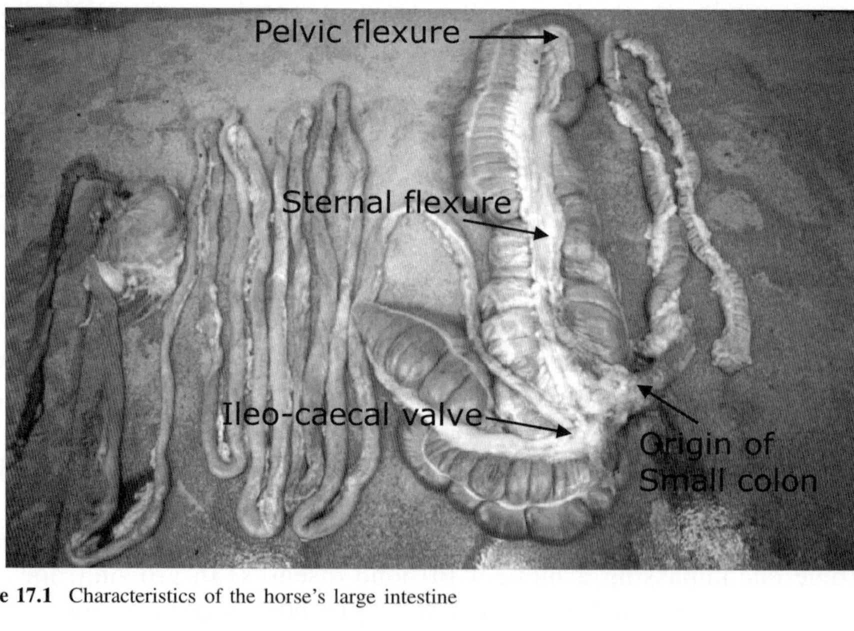


**Figure 17.1** Characteristics of the horse's large intestine

## Idiosyncrasies of the digestive system of the horse

### MOUTH PROCESSING OF FOOD

In contrast to sheep and cattle, the horse is quite different in the way that it ingests and processes its food. The horse's upper lip is analogous to the trunk of an elephant; it is extremely mobile, sensitive and strong. It is used to sort through food, select it and then manoeuvre it so that the teeth can grip it. The horse, unlike the ruminant, has both upper and lower incisors (Figure 17.2) and is thus able to bite off small pieces of food in a very selective fashion; this ability allows it to closely graze pasture. Horses are selective grazers (Archer, 1978), often rejecting food already taken into the mouth, possibly after the release of sap and other plant materials upon which the horse may judge its suitability. After the material has passed sensory evaluation, the tongue is used to manoeuvre food between the molars; these cheek teeth (Figure 17.2) crush and grind through a combination of lateral and vertical movements. The length of this process depends on the nature of the food and it is accompanied by the production of copious amounts of saliva, mostly from the parotid gland (at least 15 l may be produced in a 24-h period by a 500kg horse).

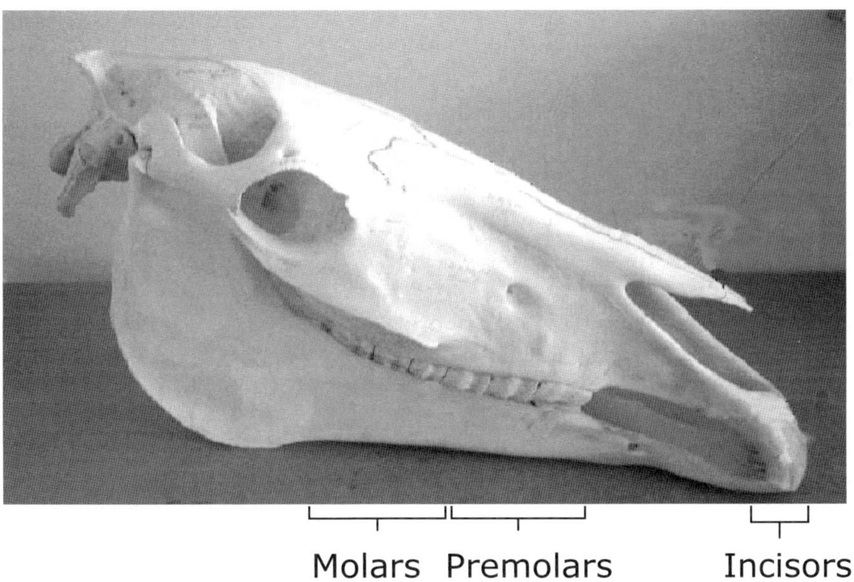


**Figure 17.2** Location of teeth

Chewing time depends on the type of food fed; saliva production only occurs when the horse is chewing so it also depends on the nature of the food. Horse saliva coats the food particles, lubricating and moistening them as they are physically broken down during the chewing process. As food particles become smaller the saliva holds them together in a bolus of "porridge-like" consistency. Horse saliva contains bicarbonate and mucus, but it has virtually no enzymatic activity. Foods that are poorly chewed will tend to be poorly buffered and poorly lubricated. A rapidly eaten meal of concentrates may lead to prolonged retention in the stomach because insufficient saliva has been added; this can lead to an abnormal fermentation, excessive gas production and colic (Frape, 1998). Furthermore, poorly-ensalivated material may lodge in the oesophagus leading to a blockage, a problem frequently associated with the consumption of sugar beet pulp products. Some feeds, such as beet pulp products and grass/lucerne nuts, can be soaked before feeding to prevent rapid consumption and to avoid oesophageal blockages. Concentrates, that are unsuitable for soaking, can be supplied as small pellets (≤3mm) to reduce the rate of consumption and also the risk of blockage. The rate of feeding can also be reduced by placing large round stones (large enough that the animal cannot consume them) in the feed receptacle, so that the horse has to move them around to seek out and retrieve its food. Feed products that are less dense than pellets, such as extrusions or coarse mixes ("mueslis") are preferable because they slow consumption rates and maximise time spent feeding.

Processing food effectively within the mouth is crucial to the well-being of the horse. Unlike ruminants that are able to re-chew regurgitated food, the horse has one opportunity to mouth-process its food effectively. A horse (500-600kg) will chew about 4000 times for every kg of hay consumed and a pony (~250kg) will chew up to 12000 times; the pony chews more because it has a much smaller mouth and therefore tooth area (molar battery). Thus, there is a general relationship between body size and time spent chewing food, although sufficient measurements have not been made to establish this precise relationship in terms of chews/kg for different feeds. Concentrate feeds may only require 800 to 1200 chews/kg by a horse and 5000 to 8000/kg by a pony (Meyer *et al.*, 1975). It is probably desirable, from the perspective of maximising surface area and 'flowability', that fibre particles are reduced to less than 2mm, but examination of horse faeces shows fibrous material up to 4cm in length, indicating that comminution of fibre in the mouth has variable results. It is debatable whether the benefits to be gained by 'fine' grinding are outweighed by the energy cost of comminution and the 'wear and tear' to the teeth.

The lower jaw is narrower than the top jaw and, as a result, the molar teeth in the lower jaw are set closer together than are those in the top jaw (Figure 17.2). The action of chewing has a shearing effect due to the lateral movement of the teeth over each other. Incomplete occlusion can create uneven wear on the crowns so that rough edges/points develop on the outer edge of the top teeth and on the inner edge on the bottom row. These points damage the cheek and tongue causing pain and, as a result, the animal drops food from its mouth (quidding). Dental problems must be addressed by rasping (filing or "floating") the teeth to remove the rough edges Mean chewing rates before and after tooth rasping were 2513 and 2195 chews/kg hay DM ($p<0.001$) respectively (Ellis *et al.*, 2000) and, as expected, there were no differences in chew rate (~one chew/second). However, the rate of DM consumption was significantly ($p<0.001$) increased from 28.5 to 32.9g DM/minute following dental treatment. Furthermore, there was a significant ($p<0.05$) increase in the proportion of faecal particles between 1000 and 250 μm, suggesting that changes in the occlusal surface following rasping had enabled a more effective comminution of fibre. Further work (Ellis *et al.*, 2001a) failed to demonstrate any differences in mean retention time (MRT) of liquid or solid phases following dental correction, although the maximum liquid outflow rate, measured using titanium dioxide, was significantly ($p<0.05$) reduced (33 to 27h). The effect of dental correction was also examined in relation to concentrate consumption (Ellis *et al.*, 2001b) and similar effects were recorded; significant ($p<0.05$) reductions in chewing rate (970 to 924 chews/kg DM), accompanied by an increase in intake (58.7g micronised barley increased to 70.7g/minute; $p<0.01$). Thus, impaired occlusion is compensated for by an increase in chewing time so that there is likely to be no overall effect on digestibility This was confirmed by Ralston, Foster, Divers and Hintz (2001), who were unable to demonstrate that dental correction significantly improved digestion of Timothy grass hay/ concentrate diet in horses The horse is so dependent on effective mouth-processing of food that regular examination of the teeth and appropriate dentistry is of paramount importance, if only from a welfare perspective.

## THE STOMACH

The cardiac sphincter (Figure 17.3) is a strong, muscular valve that acts in a unidirectional fashion; hence, regurgitation of food or gas rarely occurs from the stomach of horses. Thus, an abnormal production of gas in the stomach could lead to a severe colic because the horse cannot eructate and, in turn, the stomach may rupture. The horse's stomach is small (less than 0.10 of gut volume), particularly in comparison with other herbivores, such as the cow (the rumen is about 0.70 of gut volume). In the naturally-fed horse, which "trickle feeds" by grazing for about 16h each day (Duncan, 1985), it does not matter that the stomach is small because there is only a requirement to store a small amount of food. It rarely empties and food may remain in the stomach for as long as 3h. Food entering the stomach stimulates emptying but, when the animal drinks, the water does not wash out the contents, contrary to popular belief. Instead, most water follows the curvature of the stomach wall and passes into the duodenum (Frape, 1998). Food entering the stomach also stimulates the release of gastric juice (production can be as high as 30 l daily in a 500kg horse), but there is also a continuous low level of secretion. The saliva that enters with food buffers the acid produced in the stomach and in

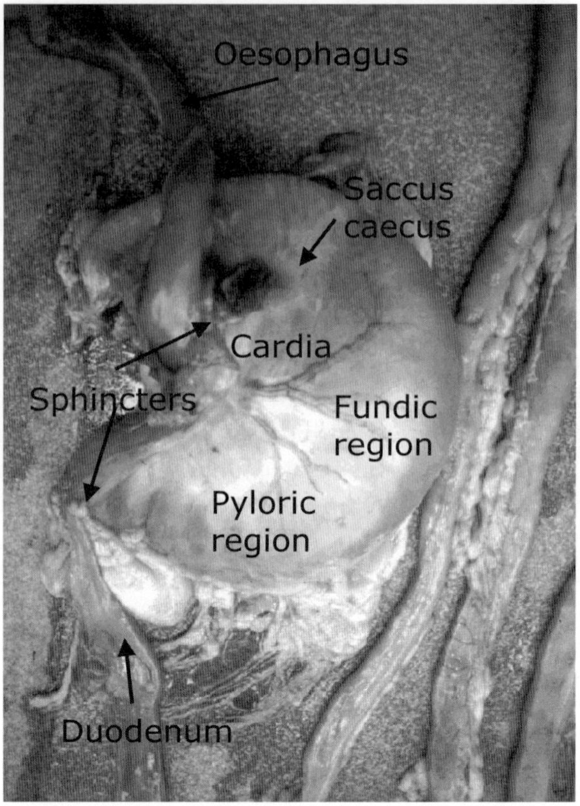


**Figure 17.3** Anatomical regions of the horse's stomach

part regulates the increase in acidity associated with the arrival of food. As a result of this, there are marked variations in the degree of acidity throughout the stomach; at the cardia the material is neutral, in the fundic area it is slightly acidic (pH5.4) and in the pyloric region it is very acidic (pH~2).

Episodic feeding of concentrates to racehorses is regarded as a cause of low inter-meal gastric pH that in turn is considered a risk factor for the formation of gastric ulcers within this population of horses (Orsini, 2000). Furthermore, horses that are unable to satisfy their feeding motivation will become frustrated and this may lead to the performance of abnormal behaviours, including stereotypies (Fraser, 1992). Apparently, the genotype of some performance horses may increase their susceptibility to the performance of such behaviours that can include "weaving" or "crib-biting" (Vecchiotti and Gainati, 1986). There is some fermentation in the oesophageal region and *saccus caecus* of the horse's stomach leading to the production of lactic acid. However, protein digestion begins in the pyloric area, although it is limited by the short time that food particles reside there.

## THE SMALL INTESTINE

Acidified material leaving the stomach stimulates a large flow of pancreatic juice (up to 20 l over a 24-h period in a 500 kg horse) and it continues at a low level in the absence of food particles. Bile release is also stimulated by acid entering the duodenum. The horse does not have a gall bladder and thus, because it cannot store bile, there is a continuous production. Although in evolutionary terms the horse would not have been exposed to high-fat foods, fat digestion in the horse seems to be fairly efficient (Hollands and Cuddeford, 1992) and it is now common practice to feed vegetable oil to horses. In a 500kg horse, the small intestine can be up to 20 m long (see Smyth, 1988 for detailed information on intestinal lengths during growth of horses) and food residues pass through it quite quickly (about 1 h). The small intestine is obviously the major site of protein, fat and hydrolysable carbohydrate digestion.

The horse has evolved to digest structural carbohydrates and not storage polysaccharides, such as starch, and the concentration of pancreatic $\alpha$-amylase in horses is far less than that found in the carnivore or omnivore. Thus, it is not surprising that the output of $\alpha$-amylase per unit weight of pancreatic tissue is only 0.05 to 0.06 of that attained in the pig (Roberts, 1974), although it was considered that this continuously secreted enzyme was probably adequate (sic) for initial starch digestion. Corring (1982) stated that "a pig of 50kg live weight produced enough amylase to hydrolyse 30kg of soluble starch daily". A pig of this weight will consume less than 1kg starch daily and thus it is producing 30-50 times too much amylase daily. In contrast, a racehorse in full training may be fed 9kg oats daily, supplying about 3.6kg starch although it will only produce enough amylase to hydrolyse 1.5kg. This assumes that the above data are reliable and that it is valid to compare species on the basis of enzyme production/unit weight of tissue. Simple sugars are rapidly absorbed and, whilst maltose can be easily digested, hydrolysis of starch to maltose is considered to be the rate-limiting step in the small intestinal degradation of starch by the horse. Cooked starch is more readily hydrolysed than raw starch (McLean *et al.*, 2000). It is undesirable for undigested starch to enter the caecum because it can be rapidly fermented to lactic acid creating an acidotic condition analogous to that sometimes seen in the rumen of cereal-fed beef cattle. Thus, large meals, rich in starch, should not be given to horses. Potter and co-workers at Texas A&M University have suggested that not more that 4g starch should be fed per kg bodyweight (W) at a meal (Potter *et al.*, 1992). However, a more conservative value of 2g/kg W/meal was proposed by Kienzle *et al.* (1992) and recently, evidence has been adduced that indicates that this value may also be too high under certain circumstances (Cuddeford, 1999).

## THE LARGE INTESTINE

The physical shape and arrangement of the large intestine (Figure 17.4) of the horse slows down the rate of passage of food particles. However, there is no structure analogous to the reticulo-omasal orifice of ruminants, which places a size limit on food residues, that prevents their aboral flow. Limiting flow and increasing residence time in the large intestine of the horse is crucial to the effective breakdown of the plant cell wall materials remaining after enzymatic pre-digestion in the stomach and small intestine.

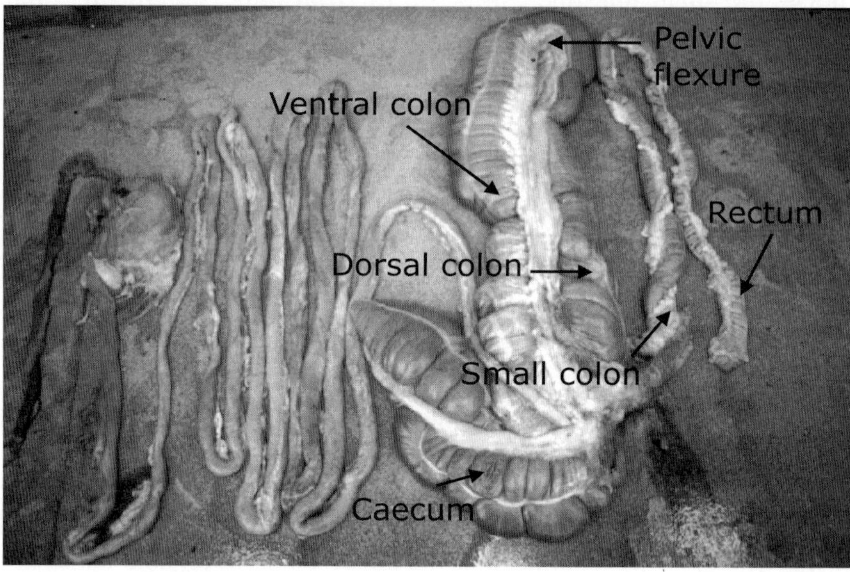


**Figure 17.4** Anatomical regions of the horse's large intestine

The caecum is entered from the ileum via the ileo-caecal valve and is a large blind sac. In a mature, 450/500 kg horse it would be about 1 m long, having a capacity of approximately 30 l and accounting for about 0.15 of total gut volume. The caecum exits to the ventral colon via the caecal-ventral colonic valve, located near to the entrance valve, so material enters and leaves the caecum at nearly the same place. The large colon is just over 3 m long and has about twice the capacity of the caecum and thus represents over 0.30 of the total gut volume. Bends or flexures separate the different regions of the large colon; the dorsal and ventral colons are separated by the pelvic flexure (Figure 17.1). In addition, there are the sternal and diaphragmatic flexures. Parts of the dorsal colon can be as much as half a metre in diameter before reducing in size to join the small colon at the dorsal colonic junction. The small colon is about 3 m long and represents about 0.10 of total gut volume. This organ terminates in the rectum that is only 30cm long and thus has limited storage capacity. Food residues move from one compartment to another with very little mixing between compartments or with any retrograde flow, although considerable mixing occurs within each compartment. The muscular valves and flexures minimise backflow of material and achieve separation between compartments. Furthermore, onward passage to the rectum is increasingly resisted such that large food particles (>1cm) are held back. The purpose of this resistance to flow is to ensure that the micro-organisms have sufficient time to ferment plant cell wall residues. This occurs at different sites within the large intestine - the caecum, the ventral colon and the ventral-dorsal colonic junction - that act as the major barriers to the flow of coarse particles. Fluid and small particles (<2mm) are preferentially retained at the interface of the dorsal and distal colon (Sperber *et al.*, 1992); this mechanism is known as the "colonic separation mechanism" and it operates in other post-gastric fermenters. This complex series of valves and flexures, whilst benefiting the horse in terms of digestive efficiency, represent risk areas for the horse if the diet is mismanaged. The "plumbing" was designed for a grazing animal consuming forage DM over extended periods of time, not for an animal fed large, distinct meals of high dry matter forage, or forage and concentrate. Entrapment of gas and impactions within the large intestine of equids are quite common in housed animals, meal-fed dry diets.

It may take up to 65 h for 0.95 of all of the waste materials from a grain diet to be voided by ponies (Frape, 1998), but the exact time depends on the nature of the diet and the amount consumed. For example, ponies fed *ad libitum* lucerne (443g neutral detergent fibre [NDF]/kgDM) or oat straw (715 gNDF/ kgDM) had respective mean retention times (MRTs) for chromium-fibre of 21.3 and 31.5h. When intake was restricted (0.70 of *ad libitum* intake), MRTs were, respectively, 30.5 and 36.0h (Pearson, Archibald and Muirhead, 2001). Thus, it seems that poorer quality forages are retained longer in the GIT and that limitation of intake will have a similar effect. Most of the digesta from a meal remains in the stomach and small intestine for no more than about 3h and thus, feed residues spend most of their time in the large intestine. Residues from a lucerne/cocksfoot hay that was ground and pelleted were retained longer ($p<0.05$) in the GIT than those from chopped hay (Drogoul *et al.*, 2000a); animals were fed at maintenance and DMI (1.7 kgDM/100 kgW) was equalised. However, there was no significant difference between the apparent digestibility coefficients (ADCs) of the main components of the two physical forms of the diets. The authors concluded that, since the residues from the ground and pelleted diet were retained for longer in the colon and that there were no differences in apparent digestibility of fibre fractions, then the rate of fibre degradation must have been reduced. These results are at variance with those of earlier workers (for example Wolter *et al.*, 1974) who demonstrated that digesta of horses given ground grass hay, passed more rapidly through the GIT with a resultant reduction in fibre ADC, although DMIs were the same. In *ad libitum* feeding experiments, it was shown that as DMI of ground, pelleted forage increased, digestion of fibre declined (Todd *et al.*, 1995). Further work by Drogoul *et al.*, (2000b) demonstrated that the *in situ* degradation of NDF was significantly ($p<0.001$) less in both the caecum and colon (in terms of both rate and extent) of animals fed ground pelleted hay than in those fed chopped hay. Although the surface area available to cellulolytic degradation would be increased by fine grinding, it appeared that substrate fermentation rate was reduced and that there was an increase in lag times. Artefacts due to the physical consistency of the sample within incubation bags cannot be ignored. Clearly, the exact relationship between particle size, MRT and rate of fermentation remains to be explored in terms of defining the extent of fibre degradation in the horse's large intestine.

Organic matter (OM) and NDF were better digested by donkeys, compared with both ponies and thoroughbred horses; differences that probably reflected the relative sizes of the large intestine and thus, the residence time of feed residues (Cuddeford *et al.*, 1995). Although it is commonly accepted that ruminants digest fibrous feeds more effectively than equids, it is not because the latter are less able to ferment feed residues. For example, an *in situ* experiment compared the degradation of acid detergent fibre (ADF) and crude protein (CP) in the caecum of the pony with that in the rumen of the steer over a 12 to 48h period. There were no significant differences although, the degradation of sugar beet pulp and hay was greater in the pony caecum at 12h (Hyslop *et al.*, 1997).

Fermentation results in the production of large volumes of gas that have to be removed from the lumen of the gut, otherwise the horse may develop colic. Gut movement helps gas removal; large volumes (150 l) may be absorbed into the blood, carried to the lungs and, following diffusion out of the blood, exhaled. In addition, gas will be expelled from the anus. Whilst microbial populations are changing in response to dietary change, fermentation will be at a sub-optimal level. For example, caecal bacteria from horses fed cereal are less efficient at fermenting hay than bacteria from hay-fed horses and vice-versa (Frape, 1998). Meal-fed horses experience large fluctuations in the microbial population in their large intestine (by a factor of 100). Thus, speed of dietary change and frequency of feeding can have a large effect on hindgut function and on the occurrence of digestive disorders. The overall digestibility of the feed may be little altered, although the well-being of the horse can be seriously jeopardised. Changes in hay:cereal ratios have both qualitative and quantitative effects on the species of organism present in the large intestine in the same way as rumen micro-organisms are affected. Hintz *et al.* (1971) showed that varying forage:concentrate ratios affected the relative production of volatile fatty acids (VFAs); more propionate being produced when cereal was fed. Of course, if small intestinal hydrolysis of starch was complete, feeding of cereal should not affect caecal fermentation patterns. However, it was recently shown (McLean *et al.*, 2000) that feeding a small meal of raw barley (2.1g starch/kg W – close to the 'safe' value of 2g/kgW proposed by Kienzle *et al.*, 1992) resulted in significant ($p<0.05$) changes in the caecal environment. There was an increase in propionate, a reduction in acetate and an increase in lactate.

The whole process of protein breakdown, microbial protein formation and the contribution that micro-organisms make to the nitrogen economy of the horse are poorly understood. Frape (1998) has stated that more than half the dry weight of horse faeces is bacteria and thus, their protein will only benefit the roses or earthworms. Furthermore, although significant vitamin formation occurs in the large intestine, it is questionable as to how much of these vitamins are available to the host animal, particularly in animals fed high-cereal diets and when, as a consequence, there is a less active fermentation in the large intestine.

## CONCLUSION

A grazing horse in the "wild" would experience qualitative differences between mouthfuls of food ingested throughout each day. However, since each mouthful would only represent a few grams of forage, this would mix with other mouthfuls in the stomach to present the duodenum with a fairly homogenous digesta stream. This situation should be emulated when feeding domesticated horses. Dietary components, that separately are very different in terms of nutrient concentration and source, should be mixed together in order to produce a total mixed ration (TMR) that is available *ad libitum.* This will give rise to a stable flora and fauna in the large intestine; episodic feeding (meals) should be avoided. The provision of high dry matter food appears to be unavoidable at certain times of year (e.g. winter) and in certain situations (e.g. racing establishments), although the increasing use of high dry matter silage products ("haylages") contributes to reducing the overall ration dry matter. It is unlikely, however, that the dependency on cereal starch as a source of energy will lessen, albeit that more will be in a cooked form. Whilst oil is vigorously promoted as an alternative energy source for horses, it is likely that its use will always be limited to less than 0.15 of the daily DMI. Fat-rich feeds, such as full-fat soya or naked oats, are a means of providing additional supplies of energy. More recently, rice bran has been promoted for use in horse diets, although it is unlikely to be used in the UK because it contains γ-oryzynol, a substance credited with anabolic activities and thus likely to attract the ire of the Jockey Club.

## Voluntary food intake by horses

### CONTROLS

It is not known whether the controls of intake are the same for horses and ponies, different sexes or for different breed types. Given the opportunity, non-working horses and ponies will eat in excess of their energy needs and, as a result, become obese. Ralston (1992) reported an attempt to stabilise intake and body weight in horse mares fed a pelleted diet *ad libitum.* However, animals continued to gain weight and consume all feed offered over a five-week period, so the experiment was terminated on the grounds that the animals were becoming obese. There appears to be some sensitivity to energy intake in that ponies ate larger meals more frequently when offered a pelleted diet of a reduced energy concentration (Laut *et al.*, 1985) than when they were fed a standard pelleted diet. The ponies' response to changes in dietary energy concentration took between two and 14 days to stabilise, indicating a less precise mechanism than that present in other species (rats and monkeys), where compensation occurs in less than 24 h (Gibbs and Smith, 1978). However, ponies were able to compensate intake of the pelleted diet that they were accustomed to when given additional intragastric inputs of energy in the form of glucose, maize oil or α-cellulose accurately, within a 24 h period (Ralston and Baile, 1982b; 1983).

Some feedback mechanisms appear to affect food intake by ponies. Ralston and Baile (1983) showed that reductions in intake occurred at times that would reflect the post-absorptive state; 10 to 15 minutes for glucose and 4 to 6h for cellulose. An intra-gastric load of maize oil immediately after a 4h fast, and before a meal, did not affect consumption of the meal, but did reduce subsequent intake by tripling the normal inter-meal interval. This could have resulted from metabolic feedback or a reduced rate of gastric emptying. Ralston and Baile (1982a) concluded that elevated levels of plasma glucose and insulin do not immediately generate satiety cues in ponies, although this view was based on glucose infusions via the jugular vein. Such an infusion would enable utilisation of the metabolite and, possibly, reduce effects at receptor sites. It is noteworthy that the glucose would probably have by-passed liver receptors as well.

The effect of gut fill on intake is equivocal. Intra-gastric infusions of kaolin had no significant effect on DMI or feeding behaviour of ponies, when compared with control animals (Ralston and Baile, 1982b). These authors suggested that stomach fill had no effect on intake although this ignores the fact that kaolin is inert and that it would not generate stimuli analogous to those produced by feed residues. Removal of 1.2 to 1.5 l of caecal contents (equivalent to 0.22 of total caecal content of a 200kg pony) also had no effect on subsequent feeding behaviour of ponies (Ralston *et al.*, 1983). However, intra-gastric infusions of α-cellulose significantly ($p<0.05$) reduced total DMI after 3 to 18 h post-infusion (Ralston and Baile, 1982b). Both of these results need to be interpreted with care because removal of a small amount of digesta is unlikely to have had much effect on intake and, in the case of α-cellulose, it could have had a "fill" effect, a metabolite effect or both. In fact, Ralston and Baile (1982) suggested that intra-gastric loads of nutrients generate satiety cues in ponies that are not related to the volume or bulk of the treatment. For example, a control infusion of 2 l of water had no effect on feeding behaviour, whereas 2 l of water containing 300g of dissolved glucose decreased intakes 0 to 3 h post-treatment. This probably represents a post-absorptive effect, rather than a localised gastric response, because of its duration. However, the tonicity of the solution would have affected fluid balance that, in itself, could have had an effect. NDF apparent digestibility and NDF content of feed are not reliable predictors of DMI ($r^2 = 0.266$) in horses (Cymbaluk, 1990) suggesting that physical capacity of the large intestine is unlikely to limit feed intake. However, if faecal output is a determinant of DMI, then large intestinal capacity may have a role in controlling intake. The flow of digesta through the horse's GIT is slowed but it is not limited by particle size in the same way as it is in ruminants since there is no analogous structure to the reticulo-omasal orifice. Thus, digesta cannot be retained in the horse's GIT in the same way that it can in ruminants and, therefore, there is less likelihood of "fill" negatively affecting intake.

Intra-gastric infusion of acetate (0.75mmol/kg W) caused ponies to increase feed intake ($p<0.05$) by reducing the duration of the first inter-meal interval (Ralston *et al.*, 1983). Intravenous studies with short chain, volatile fatty acids have not been undertaken and, as a result, it is not known how circulating levels of these acids may affect voluntary feed intake. Following a 4 h fast, above normal levels of acetate (1.0 and 1.25mmol/kg W) and propionate (0.75mmol/kg W) were introduced as a bolus into the caecum of ponies and reduced feed intake, manifest by prolonging the first inter-meal interval (Ralston *et al.*, 1983). An intra-caecal infusion of 0.4mmol propionate/kg W significantly ($p<0.05$) increased total feed intake by 1.075 relative to control values. In contrast, an infusion of 1mmol propionate/kg W significantly ($p<0.01$) reduced, by 0.22, the size of the first meal consumed, without affecting subsequent feeding behaviours. However, the relevance of this type of research, which relied on the provision of complete pelleted diets fed *ad libitum* and consumed in 10/11 meals/24h, to the intake of an *ad libitum* forage-fed horse or pony is questionable.

In summary, there is a dearth of facts relating to intake controls in horses, although Ralston (1984) concluded that horses rely primarily on oro-pharyngeal and external stimuli to control the size and duration of an isolated meal; it was considered that meal frequency is regulated by the presence and/or absorption of the products of digestion, together with metabolic cues that may reflect body energy stores. However, the influence of the latter may be deemed weak, in view of the fact that fat ponies tend to get fatter.

## ESTIMATES OF FEED INTAKE

Various attempts have made to measure the voluntary intake of different feeds by horses and ponies and to derive means whereby intake may be predicted. The foregoing represents a summary of this work and serves to illustrate how the equid responds to the different forms and characteristics of feed in a way that is quite different from that of ruminants.

### *Hay*

The voluntary DMI of a wide variety of hays have been measured and attempts made to establish the relationship between hay type, fibre content (defined as NDF and ADF) and voluntary DMI (Table 17.1). Aiken *et al.* (1989) fed Coastal Bermuda grass to both yearlings and mature geldings, and suggested that food intake was regulated by energy requirement, rather than by gut capacity. This was based on the fact that the yearlings, with higher nutrient need, consumed more DM *pro rata* than the mature horses; 0.025 versus 0.02 of body weight. This is in keeping with the view proposed by Frape *et al.* (1982), based on a comparitive study with a pony, horse and white rhino, that voluntary DMI was proportionate to energy requirement rather than gut volume.

Comparisons of the voluntary DMI of chopped hays (legume and grass) by Arabian geldings (Crozier *et al.*, 1997) led to the conclusion that the higher intakes ($p<0.05$) of legume hay, compared with grass hays, were a reflection of its significantly higher ($p<0.01$) dry matter digestibility.

Cymbaluk (1990) compared a number of Canadian grass hays, fed *ad libitum* to horses, with long alfalfa hay and dehydrated alfalfa pellets. It appeared that horses voluntarily consumed more alfalfa hay than grass hay although there was no explanation for this phenomenon. Ponies offered *ad libitum* mature, threshed grass hay by Hyslop *et al.* (1998) were able to consume relatively large amounts of dry matter, even though this hay was of very poor quality (coefficient of dry matter digestibility [DMD], 0.30). These results

**Table 17.1** RELATIONSHIP BETWEEN HAY TYPE, FIBRE CONTENT AND VOLUNTARY DRY MATTER INTAKE OF HORSES

| *Hay Type* | *Horse type* | *Content (g/kg DM)* | | *Voluntary Dry Matter Intake* | *Apparent digestibility coefficient* | | *Reference* |
|---|---|---|---|---|---|---|---|
| | | *NDF* | *ADF* | *(g/kg $W^{0.75}$)* | *NDF* | *ADF* | |
| Coastal bermuda grass | Yearlings | 704.5 | 319.0 | 111.5 | 0.45 | 0.40 | Aitken *et al.* (1989) |
| | Mature geldings | | | 95.6 | 0.46 | 0.36 | |
| Alfalfa | Arabian geldings | 550 | 430 | 122 | 0.47 | 0.45 | Crozier *et al.* (1997) |
| Tall fescue | | 720 | 400 | 111 | 0.44 | 0.37 | |
| Caucasian bluestem | | 730 | 390 | 102 | 0.41 | 0.33 | |
| Altai wildrye | | 749 | - | 81.2 | - | - | |
| Bromegrass | | 595 | - | 113.6 | - | - | |
| Crested wheatgrass | | 689 | - | 85.0 | - | - | |
| Kentucky bluegrass | | 727 | - | 82.3 | - | - | |
| Oat hay | Mature horses | 685 | - | 81.2 | - | - | Cymbaluk (1990) |
| Reed canary grass | | 655 | - | 99.4 | - | - | |
| Long alfalfa hay | | 414 | - | 114.4 | - | - | |
| Dehydrated alfalfa pellets | | 439 | - | 97.9 | - | - | |

**Table 17.1** CONTD.

| *Hay Type* | *Horse type* | *Content (g/kg DM)* *NDF* | *ADF* | *Voluntary Dry Matter Intake ($g/kg\ W^{0.75}$)* | *Apparent digestibility coefficient* *NDF* | *ADF* | *Reference* |
|---|---|---|---|---|---|---|---|
| Mature, threshed grass hay | Ponies | 796 | 488 | 95.6 | 0.28 | 0.30 | Hyslop *et al.* (1998) |
| High temperature | Mature | | | | | | Hyslop *et al.* (1998) |
| dehydrated grass | ponies | 677 | 300 | 110 | 0.51 | 0.34 | |
| Hay | | 695 | 332 | 113 | 0.40 | 0.26 | |
| Alfalfa | | 535 | | 111 | | | |
| | | 563 | | 92 | | | |
| Regrowth grass | Mature | 641 | | 110 | | | Dulphy *et al.* (1997) |
| | horse | 672 | | 95 | | | |
| Early cut grass hay | geldings | 665 | | 115 | | | |
| | | 628 | | 104 | | | |
| Normal cut grass hay | | 663 | | 111 | | | |
| | | 655 | | 99 | | | |
| Late cut grass hay | | 702 | | 102 | | | |
| | | 709 | | 100 | | | |

support the view that there is a poor relationship between intake and the cell wall content of hays. A further experiment (Hyslop *et al.*, 1998) examined the effect of the method of conservation on the voluntary feed intake of grass products by mature ponies. Although the hay was of poorer quality, more was consumed; the difference in intake was non-significant but the difference in NDF digestibility was ($p<0.01$). A comparative study in France (Dulphy *et al.*, 1997) with mature horse geldings showed very similar voluntary DMI for different hays. Alfalfa, re-growth grass, early cut, normal cut and late cut grass hays were fed in two trials. The authors concluded that because the horses consumed the different hays in practically the same amounts, it would be difficult to define precise criteria whereby it would be possible to predict likely intakes of dry forages by horses. A retrospective analysis of data obtained by INRA (Theix) and of values taken from published papers provided a data set for assessing voluntary DMI of horses fed different dry forages (Dulphy *et al.*, 1997). The pooled results for horses gave DMIs for legumes (n=12), grasses (n=38) and re-growth grass hays (n=7) of 108, 93 and 98g/kg $W^{0.75}$ respectively; the only significant ($p<0.05$) difference was between legume and grass hay. The authors concluded that voluntary intake of horses was not influenced by either the CP, crude fibre (CF) or NDF content of the forage. Multiple regression analysis yielded $r^2$ values between 0.11 and 0.13; in contrast, $r^2$ values for sheep calculated under similar conditions produced significant correlations of 0.78 to 0.84. Thus, it is impossible to reliably predict the intake of dry hays by horses based on forage analysis in contrast to ruminants, where effective equations have been derived and are based primarily on fibre content. Thus, Dulphy *et al.*, (1997) have proposed that the voluntary intake of hays by housed, mature light horses will be in the range 19-22, 18-21 and 22-25g/kg W for grass, re-growth grass and alfalfa hays respectively. These values may be regarded as conservative estimates of voluntary DMI by horses. It seems to be a consistent finding that the intakes of legume hays are higher than that of grass hays and this may be for the reasons proposed by Minson (1990) to account for the higher intake of legumes by ruminants; it was proposed that legumes had lower values for resistance to physical breakdown, percentage of cell wall, length-to-width ratios of fibres and energy required for mastication compared to grasses. It is noteworthy that the inclusion of soaked unmolassed sugar beet pulp in a daily ration can significantly ($p<0.05$) depress the voluntary intake of hay by ponies so that the maximum recommended inclusion of dry product is 0.3kg/day/100kg W (Hyslop and Cuddeford, 1999). The nature of this interaction is not known.

A recent review (Lawrence, Lawrence and Coleman, 2001) of published studies that reported both NDF and voluntary DMI (VDMI) in mature horses fed long stem grass hays *ad libitum* concluded that there was a good relationship between the two parameters, represented by:

$$VDMI(y)=124.55+0.0155x^2-2.5742x \ (r^2=0.67,\ p<0.001) \quad \text{(Equation 17.1)}$$
$$(x=\%NDF;\ y=g/kg\ W/day)$$

The reliability of this equation was tested in terms of predicting intake by feeding two orchard grass and two timothy hays to 4 mature equids (278-705kg). Predicted daily intakes were not significantly different from actual intakes and, in fact, the two were highly correlated ($r^2=0.86$, $p<0.001$). Incorporation of the experimental data into those derived from the literature (Equation 17.1) yielded:

$$VDMI(y)=80.954+0.0073x^2-1.3677x \ (r^2=0.50,\ p<0.01;\ n=21) \text{(Equation 17.2)}$$

It is apparent from these data that, whilst NDF may have a role in determining *ad libitum* intake of hays, there are clearly other factors involved.

***Fresh herbage***

There is a paucity of information in relation to the voluntary intake of fresh forage by horses, but that which is available is detailed in Table 17.2.

**Table 17.2** ESTIMATES OF VOLUNTARY DRY MATTER INTAKE OF PASTURE BY HORSES

| *Pasture* | *Horse type* | *NDF Content (g/kg DM)* | *Voluntary dry matter intake* | *Reference* |
|---|---|---|---|---|
| Fresh forage | Horses | 300 – 611 | 97 g/kg $W^{0.75}$ | Dulphy *et al.* (1997) |
| Fresh forages | | - | 105 g/kg $W^{0.75}$ | Dulphy *et al.* (1997) |
| Fresh grass (predicted) | | - | 19 – 22 g DM/kg W | |
| Pasture, grazed | Yearlings | - | 85g/kg $W^{0.75}$ | Grace *et al.* (2002) |
| | Lactating, brood mares | - | 118 g/kg $W^{0.75}$ | |
| Pasture | Australian stockhorse weanlings | - | 20 – 30 g DM/kg W | McMeniman (2000) |
| Pasture | Thoroughbred weanlings | | 100g OM/kg W | Friend and Nash (2000) |

Dulphy *et al.*, (1997), in a review, included data for 16 fresh forages (covering a range of NDF from 300 to 611g/kg DM) and obtained a mean intake figure similar to that for grass hays whose NDF content varied from 495 to 709g/kg DM. Published values for fresh forages (examined by Dulphy *et al.*, 1997) varied between 90 and 117, with a mean of 105gDM/kg $W^{0.75}$. As a result of analysing INRA data, these authors suggested a probable fresh forage (grass) voluntary intake of 19-22gDM/kg W.

An interesting aspect of recent work in New Zealand (Grace *et al.*, 2002; Grace, personal communication), was that when pasture was cut and fed to horses in order to measure apparent DM digestibility *in vivo*, DMI was lower than when grazing. The depression was 10-15% in stalled yearlings and 5-8% in corralled mares; both groups were offered about 30% excess herbage. This work investigated the pasture intakes of yearlings and lactating brood mares and was based on faecal collection off the pasture and an *in vivo* assessment of pasture digestibility. This outcome illustrated the importance of grazing preference and its effect on voluntary DMI. Pasture intake data obtained in Australia (McMeniman, 2000) using alkane markers and Australian Stockhorse weanlings, produced similar results to those obtained in New Zealand. Further Australian work with thoroughbred weanlings (Friend and Nash, 2000) used similar markers but obtained unreliable estimates of intake (100gOM/kg W). These overestimates were thought to be as a result of pasture sampling errors but were probably also a result of too infrequent dosing of alkane. These types of problem further highlight the difficulty of conducting pasture intake studies.

***Straws***

The relationship between straw type, fibre content and DMI of horses has been estimated by a number of workers, and comparisons drawn between the DMI of straws and other forages (Table 17.3).

**Table 17.3** RELATIONSHIP BETWEEN STRAW TYPE, FIBRE CONTENT AND VOLUNTARY DRY MATTER INTAKE OF HORSES

| *Straw type* | *Horse type* | *NDF Content (g/kg DM)* | *Voluntary dry matter intake* | *Reference* |
|---|---|---|---|---|
| Barley straw | Mature gelded horses | 817 - 830 | 43 –46 g DM/kg W $^{0.75}$ | Dulphy *et al.*, (1997) |
| Straws | - | - | 61 gDM/kg W $^{0.75}$ | Dulphy *et al.*, (1997) |
| Straw | Adult, light horses at maintenance | | 11 – 14 gDM/kg W | Dulphy *et al.*, (1997) |
| Alfalfa | | | 79.5 gDM/kg W $^{0.75}$ | |
| Alfalfa/oat straw | | | 73.3 gDM/kg W $^{0.75}$ | Hyslop and Calder, 2001 |
| Alfalfa/oil/yeast | | | 77.7 gDM/kg W $^{0.75}$ | |

Dulphy *et al*., (1997) measured the voluntary DMI of barley straw by mature, gelded horses to be approximately half that of grass hays. Pearson and Merritt (1991) had previously reported a similar situation in resting donkeys; 80.9 and 36.8g DM/kg $W^{.75}$/day respectively for hay and barley straw. However, the difference was not so great in resting ponies (99.1 and 59.8) and, surprisingly, the ponies appeared to be better able to compensate for the poor quality forage offered. Pearson *et al.* (2001) reported that the voluntary DMI of oat straw by ponies was reduced by about 40% compared to when the ponies were fed *ad libitum* artificially dehydrated alfalfa. Similarly, Dulphy *et al*., (1997) reported a pooled intake value for undefined straws by adult light horses at maintenance that was rather lower than that reported for other dry forages.

Thus, horses do not appear to be able to effectively compensate for lower feed energy concentrations by eating more, although there is no evidence to support the view that intake is limited by the capacity of the GIT. Longer MRTs may inhibit intake although they may in themselves be a result of low intakes. Furthermore, rate of elimination from the hindgut may have an impact on intake. Low intake of "cereal straw" must be influenced by its low palatability, a complex of organoleptic qualities including taste, structure, texture and smell. However, results recently reported by Hyslop and Calder (2001) showed that the inclusion of approximately 0.50 oat straw in a short-chopped, dehydrated and molassed alfalfa diet had very little effect on total DMI. Thus, it would seem that the voluntary intake of straw by horses can be markedly affected by the inclusion of other dietary ingredients (perhaps supplying fermentable energy and nitrogen) and that the type of straw may also have an impact on intake. An alternative explanation for low intakes of straw could be that the rate of comminution falls as the quality of the diet declines (Forbes, 1988), so a poorer quality diet, such as straw, takes longer to eat. In addition, longer inter-meal intervals are required and, if time spent feeding is an important feedback mechanism in intake control, then it is understandable that horses have reduced intakes of straw.

### *Silages*

The use of ensiled forage is becoming increasingly popular for horse and pony feeding, and recent research has examined the relationship between the dry matter content of different silages, and the voluntary DMI of these materials (Table 17.4).

The intakes of ponies fed limited amounts (1.65kg DM/100kg W) of grass-derived products, hay, haylage, big-bale silage and clamp silage were significantly ($p<0.05$) different (Moore-Colyer and Longland, 2000). Similar, but lower, intakes of both long and short chopped big bale silage have been

**Table 17.4** RELATIONSHIP BETWEEN SILAGE TYPE, DRY MATTER CONTENT AND VOLUNTARY DRY MATTER INTAKE OF HORSES

| *Silage type* | *Horse type* | *DM content (g/kg)* | *Voluntary dry matter intake* | *Reference* |
|---|---|---|---|---|
| Hay | | 922 | 62.9g DM/kg $W^{0.75}$ | |
| Haylage | | 676 | 79.2g DM/kg $W^{0.75}$ | Moore-Colyer and |
| Big-bale silage | Limit-fed | 500 | 74.6g DM/kg $W^{0.75}$ | Longland (2000) |
| Clamp silage | ponies | 337 | 38.8g DM/kg $W^{0.75}$ | |
| Big-bale silage, long chop and short chop | - | - | 63g DM/kg $W^{0.75}$ | Morrow *et al.* (1999) |
| Big-bale grass | | 371 | 6.13 kg DM/d | |
| Big-bale red clover | Ponies | 268 | 7.2 kg DM/d | Hale and Moore- |
| Grass hay | | 852 | 5.5 kgDM/d | Colyer (2001) |

reported elsewhere (Morrow, Moore-Colyer and Longland, 1999). It appears that the type of forage ensiled in bales has a major impact on intake. For example, Hale and Moore-Colyer (2001) measured the voluntary intakes of big-bale grass and big-bale red clover silages, compared with grass hay. Ponies consumed significantly ($p<0.05$) more red clover silage than hay; grass silage intakes were intermediate; it was argued that maintenance of constant body weight implied some degree of intake regulation, although the short duration of the trial makes this conclusion uncertain. Low intakes of clamp grass silage (<50% of hay intake) by horses have been previously reported by others (McLean *et al.*, 1995). These low intakes were associated with significantly ($p<0.01$) longer MRT compared with a hay diet; 51.7h compared with 36.8h using either chromium-mordanted hay or C32 alkane (McLean, 2001). Since physical regulation of intake appears to be unimportant in the horse, dry matter content of the forage cannot account for these measured differences although intake of maize silage has been shown to fall as dry matter content falls (Agabriel *et al.*, 1982). However, the nature of the conservation process is usually less good in low dry matter silages; fermentation characteristics of clamp silage have long been known to affect its intake by ruminants (for example see McCullough, 1966) and perhaps they also affect the DMI of horses. *Ad libitum* feeding of maize silage (DM:315g/kg) to horses resulted in very low intakes (40.6g/kg $W^{0.75}$) and considerable refusals although conservation quality was satisfactory (Martin-Rosset and Dulphy, 1987). This contrasted with *ad libitum* hay intakes in the same study of 99.1g DM/kg $W^{0.75}$.

***Concentrates***

Horses are rarely allowed *ad libitum* access to concentrated feed. One study was reported (Cuddeford and Hyslop, 1996) in which ponies were offered a high-fibre feed (418g NDF/kg DM; 166g CP/kg DM) and consumed between 76 and 137 (mean 104) g DM/kg $W^{0.75}$. On average, the animals consumed in excess of three times their calculated digestible energy (DE) requirement, thereby indicating that equids fail to regulate their energy intake, at least in the short term. A more recent study (Argo, Fuller and Cox, 2001) compared the DE intakes of pony mares offered *ad libitum* access to the same complete diet in a pelleted or chaff form. Mean DE intakes of chaff and pellets increased ($p<0.01$) to attain maxima of 1.15 (0.11) and 1.76 (0.25) MJ/kg $W^{0.75}$ on days 25 and 26 respectively. During this period of time, intakes of chaff-fed animals were only 73% ($p<0.001$) of pellet-fed DE intake and during a second period (days 35 to 63), it was 79% ($p<0.01$). By the end of this second period, the coefficients of digestibility for measured parameters significantly declined ($p<0.001$) for both diets (GE by 0.16 and NDF by 0.28) and, as a consequence, chaff DE intake was reduced to 0.68 (0.07) MJ/kg $W^{0.75}$. Although condition score and average daily gain increased over the first 4 weeks, growth and appetite returned to near maintenance values within 9 weeks. The authors concluded that nutritional characterisation of *ad libitum* diets must account for physiological adaptation that in this case, took some 35 days; Ralston (1992) abandoned an *ad libitum* experiment after 5 weeks possibly just when intakes might have stabilised or reduced. In view of the fact that most Latin Square experiments utilise 21-day periods, intake data obtained from *ad libitum* feeding experiments under these circumstances would be of questionable validity.

***Conclusion***

It would appear that many of the data reported have been from short-term experiments using classical experimental designs (e.g. Latin squares) that do not allow sufficient time for physiological adaptation to enable true measures of intake. However, it seems clear, that in equids, there is not the strong relationship, measured in ruminants, between NDF content and intake. Perhaps this is simply due to the absence of a metering device in the horse that is analogous to the reticulo-omasal orifice. Alternatively, perhaps the horse responds to the "bulkiness" of the food on offer. Kyriazakis and Emmans (1995) proposed that, in pigs, water-holding capacity (WHC) limited the intake of "bulky" foods rather than fibre content *per se*. Tsaras *et al.* (1998) tested the proposal that WHC of a food was an adequate descriptor of its "bulk" and concluded that it accounts for the effects of different foods on voluntary food intake of pigs. In contrast, CF, ADF and NDF of feeds were inadequate in this respect. In view of the fact that sugar beet pulp has been shown to depress voluntary food intake by horses (Hyslop, Roy and Cuddeford, 1998; Hyslop and Cuddeford, 1999), perhaps the WHC of horse feeds should be assessed. This could then be related to intake rather than continue to seek a relationship between fibre content *per se* and intake. It is clear that equids are more sensitive to the feel, smell and taste of their food than are ruminants and, thus, oro-pharyngeal monitoring is more important in this species. Horse feed manufacturers recognise the importance of the organoleptic qualities of their products and this is apparent by their liberal use of syrups/molasses etc., metaphorically to "sweeten the pill".

## INFLUENCE OF BREED AND PHYSIOLOGICAL STATUS ON INTAKE

A diet of 0.85 meadow hay and 0.15 concentrate was fed *ad libitum* to dry, pregnant and lactating heavy horse (Comtois and Breton) breeds; their respective DMIs were 117, 113 and 162g/kg $W^{0.75}$ (Martin-Rosset *et al.*, 1990). In the same study, light horse geldings consumed 100g DM/kg $W^{0.75}$; this was significantly less ($p<0.02$) than that of the dry mares. The voluntary food intakes of heavy breeds and lactating mares were respectively significantly greater than light breeds and non- lactating mares.

## EFFECT OF PROCESSING FORAGE ON ITS INTAKE BY HORSES

The physical form of the forage is important because it affects the rate at which the horse can consume its feed; the quantity of fibre (for example g NDF/kg DM) *per se* is meaningless in this context. Grass can be presented to a performance horse in at least five forms; fresh, ensiled, artificially dehydrated, sun-cured or dried, ground and then pelleted. The rate at which dry matter is consumed will be lowest with the fresh grass and highest with the pellets because the concentration of DM (g DM/kg) in the latter will be about five times greater than it is in the grass. An early experiment (Haenlein *et al.*, 1966) demonstrated that three different physical forms of alfalfa hay (loose, wafered and pelleted) were consumed in different amounts. Whilst the three different diets were similar in chemical composition, they differed significantly in density and in mean particle size. Horses consumed 17% more wafers and 24% more pellets than loose hay. The CF of the pellets was significantly ($p<0.01$) less well digested than that of the loose hay, presumably reflecting a more rapid rate of passage through the gut. Todd *et al.*, (1995) obtained similar results when feeding different forms of alfalfa to horses. When alfalfa-based forages are fed *ad libitum,* the ranges of voluntary DMIs (g DM/kg $W^{0.75}$) reported in the literature are 75.3 to 122.0 for hays (Haenlein *et al.*, 1966; Cymbaluk, 1990; Crozier *et al.*, 1997; Dulphy *et al.*, 1997), 88.3 to 138.8 for dried wafers, cubes or pellets (Haenlein *et al.*, 1966; Cymbaluk, 1990; Todd *et al.*, 1995) and 100.0 to 155.0 for short-chopped, artificially dried material (Pearson *et al.*, 1998).

The rapid consumption of pelleted feed is often associated with the development of abnormal behaviours such as wood chewing (Haenlein *et al.*, 1966) and, possibly, the onset of disease (Frape, 1998). Although the rate of consumption can be affected by modifying the physical form of forage with a resultant increase in total voluntary food intake, this is not always the case. For example, *ad libitum* provision of short-chop, dehydrated grass or traditional grass hay, both made from the same, second cut perennial ryegrass sward cut on the same day, resulted in similar intakes by ponies (Hyslop *et al.*, 1998). Earlier Gallagher, Hintz and Schryver (1984) had shown that chopping hay into a chaff form did not influence the digestibility of OM or ADF. Furthermore, Morrow *et al.*, (1999) measured no difference in nutrient digestibility or digesta passage rate when ponies were fed hay, either in long (18cm) or short-chop (5.3cm) form; it was also observed that long and short-chop (29.3 and 6.8cm respectively) forms of big bale silage did not differ in these respects. Thus, the extent of physical treatment of forage will affect whether or not DM intake changes and whether digestibility parameters remain the same. Forages produced for admixture with concentrates, compounds or cereals are normally sold as “chops” or “chaffs”; the nutrient digestibilty and digesta passage rates for these materials should be the same as if the unprocessed forage were fed.

## CONCLUSION

The animal’s daily rate of nutrient extraction from forages is a product of the animal’s daily food intake and the digestibility of the ingested forage. The latter will depend on fibre content and the rate of passage of forage through the GIT. The strategy adopted by hind-gut fermenters is to eat relatively more than ruminants (Janis, 1976), especially of high fibre foods because, without a selective delaying mechanism for large particles, digesta passes quickly through the fermentation zone (caecum and colon). Equids are capable of extracting more nutrients per day from *ad libitum* forage diets than bovids (Duncan, Foose, Gordon, Gakahu and Lloyd, 1990) although perhaps the daily energetic costs of the extra grazing (~5h longer) outweigh the benefits. It is clear that the maximisation of DMI is critical to the adequate supply of nutrients to the horse. However, experiments that have measured straw intakes suggest that the model proposed for the horse does not hold true. Ponies fed *ad libitum* artificially dehydrated lucerne or oat straw consumed respectively, 155.0 or 94.7g DM/kg $W^{0.75}$ and when restricted to 0.70 of *ad libitum intake*, the equivalent figures were 70.2 or 67.5g DM/kg $W^{0.75}$ (Pearson *et al.*, 2001). Both the *ad libitum* intakes of lucerne and oat straw exceeded previously published values (see above) although this could have been a seasonal effect, resulting from the extended photoperiod during the summer months of the experiment. This would agree with the observations of Fuller, Cox and Argo (1998) that ponies had higher digestible energy intakes on long 'day-lengths' than on short 'day-lengths'. Apart from the apparent seasonal effect, ponies consumed less straw than lucerne and chromium-fibre MRTs were longer for the straw diets when compared with the respective lucerne diets (Pearson *et al.*, 2001). This raises the question of whether the longer MRT of oat straw is a reflection of its lower intake, lower digestibility, slower rate of emptying from the colon or its lower CP content. Further questions could be whether the lower voluntary DMI of oat straw relative to lucerne is a reflection of its higher NDF content (715 vs. 443g/kg DM), lower OM digestibility (0.44 vs. 0.58), longer MRT of chromium-fibre (*ad libitum*, 31.5 vs. 21.3; restricted, 36.0 vs. 30.5h), lower CP content (38.8 vs. 146g/kg DM) or just greater faecal bulk? These questions remain to be answered..

## Feed interactions

In two feeding trials, horses were fed long grass hay and hay plus 0.30 or 0.60 concentrate in the DM or maize silage supplemented with 0, 0.30, 0.60 and 0.90 concentrate (Martin-Rosset and Dulphy, 1987); in both trials, animals were fed at maintenance (M), 1.4 times M and *ad libitum*. Associative effects between concentrate and forage were considered by the authors to be negligible and forage digestibility appeared to be unaffected by level of concentrate inclusion in the diet. This was in direct contrast to the negative associative effects measured in sheep fed the same diets in a concurrent feeding trial. The influence of feeding level (maintenance and 3xM) and different levels of barley meal inclusion on apparent digestibility of the gross energy of pig diets have been investigated (Peers *et al.*, 1977). It was observed that, as with the horse experiment of Martin-Rosset and Dulphy (1987), there were no interactions between level of intake and diet; however, the levels of CF in the pig diets were low, ranging from 20 to 50g/kg diet. In an experiment (Cunningham *et al.*, 1962) where CF was increased from 40 to 200g/kg diet, it was shown that level of feeding had a considerable effect on apparent digestibility. Thus, it may be concluded that, for pigs at least, the influence of level of feeding on the energy value of a feed will depend entirely on the fibre content of the diet in which it is included. The horses used by Martin-Rosset and Dulphy (1987) were immature (<one year) although the authors claimed there were no differences between mature and immature horses in terms of measuring digestibility. However, there is evidence for higher intakes by growing horses (Aiken *et al.*, 1989) that might negatively affect total ration digestibility. Thus, Martin-Rosset and Dulphy (1987) consider that experiments designed to measure apparent digestibility need not take feeding level into consideration and that valid digestibility values can be assessed by difference. However, Pearson *et al.*, (2001) showed that there was an effect of feeding level on digestibility of feed by donkeys and ponies and that the precise effect was influenced by the type of forage that was fed. For example, the apparent digestibility coefficient (ADC) of oat straw DM was higher when it was fed *ad libitum* than when it was fed in restricted amounts. In contrast, the ADC of alfalfa DM was higher when intake was restricted; the effects were most marked in donkeys. The effect with straw probably resulted from the animals being able to select better quality material whereas with the alfalfa, a reduced intake would slow rate of passage and thereby enable a more complete fermentation.

Further experiments by Martin-Rosset *et al.*, (1990) measured the influence of feeding level on digestibility estimates in mature horses. Increasing the feeding level from M to *ad libitum* did not significantly change diet digestibility in these animals. More recent work in Sweden (Palmgren Karlsson *et al.*, 2000) pointed to there being associative effects on total tract digestibility in horses fed different ratios of grass hay and whole oats. This conclusion was based on an apparent curvilinear relationship between digestibilities of dietary fibre (NDF, ADF, CF) with increasing levels of oat inclusion; it was considered that this indicated negative associative effects between the two dietary components. However, this conclusion might be regarded as naïve because it assumes that oat fibre should be as digestible as hay fibre; it is not, because they are not the same chemical entities. Furthermore, these authors failed to predict the likely digestibility of the fibrous components of the diet and then to test whether or not the measured values were significantly different from the predicted values. A rather similar study substituted naked oats for alfalfa on a w/w basis at 0, 0.20, 0.40 and 0.60 of the total dry diet (Cuddeford *et al.*, 1992) and showed a non-linear increase in the ADC of ration gross energy. This suggested a synergistic interactive effect between the high level of oat feeding and the forage, possibly manifest through a reduced rate of passage; the 0.60 oat diet had the slowest rate of passage but the differences were non-significant. There were no significant differences measured between the ADCs of ADF or NDF at different levels of oat inclusion, conflicting with the views advanced by the Swedish workers (Palmgren Karlsson *et al.*, 2000). An associative effect, independent of rate of passage, was reported by Moore-Colyer and Longland (2001) when a 70:30 mix of hay and plain sugar beet pulp was fed to ponies at 1.65kg DM/ 100kg W. A strong associative effect on the degradation of non-starch polysaccharide (NSP) was also noted, as well as the ADCs for OM, ADF, and NDF of the beet pulp being 10 to 30% higher than values measured previously (Moore-Colyer, 2000).

Thus, there is enough evidence to suggest that feed interactions do in fact occur in the horse and that, perhaps, the assertions of Martin-Rosset and Dulphy (1987) need re-examination.

## Some mineralogical quirks

### COBALT

An obvious deficiency has not been produced in horses. They apparently thrive in those areas of the country where ruminants show clinical signs of cobalt deficiency-"pining". It is assumed that cobalt is necessary for the synthesis of $B_{12}$ in horses and NRC (1989) recommends a dietary inclusion of 0.1mg/kg dietary DM to safeguard intestinal synthesis of the vitamin. In situations where the metabolic demand for $B_{12}$ or its metabolites are high and where intestinal synthesis may be compromised, cobalt supplementation may be required. However, if this is the case, it would probably be better to provide a dietary supply of the vitamin, thus circumventing the need for synthesis; the efficacy of this synthetic process in the horse is not known. Racehorses fed high levels of cereal are unlikely to be able to hydrolyse all the starch available and, thus, some will pass to the caecum with the resultant production of propionate. Under these circumstances, the fermentative process would be less pronounced due to very low fibre inputs and additional $B_{12}$ would be required to assist in the metabolism of propionate. It is specifically required to convert methylmalonyl-coenzyme A to succinyl-coenzyme A.

### COPPER, MOLYBDENUM, SULPHATE INTERACTION

Hypocupraemia in ruminants can result either from low herbage copper *per se* or high herbage molybdenum (20 to 100mg/kg DM); there are areas within the UK, known as "teart" pastures, where this commonly occurs. Molybdenum exerts its effects on copper in ruminants only in the presence of sulphur, forming insoluble copper thiomolybdate, thereby limiting the uptake of copper; in excess, this complex may be absorbed and exert a systemic effect on copper. This process depends on the formation of sulphide by the reduction of sulphate or organic sulphur compounds in the rumen. The interaction does not appear to occur in horses (Strickland, Smith, Woods and Mason, 1987), probably because the environment in which the sulphate is reduced is distal to the site of copper absorption.

There is debate about the occurrence of simple copper deficiency in horses. Clinical signs are not as clear as they are in ruminants and there is a dispute about the interpretation of serum copper levels. Suttle *et al.* (1996) determined a linear relationship between serum copper and liver stores in 44 horses in contrast to the curvilinear relationship measured in ruminants; it was concluded that adequate liver stores could be achieved by feeding 20mg copper/kg dietary DM. They proposed that 16μmol/l be used as a threshold value to distinguish between normal and subnormal serum values (a value below the often quoted range of 18-28μmol/l); a serum level of 11.5μmol/l was used to distinguish deficient from marginal liver stores. However, serum copper in the horse is affected by other factors not related to diet (e.g. inflammation) and liver samples are probably the only way of obtaining unequivocal data on horse copper status. Recently, this notion has been challenged (Gee *et al.*, 2000) and the relationship between plasma copper and liver copper is deemed to be poor; it was considered that there are insufficient data to establish reference ranges for adequacy and deficiency so that tissue copper concentrations cannot be used as an indicator of copper status in horses. There is an interesting contrast between ruminants and horses in terms of the significance of liver copper stores. Liver copper levels between 15 and 25mg/kg DM (59-100μmol/kg fresh tissue) are in the deficient range for ruminants. They are associated with serum levels of <0.5mg/l (8μmol/l) whereas the same liver levels in horses are considered normal and are associated with serum levels >1.0mg/l (15μmol/l). Copper supplementation has only been shown to affect liver copper stores in weanling horses (N. Grace-personal communication) whereas similar supplements have significant effects on the liver copper stores of ruminants. The dietary copper absorption coefficient in horses is ~0.30, in contrast to ruminants where it is only ~0.05. Ruminant serum copper levels remain fairly constant until liver stores become depleted and then, there is a linear relationship between liver and serum copper levels. Thus, since the horses examined by Suttle *et al.*, (1996) appeared to have adequate liver copper reserves, it is difficult to explain the apparent relationship between serum and liver copper levels (N. Grace-personal communication). However, it is noteworthy that horse data are very limited and nobody has simultaneously measured serum and liver copper sequentially from copper-deficient animals (1.6μmol copper/l serum) through to copper-sufficient horses (>12μmol copper/l serum). In contrast, ruminant data sets are available over the ranges 2 to 20μmol copper/l serum and 25 to 1000μmol copper/kg fresh liver tissue.

NRC (1989) suggested a dietary copper concentration of 10mg/kg DM, although there is a trend to use much higher levels of dietary copper following the publication of some data by Knight *et al.* (1990). There is no doubt that trace minerals, such as copper, play a pivotal role in the formation of cartilage, but the design and the results of Knight *et al.* (1990) did not convince NRC to amend their recommendations. Furthermore, subsequent experimentation using elevated levels of dietary copper have failed to demonstrate that the extra copper was beneficial in any way for breeding mares (Pearce *et al.*, 1998) or for growing, thoroughbred yearlings (Grace *et al.*, 2002). However, copper continues to be supplemented to high levels in breeding and growing horse diets. It is perhaps fortunate that the horse is more resistant to copper toxicity than even the pig. Ponies have been shown (Smith *et al.,* 1975) to tolerate levels of 791mg copper/kg DM, fed over a period of 6 months, without any apparent ill effect.

## DIETARY CATION/ANION BALANCE (DCAB)

This feature of a diet has been shown to be important in terms of disease prevention and also, in terms of farm animal production. For example, its significance has been shown in the aetiology of hypocalcaemia in dairy cattle (see for example Block, 1991; Byers, 1994) and as affecting pig growth rates (Cole *et al.*, 1992). It has been suggested that inadequate bone mineralisation might be associated with the high incidence of bone fractures in young racehorses (Porr *et al.*, 1997) because bone mineral content has been shown to affect both bone breaking load and strength (Lawrence *et al.*, 1994). Consequently, the effects of different dietary DCABs on mineral metabolism have been investigated in horses. Increases in bone mineral content (BMC) were achieved in animals fed approximately twice recommended dietary levels of calcium (NRC, 1989) but DCAB *per se* appeared to have no effect on BMC in this particular experiment (Porr *et al.*, 2000). Horses in peak training condition are fed diets that can contain up to 700g cereal/kg. In view of the fact that the DCAB of oats is about 90mequiv/kg DM and that of "a racehorse hay" may be 400 at the most, the overall dietary DCAB will only be 183mequiv/kg DM based on a 70:30 mix of cereal and hay. This would be regarded as acidogenic and likely to have a negative effect on calcium balance as evidenced by the work at Oklahoma State University; urinary calcium excretion increased significantly ($p<0.05$) as DCAB decreased from 350 to 231mequiv/kg DM (Baker *et al.*, 1993); these changes can contribute to a negative calcium balance. This relationship was confirmed by Wall, Topliff, Freeman, Breazile, Wagner and Stutz (1993) who showed that calcium balance was significantly ($p<0.05$) less when horses were fed a highly anionic diet.

Dietary chloride has little or no direct effect on bone but it can exert an indirect effect as an anion in DCAB. In contrast, dietary calcium can both affect bone indirectly as a cation in DCAB or directly through its incorporation into hydroxyapatite. Racehorses whose future is in flat racing begin training when they are still growing at around 15 months of age and, unlike farm animals, their bones are subjected to great stress. It is estimated that up to 70% of horses in training suffer from "bucked shins", a condition that involves periostitis of the third metacarpal and sometimes microfractures (Nunamaker, 1986). Once training begins, there is a loss of BMC over a period of time that is then followed by a period of mineralisation. It appears that supplementary dietary calcium, phosphorus and magnesium at respectively 1.7, 1.3 and 1.7 times NRC (1989) values reduces bone mineral loss in the early stages of training (Nolan *et al.*, 2001). Thus, it seems that in horses entering training, supplementary dietary minerals, in particular calcium, are beneficial to bone structure and in reducing the risk of injury. Again, this represents a situation that is peculiar to horses and where there is no parallel amongst farmed animals, other than perhaps racing ostriches and camels.

## CONCLUSION

Horses show remarkable tolerances to both shortages and excesses of trace elements that would, in themselves, create clinical disease in ruminant animals. This may be partly explained on the basis that the horse is a post-gastric fermenter and, as a consequence, hydrolysis of food and absorption of subsequent end products occurs prior to the reducing medium located at the major site of fermentation in the large intestine. The disadvantage, however, is that the horse is extremely sensitive to food-borne toxins, such as botulinum (Ricketts *et al.*, 1984). The horse's apparent low dietary requirement for cobalt and its tolerance of very high dietary levels of copper remain unexplained although, in the latter case, it is probably fortuitous in view of the frequency of over supplementation. The significance of DCAB in relation to adequate mineralisation of bone has become well established although feed manufacturers seem, as yet, reluctant to optimise their products in these terms. Equally, the increased need for calcium by horses entering training has not yet been fully realised.

# Nitrogen metabolism in the horse

The activity of the microbial population in the large intestine of equids is likely to be limited by an undersupply of fermentable energy sources and nitrogen because, unlike the ruminant, a lot of dietary protein nitrogen and hydrolysable carbohydrate will have been digested prior to the site of fermentation. This situation is exacerbated by low dietary levels of protein, of low quality, that are contained in relatively indigestible, high fibre diets; mature ponies and horses at maintenance appear able to tolerate these circumstances. For example, mature animals may be over wintered on hay containing only 60g CP/ kg DM and yet do not apparently manifest signs of protein malnutrition. It has been suggested (Martin *et al.*, 1996) that, when horses are fed low nitrogen diets, renal conservation of nitrogen occurs. Furthermore, more urea is lost from the blood and degraded in the digestive tract, suggesting a compensatory source of nitrogen when horses are fed these low nitrogen diets. Frape (1998) describes the extent of nitrogen recycling in a 150kg pony to be equivalent to an intake of 54 to 154g CP daily. This was based on ponies that were given diets containing 60 to 180g CP/kg, recycling and degrading in the GIT between 200 and 574mg urea nitrogen/kg $W^{0.75}$ daily. In contrast, there is evidence that growing horses can be affected by protein of sub-optimal quality. There are numerous reports (see for example Hintz *et al.*, 1971; Barton *et al.*, 1973; Ott *et al.*, 1979) that indicate that poor quality proteins, such as linseed meal, do not support such a high rate of growth as do better quality proteins. Addition of lysine to low quality protein resulted in live-weight gains comparable to those achieved by feeding milk or soya protein. Apart from this type of work and the demonstrable need for lysine, there are very few data on the effect of protein quality and thus, NRC (1989) considered it was impractical to suggest a requirement in these terms. Whilst it would appear that mature horses are unaffected by protein quality, there is a difference between protein sources in terms of their ability to meet the protein needs of the animal (NRC, 1989). However, this is probably a reflection of variations in protein digestibility between different protein sources (Reitnour and Salsbury, 1976) and of the protein content of the diet rather than of its quality *per se*. NRC (1989) concluded that there are inadequate data on protein digestibility and, since the site of protein degradation greatly affects the efficiency of its utilisation, crude protein should be used. However, the French have taken a different view on this and have coined the term “Matières Azotées Digestibles Cheval” or MADC. This is the digestible crude protein (DCP) corrected for that part of the CP that does not supply amino acid to the animal. The MADC is the sum of the feed and microbial amino acids absorbed from the small and large intestine respectively; the former has been measured and the latter assumed – probably incorrectly. Comparing MADC with DCP values shows that the latter over-values forages by 10 to 30% (Martin-Rosset *et al.*, 1994). Thus, appropriate MADC values are calculated from the DCP of forages by multiplying by a factor K, which is 0.90, 0.85 0.80 and 0.70 for green forages, hay/dehydrated forages, straws and good quality, grass silages respectively. The DCP value of concentrates, cereals etc., is equivalent to MADC.

In most cases, DCP is predicted from CP (Table 17.5).

**Table 17.5** PREDICTION OF DCP (g /KG DM)

| *Feed Type* | *Equation* | $r^2$ |
|---|---|---|
| Fresh forage | = -74.52 + 0.9568 CP + 0.1167 CF | 0.980 |
| Grass hay | = -25.96 + 0.8357 CP | 0.968 |
| Legume hay | = -29.95 + 0.8673 CP | 0.933 |
| All forages | = -27.57+ 0.8441 CP | 0.964 |
| Cereals | = -4.94 + 0.8533 CP | 0.931 |

(Adapted from Martin-Rosset, Vermorel, Doreau, Tisserand and Andrieu, 1994)

Apparent digestibility data give no indication of the site of digestion or of the nutrients absorbed. It is more beneficial to the horse if the crude protein contains little non-protein nitrogen (NPN) and that it is digested pre-caecally, so that amino acids may be absorbed from the small intestine. Martin-Rosset *et al.*, (1994) assume that endogenous nitrogen entering the caecum amounts to 5 g /kg DMI and that lost in the faeces equates to 3 g /kg DMI. These data, together with that obtained from fistulated animals, enable the calculation of the true pre-caecal digestibility of nitrogen. Jarrige and Tisserand (1984) have estimated coefficients of 0.45, 0.70 and 0.85 for grass hay, fresh grass and concentrate, respectively. Clearly, the stage of growth at which roughages are harvested will affect how much protein-N is degraded pre-caecally. Studies using either illeally-fistulated ponies (Potter *et al.*, 1992) or the mobile-bag technique in horses (Macheboeuf *et al.*, 1995), have confirmed the estimates of Jarrige and Tisserand (1984). More recent work (Moore-Colyer *et al.*, 1998), has shown pre-caecal CP disappearances of 0.77, 0.52, 0.60 and 0.30 for an oat hull/naked oat mixture (2:1), hay, soya hulls and sugar beet pulp; the proportional disappearance depending on the botanical source of material.

Some feed protein and endogenous nitrogen will pass into the large intestine where some will be degraded and the end products incorporated into microbial protein. Faecal nitrogen will be composed of indigestible feed nitrogen mostly bound to fibre, the so-called acid-detergent, insoluble nitrogen (ADIN), microbial protein nitrogen and endogenous nitrogen. The different origins of faecal nitrogen make the estimation of the large intestinal contribution to absorbed nitrogen complex. However, Jarrige and Tisserand (1984) calculated large intestinal true protein digestibility to be 0.90 for concentrates, 0.80 for fresh grass and 0.75 for hays and silages. It was assumed that 15% of the digested protein was absorbed as amino acids. However, it appears that this assumption is flawed because *in vitro* studies (Bochröder, Schubert and Bödeker, 1994) have failed to demonstrate a transmucosal flux of lysine, histidine and arginine across colonic tissue. If these amino acids are released in the lumen of the large intestine by microbial activity, they will not be able to contribute to the plasma amino acid pool. These findings confirm those of others (Wysocki and Baker, 1975; Freeman *et al.*, 1989; Freeman and Donawick, 1991), but are at variance with the results of Slade *et al.* (1971). The latter group of workers suggested that lysine in particular, was rapidly absorbed from the large intestine; however, the nature of their experiment would have allowed $^{15}N$ enrichment of ammonia which could have been absorbed from the caecum and colon and could then have subsequently labelled circulating lysine giving the impression that lysine had, in fact, been absorbed from the lumen of the gut. It is noteworthy that ammonia is transported across the colonic mucosa at rates equal to, or greater than, those measured with sheep ruminal mucosa (Bochröder *et al.*, 1994) and will be available for incorporation into non-essential amino acids in the liver of the horse.

## The impact of feeding routines

Traditionally, dairy cattle were fed roughages and concentrates separately; this practice resulted in large fluctuations in populations of organisms within the reticulo-rumen. Part of the success of complete diets or Total Mixed Rations (TMRs) is that rumen microbial populations remain more stable (both in terms of numbers and activity), leading to a more effective fermentation and, thus, benefiting health and production. Separate feeding of roughage and concentrate to horses does not have the direct impact seen in ruminants, since there is the opportunity for both pre-digestion and digesta mixing prior to its arrival at the site of fermentation in the horse. However, in view of the fact that those horses being fed concentrate are "working" or "performing" in some way, it adds another dimension when considering the effects of feeding. Horses can be undergoing aerobic or anaerobic work or, a combination of both, and the glycaemic response to feeding is important because it can impair their ability to perform work. A hyperglycaemic response occurs when horses are fed a concentrate meal and this will be accompanied by an increase in plasma insulin levels. These post-feeding changes can have an impact on the horse's ability to perform work as shown by Pagan *et al.* (1996). It was shown that, 3h after a grain-based meal, there was a large reduction in blood glucose in horses performing an exercise test; this change was interpreted as an undesirable effect. It was proposed that insulin levels were high at the onset of the exercise period and that this increased the uptake of glucose by the muscles. Horses that worked 8h after a meal, or after an overnight fast, began exercise with resting levels of both glucose and insulin. During exercise, blood glucose increased in these horses suggesting that they were mobilising liver glycogen more rapidly and releasing glucose more quickly than it could be cleared from the blood. In contrast, less insulin was produced in response to a grain meal and blood glucose was lower (Pagan, Rotmensen and Jackson, 1995), following supplementation with trivalent chromium in the form of chromium yeast; on this basis, it was suggested that the metabolic response of the horse to a supply of sugar (as starch or water soluble carbohydrates (WSC)) could be moderated. Pagan *et al.* (1999) have demonstrated that both feed type and level of intake can affect the glycaemic response of thoroughbred horses although, the exact relevance of the change in this response to a horse's performance or behaviour, has as yet to be fully determined.

Pre-feeding a horse with roughage prior to a meal of concentrate would create a state of partial satiety in the horse so that, when confronted with a meal, its appetite drive would be reduced and, thus, its rate of consumption of the subsequent starch-rich meal would be slower. This effect of roughage pre-feeding on concentrate consumption rates is observed in practice, but its desirability is questionable. Obviously, the longer starch is exposed to hydrolytic enzyme activity in the small intestine the more complete starch degradation will be, so that, at least superficially, slow ingestion of concentrate is desirable. However, Pagan (1999) has shown that feeding hay 2h before a grain meal significantly reduced ('P' value not given) the horse's glycaemic response. This was associated with less insulin being produced and an increase in plasma protein; the latter was interpreted as signifying a hypovolaemic state. Horses produce about twice as much saliva when fed hay compared to when they are fed concentrate and Meyer *et al.* (1985) have quoted figures of 400/480g saliva/100g hay DM compared to only 206g/100g concentrate DM. Blood volume will be affected by the quantity of liquid secreted into the gut. Pagan (1999) considered that this might generate a thirst response, since a large increase in water consumption was recorded following hay feeding. The increase in digesta volume would hasten the rate of passage; although, since this effect should precede the meal, it is difficult to envisage how pre-caecal starch digestion of the following meal would be affected. Unpublished work from Edinburgh has shown that the passage rate of markers bound to both concentrate and forage, as well as a liquid phase marker, was faster when concentrate was fed 2h after a forage meal compared to feeding concentrate with or before a forage meal. However, this result may have been confounded since the animals were still eating forage when offered the concentrate; the concentrate and forage meals were not discrete in this instance. Pagan (1999) does not indicate if, when forage was pre-fed, all the forage was consumed prior to offering the meal of concentrate. This could clearly have a large effect on the outcome of the experiment.

Forage is often chaffed and mixed into a concentrate meal in order to reduce the rate of consumption of that meal; the rest of the forage allocation is fed separately. Harris (1999) noted that adding chaff to pellets reduced consumption rate of pellets by 46% in horses and 43% in ponies when compared with feeding pellets alone, although there is no knowledge of this effect on subsequent small intestinal starch digestion. Pagan (1999) recorded similar physiological changes in horses that were fed hay with their concentrates to those in horses that were pre-fed hay; it was suggested that increased rate of passage reduced pre-caecal starch digestion, resulting in starch flowing into the caecum; this might have accounted for a rise in plasma lactate measured 3h after the grain meal. It is naïve to expect that starch sources will be degraded in a constant way in the small intestine irrespective of the basal diet simply, because feeds interact in the lumen of the gut. For example, Meyer *et al.,* (1993) demonstrated that the pre-ileal digestibility of ground maize was reduced by substituting ground lucerne meal for hay in a mixed ration fed to horses. Kleffken (1993) showed that this substitution altered the rate of passage of the ground maize through the small intestine, thereby accounting for the differences measured by Meyer *et al.,* (1993). Recent, unpublished work at Edinburgh confirmed that the nature of the basal forage can affect the passage rate of the components of mixed diets; oat straw residues passed through the digestive tract more slowly than haylage residues. Concentrate particles were retained for less time in the digestive tract of straw-fed animals than were forage particles (according to expectation); however, when haylage was the basal forage, the converse was true. Thus, the nature of any chaff that is mixed into a concentrate meal, together with the type of basal forage fed, may have far-reaching effects on the efficacy of pre-caecal starch digestibility. Of course, the extent of these effects will depend on the size of the concentrate meal offered so that, in general, provision of small meals of starch are unlikely to lead to significant quantities of starch entering the caecum, irrespective of the type of chaff or basal forage used. Feeding forage after a concentrate meal is likely to accelerate the rate of passage of the digesta thereby reducing pre-caecal starch degradation. Whilst there is little evidence to indicate that overall diet digestibility is negatively affected by feeding protocols, it seems likely that pre-caecal starch digestion could be compromised, based on circumstantial evidence provided by changes in blood parameters (Pagan, 1999). Thus, it would seem wise to feed forage after concentrate meals, having allowed sufficient time (~2h) for most of the residues of the meal to pass through the stomach and small intestine. However, it is still likely that, initially, some starch from a meal fed after a fast will arrive in the caecum undigested because passage rate will be rapid at this stage in the meal.

## Effect of exercise on digestibility

In contrast to most ruminants, horses are kept for their athletic ability and thus perform some form of work. In their seminal review of the literature on the nutrition of the horse, Olsson and Ruudvere (1955) concluded that "light exercise" may improve digestibility of a ration and that "heavy work" may depress it. This conclusion was based on results obtained with three geldings in an experiment conducted in 1888 (Grandeau and LeClerc, 1888). More recent Australian work (Orton *et al.*, 1985a; 1985b) compared exercised (12km/h for 1h) and non-exercised horses fed two levels of protein (60 to 80 or 120 to 140 g/kg). Exercise increased voluntary feed intake and apparent DM digestibility although the MRT of particulate matter was reduced ($p<0.05$); MRT of the fluid marker was increased ($p<0.05$). The former was probably a reflection of increased intake. Pearson and Merritt (1991) did not measure an increase in DMI in exercised donkeys perhaps, because intake was limited by faecal mass and its rate of elimination from the rectum. Hintz (1988) summarised these experiments and concluded that the average ADC for DM in exercised horses was 0.81 and that it represented 119% of the value measured in control animals. ADC for protein was slightly higher at 0.85, representing 114% of control values. Worth, Fontenot and Meacham (1987) paired 8 mature geldings according to weight and one member of each pair underwent a 60-day course of exercise training for 2h/day, 5 days/week. Average ADC for DM in the exercised group was 0.65, equivalent to 107% of the control group values, whereas ADC for protein was 109% of control group values. More recently, Pearson and Merritt (1991) were able to confirm that digestibility coefficients were higher in exercised donkeys although the effect was not significant. There is no apparent parallel in working ruminants (Pearson and Lawrence, 1992). There appears to be sufficient evidence to support the view that light exercise by equids increases DM digestibility, as originally suggested in the late 19$^{th}$ Century, but the reasons for this remain obscure.

## Fermentation stimulants

There is considerable information on the use of substances that modify activity within the reticulo-rumen of ruminants and there has been a focus on the use of probiotics, mostly in terms of the use of yeast or yeast culture. As early as 1925, Eckles and Williams (1925) described the use of yeast as a supplementary feed for lactating dairy cows and, since then, there has been a massive expansion in research that has focussed on the use of yeast or yeast culture in animal diets. Strains of *Saccharomyces cerevisiae* have received the most attention and their effect seems to be indirect in that improved production is as a result of increased intake. Effects have been ascribed to nutrient provision (e.g. growth factors, vitamins and minerals), stimulation of lactate uptake and/or oxygen scavenging (although unlikely in the large intestine of the horse).

The latter requires that the yeast is alive and metabolically active so the provision of yeast culture or dead cells would not be effective in this context. The inescapable fact is that relatively small amounts of yeast culture (10g/dairy cow/day) appear to have a significant effect on rumen fermentation (see, for example, Erasmus *et al.*, 1992). Horses are post-gastric fermenters, so the yeast has to survive the gastric phase of digestion that involves exposure to acid-pepsin hydrolysis if the effect of the yeast depends on the delivery of viable organisms to the site of activity, namely the caecum and colon. A review of the role of yeast culture in equine nutrition and physiology (Hill *et al.*, 2001) focussed on the role of *S. cerevisiae*[1026]. A tentative model was suggested to define the mode of action of yeast culture in the horse's digestive tract. Microbial action on the diet was proposed to occur in the fundic region of the stomach or in the upper duodenum to partially explain increases in the apparent absorption of calcium and phosphorus and maybe other nutrients (not specified). This is confusing, since the authors acknowledge that most phosphorus is absorbed from the large intestine (Frape, 1998). Further, Hill *et al.* (2001) indicated that there are many studies in horses that failed to demonstrate any beneficial effect following dietary supplementation with *S. cerevisiae*[1026]. The varied results following oral supplementation possibly reflect differences in the survivability of this strain throughout the digestive tract of the horse and the variability in the nature of the diets fed. Recently, Medina *et al.* (2000) reported that the dietary addition (10g/day) of *S. cerevisiae*[1026] to a high starch diet (359g starch/kg) depressed the apparent digestibility of DM, OM, NDF and ADF. This is surprising since, in ruminants, *S. cerevisiae*[1026] is credited with beneficial effects, particularly when a lot of starch is fed and when enhancement of lactate utilisation is critically important. Medina *et al.* (2000) concluded that the yeast culture stimulated fibrolytic activity in the large intestine of horses fed high fibre (341g NDF/kg) rations although, according to the data presented, it certainly appears to have the opposite effect in horses fed lower fibre (218g NDF/kg) diets. In contrast, Hill and Gutsell (1998) demonstrated that the same level of supplementation increased the apparent digestibility coefficients for the feed components of a mixed diet (0.82 hay, 0.18 concentrates), but only significantly for NDF ($p<0.05$). Interestingly, Hill *et al.*, (2001) reported no effect in animals fed 0.95 hay and 0.05 concentrates.

Variable results obtained in *in vivo* trials may be a reflection of the varied survival of yeast in feeds following pelleting; few data are available to quantify the survival of yeast during this process. The high temperature and moisture during processing are likely to have adverse effects on the viability of unprotected yeast. Some work at Kansas State University (Maloney *et al.*, 1998) demonstrated that *S. cerevisiae*[47] survived steam conditioning (~10 seconds at 80$^{0}$C) and the pelleting process used to produce diets for piglets.

The yeast was in the form of a heat stable product (Biosaf Sc47) and appeared to be unaffected by these processing conditions. Furthermore, when fed to piglets, viable *S. cerevisiae*$^{47}$ were recovered from the faeces. These results demonstrate that this form of yeast (Biosaf Sc47) was not only able to withstand the commercial pelleting process, but was also able to survive the gastric and intestinal phases of digestion in the pig. Published information is available on the faecal recovery of viable forms of yeast following oral administration of *S. cerevisiae*$^{47}$ (Biosaf Sc47) to sheep (Fiems *et al.*, 1993). It is apparent that at least this commercial form of the strain is also capable of withstanding exposure to both fermentative and hydrolytic environments within the GIT. Recently completed, but unpublished, work at Edinburgh has shown that this strain of yeast also survives exposure to acid/pepsin hydrolysis *in vitro* and pelleting at 70$^0$C. Furthermore, oral dosing of horses with Biosaf Sc47 enabled the recovery of viable organisms from the faeces although this is not surprising in view of the results obtained with pigs. Thus, this particular form of heat stable *S. cerevisiae*$^{47}$ (Biosaf Sc47) remains viable throughout the GIT of the horse and can thus perform functions in the horse's large intestine analogous to those of yeast strains given orally to ruminants. However, if some of the activity of *S. cerevisiae* depends on non-viable cells providing nutritional support to the caecal/colonic microflora, then its survivability is less important. Newman and Spring (1994) have shown that different strains of yeast (*S. cerevisiae*$^{1026}$ and *S. cerevisiae*$^{38618}$) have different effects *in vitro* on ruminal and caecal fermentations although the responses in the different media were very similar suggesting a common mode of action. Lyons (1994) has also pointed out that different strains possess different activities and that, in the future, specific strains may be developed for defined purposes. There are no "live" products that are currently licensed for use in the UK, although several are apparently incorporated into horse compounds, or are sold as supplements.

## Summary

The horse presents a challenge to the nutritionist who has to sift the fact from the fantasy in terms of deciding effective feeding protocols. The anatomical features of the horse's gut, together with a post-gastric fermentation, make the horse particularly vulnerable to dietary mis-management in a way not seen in ruminants. The digesta must be of low dry matter in order to flow through the complicated and convoluted large intestine that is specifically designed to arrest a liquid flow to enable a satisfactory fermentation. Grass-fed horses epitomise the ideal situation and rarely experience situations in which impaired digesta flow leads to gut-related problems. Much research with horses has not been exposed to the same degree of rigorous appraisal that so much ruminant research has endured. Effects are looked for, rather than measured and, as a consequence, hard scientific facts tend to be ignored, or are not available. A classic example is that of copper supplementation where one publication has led to the common-place usage of high levels of dietary copper for young, growing animals and mares, yet the scientific committee of the NRC (1989), who reviewed the available evidence, could not recommend these levels. Recent work from New Zealand (Grace *et al.*, 2002), however, confirms the wisdom of the NRC committee with respect to the "benefits" of copper supplementation. Unfortunately, horse nutritional research is not a topical area for rigorous scientific research because there is not a simple cause and effect relationship. Coughing racehorses cannot race, but inadequately fed horses have to and, until someone takes the wider view, it is unlikely that the subject will develop apace. However, the nutrition of horses is both interesting and challenging, in part because of their unique features, some of which are outlined in this chapter, but also because there is no simple production parameter whereby adequacy can be assessed.

## Acknowledgements

Thanks are due to Colin Morgan, David Smith and Helen Stebbens for their critical and constructive inputs.

## References

Agabriel, J., Trillaud-Geyl, C., Martin-Rosset, M. and Jussiaux, M. (1982) Utilisation de l'ensilage de mais par le poulain de boucherie. *Bulletin Technical* CRZV Theix, INRA, **49**, 5-13.

Aiken, G.E., Potter, G.D., Conrad, B.E. and Evans, J.W. (1989) Voluntary intake and digestion of Coastal Bermuda grass hay by yearling and mature horses. *Equine Veterinary Science*, **9**, 262-264.

Archer, M. (1978) Further studies on palatability of grasses to horses. *Journal of the British Grassland Society*, **33**, 239-243.

Argenzio, R.A., Lowe, J.E., Pickard, D.W. and Stevens, C.E. (1974) Digesta passage and water exchange in the equine large intestine. *American Journal of Physiology*, **226**, 1035-1042.

Argo, C.McG., Fuller, Z. and Cox, J.E. (2001) Digestible energy intakes, growth and feeding behaviour of pony mares offered *ad libitum* access to a complete diet in a pelleted or chaff-based form. *Proceedings of the 17th Equine Nutrition and Physiology Symposium*, Kentucky, USA. p.171-173.

Baker, L.A., Topliff, D.R., Freeman, D.W., Teeter, R.G. and Breazile, J.E. (1993) Effect of dietary cation-anion balance on urinary mineral excretion in horses. *Proceedings of the 13th Equine Nutrition and Physiology Symposium*, Gainesville, USA. p.44-49.

Barton, A., Anderson, D.L. and Lyford, S. (1973) Studies of protein quality and quantity in the early weaned foal. *Proceedings of the 3rd Equine Nutrition and Physiology Symposium*, Gainesville, USA. p.19.

Block, E. (1991) Anion-cation balance and its effect on the performance of ruminants. In: *Recent Advances in Animal Nutrition*, eds. W. Haresign and D.J.A.Cole, Butterworths Heinemann, p.163-179.

Bochröder, B., Schubert, R. and Bödeker, D. (1994) Studies on the transport *in vitro* of lysine, histidine, arginine and ammonia across the mucosa of the equine colon. *Equine Veterinary Journal*, **26**, 131-133.

Byers, D.I. (1994) Management considerations for successful use of anionic salts in dry-cow diets. *Compendium on Continuing Education for the Practicing Veterinarian*, **16**, 237-242.

Cole, D.J.A., Wiseman, J., Davies, J., Partridge, G.C. and Reeve, A. (1992) The effect of dietary electrolyte balance on the performance of growing pigs. *Animal Production*, **54**, 485.

Corring, T. (1982) Enzyme digestion in the proximal digestive tract of the pig: a review. *Livestock Production Science*, **9**, 581-590.

Crozier, J.A., Allen, V.G., Jack, N.E., Fontenot, J.P. and Cochran, M.A. (1997) Digestibility, apparent mineral absorption and voluntary intake by horses fed alfalfa, tall fescue and caucasian bluestem. *Journal of Animal Science*, **75**, 1651-1658.

Cuddeford, D. (1999) Recent advances in equine nutrition. *Recent Advances in Animal Nutrition in Australia*, **12**, 99-105.

Cuddeford, D., and Hyslop, J.J. (1996). Intake and digestibility of a high fibre concentrate offered *ad libitum* to ponies and donkeys. Proceedings of the 47th Annual Meeting of the EAAP, Lillehammer, Norway, p.296(a).

Cuddeford, D., Khan, N. and Muirhead, R. (1992) Naked oats-an alternative energy source for performance horses. *Proceedings of the 4th International Oat Conference*, Adelaide, Australia. p.42-50.

Cuddeford, D., Pearson, R.A., Archibald, R.F. and Muirhead, R.H. (1995) Digestibility and gastrointestinal transit time of diets containing different proportions of alfalfa and oat straw given to Thoroughbreds, Shetland ponies, Highland ponies and donkeys. *Animal Science*, **61**, 407-417.

Cunningham, H.M., Friend, D.W. and Nicholson, J.W.G. (1962) The effect of age, body weight, feed intake and adaptability of pigs on the digestibility and nutritive value of cellulose. *Canadian Journal of Animal Science*, **42**, 167-175.

Cymbaluk, N.F. (1990) Comparison of forage digestion by cattle and horses.

*Canadian Journal of Animal Science*, **70**, 601-610.

Drogoul, C., Poncet, C. and Tisserand, J.L. (2000a) Feeding ground and pelleted hay rather than chopped hay to ponies. 1. Consequences for *in vivo* digestibility and rate of passage of digesta. *Animal Feed Science and Technology*, **10547**, 1-14.

Drogoul, C., Poncet, C. and Tisserand, J.L. (2000b) Feeding ground and pelleted hay rather than chopped hay to ponies. 2. Consequences on fibre degradation in the caecum and colon. *Animal Feed Science and Technology*, **10548**, 1-15.

Dulphy, J.P., Martin-Rosset, W., Dubroeucq, H. and Jailler, M. (1997) Evaluation of voluntary intake of forage trough-fed to light horses. Comparison with sheep. Factors of variation and prediction. *Livestock Production Science*, **52**, 97-104.

Dulphy, J.P., Martin-Rosset, W., Dubroeucq, H., Ballet, J.M., Detour, A. and Jailler, M. (1997) Compared feeding patterns in *ad libitum* intake of dry forages by horses and sheep. *Livestock Production Science*, **52**, 49-56.

Duncan, P. (1985) Time-budgets of Camargue horses. 1. Environmental influences. *Behaviour*, **92**, 188-208.

Duncan, P., Foose, T.J., Gordon, I.J., Gakahu, C.G. and lloyd, M. (1990) Comparative nutrient extraction from forages by grazing bovids and equids: a test of the nutritional model of equid/bovid competition and coexistence. *Oecologia*, **84**, 411-418.

Eckles, C.H. and Williams, V.M. (1925) Yeast as a supplementary feed for lactating cows. *Journal of Dairy Science*, **8**, 89-93.

Ellis, A.D., Fagence, K., Warr, E.M. and Hill, J. (2000) Effect of dental condition on short term intake rates and faecal particle size in adult horses. *Proceedings of the 51st Annual Meeting of the European Association of Animal Production*, Wageningen Pers, p. 375.

Ellis, A.D., Warr, E.M. and Hill, J. (2001a) Kinetics of forage feed particles in horses before and after dental treatment. *Proceedings of the 52nd Annual Meeting of the European Association of Animal Production*, Wageningen Pers, p. 339.

Ellis, A.D., Warr, E.M. and Hill, J. (2001b) Effect of dental condition and types of concentrates on intake behaviour of horses. *Proceedings of the 52nd Annual Meeting of the European Association of Animal Production*, Wageningen Pers, p. 340.

Erasmus, L.J., Botha, P.M. and Kistner, A. (1992) Effect of yeast culture supplement on production, rumen fermentation and duodenal nitrogen flow in dairy cows. *Journal of Dairy Science*, **75**, 3056-3065.

Fiems, L.O., Cottyn, B.G., Dussert, L. and Vanacker, J.M. (1993) Effect of a viable yeast culture on digestibility and rumen fermentation in sheep fed different types of diets. *Reproduction and Nutrition Developments*, **33**, 43-49.

Frape, D. (1998) *Equine Nutrition and Feeding*. Second edition, Blackwell Science Ltd., Oxford, UK.

Frape, D.L., Tuck, M.G., Sutcliffe, N.H. and Jones, D.B. (1982) The use of inert markers in the measurement of the digestibility of cubed concentrate and of hay given in several proportions to the pony, horse and white rhinoceros (*Diceros simus*). *Comparative Biochemistry and Physiology*, **72A**, 77-83.

Fraser, A.F. (1992). *The Behaviour of the Horse*. CAB International, Wallingford, Oxfordshire, UK.

Freeman, D.E. and Donawick, W.J. (1991) *In vitro* transport of cycloleucine by equine cecal mucosa. *American Journal of Veterinary Research*, **52**, 539-542.

Freeman, D.E., Kleinzeller, A., Donawick, W.J. and Topkis, V.A. (1989) *In vitro* transport of L-alanine by equine cecal mucosa. *American Journal of Veterinary Research*, **50**, 2138-2144.

Friend, M.A. and Nash, D. (2000) Pasture intake by grazing horses. *RIRDC Publication No 00/. Project No UCS-22A*. Rural Industries Research and Development Corporation, Australia.

Forbes, J.M. (1988) Metabolic aspects of the regulation of voluntary food intake and appetite. In: *Nutrition Research Reviews 1*. Cambridge University Press, Cambridge.

Fuller, Z., Cox, J.E. and Argo, C.McG. (1998) Photoperiodic entrainment of seasonal changes in appetite and growth in pony colts. In: *Proceedings of the British Society for Animal Science. P133.*

Gallagher, J.R., Hintz, H. and Schryver, H.F. (1984) A nutritional evaluation of chopped hay for equines. *Animal Production in Australia*, **15**, 349-352.

Gee, E.K., Grace, N.D., Firth, E.C. and Fennessy, P.F. (2000) The change in liver copper concentrations of thoroughbred foals from birth to 160 days of age, and the effect of prenatal mare copper supplementation. *Australian Veterinary Journal*, **78**, 18-24.

Gibbs, J. and Smith, G.P. (1978) The gut and preabsorptive satiety. *Acta-Hepato-Gastroenterology*, **25**, 413-416.

Glade, M.J. and Reimers, T.J. (1985) Effects of dietary energy supply on serum thyroxine, triiodothyronine and insulin concentrations in young horses. *Journal of Endocrinology*, **104**, 93-98.

Grace, N.D., Gee, E.K., Firth, E.C. and Shaw, H.L. (2002) Digestible energy intake, dry matter digestibility and mineral status of grazing New Zealand thoroughbred yearlings. *New Zealand Veterinary Journal*, **49**, (In press).

Grandeau, L. and LeClerc, A. (1888) Alimentation du Cheval de Tract. *Annales du Science et du Agronomie, Paris*, **5**, 211-221.

Haenlein, G.F., Holdren, R.D. and Yoon, Y.M. (1966) Comparative responses of horses and sheep to different physical forms of alfalfa. *Journal of Animal Science*, **25**, 740-743.

Hale, C.E. and Moore-Colyer, M.J.S. (2001) Voluntary food intake and apparent digestibilities of hay, big-bale grass silage and red clover silage by ponies. *Proceedings of the 17th Equine Nutrition and Physiology Symposium*, Kentucky, USA. p.468-469.

Hill, J. and Gutsell, S. (1998) Effect of supplementation of a hay and concentrate diet with live yeast culture on the digestibility of nutrients in 2 and 3 year old riding school horses. *Proceedings of the British Society of Animal Science*, p.128.

Hill, J., Tracey, S.V., Willis, M., Jones, L. and Ellis, A.D. (2001) Yeast culture in equine nutrition and physiology. *Proceedings of the 17th Annual Symposium on Biotechnology in the Feed Industry*, p.97-114.

Harris, P.A. (1999) How understanding the digestive process can help minimise digestive disturbances due to diet and feeding practices. *Proceedings of the BEVA Specialist days on Behaviour and Nutrition*, September 1999. Equine Veterinary Journal Ltd., Suffolk. p.45-49.

Hintz, H. (1988) Effect of exercise on digestibility. *Equine Practice*, **10**, 5-6.

Hintz, H.F., Argenzio, R.A. and Schryver, H.F. (1971) Digestion coefficients, blood glucose levels and molar percentages of volatile fatty acids in intestinal fluid of ponies fed varying forage:grain ratios. *Journal of Animal Science*, **33**, 992-995.

Hintz, H.F., Schryver, H.F. and Lowe, J.E. (1971) Comparison of a blend of milk products and linseed meal as protein supplements for young growing horses. *Journal of Animal Science*, **33**, 1274-1277.

Hollands, T. and Cuddeford, D. (1992) Effect of supplementary soya oil on the digestibility of nutrients contained in a 40:60 roughage/concentrate diet fed to horses. *Pferdeheilkunde*, p. 128-132.

Hyslop, J.J. and Calder, S. (2001) Voluntary intake and apparent digestibility in ponies offered alfalfa based forages *ad libitum*. *Proceedings of the British Society of Animal Science*, p. 90.

Hyslop, J.J. and Cuddeford, D. (1999) Soaked unmolassed sugar beet pulp as a partial forage replacer in equine diets when ponies are offered grass hay *ad libitum*. *Proceedings of the British Society of Animal Science*, p.140.

Hyslop, J.J., Bayley, A., Tomlinson, A.L. and Cuddeford, D. (1998) Voluntary feed intake and apparent digestibility *in vivo* in ponies given *ad libitum* access to dehydrated grass or hay harvested from the same grass crop. *Proceedings of the British Society of Animal Science*, p.131.

Hyslop, J.J., Jessop, N.S., Stefansdottir, G.J. and Cuddeford, D. (1997) Comparitive protein and fibre degradation measured *in situ* in the caecum of ponies and in the rumen of steers. *Proceedings of the British Society of Animal Science*, p.121.

Hyslop, J.J., Roy, S. and Cuddeford, D. (1998) *Ad libitum* sugar beet pulp as the major fibre source in equine diets when ponies are offered a restricted amount of mature grass hay. *Proceedings of the British Society of Animal Science*, p. 132.

Hyslop, J.J., Tomlinson, A.L., Bayley, A. and Cuddeford, D. (1998) Voluntary feed intake and apparent digestibility *in vivo* in ponies offered a mature threshed grass hay *ad libitum*. *Proceedings of the British Society of Animal Science*, p.130.

Janis, C.M. (1976) The evolutionary strategy of the Equidae and the origins of rumen and caecal digestion. *Evolution*, **30**, 757-774.

Jarrige, R. and Tisserand, J.L. (1984) Métabolisme, besoins et alimentation azotée du cheval. In: R. Jarrige and W. Martin-Rosset (Editors), *Le Cheval, Reproduction, Sélection, Alimentation, Exploitation*. INRA Publications, Route de St Cyr, 78000 Versailles, pp.277-302.

Kienzle, E., Radicke, S., Wilke, S., Landes, E. and Meyer, H. (1992) Praeileale Starkeverdauung in Abhangigheit von Starkeart und –zubereitung. *Pferdeheilkunde*, p. 103-106.

Kleffken, D. (1993) Praeileale Verdauung von Getreidestärke (Gerste/Mais) in Abhangigkeit von Zubereitung, Rauhfutterangebot und Amylasezusatz beim Pferd. Tierärztlische Hochschule, Hannover, Dissertation.

Knight, D.A., Weisbrode, S.E., Schmall, L.M., Reed, S.M., Gabel, A.A., Bramlage, L.R. and Tyznik, W.I. (1990) The effects of copper supplementation on the prevalence of cartilage lesions in foals. *Equine Veterinary Journal*, **22**, 426-432.

Kyriazakis, I. and Emmans, G.C. (1995) The voluntary food intake of pigs given feeds based on wheat bran, dried citrus pulp and grass meal, in relation to measurements of food bulk. *British Journal of Nutrition*, **73**, 191-207.

Laut, J.E., Houpt, K.A., Hintz, H.F. and Houpt, T.R. (1985) The effects of caloric dilution on meal patterns and feed intake in ponies. *Physiology and Behaviour*, **35**, 549-554.

Lawrence, A.C.St., Lawrence, L.M. and Coleman, R.J. (2001) Using an empirical equation to predict voluntary intake of grass hays by mature equids. *Proceedings of the 17th Equine Nutrition and Physiology Symposium*, Kentucky, USA. p.99-100.

Lawrence, L.A., Ott, E.A., Miller, G.J., Poulos, J.W., Pietrowski, G. and Asquith, R.L. (1994) The mechanical properties of equine third metacarpal as affected by age. *Journal of Animal Science*, **72**, 2617-2623.

Lyons, T.P. (1994) Biotechnology in the feed industry: 1994 and beyond. *Proceedings of the 10th Annual Symposium on Biotechnology in the Feed Industry*, Lexington, Kentucky.p.1-50.

Macheboeuf, D., Marangi, M., Poncet, C. and Martin-Rosset, W. (1995) Study of nitrogen digestion from different hays by the mobile nylon bag technique in horses. *Annales Zootechnie*, **44**, 219.

Mair, T.S. and Hillyer, M.H. (1997) Chronic colic in the mature horse: A retrospective review of 106 cases. *Equine Veterinary Journal*, **29**, 415-420.

Maloney, C.A., Hancock, J.D., Hines, R.H., Cao, H., Nemecek, C.S. and Park, J.S. (1998) Effect of a heat stable yeast product in pelleted diets for weanling pigs. *Kansas State University Occasional Publications, Swine*. p.62-66.

Martin, R.G., McMeniman, N.P., Norton, B.W. and Dowsett, K.F. (1996) Utilisation of endogenous and dietary urea in the large intestine of the mature horse. *British Journal of Nutrition*, **76**, 373-386.

Martin-Rosset, W. and Dulphy, J.P. (1987) Digestibility interactions between forages and concentrates in horses: influence of feeding level-comparison with sheep. *Livestock Production Science*, **17**, 263-276.

Martin-Rosset, W., Doreau, M., Boulot, S. and Miraglia, N. (1990) Influence of level of feeding and physiological state on diet digestibility in light and heavy breed horses. *Livestock Production Science*, **25**, 257-264.

Martin-Rosset, W., Vermorel, N., Doreau, M., Tisserand, J.L. and Andrieu, J. (1994) The French horse feed evaluation systems and recommended allowances for energy and protein. *Livestock Production Science*, **40**, 37-56.

McCullough, M.E. (1966) The nutritive value of silage as influenced by silage fermentation and ration supplementation. *Proceedings of the 10th International Grassland Conference*, Helsinki, p.581.

McLean, B.M.L. (2001) Estimating digesta passage rate of forage based diets in horses using N-alkanes. *Proceedings of the* 17th *Equine Nutrition and Physiology Symposium*, Kentucky, USA. p.192-194.

McLean, B.M.L., Afzalzadeh, A., Bates, L., Mayes, R.W. and Hovell, F.D. DeB. (1995) Voluntary intake, digestibility and rate of passage of a hay and a silage fed to horses and to cattle. *Animal Science*, **60**, 555.

McLean, B.M.L., Hyslop, J.J., Longland, A.C., Cuddeford, D. and Hollands, T. (2000) Physical processing of barley and its effects on intra-caecal fermentation parameters. *Animal Feed Science and Technology*, **85**, 79-87.

McMeniman, N.P. (2000) Nutrition of grazing broodmares, their foals and young horses. *RIRDC Publication No 00/28. Project No UQ-45A*. Rural Industries Research and Development Corporation, Australia.

Medina, B., Poillon,D., Power, R. and Julliand, V. (2000) Effect of a dried yeast culture on *in vivo* apparent digestibility and on *in vitro* fibrolytic activity of large intestine fluid contents in horses fed high fibre or high starch pelleted feeds. *Proceedings of the British Society of Animal Science*. p.58.

Meyer, H., Ahlswede, L. and Reinhardt, H.J. (1975) Untersuchungen uber Freßdauer, Kaufrequenz und Futterzerkleinerung beim Pferd. *Deutsch Tierärztliche Wochenschrift*, **82**, 49-96.

Meyer, H., Coenen, M. and Gurer, C. (1985). Investigations of saliva production and chewing in horses fed various feeds. In: *Proceedings of the 9th Equine Nutrition and Physiology Symposium*, East Lansing, Michigan. p. 38-41.

Minson, D.J. (1990) *Forage in Ruminant Nutrition*. Academic Press, New York.

Moore-Colyer, M.J.S. (2000) Studies on the degradation kinetics of botanically diverse fibrous feeds and their apparent digestibility and rate of passage when fed to ponies. *PhD thesis*, University of Edinburgh.

Moore-Colyer, M.J.S. and Longland, A.C. (2000) Intakes and *in vivo* apparent digestibilities of four types of conserved grass forage by ponies. *Animal Science*, **71**, 527-534.

Moore-Colyer, M.J.S. and Longland, A.C. (2001) The effect of plain sugar beet pulp on the *in vitro* gas production and *in vivo* apparent digestibility of hay when offered to ponies. *Proceedings of the 17th Equine Nutrition and Physiology Symposium*, Kentucky, USA. p. 145-147.

Moore-Colyer, M.J.S., Longland, A.C., Hyslop, J.J. and Cuddeford, D. (1998) The degradation of protein and non-starch polysaccharides (NSP) from botanically diverse sources of dietary fibre by ponies as measured by the mobile bag technique. In: "*In vitro Techniques for Measuring Nutrient Supply to Ruminants*. Occasional Publication No. 22, BSAS, Penicuik, Edinburgh.

Morrow, H.J., Moore-Colyer, M.J.S. and Longland, A.C. (1999) The apparent digestibilities and rates of passage of two chop lengths of big bale silage and hay in ponies. *Proceedings of the British Society of Animal Science*, BSAS, P.O. Box 3, Penicuik, Midlothian, EH26 0RZ, UK. p.142.

Newman, K.E. and Spring, P. (1994) A comparison of two different strains of yeast in their ability to alter ruminal and cecal fermentations. *Proceedings of the 10th Annual Symposium on Biotechnology in the Feed Industry*, Lexington, Kentucky. Poster presentation.

Nolan, M.M., Potter, G.D., Mathiason, K.J., Gibbs, P.G., Morris, E.L., Greene, L.W. and Topliff, D. (2001) Bone density in the juvenile racehorse fed differing levels of minerals. *Proceedings of the 17th Equine Nutrition and Physiology Symposium*, Kentucky, USA. p.33-38.

NRC (1989) *Nutrient requirements of horses*, 5th edition. National Academy Press, Washington, D.C.

Nunamaker, D.M. (1986) The bucked shin complex. *Proceedings of the American Association of Equine Practitioners*, p.457-460.

Olsson, N.A. and Ruudvere, A. (1955) The nutrition of the horse. *Nutrition Abstracts and Reviews*, **25**, 1-18.

Orsini, J. (2000) Gastric ulceration in the mature horse: a review. *Equine Veterinary Education*, **12**, 24-27.

Orton, R.K., Hume, I.D. and Leng, R.A. (1985a) Effects of level of dietary protein and exercise on growth rates of horses. *Equine Veterinary Journal*, **17**, 381-385.

Orton, R.K., Hume, I.D. and Leng, R.A. (1985b) Effects of exercise and level of dietary protein on digestive function in horses. *Equine Veterinary Journal*, **17**, 386-390.

Ott, E.A., Asquith, R.L., Feaster, J.P. and Martin, F.G. (1979) Influence of protein level and quality on the growth and development of yearling foals. *Journal of Animal Science*, **49**, 620-628.

Pagan, J.D. (1999). Time of feeding critical for performance. In: *Advances in equine nutrition*. Proceedings of the 1999 Equine Nutrition Conference for Feed Manufacturers, Kentucky Equine Research, Versailles, Kentucky. p 117-125.

Pagan, J.D., Burger, I. and Jackson, S.G. (1996). The influence of time of feeding on exercise response in Thoroughbreds fed a fat supplemented or high carbohydrate diet. *World Equine Veterinary Review*, **1**: 43-44.

Pagan, J.D., Harris, P.A., Kennedy, M.A.P., Davidson, N. and Hoekstra, K.E. (1999). Feed type and intake affect glycaemic response in Thoroughbred horses. *Proceedings for the 1999 Equine Nutrition Conference for Feed Manufacturers*, KER, Lexington, Kentucky.p.147-150.

Pagan, J.D., Rotmensen, T. and Jackson, S.G. (1995). The effect of chromium supplementation on metabolic response to exercise in Thoroughbred horses. *Proceedings of the 14th Equine Nutrition and Physiology Symposium*, Ontario, Canada.p.96-101.

Palmgren Karlsson, C., Lindberg, J.E. and Rundberg, M. (2000) Associative effects on total tract digestibility in horses fed different ratios of grass hay and whole oats. *Livestock Production Science*, **65**, 143-153.

Pearce, S.G., Grace, N.D., Witchel, J.J., Firth, E.C. and Fennessy, P.F. (1998) Effect of copper supplementation on copper status of pregnant mares and foals. *Equine Veterinary Journal*, **30**, 200-203.

Pearson, R.A., Archibald, R.F. and Muirhead, R.H. (2001) The effect of forage quality and level of feeding on digestibility and gastrointestinal transit time of oat straw and alfalfa given to ponies and donkeys. *British Journal of Nutrition*, **85**, 599-606.

Pearson, R.A. and Lawrence, P.R. (1992) Intake, digestion, gastro-intestinal transit time and nitrogen balance in working oxen: studies in Costa Rica and Nepal. *Animal Production*, **55**, 361-370.

Pearson, R.A. and Merritt, J.B. (1991) Intake, digestion and gastrointestinal transit time in resting donkeys and ponies and exercised donkeys given *ad libitum* hay and straw. *Equine Veterinary Journal*, **23**, 339-343.

Peers, D.G., Taylor, A.G. and Whittemore, C.T. (1977) The influence of feeding level and level of dietary inclusion on the digestibility of barley meal in the pig. *Animal Feed Science and Technology*, **2**, 41-47.

Porr, C.A.S., Kronfeld, D.S., Lawrence, L.A., Pleasant, R.S. and Harris, P. (2000) Diet and conditioning influence bone development. *Equine Practice*, **22**, 18-21.

Porr, C.A.S., Ott, E.A., Johnson, E.L. and Madison, J.B. (1997) Bone mineral in young thoroughbred horses is affected by training. *Equine Practice*, **19**, 28-31.

Potter, G.D., Arnold, F.F., Householder, D.D., Hansen, D.H. and Brown, K.M. (1992) Digestion of starch in the small or large intestine of the equine. *Pferdeheilkunde*, p.107-111.

Potter, G.D., Gibbs, P.G., Haley, R.G. and Klenshoj, C. (1992) Digestion of protein in the small and large intestine of equines fed mixed diets. *Pferdeheilkunde*, p.140-143.

Ralston, S.L. (1984) Controls of feeding in horses. *Journal of Animal Science*, **59**, 1354-1361.

Ralston, S.L. (1992) Regulation of feed intake in the horse in relation to gastrointestinal disease. *Pferdeheilkunde*, p.15-18.

Ralston, S.L. and Baile, C.A. (1982a) Plasma glucose and insulin concentrations and feeding behaviour in ponies. *Journal of Animal Science*, **54**, 1132-1137.

Ralston, S.L. and Baile, C.A. (1982b) Gastrointestinal stimuli in the control of feed intake in ponies. *Journal of Animal Science*, **55**, 243-253.

Ralston, S.L. and Baile, C.A. (1983) Effects of intragastric xylose, sodium chloride and corn oil on feeding behaviour of ponies. *Journal of Animal Science*, **56**, 302-308.

Ralston, S.L., Foster, D.L., Divers, T. and Hintz, H.F. (2001) Effect of dental correction on feed digestibility in horses. *Equine Veterinary Journal*, **33**, 390-393.

Ralston, S.L., Freeman, D.E. and Baile, C.A. (1983) Volatile fatty acids and the role of the large intestine in the control of feed intake in ponies. *Journal of Animal Science*, **57**, 815-820.

Reitnour, C.M. and Salsbury, R.L. (1976) Utilisation of proteins by the equine species. *American Journal of Veterinary Research*, 37, 1065-1067.

Ricketts, S.W., Greet, T.R.C., Glyn, P.J., Ginnet, C.D.R., McAllister, E.P., McCaig, J., Skinner, P.H., Webbon, P.M., Frape, D.L., Smith, G.R. and Murray, L.G. (1984) Thirteen cases of botulism in horses fed big bale silage. *Equine Veterinary Journal*, **16**, 515-518.

Roberts, M.C. (1974) Amylase activity in the small intestine of the horse. *Research in Veterinary Science*, **17**, 400-401.

Slade, L.M., Bishop, R., Morris, J.G. and Robinson, D.W. (1971) Digestion and absorption of $N^{15}$-labelled microbial protein in the large intestine of the horse. *British Veterinary Journal*, **127**, 11-13.

Smith, J.D., Jordan, R.M. and Nelson, M.L. (1975) Tolerance of ponies to high levels of dietary copper. *Journal of Animal Science*, **41**, 1645-1649.

Smyth, G.B. (1988) Effects of age, sex, and post mortem interval on intestinal lengths of horses during development. *Equine Veterinary Journal*, **20**, 104-108.

Sperber, I., Bjornhag, G. and Holtenius, K. (1992) A separation mechanism and fluid flow in the large intestine of the horse. *Pferdeheilkunde*. p.29-32.

Strickland, K., Smith, F., Woods, M. and Mason, J. (1987) Dietary molybdenum as a putative copper antagonist in the horse. *Equine Veterinary Journal*, **19**, 50-54.

Suttle, N.F., Small, J.N.W., Collins, E.A., Mason, D.K. and Watkins, K.L. (1996) Serum and hepatic copper concentrations used to define normal, marginal and deficient copper status in horses. *Equine Veterinary Journal*, **28**, 497-499.

Todd, L., Sauer, W.C., Christopherson, R.J., Coleman, R.J. and Caine, W.R. (1995) The effect of feeding different forms of alfalfa on nutrient digestibility and voluntary intake in mature horses. *Journal of Animal Physiology and Animal Nutrition*, **73**, 1-8.

Tsaras, L.N., Kyriazakis, I. and Emmans, G.C. (1998) The prediction of the voluntary food intake of pigs on poor quality foods. *Animal Science*, **66**, 713-723.

Vecchiotti, G.G. and Gainati, R. (1986). Evidence of heredity of cribbing, weaving and stall-walking in Thoroughbred horses. *Livestock Production Science*, **14,** 91-95.

Wall, D.L., Topliff, D.R., Freeman, D.W., Breazile, J.E., Wagner, D.G. and Stutz, W.A. (1993) The effect of dietary cation-anion balance on mineral balance in the anaerobically exercised horse. *Proceedings of the 13th Equine Nutrition and Physiology Symposium*, Gainesville, USA.p.50-55.

Wolter, R., Durix, A. and Letourneau, J.C. (1974) Influence du mode de présentation du fourrage sur la vitesse du transit digéstif chez le poney. *Annales de Zootechnologie*, **23**, 293-300.

Worth, M.J., Fontenot, J.P. and Meacham, T.N. (1987) Physiological effects of exercise and diet on metabolism in the equine. *Proceedings of the 10th Equine Nutrition and Physiology Symposium*, Colorado State University, Fort Collins, p. 145-151.

Wysocki, A.A. and Baker, J.P. (1975) Utilisation of bacterial protein from the lower gut of the horse. *Proceedings of the 4th Equine Nutrition and Physiology Symposium*, Davis, California. p. 21-43.

*This paper was first published in 2002*

18

# COMPANION ANIMAL NUTRITION

EDWARD ROWE
*Head of Nutrition, Nestlé Purina R&D Centre, Amiens, 80800 Aubigny, France*

## Introduction

Earle (2001) summarised the directions being taken by recent advances in companion animal (pet) nutrition. These advances are focused on several topics designed to extend the duration of optimal health of pets and take advantage of the developing knowledge of functional nutrition. Additionally, researchers are addressing some specific peculiarities of pet health and metabolism, and pet feeding practices.

The following are currently active areas of research in pet nutrition:

- Intestinal health
- Immunity, Natural defences and Ageing
- Skin and coat health
- Urinary tract health
- Oral health
- Energy metabolism

The most important factor specific to the pet is the often-total dependence on foods provided by the owner, which may extend to all feeding occasions, throughout the entire life of the animal. Food manufacturers meet this challenge by providing nutritionally complete diets, designed to be fed exclusively and on a continuous basis. It is important to make the distinction between nutritional objectives of pet food manufacturers and the manufacturers of food for production animals. The former aim to maximise the duration of the pet's healthy condition and to optimise health and quality of life. Maximised weight gain, production efficiencies of animals and food conversion ratios are not objectives. Therefore, nutrition of companion animals has more affinity with human than with production animal nutrition. The structure and the relatively short residence time of food in the pet's non-ruminant digestive system places a greater onus on the food, with little assistance from fermentation processes, to supply the majority of the energy and nutrient requirements. However, as discussed in this chapter, even in a non-ruminant digestive system, there is increasing recognition of the importance of gut bacteria for healthy digestion.

Official, globally recognised nutrient recommendations have existed for almost 30 years. Early data normally expressed nutrient levels as units required per kg body weight (NRC, 1974). This, and subsequent publications of the NRC, were based on the collation of studies using predominantly purified diets demonstrating the levels of nutrients required to prevent symptoms of nutrient deficiency. While NRC (1985) for dogs contained updated information on nutrient requirements, it made no allowance for the digestibility of typical petfood ingredients. Consequently, AAFCO (Association of American Feed Control Officials, 1992) published dietary recommendations, updating the NRC levels in light of current knowledge and nutrient bioavailability from practical food ingredients. More recently, FEDIAF (2000) have published feeding recommendations and nutrient tables for Europe based on the AAFCO tables.

Formulation of diets for companion animals involves combining meats and meat off-cuts, or cereals and vegetables, together with fats and oils, to provide the correct balance of all the essential nutrients. Supplementary vitamins and minerals are added to meet the requirements for these nutrients and to cover losses associated with processing or extended storage. Processing ensures adequate cooking of the raw materials, giving improved digestibility and preservation for long-term storage. By adjusting the levels of the essential nutrients to the energy value of the food, rather than by simple concentration, it is possible to ensure that, for whatever type of food is used, the animal will obtain the correct level of every nutrient, provided it consumes its daily energy requirement. Therefore, the official tables of nutrient requirements express the data in terms of concentration in the dry matter of the product, or the conceptually easier, 'grams (or milligrams, or I.U) of nutrient required in 1000 kcals (4.184 MJ) of metabolisable energy '.

It has often been stated that pets will not benefit from diets if they do not consume their daily individual energy requirement. Accordingly, companies conduct significant research into diet palatability, which is affected by variations in taste and flavour, which make up the product range, and also by various textures.

Product textures define the categories of commercial petfoods: wet, semi-moist, and dry. These categories differ in moisture content, ranging from 820 to 80 g/kg, and an inverse relationship exists between dietary energy value and product moisture content. By linking the concentration of the essential nutrients in the food to energy concentration, whatever combination of varieties or textures the animal is fed, it will obtain all the essential nutrients at the correct level. Of course it is not possible to account fully for the tendency of most owners to give human food left-overs, which are usually nutritionally imbalanced for the cat or dog. Accordingly, complete diets are normally formulated to provide more than the minimum nutrient requirements, especially for the trace minerals and vitamins, which are required in minute quantities on a continuous basis. Some non-complete categories of petfoods fed primarily for pet enjoyment, such as some brands of biscuits and treats, are fortified with vitamins and minerals to keep the total diet in nutrient balance. However, feeding recommendations typically restrict the use of these products to 10-25% of the pet's daily energy requirement.

The purpose of this chapter is to review recent research findings that have had an impact on the nutritional profile of commercial cat and dog food.

Nutrient recommendations have been modified with the advance of knowledge to enhance the health and vitality of pets beyond basic protection from nutrient deficiency. This has occurred over the past 40 years at the level of species, breed, lifestage and, lastly, lifestyle. Genetic research holds the promise of future individual definition of nutritional needs for prevention of disease (Earle, 2001). Petfood developments for the dietary management of disease, which are prescribed and monitored by veterinarians, are outside of the scope of this review.

## Comparative canine and feline nutrition

Cats and dogs differ in the classification of their dietary habits: dogs are true omnivores and can survive on a predominantly vegetarian diet; cats are true (obligate) carnivores and their diet must contain a number of nutrients that can only be found in meat. This feline carnivorous habit is accompanied by several nutritional peculiarities of the cat caused by increases or decreases in the activities of specific metabolic enzymes (Czarnecki-Maulden, 1986).

### PROTEIN

Cats preferentially metabolise protein for energy, exhibiting a high rate of gluconeogenesis in the liver, irrespective of the level of dietary protein (Rogers *et al.*, 1977). Dogs, by contrast, adapt protein metabolism to conserve protein during dietary protein deficit. Cats must also, of course, be supplied with sufficient protein for maintenance of body structure and for enzyme and humoral functions. Therefore, on an energy-equivalent basis, cats require more protein than dogs: the adult cat requires 26% more protein than the adult dog; the kitten requires 19% more protein than the puppy (AAFCO, 2001). Thus, for an adult cat, a diet containing 260 g protein/kg on a dry matter basis is required. However, recent studies, while confirming that this level was more than adequate for protection of body protein stores, showed that 300 g protein/kg is required to maintain lean muscle mass, and therefore to maintain optimal body condition (Hannah and Laflamme, 1996). Even more recently, Yu *et al.* (2001) investigated an occasionally observed phenomenon that black cats develop a brown-red coat coloration. This is actually caused by low production of coat pigment (melanin) because of inadequate levels of the precursor amino acids (tyrosine & phenylalanine). The minimum AAFCO requirement for Phe + Tyr to support health and growth of kittens is 8.5 g/kg. However, black cats consuming a diet containing 17 g/kg of Phe + Tyr developed the red coat, while those eating 24 g/kg maintained black coats.

The specific requirement of the cat for the free sulphonated amino acid taurine has been well documented (Hayes *et al.*, 1975; Burger and Barnett, 1982). The NRC (1986) recommendation for a dietary level of 0.4 g taurine/kg to protect retinal integrity, was modified following studies showing that higher levels are required to protect cats from cardiac myopathy (Pion *et al.*, 1989) and kitten growth abnormalities (Sturman *et al.*, 1986). Accordingly, the taurine requirement was increased to 1 g/kg dry foods and 2.5 g/kg in canned foods (Earle and Smith, 1991). Differences in gut microflora patterns between cats fed dry and canned foods probably explain the greater requirement in wet foods (Fay *et al.*, 1998). Cats also require greater amounts of other sulphur amino acids (methionine and cystine) than dogs (NRC, 1986). There are several possible explanations for this, including some synthesis, albeit weak in the cat, of taurine from methionine; the production of the urinary pheromone felinine from sulphur amino acids; or keratin production for the cat's thick coat. The other essential amino acids of cats and dogs are arginine, histidine, isoleucine, leucine, lysine, threonine, tryptophan and valine (NRC, 1986).

Proteins are well digested by cats and dogs, depending on the source and quality, and typically more than 80% of dietary protein is absorbed. Undigested protein can be fermented in the colon by bacteria to toxic nitrogenous compounds, which may be absorbed, and may also cause diarrhoea (Macfarlane and Cummings, 1991).

## FATS AND FATTY ACIDS

It has long been recognised that the cat has a requirement for animal-based fats to supply the derived polyunsaturated arachidonic acid (Hassam *et al.*, 1977). The dog has retained the ability to desaturate linoleic acid from plant oils to the derived homologues. In spite of its deficiencies in desaturase enzymes, the cat has a requirement for linoleic acid, which functions in the maintenance of epidermal integrity (Sinclair *et al.*, 1979). While it is well established that the cat and dog have nutritional requirements for these omega-6 polyunsaturated fatty acids (linoleic acid for the dog, linoleic acid and arachidonic acid for the cat), it is still unclear to what extent they have a requirement for the omega-3 polyunsaturated fatty acids (AAFCO, 2001). These EFAs, originating from marine oils, form separate series of prostaglandins from the omega-6 EFAs and are metabolically only weakly inflammatory, while arachidonic acid is metabolised to strongly pro-inflammatory eicosanoids (Codner and Thatcher, 1993). Furthermore, there is competition between the omega-6 and the omega-3 series for enzymes in the production of derived EFAs.

Studies of blood cells *in vitro* have suggested a ratio of omega-6 to omega-3 of between 5:1 and 10:1 for optimal inflammatory response (Boudreaux *et al.*, 1997). Improved coat quality in dogs was claimed for a diet with these ratios of omega-6 to omega-3 fatty acids, when compared with diet that had a higher ratio (Davenport, 2000). It should be noted that several other nutrient differences existed between the foods in this study. The diet resulting in poor coat quality was formulated close to the AAFCO minimum, while the diet resulting in improved coat quality contained excesses of several nutrients implicated in skin and coat integrity. It should also be noted that studies of skin and coat condition are difficult to interpret, with local conditions, including animal individuality, and seasonal changes affecting both physical and sensory evaluations. Furthermore, a separate study of higher quality foods differing in omega-6 to 3 ratios failed to demonstrate effects on coat quality. Therefore, it is not yet clear whether cats or dogs have specific requirements for omega-3 fatty acids, or whether there is an optimal ratio between omega-6 and omega-3 (Cambell *et al.*, 2000). Large amounts of linoleic acid, together with high levels of zinc and/or B vitamins apparently lead to improvements in coat condition, again by comparison with products formulated to AAFCO minimum nutrient levels (Marsh *et al.*, 2000). It is therefore to be expected that, whilst not showing gross deficiency effects, the coat condition of cats and dogs fed an AAFCO-minimum diet can be improved by a diet with higher levels of essential nutrients.

Fats are normally extremely well digested in cats and dogs unless rancid, typically with over 90 % absorbed. Poor fat absorption leads to steatorrhoea.

## CARBOHYDRATES

Carbohydrates are not essential dietary components for cats and dogs, but cooked cereal starches are digested and provide major contributions as energy sources in dry products. Dogs can cope with up to 70 per cent of the energy of a diet as carbohydrate, whereas the cat is limited to 45 per cent. Cats also have low levels of pancreatic amylase (only 5% of that of the dog), that do not adapt to changes in dietary carbohydrate level (Kienzle, 1993a). In the cat, sugar-digesting intestinal disaccharidases have only 40% of the activity of those in the dog (Kienzle, 1993b) and also do not adapt to dietary change. The cat has a limited ability to metabolise glucose arriving at the liver from the portal vein; the lack of active glucokinase in the cat liver prevents the cat from responding to increases in dietary levels of carbohydrate (Ballard, 1965). These enzyme limitations in the cat dictate that, although many cats thrive on a mixed feeding regime of wet and dry foods, they are less tolerant than dogs of large changes in dietary carbohydrate levels.

Cooked starches are well digested by cats and dogs, typically in excess of 80% digestibility, but subject to the limitations of starch content described above. Undigested starch can lead to osmotic diarrhoea.

## FIBRE

There are no official recommendations for fibre level in cat and dog foods, but both insoluble and soluble fibres are beneficial for digestive health. Insoluble fibre (e.g. cellulose) provides bulk to faeces and aids passage of the bolus through the digestive system. Unlike humans, dogs are not considered to suffer from diverticulosis, but this may partly be attributable to the indigestible fibre levels in typical dog foods (25 g/kg). Soluble fibre is also beneficial by attracting water, thus improving faecal consistency when watery faeces are caused by other factors.

The most interesting properties of fibre concern their fermentability by gut bacteria. The non-digestible oligosaccharide, inulin, contains nutritive fractions for beneficial colonic bacteria (*Bifidobacteria, Lactobacillus*). Inulin is a fructo-oligosaccharide (FOS), consisting of one fructose and three glucose sub-units connected by beta links. The beta link is indigestible by mammals, hence inulin reaches the colon intact. *Bifidobacteria* metabolise inulin, releasing short-chain fatty acids which nourish gut endothelial cells, reduce colonic pH, inhibit the proliferation of potentially pathogenic gut bacteria (*Clostridia*), and provide an improved medium for mineral absorption (Czarnecki-Maulden and Russell, 2000a and b). Stimulation of *Bifidobacteria* may have two further benefits: *Bifidobacteria* are known to produce B vitamins and may also improve the pet's resistance to disease (Earle, 2001). Both cats and dogs benefit from inulin prebiotics (Patil, Carrion and Holmes, 2001).

## VITAMINS

There are two documented peculiarities of vitamin metabolism in the cat. Dogs can synthesise niacin from tryptophan to supplement dietary sources. An alternative metabolic pathway of tryptophan metabolism in the cat is highly active and necessitates that sufficient niacin is added to the diet to meet requirements (Ikeda *et al.*, 1965). Dogs can synthesise vitamin A from beta-carotene present in plant materials at the intestinal wall. The cat has very low activity of this enzyme and must be provided with pre-formed vitamin A in the diet (Gershoff *et al.*, 1957). Accordingly, the cat has higher requirements for vitamin A and niacin than the dog. Caution must be exercised for both cat foods and dog foods in the levels of the fat soluble vitamins, especially Vitamin A (Cline *et al.*, 1995) and Vitamin D which, if consumed in excessive amounts, become toxic. Vitamin C is not recognised as an essential nutrient for cats and dogs as sufficient quantities are synthesised from glucose.

Recently high doses of antioxidant vitamins, many times in excess of the minimum requirement (Vitamin E) plus Vitamin C, and other anti-oxidants have been shown to stimulate some aspects of the natural defences of cats and dogs. For example, an improved antibody response to vaccination was observed when high levels of antioxidant nutrients were fed (Chew *et al.*, 2000; Devlin *et al.*, 2000). Additionally, *in vitro* models suggest greater protection of DNA with antioxidant nutrient feeding (Heaton, 2001). The proposed mechanism for these effects is by absorption of free radicals generated by oxidative metabolism and stress. These results have been extrapolated to possible long-term benefits, including an enhanced immune system, increased protection from cancer and greater longevity. Proof of such long-term benefits remains to be substantiated. It is also possible that these results, showing a positive influence of vitamin E on immune function, simply reflect a higher requirement for Vitamin E for optimal immune function, relative to the level required to prevent deficiency signs.

It should be noted that manufacturers have to exercise caution when undertaking super-supplementation of vitamins and minerals: minerals can interact competitively, causing deficiencies; and fat soluble vitamins in excess can be toxic (NRC, 1986).

## MINERALS

Chemical form and balance are the keys to the correct uptake of minerals. Increases over earlier recommendations (NRC, 1974; 1985; 1986) have been made in light of new evidence for iron (Chausow and Czarnecki-Maulden, 1987), copper (Czarnecki-Maulden *et al.*, 1993), and zinc (Sanecki *et al.*, 1982). These studies highlight an evolving knowledge of the nutrient requirements of dogs and cats. The fundamental studies have rarely been designed to compare directly, or even determine precise minimum requirements of cats and dogs. Therefore, while the AAFCO recommended levels of many minerals differ between cats and dogs, it is not always correct to conclude proven differences in requirements between the species.

Incorrect mineral balance leads to problems with bioavailability and apparent deficits in both species. The dietary balance of cationic and anionic minerals is especially important in the cat, as the excretion of excess ions to maintain acid-base homeostasis changes the pH of urine and can allow crystallisation of urinary complexes, leading to potentially fatal blockage of the urinary tract (Osborne, 1982). This condition, called FLUTD (Feline lower urinary tract disease), was formerly characterised by struvite (magnesium ammonium phosphate) crystallising at a urinary pH more alkaline than pH 6.4. Pet food manufacturers controlled the mineral balance of dry pet foods to ensure slightly acid urine to help prevent crystal formation. However, in more recent years, while the incidence of struvite in referred clinical cases has declined, there has been an increase in crystallisation of calcium oxalate crystals, which precipitate at acid pH (below 6.0) (Buffington, 1993). Current best practice is to ensure that the mineral balance of dry products produces cat urine between pH 6.0 and 6.4. More recently, researchers have tried to apply human models of urinary super-saturation. Attempts are made to measure the physico-chemical activities of all relevant solutes and their interactions, to predict the tendency for cat urine to precipitate struvite or oxalate crystals (Smith *et al.*, 1997). It is not yet clear whether this technique can be successfully applied to cat urine.

## ENERGY

Cats have a somewhat lower energy requirement than dogs of the same body weight, and there has been a tendency over time to reduce the recommended daily energy needs for both species in light of new developments.

The energy equation for adult cats (NRC, 1986):

$$\text{Maintenance energy requirement (kcals per day)} = 70 \times \text{Body weight (kg)}$$
$$(100 \text{ kcals} = 0.4184 \text{ MJ})$$

has been modified by most manufacturers in light of the high digestibility of cat foods today, and energy balance studies *in vivo*. These studies support the following energy equation:

$$\text{Maintenance energy requirement (kcals per day)} = 57 \times \text{Body weight (kg)}$$
$$(100 \text{ kcals} = 0.4184 \text{ MJ})$$

which has now been adopted in the FEDIAF recommendations (FEDIAF, 2000).

A similar pattern of events has followed the changes in dog feeding recommendations. Maintenance energy requirements (kcals) were set by NRC

(1985) and followed by AAFCO at 132 x Body weight$^{0.75}$, this value was determined by energy balance studies of dogs *in vivo*. Studies of the feeding requirements for weight maintenance of domestic dogs in homes, which are typically more sedentary than colony dogs, produces feeding equation factors of approximately 110 (Patil and Bisby, 2001; Wichert *et al.*, 2000). Several companies have now adopted this factor in the calculation of feeding rations, with FEDIAF also proposing similar factors with adjustments for level of activity. It is notable that in both colony and domestic studies of pets, there is considerable individual variation in energy requirements. This is partly attributable to individual variations in exercise, coat length, exposure to external climate, plus differences in metabolic efficiency and digestibility. For this reason, feeding recommendations should always include advice to adjust diets in order to keep the animal in optimal lean condition.

Energy requirements also vary with age and physiological function. Gestating females need increasing intakes of energy from mid-term to parturition when they are fed 60 per cent more food than at mating. Lactating females require up to four times their maintenance energy requirement, while pets at maximal growth rate require up to twice their adult requirement on a unit bodyweight basis. Senior cat foods require at least the same energy level as adult cat foods, not less, as has been previously supposed, as geriatric cats suffer from reduced digestibility. Senior dog foods require slightly less energy than adult dog foods (by 10%) because of a reduction in activity of senior dogs.

## Diet related health issues in pets

Pet foods can have benefits beyond the immediate supply of energy and essential nutrients. Pet foods can, by enhancing natural protective mechanisms, help to prevent or delay the onset of various ailments resulting from external stresses and pathogens, and can help to overcome individual metabolic deficits.

### INTESTINAL HEALTH

Some large breeds of dog tend to produce softer faeces with a higher water content than small breeds (Meyer *et al.*, 1999), possibly because large breeds have a relatively smaller digestive system than small breeds and may have a lower digestive capacity. Some table scraps fed to dogs may be of poor digestibility. Certain individuals among the 'sensitive' breeds may also have clinical or sub-clinical deficiencies in digestive function. Exocrine pancreatic insufficiency occurs in some German Shepherd Dogs and also Rough–Coated Collies (Westermarck, 1980). One effect of the arrival of poorly digested components, particularly protein, in the colon is the stimulation of growth of Clostridia, with consequent diarrhoea and production of enterotoxins.

Dogs are also prone to 'morbid habits', including copraphagy of canine and other species' faecal material, delivering a large microbial load to the large intestine.

## ALLERGY, IMMUNITY AND INFLAMMATION

Selective immune (IgA) deficiency has been reported in individual Beagles, Shar Pei, Irish Wolfhound, Cocker Spaniels and may be implicated in German Shepherds with small-intestinal bacterial overgrowth (German *et al.*, 2000).

Inflammatory joint disease (arthritis) affects many ageing dogs, with immobilising effects. Supplementation of pet foods using collagen precursors (glucosamine and chondroitin sulphate) and anti-inflammatory substances proposed for joint problems (fish oils and green-lipped mussel extract) follow trends in health food shops for people (Bui *et al.*, 2001).

Environmental allergens affect up to 10% of the pet population; air borne and flea allergies being the most prevalent. True food allergies account for only 10% of the total and generally manifest as deterioration in coat condition and stool consistency. Truly food-allergic animals require specialised diets.

Modulation of both the pet's inflammatory response and enhancement of the pet's immune response are both future goals of pet nutrition research.

## URINARY TRACT HEALTH

FLUTD affects about 1% of cats (Lawlor *et al.*, 1985). Wet foods are not generally implicated because of their high water content, which promotes urination. There are several non-dietary risk factors leading to blockage of the urinary tract, including mucus production in urinary infections, obesity, stress and litter tray usage (perhaps increasing urine residence time in the bladder). Correct mineral balance of dry foods minimises the precipitation of mineral crystals and modulates urine pH.

Renal disease is a common cause of fatality in pets and most senior pets will have some degree of reduction in renal capacity, even though it may be asymptomatic. High phosphorus levels are cytotoxic to the kidneys and senior diets normally have lower phosphorus levels than adult foods. Protein level, once believed also to require reduction in senior products, is now maintained at adult levels as reduced protein digestibility and loss of lean mass is a consequence of ageing. Protein is not now implicated as a cause of renal insufficiency in healthy animals. Animals diagnosed with kidney disease are typically fed a therapeutic diet with restricted phosphorus and high quality protein

## ORAL HEALTH

Inadequate teeth cleaning of pets by their owners makes oral hygiene an important cause of ill health in pets, with over 80 per cent of adult cats having some form of periodontal disease (Watson, 1997). While pets do not suffer from dental caries, plaque deposition produced by oral streptococcal bacteria leads to gum inflammation, with bacterial ingress and eventual tooth loss. Tartar formation by the calcification of plaque and the production of odorous sulphides are perceived by owners. Dry foods provide an abrasive action on the tooth surface and can reduce the degree of deposition of plaque and tartar compared with softer foods.

## ENERGY AND WEIGHT CONTROL

Obesity is relatively common in pets, affecting between 25 and 40% of dogs and cats. Obesity has deleterious effects on mobility and grooming and increased incidence of painful joint problems, diabetes, potentially fatal ‘fatty liver’ in cats, pancreatic disease and urinary tract disease are all potential consequences of obesity. Various cancers may also be associated with obesity, although high blood pressure, which is a major consequence of obesity in humans, is not common in pets. Mobility is decreased in obese cats and they tend to have poorer coats. Mortality is increased in obese middle-age pets.

For dogs, the underlying cause of obesity is a combination of frequently available foods together with a relatively sedentary lifestyle. The dog has evolved to expend considerable energy in finding food and from a scavenging habit to eat whenever it comes upon food. Cats have traditionally been excellent weight managers, able to control energy intake by hunting when needing to satisfy an energy deficit. Two factors have increased the incidence of obesity in cats: the domestic life of the cat is now more sedentary (leading to boredom and overeating) and the common practice of neutering, which reduces the energy needs of cats.

Using the developing knowledge of the physiology of obesity, various compounds that may be involved metabolically in weight control are being tested in weight-reduction diets. These include supplementation of L-carnitine (Sunvold *et al.*, 1999), which is involved in cellular oxidation of fatty acids, and slow-release starch sources (e.g. barley) to minimise post-prandial increases in blood sugars (Bouchard and Sunvold, 2000).

Obesity results when energy intake exceeds energy expenditure. This is exacerbated by a diet with components varying in energy concentration, especially when the mixed diet contains high-energy components that are also very palatable – a combination that can over-ride normal satiety mechanisms (Rolls, Rowe, and Turner, 1980). Over and above this effect of over consumption of energy, the ratio of the energy sources in the food is also important in influencing obesity. A diet which has a high concentration of energy, but also has a high fat concentration, will both increase the risk of over consumption through enhanced palatability (fat is palatable to pets) and owner-overfeeding. Fat is also the most digestible of energy sources and is the most efficiently metabolised. In circumstances of energy surplus, poultry data show that lipid synthesis from dietary fat is 90% efficient, while lipid synthesis from dietary starch is 74% efficient and lipid synthesis from protein is only 53% efficient (Verstegen, 2000).

Over 30 years ago, Romsos *et al.* (1978) showed that dogs fed high-fat diets laid down more body fat than dogs fed high carbohydrate diets. This could not be explained in terms of a small difference in energy intake between the foods. More recently, increased fat deposition was caused in kittens on a diet richer in fat, even though energy intakes and weight gains were similar (Patil: Personal communication). It remains to be determined whether such kittens grow up to become obese cats.

## Trends in nutrition of pets

Both dog food and cat food purchases have shown an increase in complete dry pet foods over the past decade. As noted earlier, providing the pet is fed to its individual energy requirements it will gain sufficient nourishment and all its essential nutrients whatever combination of wet and dry foods are used.

In recent years a new product sector has opened up, the super-premium dry sector. These products are formulated from more expensive and more digestible ingredients. They serve a need for animals with increased energy requirements, either through inefficiencies of digestion or metabolism, or through excessive energy expenditure. Such products normally have an increased fat content, which helps to provide the high digestibility and palatability of these products. At the extreme, certain super premium products exist with over 200 g fat/kg, and with over 46% of the dietary energy coming from fat. While suitable for endurance and hard-working animals, this fat level is excessive for the typical household pet and, linked with the high acceptance and digestibility of these products, increases the risk that pets will become obese. Such high fat products may also lose the dental efficacy of dry foods, with a loss of 'crunch'. Frequently, such kibbles are swallowed whole without any chewing.

In order to address the problem of oral hygiene, complete pet foods of unique texture and increased kibble size have been developed which further enhance the cleaning efficacy of dry foods by allowing the tooth to penetrate before the kibble shatters. This has an extra abrasive effect on the tooth surface and can reduce plaque and tartar accretion over only a few weeks, by over 20% compared to standard kibbles. Up to 50% tartar reduction is achieved over 6 months. Such large kibbles also develop a more controlled feeding style in the pet, with each separate kibble properly chewed and with easier digestion than with kibbles swallowed whole (Cupp, 1999)

Biscuits of the correct texture also help clean the teeth, and reduce the accretion of plaque and tartar of dogs eating only wet foods.

Protection and enhancement of digestion have been achieved in dogs and cats by the use of prebiotics. Chicory is an excellent source of inulin, and causes increases in Bifidobacteria while reducing levels of Clostridia. Chicory is used across the range of pet foods, wet and dry, standard and super-premium, and across the life stage products. It is also available in biscuit form to ensure an undiluted level and the intended efficacy, regardless of the variety or texture of product used.

## Optimal nutritional profiles and lifestage

Energy and nutrient needs can be met with a combination of the product nutrient concentration and adjustment of the quantity fed. In view of the high incidence of obesity among pets, a primary objective is to maintain or grow lean, lively and healthy animals, while adapting products to situations that require greater energy levels or nutrient concentration.

Wet foods provide all the essential nutrients of pets, which will thrive on canned foods as the sole source of nourishment for their whole lives. Although such products have a high proportion of energy as fat (all-meat products have almost no carbohydrate), they are of relatively low energy concentration and may be less implicated as risk factors in obesity than dry foods (Donoghue and Scarlett, 1998). Wet kitten and puppy foods are of slightly lower moisture content and higher energy concentration than adult foods to minimise the volume of foods required to meet the energy needs for growth. Increased levels of vitamins and minerals are also formulated in products designed for growing animals.

High fat foods are, however, implicated as a risk factor in obesity (Donoghue and Scarlett, 1998). To achieve a balance of macro-nutrients to maintain lean body condition, fat levels for cats can be between 100 and 160 g/kg. Diets designed to help owners control the weight of their pets ("light diets") benefit from an increase in protein content, and a fat content of 80 g/kg, which will still meet the AAFCO requirements for fats and fatty acids. If used for a weight reduction programme, light diets should have an increase in vitamins and minerals to maintain micro-nutrient supply with reduced intakes. In any case intake reduction should be limited to 15 per cent in dieting obese cats to avoid the risk of development of hepatic lipidosis. Senior diets should also have increased levels of vitamins and minerals, but reduced phosphorus compared with adult foods.

For dog foods, products are now orientated to breed size and lifestyle. The 'average' normally active pet dog does not require the high fat and high protein content of some of the super-premium products. A useful profile of 200 g protein/kg and 100 g fat/kg will meet all of requirements and keep the dog in good condition. Small dogs form a highly heterogeneous group. Many small dogs have long coats, and can benefit from more protein (e.g. 250 g/kg fresh weight). Many terrier breeds are highly active, for which an increase in fat content and energy concentration is indicated. Large breeds benefit from an increase in protein content (250 g/kg fresh weight) to maintain their increased body mass, while more active pet dogs require increased protein and energy concentrations. This energy increase is best achieved by adjusting feed intake, rather than a fat increase, in order to keep the pet in lean condition. Working dogs require increased feed intakes and concentrations of protein and fat (300 g protein/kg and 200 g fat/kg) for heavy endurance work, not just to meet increased energy requirements, but because fatty acids are a primary metabolic fuel under endurance work in dogs (Hammel *et al.*, 1976). Senior dog foods also require an increase in micro-nutrients but a decrease in phosphorus. While puppy foods require increased protein, fat, vitamins and minerals, high energy and high calcium intakes can impair optimal growth in large breeds, with the body mass outgrowing the skeleton. (Hedhammer *et al.*, 1974). Puppy foods should be formulated to accommodate the reduced needs of these large breeds (up to 270-320 g protein and 120-160 g fat/kg).

## Conclusion

The existing nutrient recommendations for cats and dogs (e.g. AAFCO, 2001) provide the bases to ensure that all of the pets needs are met by manufactured diets. Research over the past 30 years has refined and modified these recommendations for practical petfood ingredients and their interactions, and this will continue in the light of the available petfood ingredients for the petfood industry.

The goal of a dietary basis for optimised health in pets is being achieved by the application of functional nutrition to petfoods. The immediate further steps to long-term improvements in pet health involve the optimisation of gut flora by the use of prebiotics, improvements in oral health by the enhancement of dental cleaning efficacy, and control of energy concentration in products to suit the pets energy needs by limiting fat content. Future developments in the areas of functional nutrition, and exploitation of new research findings in such areas of natural defences and longevity will follow.

## References

AAFCO (2001). Official Publication of the Association of American Feed Control Officials. Oxford, IN, USA.

Ballard, F.J. (1965): Glucose utilisation in mammalian liver, *Comparative Biochemistry and Physiology,* **14**: 437-443.

Buffington, C.A. (1993). Acid questions, potential dangers associated with cat food acification. *Pet Food Industry*, Sept/Oct pp 4-8.

Bui, L.M., Pawlowski, K. and Bierer, T.L. (2001). The influence of green –lipped mussel powder on allevaiting arthritic signs in dogs. *FASEB* [Further details needed]

Burger, I.H. and. Barnett K.C. (1982). The taurine requirement of the adult cat. *Journal of Small Animal Practice*, **23**, 533.

Bouchard, G.F. and Sunvold, G.D. (2000). Effects of dietary carbohydrate source on postprandial plasma glucose and insulin concentrations in cats. In : *Recent Advances in Canine and Feline Nutritional Research: Proceedings of the Iams Nutritional Symposium*, **111**, 123-130.

Boudreaux, M.K., Reinhart, G.A., Vaughn, D.M., Spano, J.S. and Mooney, M. (1997). The effects of varying omega 6:omega 3 fatty acid ratios on platelet reactivity, coagulation screening assays and antithrombin III activity in dogs. *Journal of the American Animal Hospital Association*, **33,** 235- 243.

Campbell, K.L., LaFlamme, D.P. and Harrison, J. (2000). Seasonal variations in skin surface pH, skin hydration, and hair epilation of normal dogs in Midwestern United States climate. *Veterinary Dermatology*, **11**, (Suppl. 1), FC-16, 19.

Chausow, D.G., Czarnecki-Maulden, G.L. (1987). Estimation of the dietary iron requirement for the weanling puppy and kitten. *Journal of Nutrition*, **117**, 928-932.

Chew, B.P., Park, J.S., Wong, T.S., Kim, H.W., Weng, B.B., Byrne, K.M., Hayek, M.G. and Reinhart, G.A. (2000). Dietary beta-carotene stimulates cell-mediated humoral immune response in dogs. *Journal of Nutrition*, **130(8)**, 1910-1913.

Cline, J.L., Czarnecki-Maulden, G.L., Losonsky, J.M. and Easter, R.A. (1995). Effect of Vitamin A on bone density and mucosal epithelium in dogs. *Journal of Animal Science,* **73 (suppl 1**), 192 (abs).

Codner, E.C. and Thatcher, C.D. (1993). Nutritional management of skin diseases. *Compendium on Continuing Education for the Practicing* Veterinarian, **15**, 411-424.

Cupp, C.J. (1999). Reduction of plaque and calculus build up in cats fed a specially formulated dry cat food. *Veterinary International*, **11(2)**, 25-30.

Czarnecki-Maulden, G.L. (1986). Nutritional idiosyncracies of the cat. *Proceedings of the Annual Meeting of the American Association of Zoo Veterinarians*,

Nov 2-6, Chicago

Czarnecki-Maulden, G.L., Rudnick, R.C., Chausow, D.G. (1993). Copper bioavailability and requirement in the dog: comparison of copper oxide and copper sulfate *Federation American Society Experimental Biology Journal* **7** **(3)**, A306

Czarnecki-Maulden, G.L. and Russell, T.J. (2000a). Effect of chicory on fecal microflora in dogs fed soy-containing or soy-free diets. *Federation American Society Experimental Biology Journal*, **14(4)**, A488.

Czarnecki-Maulden, G.L. and Russell, T.J. (2000b). Effect of diet type on fecal microflora in dogs. *Federation American Society Experimental Biology Journal*, **14(4)**, A488.

Davenport, G.M. (2000). The impact of nutrition on skin and hair coat. *Presented at 4th World Congress of Veterinary Dermatology 2000.* Published in: *Current Research in Canine Dermatology.* The Iams Company, Dayton, OH. P.4-9.

Devlin, P., Koelsch, S., Heaton, P.R., Charlton, C.J., O'Reilly, J.D., Smith, B.E. and Harper, J. (2000). Effects of antioxidant supplementation on the immune response in weaned puppies. *Proceedings of 18th ACVIM*, Seattle, May 2000, abs. 136.

Donoghue, S. and Scarlett, J.M. (1998). Diet and feline obesity. *Journal of Nutrition*, **128**, 2776S-2778S.

Earle, K.E. (2001). Recent advances in pet nutrition (2). *Food Technology*, **5**, 4.

Earle, K.E. and Smith, P.M. (1991). The effect of dietary taurine content on the plasma taurine concentration of the cat. *British Journal of Nutrition,* **66**, 227-235.

Fay, L.B., Metairon, S., Montigon, F. and Ballevre, O. (1998). Evaluation of taurine metabolism in cats by dual stable isotope analysis. *Analytical Chemistry*, **260**, 85-91.

German, A.J., Hall, E.J. and Day, M.J. (2000). Relative deficiency in IgA production by duodenal explants from German Shepherd Dogs with small intestinal disease. *Veterinary Immunology and Immunopathology*, **76**, 25-43.

Gershoff, S.N., Andrus, S.B. and Hegsted, D.M. (1957). Vitamin A deficiency in cats. *Laboratory Investigation*, **6**, 227-239.

Hammel, E.P., Kronfeld, D.S. and Ganjam, V.K. (1976). Metabolic responses to exhaustive exercise in racing sledge dogs fed diets containing medium, low and zero carbohydrate. *American Journal of Clinical Nutrition*, **30**, 409-418.

Hannah, S.S. and Laflamme, D.P. (1996). *Veterinary Clinical Nutrition*, **3**, 30.

Hassam, A.G., Rivers, J.P.W. and Crawford, M.A. (1977). The failure of the cat to desaturate linoleic acid: its nutritional implications, *Nutrition and Metabolism*, **21**, 321-328.

Hayes, K.C., Carey, R.E. and Schmidt, S.Y. (1975). Retinal degeneration associated with taurine deficiency in the cat. *Science*, **188**, 949.

Heaton, P. (2001.) The comet assay: A measure of DNA damage validated in the cat and dog for nutritional studies. (abs) Waltham Symposium, Vancouver.

Hedhammer, A.F., Wu, F., Krook, L., Schryer, H.F., de Lahunta, A., Whalen, J.P., Kallfelz, F.A., Nunez, E.A., Hintz, H.F., Sheffy, B.E. and Ryan, G.D. (1974). Overnutrition and skeletal disease: An experimental study in growing Great Dane dogs. *Cornell Veterinarian*, **64 (suppl 5)**

Ikeda, M., Tsuji, H., Nakasuma, S. (1965). Studies on the biosynthesis of nicotinamide adenine dinucleotide. II A role of picolinic carboxylase in the biosynthesis of nicotinamide adenine dinucleotide from typtophan in mammals. *Journal of Biological Chemistry*, **240**, 1395-1401.

Kienzle, E. (1993a). Carbohydrate metabolism in the cat 1. Activity of amylase in the gastrointestinal tract of the cat. *Journal of Animal Physiology and Animal Nutrition*, **69**, 92-101.

Kienzle, E. (1993b). Carbohydrate metabolism in the cat 3. Digestion of sugars. *Journal of Animal Physiology and Animal Nutrition*, **69**, 203-210.

Lawlor, D.F., Sjolin, D.W. and Collins, J.E. (1985). Incidence rates of lower feline urinary tract disease in the United States. *Feline Practice*, **15**, 13-16.

Marsh, K.A., Ruedisueli, F.L., Coe, S L. and Watson, T.G. (2000). Effects of zinc and linoleic acid supplementation on the skin and coat quality of dogs receiving a complete and balanced diet. *Veterinary Dermatology*, **11(4)**, 277.

Meyer, H., Zentek, J., Harernoll, H. and Maskell, I. (1999). Digestibility and compatability of mixed diets and faecal consistency in different breeds of dog. *Journal of Veterinary Medicine*, **A 46** 155-165.

McFarlane, G.T. and Cummings, J.H. (1991). The colonic flora, fermentation, and large bowel digestive function. In S.F. Phillips, J.H. Pemberton and R.G. Shorter (Eds) *The Large Intestine: Physiology, Pathophysiology and Disease*. Pp.51 Raven Press, New York

NRC (1985). *Nutrient Requirements of Dogs*, National Academy Press, Washington DC

NRC (1986). *Nutrient Requirements of Cats*, National Academy Press, Washington DC

Osborne, C.A. (1992). Feline lower urinary tract disease: state of the science. *Proceedings of the Kal Kan Symposium for the Treatment of Dog and Cat Diseases*. Kal Kan foods, Vernon, California p 89.

Patil, A.R., Carrion, P.A. and Holmes, A.K. (2001). Effect of chicory supplementation on fecal microflora of cats. *Federation American Society Experimental Biology Journal*, **15(4)**, A288.

Patil, A.R. and Bisby, T.M. (2001). Comparison of energy requirement of client-owned dogs and kennel dogs. *Purina Nutrition Forum*, St. Louis MO

Pion, P.D., Kittleson, M.D. and Rogers, Q.R. (1989). Cardiomyopathy in cats and its relation to taurine deficiency. In *Current Veterinary Therapy, Vol. 10*. Ed.

R. W. Kirk. p.251-262. Philadelphia, W. B. Saunders.

Rogers, Q.R., Morris, J.G., Freedland, R.A. (1977). Lack of enzymatic adaptation to low and high levels of dietary protein in the adult cat. *Enzyme*, **22**, 348-356.

Rolls, B.J., Rowe, E.A. and Turner, R.C. (1980). Persisitent obesity in rats following a period of consumption of a mixed high energy diet. *Journal of Physiology (London)*, **298**, 415-427.

Romsos, D.R., Hornshuh, M.J. and Leveille, G.A. (1978). Influence of dietary fat and carbohydrate on food intake, bodyweight, and body fat of adult dogs. *Proceedings of the Society for Experimental Biological Medicine*, **157**, 278-281.

Sanecki, R.K., Corbin, J.E. and Forbes, R.M. (1982). Tissue changes in dogs fed a zinc-deficient ration. *American Journal of Veterinary Research*, **43 (9)**, 1642-1646.

Sinclair, A.J., Mclean, J.G. and Monger, E.A. (1979). Metabolism of linoleic acid in the cat. *Lipids*, **14**, 932-936.

Smith, B.H.E., Stevenson, A.E. and Markwell, P.J. (1997). Urinary relative supersaturation of calcium oxalate and struvite in the cat are influenced by diet. *Waltham Syposium*, Orlando Florida (abs) p 82.

Sturman, J. A. Gargano, A. D., Messing, J. M. and Imaki, H. (1986). Feline Maternal taurine deficiency: effect on mother and offspring. *Journal of Nutrition,* **116**, 665-667.

Sunvold, G.D., Vickers, R.J., Kelley, R.L., Tetrick, M.A., Davenport, G.M. and Bouchard, G.F. (1999). Effect of dietary carnitine during energy restriction in the canine. *Federation American Society Experimental Biology Journal*, **13**, A268.

Verstegen, M.W.A. (2000). Energy declarations from poultry research and recommendations. (abs) ESVCN, Amsterdam 2000

Watson, A.D.J. (1997) Diet and periodontal disease in dogs and cats. *Veterinary Clinical Nutrition*, **4(4)**, 135-137.

Westermarck, E. (1980). The hereditary nature of canine pancreatic degenerative atrophy in the German Shepherd Dog. *Acta Veterinaria Scandinavica*, **21**, 389-394.

Yu, S., Rogers, Q.R. and Morris, J.G. (2001). Effect of low levels of dietary tyrosine on the hair colour of cats. *Journal of Small Animal Practice*, **42**,176-180.

*This paper was first published in 2002*

19

# INTERACTIONS BETWEEN THE IMMUNE SYSTEM, NUTRITION, AND PRODUCTIVITY OF ANIMALS

ELIZABETH A. KOUTSOS AND KIRK C. KLASING

*Department of Animal Science, 1 Shields Ave., University of California, Davis, CA 95616*

## Introduction

Many important interactions exist between the nutrition of an animal and the physiological processes involved in its immune function, growth and reproduction (Figure 19.1). Understanding these interactions enables the nutritionist to contribute to the welfare of animals, reduce production costs and protect consumers from food-borne pathogens. This chapter will focus on the underlying mechanisms and practical consequences of these interactions. Much of the mechanistic information was developed in rodent models; however production animal species, especially poultry and pigs, are often used to elucidate the quantitative and practical applications of interactions between nutrition and immunity.

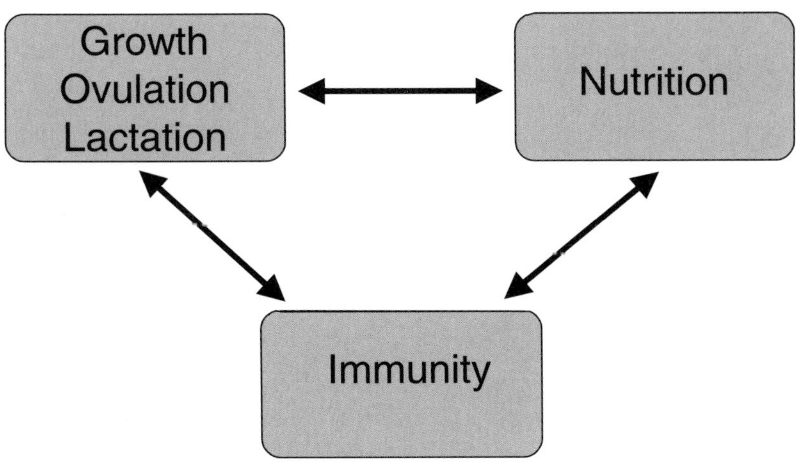


**Figure 19.1** Nutrition interacts with the physiological processes involved in immune function, growth and reproduction. For example, nutrition modulates the immune system and immune responses modulate nutritional needs.

## The systemic immune response – overview

The immune system functions to recognize the presence of macromolecules of non-self origin. Lymphocytes primarily recognize protein antigens through their cell surface receptors (e.g. membrane bound immunoglobulin), while phagocytes, such as macrophages and heterophils/neutrophils, recognize lipid and carbohydrate antigens through their surface pattern receptors. Antigen recognition results in leukocyte activation, cytokine secretion, and the engagement of effector mechanisms directed at removal of the pathogen.

The pro-inflammatory cytokines, including interleukin-1 (IL-1), IL-6, IL-8, tumour necrosis factor-α (TNFα), interferon-α (INF-α) and INF-γ act as communication molecules between immune cells and other cells of the body. Secretion of these cytokines occurs rapidly after an infectious challenge and they act locally to regulate the immune response. The pro-inflammatory cytokines reach systemically relevant levels within a few hours of a challenge. Quantitatively, their production is regulated by a complex network of co-stimulatory and feedback loops that respond to various stimuli. Among the mediators that counterbalance the pro-inflammatory cytokines are glucocorticoids, transforming growth factor-ß, receptor antagonists (e.g. IL-$1_{ra}$), soluble receptors, and acute phase proteins. In addition, some dietary factors can regulate the production of pro-inflammatory cytokines and anti-inflammatory regulators (see later).

The systemic effects of pro-inflammatory cytokines are important for coordination of the various biochemical, cellular and endocrine responses that enhance immune function and direct substrates to the immune system and other protective pathways (Table 19.1). In a homeorhetic response driven by elevated systemic levels of pro-inflammatory cytokines, nutrients are redirected from anabolic pathways related to growth, skeletal muscle accretion or reproduction towards pathways that bolster defence against pathogens. For example, nutrient repartitioning results in an increased rate of protein turnover, which leads to increased body temperature and basal metabolic rate. In addition, accelerated protein degradation may augment host defence by increasing proteosome activity and therefore enhancing expression of peptide fragments from intracellular proteins on MHC class II molecules. This process permits greater detection of intracellular pathogens and is illustrative of the heightened vigilance and activity of the immune system induced by a generalized stress state. In some tissues, such as skeletal muscle, increased proteolysis is not matched by augmented protein synthesis causing decreased tissue accretion that is manifested as impaired growth in young animals or negative nitrogen balance in mature animals. Nutrient repartitioning occurs not only with protein and amino acids, but also with virtually every other essential nutrient (Table 19.2).

**Table 19.1** EFFECTS OF PRO-INFLAMMATORY CYTOKINES ON METABOLISM AND IMMUNE FUNCTION. ADAPTED FROM (CHANG AND BISTRIAN, 1998, KLASING, 1988, LING, SCHWARTZ AND BISTRIAN, 1997).

| *Cytokine* | *Metabolic effects* | *Immune effects* |
|---|---|---|
| TNFα | ↑ weight loss<br>↑ catabolism in skeletal muscle<br>↑ lipid release by adipocytes<br>↑ osteoclast activity<br>↑ collagenase gene transcription<br>↑ resting energy expenditure<br>↓ body temperature<br>↑ hepatic cholesterol and triglyceride synthesis<br>↓ voluntary food intake<br>↓ fatty acid uptake by adipocytes | ↑ phagocytosis by neutrophils<br>↑ B cell growth/differentiation<br>↑ proliferation of fibroblasts<br>↑ cytokine production by phagocytes, endothelial cells |
| IL-1 | ↑ collagen synthesis<br>↑ bone resorption<br>↑ weight loss<br>↑ glucose oxidation<br>↑ gluconeogenesis<br>↓ voluntary food intake<br>↑ body temperature<br>↓ fatty acid uptake by tissues<br>↓ thyroxin release | ↑ intestinal mucous production<br>↑ acute phase protein (APP) production<br>↑ growth of fibroblasts, keratinocytes, glial cells<br>↑ expression of adherence molecules<br>↑ proliferation of vascular smooth muscle<br>↑ lymphocyte chemotaxis<br>↑ mediator production (IL-2, thromboxane, PGE2, histamine) |
| IL-6 | ↑ body temperature<br>↑ metallothionein production by hepatocytes<br>↓ voluntary food intake | ↑ APP production<br>↑ IL-2 production<br>↑ growth/differentiation of bone marrow stem cells, macrophages, neurons |
| IFN-γ | ↓ growth of normal/neoplastic cells | ↑ cytotoxicity of macrophages<br>↑ antigen presentation<br>↑ IL-2, IL-2R production |

## Mechanisms of the pro-inflammatory cytokines

Pro-inflammatory cytokines exert their wide-ranging actions on metabolism and tissue accretion by a multifactorial mechanism. Most cells have receptors for at least some of the pro-inflammatory cytokines and can respond directly to these mediators when their levels are sufficiently high in blood and interstitial fluids. Additionally, pro-inflammatory cytokines can stimulate neurons that innervate immune tissues such as lymph nodes, spleen, bone marrow or liver permitting communication with areas of the brain that regulate important processes such as body temperature, appetite, and behaviour (Downing and Miyan, 2000). Stimulation of local neural networks modifies vascular tone in specific tissues and, in some cases, decreases gastrointestinal motility, which affects feed intake. Pro-inflammatory cytokines can also exert their action via the endocrine system, either by modifying the release of hormones, affecting hormone receptor numbers, or impinging upon second messenger pathways. For example, the anabolic drive induced by IGF-1 and insulin is blunted by pro-inflammatory cytokines (Elsasser *et al.*, 1995).

Each pro-inflammatory cytokine has its own set of unique activities as well as a large number of actions that overlap synergistically (Paludan, 2000) with other cytokines (Table 19.1). The specific milieu of pro-inflammatory cytokines released during an infectious challenge depends upon the type of challenging pathogen and its portal of entry. For example, bacterial pathogens tend to stimulate production of IL-1, IL-6, and TNF-$\alpha$, while viral pathogens tend to stimulate the production of interferons (Fossum, 1998). Variation in the amounts and types of pro-inflammatory cytokines partially explains the wide range of specific symptoms expressed in animals with different disease challenges.

## Effect of an immune response on animal productivity

An immune response can affect production by several mechanisms, including altering metabolism, altering hormone production, and/or inducing pathology (Klasing and Johnstone, 1991). Sick animals grow slower and less efficiently, miss ovulations, or produce less milk. In the past few decades, it has become clear that a large component of this phenomenon is due to the immune response *per se*, while the pathological consequences of the invading organism are not required for impaired productivity. For this reason, farm management systems are geared toward minimizing the incidence of infectious diseases through practices such as vaccination and rigorous biosecurity programmes. Feeding growth-promoting levels of antibiotics diminishes challenges from opportunistic and commensal bacteria and consequently improves rates and efficiencies of production. With consumer and legislative pressure to minimize the use of antibiotic growth promoters, an understanding of the connections between immune responses and animal productivity becomes critical.

The immune response causes an overall change in the metabolism and behaviour of an animal. One of the most devastating impacts of this metabolic perturbance on animal performance, attributed to the effects of the pro-inflammatory cytokines, is decreased food intake (Johnson, 1998). In growing broiler chickens, the anorexia that accompanies an inflammatory response to LPS or heat-killed *Staphylococcus aureus* accounts for about 80 % of the decrease in growth rate (Klasing *et al.*, 1987). Clearly the immune response can be quite detrimental in production systems where weight gain is critical for profitability.

By altering the hormonal profile of an animal, an immune response can effectively reduce growth rates and reproductive performance (McCann, Kimura, Walczewska, Karanth, Retori and Yu, 1998). Specific binding sites for TNFα have been demonstrated in bovine pituitary, and administration of this cytokine results in a decrease in responsiveness to growth hormone releasing hormone (GHRH) and thyrotropin releasing hormone (TRH) (Elsasser *et al.*, 1997). GHRH, previously known as somatotropin releasing factor, is involved in the release of growth hormone and prolactin, while TRH stimulates the release of thyrotropin stimulating hormone, thus regulating metabolic rate, growth, and all thyroid functions. In addition to these hormones, as previously stated, the high growth rates of production animals, driven by IGF-1, are reduced by pro-inflammatory cytokine production (Elsasser, *et al.*, 1995). Obviously, reduced responsiveness to hormones can have a dramatic impact on performance.

The immune response can also inflict damage to host tissue, and this pathology is often necessary to eliminate pathogens. For example, during the innate immune response, macrophages are activated to destroy invading pathogens. The macrophage responds to cytokines and other effector molecules by producing antimicrobial factors, including reactive oxygen species and proteases. These mediators effectively destroy invading pathogens. However, host cells are also susceptible to these mediators, and therefore host pathology inevitably results as a consequence of disease. Nutritional strategies can modulate the production of cytokines and effector molecules and thus affect the level of macrophage activation and tissue pathology. However, the elimination of disease is the only mechanism by which this pathology can be completely prevented.

## Genetic implications

Given that many immune responses are associated with decreased growth and productivity, intense genetic selection for one of these processes should result in losses in the other. This negative correlation between immunity and productivity has been observed in a variety of experimental models. For example, in poultry, several long-term selection experiments based on immune response criteria have resulted in genetic lines with widely different immune responsiveness and, consequently, susceptibility to infectious disease. Selection for a high antibody response to sheep red blood cells (SRBC) over 24 generations results in a 15 % decrease in growth rate (Yang *et al.*, 2000). Conversely, selecting chickens or turkeys for high growth rates has resulted in impaired immunocompetence, disease resistance and alter pro-inflammatory cytokine release (Bayyari *et al.*, 1997, Li *et al.*, 1999, Mauldin *et al.*, 1978, Qureshi and Havenstein, 1994). For this reason, it is likely that genetic selection for performance characteristics has resulted in an increased susceptibility of today's poultry and livestock to infectious diseases compared with their ancestors. This situation heightens the need for nutritional approaches to optimise immunocompetence.

## Effect of an immune response on nutrition

Most research on nutrient requirements of animals is conducted in Federally-approved facilities that have levels of sanitation and pathogen exclusion that cannot be accomplished in real world, field conditions. Consequently, the minimal nutrient requirements summarized in the various National Research Council (NRC) publications may not be relevant to on-farm conditions where there is a prevalence of low-level non-clinical diseases and pathogenic challenges are frequent. Clearly it is of practical importance to understand the impact of these challenges on nutrient requirements.

The immune system must compete with growth and reproductive processes for nutrients, and is a component of the maintenance costs of an animal. When the immune system is engaged in defence against a pathogen, its nutrient demands are increased. Those nutrients are used as substrates for the clonal proliferation of responding lymphocytes, the production of antibodies and the hepatic secretion of acute phase proteins (Figure 19.2). Among these processes, the production of acute phase proteins quantitatively appears to be the most nutritionally demanding process (Klasing and Calvert, 2000). Consequently, the development, maintenance and use of the immune system require nutrients that must ultimately originate from the diet. Understanding the impact of disease challenges on nutrient requirements is complicated by the fact that each disease strain inflicts its own unique pathologies that have differing consequences for nutrient requirements. Those organisms that cause enteric pathology might be expected to have a large impact on digestion and absorption of nutrients, while those that inflict liver or kidney damage disproportionately impact nutrient metabolism. For this reason, it is necessary to divide the impact of infection on nutrient requirements into two components: those effects due to specific pathology and those that are due to the response of the immune system to the pathogen. Presumably, this latter component is more consistent across the multitude of different diseases and can be studied in experimental model systems.

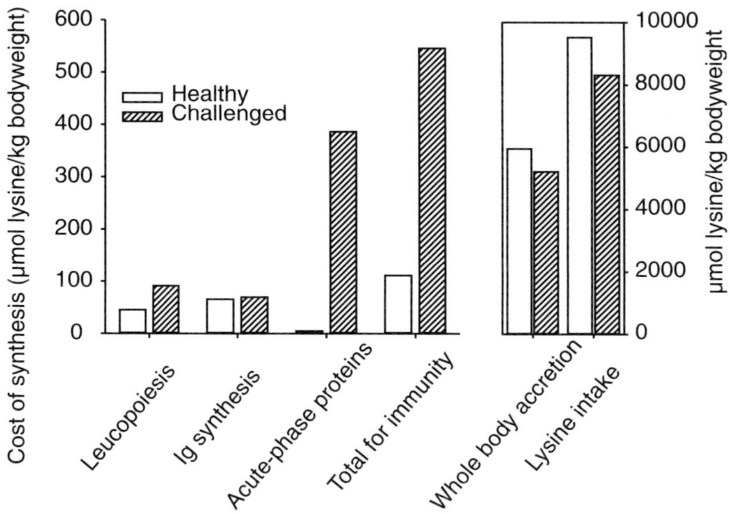


**Figure 19.2** Use of lysine for leucopoiesis, immunoglobulin (Ig) synthesis, acute-phase protein synthesis and whole-body protein accretion in 14-day broiler chicks. Chicks were in either a healthy state or challenged with lipopolysaccharide from *Salmonella typhimurium*. The proportion of lysine intake used for immunocompetence was 1.2 and 6.7 % during health and challenged states, respectively. See Klasing and Calvert (2000) for details.

The immune response to a pathogen can affect the nutrition of animals by altering digestion, absorption, metabolism, and excretion of nutrients (Table 19.2), thus affecting substrate availability and dietary requirements. Components of the immune response may increase nutrient use, such as the anabolic components of the immune response (e.g. clonal proliferation of lymphocytes, recruitment of new myeloid cells, and antibody synthesis) as well as acute phase protein production by the liver. Conversely, altered metabolism of a specific nutrient may be a consequence of the immune response, rather than an integral component of that response. For example, retinol is transported in the blood bound to retinol binding protein (RBP). During an immune response, the synthesis of RBP is dramatically reduced, resulting in decreased retinol in the blood (Rosales *et al.*, 1996). In this situation, transport of a nutrient is altered as a consequence of the acute phase response. In addition, an immune response can increase the need for some substrates. For example, an energetic cost of fever has been proposed, due to the cost of increasing body temperature (eg. shivering), the increased rates of biochemical reactions due to increased body temperature, and increased cellular utilization of ATP due to futile cycling (Baracos, Whitmore and Gale, 1987).

While the immune response may alter nutrient metabolism, lower rates of productivity during disease results in decreased nutrient needs. For example, in growing pigs and chickens, the overall requirement for lysine decreases

**Table 19.2.** EFFECT OF AN IMMUNE RESPONSE ON NUTRIENT METABOLISM

| *Nutrient* | *Immune response* | *Effect* | *Reference* |
|---|---|---|---|
| Protein | Inflammation, infection, trauma | ↑ skeletal muscle catabolism<br>↑ hepatic protein synthesis | Beisel (1977) |
| Cysteine | Acute inflammation | ↑ protein production<br>↑ glutathione production | Malmezat *et al.* (1998) |
| Glucose | Inflammation, infection, trauma | Increased turnover | Beisel (1977) |
| Lipids | Inflammation, infection | ↑ hepatic triglyceride, cholesterol synthesis<br>↓ tissue fatty acid uptake | Beisel (1977) |
| Zinc | Inflammation, infection, trauma | ↑ metallothionein<br>↓ plasma Zn | Klasing (1984) |
| Iron | Inflammation, infection, trauma | ↓ dietary Fe absorption<br>↑ ferritin, lactoferrin<br>↓ plasma Fe | Weinberg, (1999), Butler *et al.* (1973) |
| Vitamin A | Acute Inflammation | ↓ RBP synthesis<br>↓ plasma retinol | Rosales *et al.* (1996) |
| Carotenoids | Coccidiosis | ↓ absorption, pigmentation | Tyczkowski and Hamilton (1991) |

during a simulated infectious challenge (Klasing and Barnes, 1988; Webel *et al.*, 1998a; Williams *et al.*, 1997a, b; Williams *et al.*, 1997b). Presumably this is because lower rates of growth and muscle accretion decrease amino acid requirements much more than are necessary to compensate for the anabolic processes of the immune response.

Finally, some nutrients are metabolised in greater amounts during an immune response, which may increase dietary requirements during a disease state. Many effector mechanisms used by the immune system generate large amounts of reactive oxygen intermediates (ROI). Antioxidants, such as ascorbic acid and vitamin E, protect macromolecules against damage from these ROI. Evidence is accumulating that the requirements for antioxidant nutrients are greater during an inflammatory response than levels required by healthy animals (Webel *et al.*, 1998; Yoshida *et al.*, 1999). However, as previously stated, the level of nutrient intake is decreased during an immune response. Therefore, it may be necessary to increase nutrient intake prior to a disease challenge or vaccination.

In addition to conventional nutrients, other dietary factors may also be affected by an immune response. For example, during aflatoxicosis or coccidiosis in the chicken, absorption of dietary carotenoids, responsible for pigmentation of meat and eggs, is significantly decreased (Tyczkowski and Hamilton, 1987; 1991). While carotenoids are not considered essential nutrients, pigmentation of poultry products is often critical for consumer acceptance.

## Modulating the immune response via nutrition

The immune response can be modulated by nutrition in several ways. First, the nutritional status of the developing embryo has profound effects on the development of its immune system. Second, nutrients provide the substrates for proliferation of immune cells and effector molecules. On this basis, the nutritional status of an animal can dramatically affect the degree of immune cell proliferation and/or effector molecule production. Third, just as production animals require dietary nutrients, invading pathogens rely on the host for supply of many nutrients. Therefore, nutrient deficiency or excess can affect the ability of a pathogen to replicate *in vivo*. In addition, nutrients can be effective as substrates for inter- and intra-cellular communication, and their availability may be critical for an effective immune response. Finally, the pattern of nutrient intake may affect the endocrine system, which then modulates magnitude, type and/or duration of the immune response.

The time period during which immune cells differentiate and populate the tissues of the body is relatively long compared to other developmental processes and extends well beyond birth. In fact, the high rate of cell proliferation in combination with the complexity of regulatory control over the developmental events is unmatched in any other tissue of the neonate. These developmental processes require a complex series of highly regulated cellular differentiation steps followed by deletion of self-reacting clones of lymphocytes that might cause autoimmunity. For this reason, a chronic deficiency of virtually any required nutrient during the period of immune system development has negative impacts on immunocompetence. Some examples of the deleterious effects of specific nutrient deficiencies on the development of the immune system are shown in Table 19.3. In general, those required nutrients that function in regulating cell differentiation (e.g. vitamins A, D) are particularly detrimental to the development of immunocompetence.

Nutrition affects not only the development of the immune system, but also the immune response to disease. Many nutrients modulate the immune system by mechanisms related to the provision of substrates (Table 19.4). The resting immune system is probably not very nutritionally demanding, as it

**Table 19.3** EFFECT OF CHRONIC NUTRIENT DEFICIENCY ON IMMUNE SYSTEM DEVELOPMENT

| *Nutrient* | *Species* | *Effect* | *Reference* |
|---|---|---|---|
| Vitamin A | Rat | ↓ body weight | Nauss *et al.* (1985) |
| | | ↓ splenocyte # | |
| | | ↓ development/differentiation of all leukocytes | Semba (1998) |
| Vitamin D | Chicken | ↓ thymus weight | Alsam *et al.* (1998) |
| Vitamin E | Chicken | ↓ CD4-CD8+ thymocytes | Erf *et al.* (1998) |
| Magnesium | Rat | ↑ leukocyte #, 1° PMN cells | Malpuech-Brugere *et al.* (1999) |
| | | ↓ thymus weight | |
| | | ↑ thymocyte apoptosis | |
| Zinc | Mice | ↓ lymphoid organ development | Beach *et al.* (1980) |
| | | ↓ splenic RBC, leukocyte # | |
| Copper | Mice | ↓ thymus weight | Prohaska and Lukasewycz (1989) |
| | | ↓ Cu-Zn SOD activity | |
| | | ↓ ceruloplasmin activity | |
| | | ↓ Ab response to SRBC | |
| | | ↑ spleen weight | |
| | | ↑ anaemia | |

contains some of the most inactive cells of the body (e.g. resting lymphocytes). However, activation of the immune system results in some of the most metabolically active and rapidly proliferating cells of the body. This sudden burst of activity is tightly regulated and critical decisions are made at this time regarding the threshold for a response, the magnitude of the response, and the types of cells recruited for the response. Nutrients are important in supplying the substrates needed for this rapid rate of cell proliferation and the secretion of effector molecules. In fact, the pro-inflammatory response orchestrates metabolic changes, such as skeletal muscle catabolism, which provide a source of nutrients for these processes even when dietary intake is insufficient.

Just as the immune system is capable of repartitioning nutrients for cell proliferation and effector molecule production, repartitioning of some nutrients occurs as a defence mechanism against invading pathogens. Some nutrients serve as substrates for pathogens and support their proliferation and virulence. For example, iron is the limiting nutrient in the plasma and extracellular fluids of most animals. The pro-inflammatory cytokines released during a pathogen challenge mediate a shift in iron from transferrin in the extracellular fluids to ferritin located in intracellular locations (Weinberg, 1998). This change decreases the amount of iron available to pathogens and decreases their virulence. In neonatal pigs, excessive amounts of iron, provided through the diet or via injection, enhance the proliferation of several types of pathogen

**Table19.4** EFFECT OF NUTRIENT DEFICIENCY OR EXCESS ON IMMUNE FUNCTION

| *Nutrient* | *Species* | *Effect* | *Reference* |
|---|---|---|---|
| Protein Deficiency | Rat | ↓ APP production | Grimble and Grimble |
| | | ↓ NO synthesis | (1998); Wu *et al.* (1999) |
| | Pig | ↓ RBC glutathione production | Jahoor *et al.* (1995) |
| Arginine Deficiency | Rat | ↓ NO synthesis | Wu *et al.* (1999) |
| Vitamin A Deficiency | Rat | ↓ body weight | Nauss *et al.* (1985) |
| | | ↓ splenocyte mitogenesis to ConA | |
| | | ↓ Natural Killer cell #, cytotoxicity | Zhao *et al.* (1994) |
| | | ↓ neutrophil chemotaxis, adhesion, | Twining *et al.* (1997) |
| | | phagocytosis, production of | Semba (1998) |
| | | oxidative species | Krishnan *et al.* (1974) |
| | | ↓ goblet cell number | |
| | | ↓ spleen, thymus weight | |
| | Chicken | ↓ body weight | Rombout *et al.* (1992) |
| | | ↓ IgA in bile | |
| | | ↓ T lymphocyte proliferation in vitro | |
| | | ↓ antibody response to BSA | |
| | | ↑ morbidity, mortality to *E. coli* | Friedman (1989) |
| | | ↓ antibody response to *E. coli* | Friedman *et al.* (1991) |
| Vitamin A Excess | Chicken in vitro | ↓ T lymphocyte proliferation | Friedman (1989) |
| | | ↓ antibody response to BSA | |
| | | ↑ morbidity, mortality to *E. coli* | Friedman *et al.* (1991) |
| Vitamin D Deficiency | Chicken | ↓ growth, feed consumption | Alsam *et al.* (1998) |
| | | ↓ DTH response | |
| | | ↓ thymus weight | |
| Vitamin E Deficiency | Chicken | ↓ CD4-CD8+ thymocytes | Erf *et al.* (1998) |
| Vitamin E Excess | Chicken | ↓ antibody response to NDV | Friedman *et al.* (1998) |
| | Turkey | ↓ antibody response to NDV | Friedman *et al.* (1998) |
| | Rat | ↑ splenocyte, alveolar mϕ # | Moriguchi *et al.* (1990) |
| | | ↑ splenocyte mitogenesis | |
| | | ↑ NK cell activity | |
| | | ↑ phagocytosis by alveolar mϕ | |
| Pyridoxine Deficiency | Pig | ↓ hematocrit | Harmon *et al.* (1963) |
| | | ↓ Ab titre to *S. pullorum* | |
| Pantothenic Acid Deficiency | Pig | ↓ Ab titre to *S. pullorum* | Harmon *et al.* (1963) |
| Riboflavin Deficiency | Pig | ↓ Ab titre to *S. pullorum* | Harmon *et al.* (1963) |

**Table 19.4** CONTD

| *Nutrient* | *Species* | *Effect* | *Reference* |
|---|---|---|---|
| Magnesium Deficiency | Rat | ↑ plasma IL-6<br>↑ thymus TBAR | Malpuech-Brugere *et al.* (1999) |
| Zinc Deficiency | Mice | ↓ plaque forming ability to SRBC<br>↓ IgA, IgG, IgM | Beach *et al.* (1980) |
| Iron Excess | Human | ↑ lipid peroxidation<br>↑ DNA strand damage<br>↑ microbial replication | Weinberg (1999) |
| Iron Deficiency | Rat | ↓ IL-1 activity<br>↓ sIgA and IgM containing mucosal cells | Helyar and Sherman (1987) Perkkio *et al.* (1987) |

(Kadis *et al.*, 1984, Knight *et al.*, 1983). In addition to increased pathogenicity due to nutrient excess, a nutrient deficiency may also directly affect pathogens. In mice, a selenium deficiency has been demonstrated to provide a host environment in which a non-virulent strain of coxsackievirus may mutate and become virulent (Beck, 2000). The mechanism for this change in the viral genome seems to be related to antioxidant status, as vitamin E-deficiency resulted in similar observations.

In addition to the aforementioned roles, many nutrients are directly involved in, or regulate, the intracellular and intercellular communication of leukocytes (Grimble, 1998). For example, the type of dietary polyunsaturated fatty acids (PUFA) consumed by an animal is reflected in the PUFA content of cellular membranes. As PUFAs are precursors for eicosanoid synthesis, including prostaglandins and leukotrienes, the PUFA content of cellular membranes affects the types and amounts of eicosanoids released during an immune response. This change in regulatory environment is reflected in the type of immune response that predominates during an infectious challenge and in the outcome of the infection (Harbige, 1998). Specifically, feeding n-3 PUFAs of marine origin, primarily eicosapentaenoic acid (EPA; 20:5 n-3) and docosahexaenoic acid (DHA; 22:6 n-3), results in decreased production of $PGE_2$. Supplementation of EPA results in increased production of $PGE_3$, a less biologically active molecule than $PGE_2$, while enrichment with DHA causes suppression of $PGE_2$ formation via cyclooxygenase inhibition (Chapkin, McMurray and Jolly, 2000). In addition, n-3 PUFAs from marine sources have been shown to reduce IL-12 and IFN-γ release causing a shift from T-helper 1 ($T_h1$) towards $T_h2$ responses (Fritsche, Shahbazian, Feng and Berg, 1997). This modulation of the immune response causes increased susceptibility to infections that are controlled by a strong $T_h1$ response, such as *Listeria*, but an increase in resistance controlled by a strong $T_h2$ response, such as E. coli sepsis (Fritsche, Anderson and Feng, 2000). In chickens, feeding diets supplemented with n-3 fatty acids significantly decreased the incidence of septicemia by 25 %, but resulted in a 24 % increase in the incidence of tumours (Klasing and Leshchinsky, 2000). Other nutrients that modulate the communication networks within the immune system include vitamins such as A, D, and E, minerals such as iron, and volatile fatty acids like butyrate (Klasing and Leshchinsky, 2000, Säemann *et al.*, 2000, Weinberg, 2000)

Antioxidant nutrients, such as vitamin E also modulate an immune response. Reactive oxygen species are responsible for activating transcription factors, such as NF-KB, which are involved in the regulation of viral gene expression, cytokine synthesis, and the acute inflammatory reactions (Lander, 1997, Sen and Packer, 1996). Vitamin E, and other antioxidants, can inhibit the activation of these transcription factors, thus affecting the magnitude of the immune response. In addition to this role, vitamin E can affect arachidonic acid metabolism (Qureshi and Gore, 1997), thereby affecting the immune response in a similar manner to PUFAs.

Finally, the amount of diet fed, the pattern of feeding (e.g. single meal versus *ad libitum*) and the ratio between protein and energy in the diet influence the hormonal milieu. The hormonal profile in turn modulates the immune response via leukocytes, which have receptors for hormones produced by the classical endocrine system, including glucocorticoids, insulin, glucagons, growth hormone and thyroxin (Berczi *et al.*, 1998). For example, feeding protocols that result in periods of over-consumption of food impair both cell mediated and humoral indices of immunity (Klasing, 1988). Often, feeding regimens that restrict feed intake below voluntary levels result in better immunocompetence and enhanced disease resistance (BoaAmponsem *et al.*, 1997, Praharaj *et al.*, 1996, von Borell *et al.*, 1992).

## Conclusions

The immune system functions to recognise and destroy non-self molecules within the body. To maintain this function, leukocytes must proliferate, maintain receptors for recognition of foreign molecules, produce cytokines to regulate the response, and produce antibodies and other effector molecules. These functions require nutrients as substrates, without which the immune response to disease may be insufficient. In addition to the nutrient requirements of the immune system to mount an effective immune response, an immune response will affect nutrient partitioning. In general, an immune stress results in decreased nutrient intake, increased nutrient excretion, and repartitioning of nutrients away from production towards immune-related functions. In addition, production of effector molecules, such as reactive oxygen intermediates, may increase requirements for certain nutrients, such as antioxidants.

The immune response can be manipulated by nutrition. Nutritional status during embryonic development may affect immunocompetence for the life of the animal, while post-natal nutritional status may affect cell proliferation, responsiveness, phagocytic capacity, and effector molecule production. A nutrient deficiency or excess may result in increased susceptibility to disease due to these modifications. In addition, nutritional deficiency or excess may enhance the virulence or pathogenicity of certain organisms. Finally, many nutrients, specifically fatty acids and antioxidants, may modulate the immune response depending on their rate of dietary inclusion. For this reason, selection of dietary ingredients must take into account ratios of fatty acids and overall antioxidant levels. With sufficient knowledge of these interactions between nutrition and the immune response, the producer may optimise productivity and welfare while minimising disease concerns and the costs of over- or underfeeding animals.

## References

Alsam, S. M., Garlich, J. D. and Qureshi, M. A. (1998) *Poultry Science,* **77**, 842-849

Baracos, V. E., Whitmore, W. T. and Gale, R. (1987) *Can. J. Physiol. Pharmacol.,* **65**, 1248-1254

Bayyari, G. R., Huff, W. E., Rath, N. C., Balog, J. M., Newberry, L. A., Villines, J. D., Skeeles, J. K., Anthony, N. B. and Nestor, K. E. (1997) *Poultry Science,* **76**, 289-296

Beach, R. S., Gershwin, M. E., Makishima, R. K. and Hurley, L. S. (1980) *Journal of Nutrition,* **110**, 805-815

Beck, M. A. (2000) *American Journal of Clinical Nutrition,* **71**, 1676S-1679S

Beisel, W. R. (1977.) in *Advances in Nutritional Research*, vol. 1 (Draper, H. H., ed.), pp. 125-133, Plenum, New York

Berczi, I., Chow, D. A. and Sabbadini, E. R. (1998) *Domestic Animal Endocrinology,* **15**, 273-81

BoaAmponsem, K., Yang, A., Praharaj, N. K., Dunnington, E. A., Gross, W. B. and Siegel, P. B. (1997) *Journal of Applied Poultry Research,* **6**, 123-127

Butler, E. J., Curtis, M. J. and Watford, M. (1973) *Research in Veterinary Science,* **15**, 267-9

Chang, H. R. and Bistrian, B. (1998) *Journal of Parenteral and Enteral Nutrition,* **22**, 156-166

Chapkin, R. S., McMurray, D. N. and Jolly, C. A. (2000) in *Nutrition and Immunology: Principles and Practice* (Gershwin, M. E., German, J. B. and Keen, C. L., eds.), pp. 121-134, Humana Press Inc., Totowa, NJ

Downing, J. E. G. and Miyan, J. A. (2000) *Immunology Today,* **21**, 281-289
Elsasser, T. H., Caperna, T. J. and Rumsey, T. S. (1995) *Journal of Endocrinology,* **144**, 109-117
Elsasser, T. H., Kahl, S., Steele, N. C. and Rumsey, T. S. (1997) *Comparative Biochemistry and Physiology,* **116A**, 209-221
Erf, G. F., Bottje, W. G., Bersi, T. K., Headrick, M. D. and Fritts, C. A. (1998) *Poultry Science,* **77**, 529-37
Fossum, C. (1998) *Domestic Animal Endocrinology,* **15**, 439-44
Friedman, A., Bartov, I. and Sklan, D. (1998) *Poultry Science,* **77**, 956-62
Friedman, A., Meidovsky, A., Leitner, G. and Sklan, D. (1991) *Journal of Nutrition,* **121**, 395-400
Friedman, A., Sklan, D. (1989) *Journal of Nutrition,* **119**, 790-795
Fritsche, K. L., Anderson, M. and Feng, C. (2000) *Journal of Infectious Diseases,* **182 Suppl 1**, S54-61
Fritsche, K. L., Shahbazian, L. M., Feng, C. and Berg, J. N. (1997) *Clinical Science,* **92**, 95-101
Grimble, R. F. (1998) *Nutrition,* **14**, 634-40
Grimble, R. F. and Grimble, G. K. (1998) *Nutrition,* **14**, 605-610
Harbige, L. S. (1998) *Proceedings of the Nutrition Society,* **57**, 555-62
Harmon, B. G., Miller, E. R., Hoefer, J. A., Ullrey, D. E. and Luecke, R. W. (1963) *Journal of Nutrition,* **79**, 269-275
Helyar, L. and Sherman, A. R. (1987) *American Journal of Clinical Nutrition,* **46**, 346-352
Jahoor, F., Wykes, L. J., Reeds, P. J., Henry, J. F., Del Rosario, M. P. and Frazer, M. E. (1995) *Journal of Nutrition,* **125**, 1462-1472
Johnson, R. W. (1998) *Domestic Animal Endocrinology,* **15**, 309-19
Kadis, S., Udeze, F. A., Polanco, J. and Dreesen, D. W. (1984) *American Journal of Veterinary Research,* **45**, 255-9
Klasing, K. C. (1984) *American Journal of Physiology,* **247**, R901-4
Klasing, K. C. (1988) *Poultry Science* **67**, 626-34
Klasing, K. C. (1988) *Journal of Nutrition,* **118**, 1436-1446
Klasing, K. C. and Barnes, D. M. (1988) *Journal of Nutrition,* **118**, 1158-64
Klasing, K. C. and Calvert, C. C. (2000) in *Proceedings of the VIIIth International Symposium on Protein Metabolism and Nutrition* (Lobley, G. E., White, A. and MacRae, J. C., eds.), pp. 253-264, Wageningen Press, Wageningen
Klasing, K. C. and Johnstone, B. J. (1991) *Poultry Science,* **70**, 1781-1789
Klasing, K. C., Laurin, D. E., Peng, R. K. and Fry, D. M. (1987) *Journal of Nutrition,* **117**, 1629-37
Klasing, K. C. and Leshchinsky, T. V. (2000) in *Nutrition and Immunology: Principles and Practice* (Gershwin, M. E., German, J. B. and Keen, C. L., eds.), pp. 363-373, Humana Press, Inc., Totowa, NJ
Knight, C. D., Klasing, K. C. and Forsyth, D. M. (1983) *Journal of Animal Science,*

**57**, 387-95

Krishnan, S., Bhuyan, U. N., Talwar, G. P. and Ramalingaswami, V. (1974) *Immunology,* **27**, 383-393

Lander, H. M. (1997) *FASEB Journal,* **11**, 118-124

Li, Z., Nestor, K. E., Saif, Y. M., Bacon, W. L. and Anderson, J. W. (1999) *Poultry Science,* **78**, 1532-1535

Ling, P. R., Schwartz, J. H. and Bistrian, B. R. (1997) *American Journal of Physiology,* **272**, E333-339

Malmezat, T., Breuille, D., Pouyet, C., Mirand, P. P. and Obled, C. (1998) *Journal of Nutrition,* **128**, 97-105

Malpuech-Brugere, C., Nowacki, W., Gueux, E., Kuryszko, J., Rock, E., Rayssiguier, Y. and Mazur, A. (1999) *British Journal of Nutrition,* **81**, 405-411

Mauldin, J. M., Siegel, P. B. and Gross, W. B. (1978) *Poultry Science,* **57**, 1488-1492

McCann, S. M., Kimura, M., Walczewska, A., Karanth, S., Rettori, V. and Yu, W. H. (1998) *Domestic Animal Endocrinology,* **15**, 333-44

Moriguchi, S., Kobayashi, N. and Kishino, Y. (1990) *Journal of Nutrition,* **120**, 1096-1102

Nauss, K. M., Chew-Chin, P., Ambrogi, L. and Newberne, P. M. (1985) *Journal of Nutrition,* **115**, 909-918

Paludan, S. R. (2000) *Journal of Leukocyte Biology,* **67**, 18-25

Perkkio, M. V., Jansson, L. T., Dallman, P. R., Siimes, M. A. and Savilahti, E. (1987) *American Journal of Clinical Nutrition,* **46**, 341-345

Praharaj, N. K., Gross, W. B., Dunnington, E. A., Nir, I. and Siegel, P. B. (1996) *British Poultry Science,* **37**, 779-786

Prohaska, J. R. and Lukasewycz, O. A. (1989) *Journal of Nutrition,* **119**, 922-931

Qureshi, M. A. and Gore, A. B. (1997) *Immunopharmacology and Immunotoxicology,* **19**, 473-87

Qureshi, M. A. and Havenstein, G. B. (1994) *Poultry Science,* **73**, 1805-1812

Rombout, J. H. W. M., van Rens, B. T. T. M., Sitjsma, S. R., van der Weide, M. C. and West, C. E. (1992) *Veterinary Immunology and Immunopathology,* **31**, 155-166

Rosales, F. J., Ritter, S. J., Zolfaghari, R., Smith, J. E. and Ross, A. C. (1996) *Journal of Lipid Research,* **37**, 962-71

Säemann, M. D., Böhmig G. A. , Ö. C. H., Burtscher, H., Parolini, O., Diakos, C., Stöckl, J., Hörl, W. H. and Zlabinger, G. J. (2000) *FASEB Journal,* **10**, 1096

Semba, R. D. (1998) *Nutrition Reviews,* **56**, S38-S48

Sen, C. K. and Packer, L. (1996) *FASEB Journal,* **10**, 709-720

Twining, S. S., Schulte, D. P., Wilson, P. M., Fish, B. and Moulder, J. (1997) *Journal of Nutrition,* **127**, 558-565

Tyczkowski, J. K. and Hamilton, P. B. (1991) *Poultry Science,* **70**, 2074-2081

Tyczkowski, J. Z. and Hamilton, P. B. (1987) *Poultry Science,* **66**, 2011-2016
von Borell, E., Morris, J. R., Hurnik, J. F., Mallard, B. A. and Buhr, M. M. (1992) *Journal of Animal Science,* **70**, 2714-21
Webel, D. M., Johnson, R. W. and Baker, D. H. (1998a) *Journal of Nutrition,* **128**, 1760-6
Webel, D. M., Mahan, D. C., Johnson, R. W. and Baker, D. H. (1998b) *Journal of Nutrition,* **128**, 1657-60
Weinberg, E. D. (1998) *Cancer Investigation,* **16**, 291-292
Weinberg, E. D. (1999) *Emerging Infectious Diseases,* **5**, 346-352
Weinberg, E. D. (2000) *Microbes and Infection,* **2**, 85-89
Williams, N. H., Stahly, T. S. and Zimmerman, D. R. (1997a) *Journal of Animal Science,* **75**, 2463-71
Williams, N. H., Stahly, T. S. and Zimmerman, D. R. (1997b) *Journal of Animal Science,* **75**, 2481-96
Wu, G., Flynn, N. E., Flynn, S. P., Jolly, C. A. and Davis, P. K. (1999) *Journal of Nutrition,* **129**, 1347-1354
Yang, N., Larsen, C. T., Dunnington, E. A., Geraert, P. A., Picard, M. and Siegel, P. B. (2000) *Poultry Science,* **79**, 799-803
Yoshida, N., Yoshikawa, T., Manabe, H., Terasawa, Y., Kondo, M., Noguchi, N. and Niki, E. (1999) *Journal of Leukocyte Biology,* **65**, 757-63
Zhao, Z., Murasko, D. M. and Ross, A. C. (1994) *Natural Immunity,* **13**, 29-41

*This paper was first published in 2001*

20

# NUTRITION AND IMMUNITY IN FARM ANIMALS

J.C.MEIJER
*Nutreco Swine Research Centre, P.O.Box 240, 5830 AE Boxmeer, The Netherlands*

## Introduction

During the last decade the feed industry had to cope with changing rules, laws and ethical constraints on animal production. The ban on in-feed use of antibiotics for growth promoting purposes has awakened considerable interest in feed additives promising the same positive effects. As a result, many products have been promoted or claimed as the long-awaited non-antibiotic growth promoter. Among them are products that, by virtue of immune stimulation, could help animals to cope with the conditions of modern intensive animal husbandry. It is common knowledge that poorly nourished animals are more susceptible to infectious diseases. Undernutrition, as well as imbalanced nutrition, impairs the immune system, resulting in less effective protection of the host from viral and bacterial infections. In addition, the effects of infection may have a greater effect on the host when nutrition is imbalanced.

The immune system and its intricate functions play a critical role in the relationship between infection and malnutrition. This applies to all life stages but especially susceptible are very young and very old animals.

Another focus of interest and current research is the possibility of stimulating the immune system of healthy animals by nutritional means in the hope of improving health. By improving health the need for antibiotic therapy in animal production will decrease. Thus, high-health livestock will provide safe food.

Since food animals generally are short lived as a matter of economics, the effects of proper functioning of the immune system on longevity, cardiovascular disease, cancer and diseases of old age are considered less important. For companion animals, however, these aspects are extremely interesting since allergy, asthma, immune diseases, cardiovascular disease and cancer are diagnosed frequently and may have their roots in disorders of the immune system.

## The functioning of the immune system, general principles

### IMMUNITY

The animal body has several defence systems against potentially harmful foreign agents. Skin, mucous membranes and mucous secretions keep away most micro-organisms. The inner body uses the immune system to combat invaders by means of molecules, cells and tissues widely dispersed throughout the body. The lymphoid organs include the bone marrow, thymus, spleen, tonsils, lymph nodes and the aggregates of lymphoid cells known as Gut Associated Lymphoid Tissue (GALT) and Bronchus Associated Lymphoid Tissue. The GALT is of particular importance for pick-up of antigens from the gut contents and is a major lymphoid organ.

The bone marrow produces all white blood cells including lymphocytes, monocytes and granulocytes. The lymphocytes are developed further in the thymus or in the bone marrow, where they differentiate and mature into either T-cells or B-cells. In birds B-cells mature in the Bursa of Fabricius instead of the bone marrow. Monocytes develop into macrophages when they penetrate tissues. Granulocytes are phagocytes and can chemically destruct foreign material. Concentrations of immune cells are present in the lymphoid organs, and large numbers circulate through the body as white blood cells. Several types have different tasks and specializations.

T-cells destroy infected cells, carry antigen memory and regulate the activity of B-cells.They constitute cellular immunity. B-cells produce antibodies and constitute humoral immunity. T-helper 1 cells activate the generation of lymphocytes and a cellular response, T-helper 2 cells activate the B cells to produce antibodies, thus the humoral response. "Suppressor" T-cells can reduce the activity of other functional cells. The cells of the immune system communicate by means of messenger molecules, cytokines or interleukins. Th1 and Th2 cells produce different cytokines. The Th1/Th2 cytokine balance dictates the final type of immune response (Roitt *et al.*, 1985; Shearer and Clerici,1997).

#### *Non-specific immunity*

Macrophages present a primary line of defence by engulfing and chemically destroying any foreign material invading the body. These cells reside in many organs (reticulo endothelial system, Kupfer cells in the liver) or are mobile cells that are attracted to sites of inflammation. Natural killer cells are lymphocytes that recognize and kill abnormal cells.

### *Specific immunity*

Specific immunity is possible because the system can distuinguish the body's own components (self) from foreign invaders (non-self), and because the system can recognize and respond to an unlimited number of different molecules. A fast and enhanced reaction occurs upon re-exposure to a previously encountered foreign agent (the system has "memory").

Self is recognized by the presence of specific marker molecules on the surfaces of all cells in the body. In normal circumstances the cells of the immune system do not attack cells which carry these distinctive "self" molecules. An example is the bloodgroup molecules (glycoproteins) present on the surface of the red blood cells.

However, any encounter with foreign marker molecules activates cells of the immune system into a defensive response. During this response, immature immune cells are tuned to respond to the specific antigen via receptor structures that recognize and interact with the specific targets. A few of those specialized cells remain after the response to a foreign agent is completed and then function as memory cells. Thus, the next time the body encounters the same antigen, the immune system can respond to it quickly and effectively.

*Immunocompetence:* animals are born with some temporary immunity derived from maternal antibodies. Their cellular system is not yet fully differentiated but is in an active stage of development. When the immune system is able to respond to antigens with the formation of antibodies, the host is called immunocompetent. Shortly before hatching (birds) or birth most animals are immunocompetent. However, fullblown competence is normally reached when maternal immunity has subsided completely.

## RESISTANCE

Resistance to infectious diseases has many facets. Some varieties of viruses, bacteria, protozoa, helminths etc. are infectious to some species of host animals but not to others. Well-nourished animals can withstand larger numbers of pathogens. Integrity of skin, mucosa, skin pH, stomach pH, bronchial cleansing all play a part in resistance. The chemical attack of micro-organisms by enzymes and reactive molecules in tears, saliva, mucus and digestive juices also plays a significant role.

## RESILIENCE

Coping with disease is a timely process as is recovery from (sub)clinical disease.

Quick recovery and short duration of susceptibility are best. Feeding, as opposed to fasting, shortens the recovery period of hospital patients. Enhancing feed intake helps to shorten recovery time from infectious disease.

## Factors which alter the immune response: infection and nutrition

Infection and undernutrition are the interrelated major causes of disease and mortality in the developing world (Calder and Jackson, 2000). This statement is also true for animals especially very young and very old ones kept under unhygienic conditions. Undernutrition is a major risk factor for disease and mortality because many nutrients are required to fight off infections. Effective protection against invasion of the host by micro-organisms requires an intact skin and intact linings of organs in contact with the outer world. Since cell turnover rate in these linings is high, nutrients for cell replication and cell growth must be available. The immune response to infection involves a vast increase in cell replication, in the production of acute phase proteins and immunoglobulins and in the production of messenger molecules as cytokines and eicosanoids. An appropriate supply of nutrients is needed to optimize the response. Another component of the response to infection is the chemical destruction of foreign material by reactive O-species. Protection of the host from this damage requires sufficient antioxidant mechanisms, including antioxidant enzymes that all require metal ions, such as Fe, Zn, Cu, Mn, Se as active components, antioxidant vitamins, such as vitamin C and vitamin E, and glutathione. Thus, the host needs a supply of a range of nutrients to maintain protection against infective agents and to mount a succesful response if infected. Deficiencies of some vitamins and minerals impair immunity and disease resistance (Langseth, 1999: Calder and Jackson, 2000).

### INFECTION

Infections can cause malnutrition and hence deficiencies of several nutrients. The low feed intake of sick animals may be caused by the appetite depressant action of cytokines released during inflammation or an active state of the immune system (Kelley *et al.*, 1996).

High and low energy intakes as such can adversely affect the immune response. Especially weight loss or, more general, a katabolic state is associated with decreases in several measures of T-cell, B-cell and other immune cell functions. Severe malnutrition and wasting syndromes lead to impaired immune function. Wasting syndromes are often caused by viral infections, especially immunosuppressive viruses. They are more a problem of young animals under conditions of bad hygiene and high disease pressure. Chronic immune system activation as such leads to less growth and less efficient feed utilization (Williams *et al.*, 1997a,b,c; Sauber and Stahly, 1996).

## ENERGY AND FAT NUTRITION

Most defence mechanisms are impaired in protein-energy malnutrition, even if the nutritional deficiency is only moderate. T-cells are especially affected, resulting in low circulating numbers.

High energy intake results in obesity, which is also associated with impaired immune function, for example reduced responsiveness of T- and B-cells.

Too much fat in the diet can influence immune functions, possibly via a relative protein deficiency.

Animal studies indicate that diets high in fat may depress the immune response and increase the risk of infection, and high fat diets often result in diminished T-cell activity. In typical Western human diets, fat usually contributes some 40% or more of the energy intake. In humans, reduction in dietary fat intake resulted in increased T-cell responsiveness and increased capacity of natural killer cells to destroy tumour cells (Langseth, 1999).

In animal diets the fat content is usually much lower and fat contributes some 15 till 25 % of dietary energy. Obesity is not common in production animals; however, in companion animals overt obesity does occur quite frequently and is recognized as a "disease".

Fat composition in itself can influence immune function because fatty acids are structural components of cell membranes. The fluidity of membranes is affected by the chain length and degree of saturation of the incorporated fatty acids. Fluidity is important for the expression of cell surface structures such as receptors, which play crucial roles in immune function. Polyunsaturated fatty acids (PUFA) can alter the functioning of immune cells considerably. There are two classes of PUFA: the n-6 series found primarily in vegetable oils and the n-3 series found in fish oils and also in certain vegetable oils such as canola, soy, and linseed.

Immune cells use these fatty acids also to produce tissue hormones known as prostaglandins. Depending on the type of PUFA in the diet, immune cells produce different quantities and kinds of prostaglandins with very different effects on the immune response. In addition to their effects on tissue hormone levels, PUFA also exert effects by other mechanisms.

In general, diets rich in n-3 PUFA tend to inhibit the immune response, whereas those rich in n-6 PUFA tend to promote immune responses that lead to inflammation. The ratio of n-6 to n-3 PUFA may be more important than the absolute amount of each of these classes of fatty acids in the diet. This ratio can be influenced greatly by the choice of vegetable oils and animal fats in the diet of man and animal.

The ideal ratio of n-6 to n-3 PUFA is actually unknown, but estimates range from 5:1 to 10:1.

## VITAMINS

Vitamin A deficiency is associated with increased morbidity and mortality in children as well as in animals. Vitamin A deficiency is rare in animal nutrition because it is amply available and cheap Vitamin A plays a very important role in the body's defence against some viruses. An adequate supply is needed for the normal development of many types of epithelial cells and of blood cells, including lymphocytes. Networks of cytokines, which influence immune responses, may also be altered during vitamin A deficiency, and antibody responses to antigens may be modified.

Carotenoids are yellow, orange and red compounds in fruits, vegetables and some algae. Like vitamins C and E, carotenoids are antioxidants. Carotenoids increase specific subsets of lymphocytes, enhance the activity of natural killer cells, stimulate the production of cytokines and activate phagocytic cells (Kim *et al.*, 2000). Of particular interest is the capacity of lycopene to enhance the potency of the immune system.

Vitamin D is also active in the cell nucleus where its receptor is linked with the vitamin A receptor. The complex regulates RNA transcription. Immunomodulating effects of 1,25-dihydroxycholecalciferol have been reported with a shift towards a mucosal IgA response (Van der Stede et al., 2000). The use of 25-hydroxycholecalciferol ("HyD"), which displaces vitamin D3 from its carrier protein in the circulation, possibly results in more vitamin D3 entering the cell nucleus and a stronger immunomodulating effect.

Vitamin E occurs in a variety of plant foods; rich sources are wheat germ oil, maize oil and soyabean oil. Deficiency of vitamin E impairs several aspects of the immune response, including B-cell and T-cell activity. Supplementation of the diet with higher than recommended levels has been shown to enhance certain aspects of immune function in humans and animals, and to increase resistance to infectious diseases. The suggested mechanism by which vitamin E exerts its action on the immune system is by lowering of the prostaglandin synthesis and by preventing the oxidation of PUFA in cell mebranes.

Vitamin C is present in many vegetables and fruits. It is a water-soluble antioxidant, found in body fluids rather than in cellular lipids and membranes. Vitamin C acts as a major antioxidant in the aequous phase and also reinforces the effects of other antioxidants, such as vitamin E, by regenerating their active forms after they have reacted with free radicals. Certain organs in the body concentrate vitamin C to levels far higher than found in the blood. One of these organs is the thymus.

Vitamin C plays an important role in the function of phagocytes. High doses of vitamin C are often applied in an attempt to prevent respiratory infections. It is unclear whether this is effectively reducing common cold and flu.

Vitamin B6 is widely present in a variety of foods including cereals and pulses. Vitamin B6 is essential for synthesis and metabolism of amino acids and protein. Animal studies indicate that deficiencies of vitamin B6 modify T-cell activity and antibody production. High doses above the recommended daily allowance (RDA) do not seem to produce additional benefits.

## MINERALS

Zinc deficiency is associated with skin problems, respiratory infections and diarrhoea.

Cells of the immune system require many enzymes that need zinc to function, thus zinc deficiency has profound effects on immune function. Deficiency suppresses the function of the thymus and lymphocytes become less responsive to chemical signals to grow. Antibody formation and resistance to infections are impaired. Wound healing is impaired in zinc deficiency. Too much zinc also impairs immunity; both phagocytic cell and lymphocyte function are involved, but the mechanism of these effects is not clear. Iron deficiency is associated with gastrointestinal and respiratory infections. The influence of Fe status on infection is a complicated somewhat by the fact that micro-organisms also require Fe for their metabolism. Low Fe status should protect against infection, and the presence of Fe binding lactoferrin in milk probably plays a role protecting the suckling animal against bacterial infections. Thus, there is competition for Fe between the invading pathogens, the host stores and the host immune system.

Symptoms of copper deficiency are anaemia, diarrhoea, weight loss and impaired neutrophil function.

Manganese deficiency results in impaired synthesis of mucopolysaccharides and bone matrix; the mucosal barrier function can also be impaired.

Selenium activates glutathione peroxidase involved in neutralizing peroxides. Se deficiency impairs the antioxidant system of the body. Supplementation with Se and vitamin E has potential benefits but responses vary between animal species (Finch and Turner, 1996).

Some of the basic immune responses and related nutrients are presented in Table 20.1.

**Table 20.1** BASIC METABOLISM OF AN IMMUNE RESPONSE AND NUTRIENTS INVOLVED

| *Immune system* | *Response* | *Metabolic event* | *Nutrients required* |
|---|---|---|---|
| Adaptive | | | |
| Stem cells | Proliferation | Protein synthesis | Amino acids, vitamins A,D, $B_6$ |
| Lymphoid cells | Proliferation | Protein synthesis | |
| T-lymphocytes | Cytokines | Protein synthesis | |
| B-lymphocytes | Antibodies | Protein synthesis | |
| Innate system | | | |
| phagocytes | Cell activity, enzymes, cytokines, | Enzyme activity | Vitamins C,E, arginine, ornithine, Se, Cu, Zn, cofactors |
| | proliferation | Protein synthesis | |
| lysozyme | Increase | Protein synthesis | |
| plasma enzymes | Increase | Protein synthesis | |
| complement | Increase | Protein synthesis | |
| acute-phase proteins | Increase | Protein synthesis | |
| skin, mucosa | Turnover | General | Vitamin A, Zn |
| mucus, sebum, HCl | Turnover | General | |

## Immunonutrition

The use of food or feed enriched with nutrients known to be involved in protein synthesis, immunostimulation or anti-oxidant systems is called immunonutrition. The intention of immunonutrition is to back up disease resistance. The net effect on the animal is measurable, as far as disease incidence and severity are concerned, and economic aspects of growth rate and feed use can be calculated. Effects on isolated aspects of the immunological response usually cannot be used to predict the net effect on animals under conventional husbandry conditions. Therefore, most animal studies with immunomodulating products rely more on measures of animal performance and disease than on immune parameters.

Glucans have been studied in fish (Raa, 1996) as well as in pigs (Dritz *et al.*, 1995; Decuypere *et al.*, 1998; Vancaeneghem *et al.*, 2000) with promising results. Unpublished results of our own research confirm increased disease resistance in weaned piglets fed special b-glucans but not plain yeast cell walls. Herbal products receive much attention and some plant extracts and preparations certainly contain immunomodulatory components (Wills, Bone and Morgan, 2000). Evidence that these products may improve disease resistance under practical husbandry conditions is accumulating; however, reports are still largely anecdotical. Our own research indicates that some herbal products are effective in increasing feed intake and growth in weanling piglets but most of the tested products had no positive effect on either performance or disease.

Probiotics may affect the immune system (McCracken and Gaskins, 1999) but certainly not all probiotics are equally effective under current husbandry conditions. Some lactobacillus species appear to be effective as immunostimulants or as microflora-modulating probiotics. Since they are only active when alive, dry feed is not the ideal carrier because survival of lactobacilli during pelleting and drying of feed is low. Other feed ingredients containing selected strains of lactobacilli can possibly be used to good effect. Fermented feedstuffs offer promise to enhance health and to increase disease resistance.

A summary of immunonutrition is presented in Table 20.2.

**Table 20.2** PRODUCTS ELICITING NON-SPECIFIC ADJUVANT EFFECTS

| *Adjuvant effects* | *Bacterial cell wall components* | *Feed and plant components* |
|---|---|---|
| Inflammatory responses | Bacterial capsule | Glucans from yeast, fungi, grains |
| Activation of complement | Lipopolysaccharide(Gram-negative BCW) | Echinacea extracts |
| Activation of macrophages | Arabinogalactan | Ginseng extracts |
| Activation of B-cells | Peptidoglycan (murein) | Triterpene-saponins |
| Activation of T-cells | Heat stress proteins | Phorbolesters |
| Modified antigen processing | Endotoxins | Cichoric acid |

## Conclusions

Since the immune system serves to safeguard the body from any foreign invading micro-organism, it is always active. Functioning of the system requires cell proliferation, production of protein molecules and enzyme activity to destroy phagocytized material (infected body cells, bacteria, viruses). Nutrients required for the immune system and its responses are for protein synthesis and for oxidative radical production; moreover, the body requires anti-oxidants for protection. Nutrient allowances for growth are also expected to cover the metabolic needs of the immune system. Supplementing the diet with the antioxidant vitamins C and E improves resilience and is favoured whenever disease and infection are present.

In general, all cell-toxic elements will be immunosuppressive. Food should be free from lead, cadmium, mercury, mycotoxins, dioxin, pesticides and organic solvents. As several antibiotics inhibit protein synthesis, they also suppress the immune system; tetracyclines and chloramphenicol are examples, and they should not be used as feed ingredients.

Feed will contain a number of immunomodulators including ß-glucans and arabino(rhamno)galactans of plant, fungal, yeast or microbial origin, saponins and phenolic derivatives. ß-glucans are taken up by M-cells in the gut and stimulate macrophages as well as the complement system. Thus, selected feed ingredients as well as herbal extracts may enhance or modulate immune responses.

The balance between cellular and humoral responses can be altered by feed components; vitamin D may shift the response towards humoral; enhanced cellular activity may result from selected plant extracts. This area offers potential for special feeds for young animals in a stage of imbalance between acquired and maternal immunity, i.e. around weaning when activation of the innate system may increase disease resistance.

The gut microflora is an ever-present source of microbial antigens and adjuvant-active components. Segmented filamentous bacteria stimulate immunity and become part of the flora after weaning to solid food (Snel, 1997). Once established, the complex intestinal ecological system is highly stable and resists establisment of newly introduced organisms. Probiotics may enhance macrophage activity of the innate immune system and the response to particular antigens through adjuvant activity after lysis of the cells. The potential for probiotics is in the period of weaning and, in cases of disturbed intestinal ecology, following oral antibiotic treatment.

Well-balanced quality nutrition is of the utmost importance for disease resistance and the underlying immune processes but cannot compensate for bad husbandry. Hygiene can significantly contribute to better animal performance by reducing the need of the animal for immune responses and the associated metabolic needs (Toussaint *et al.*, 2001).

## References

Calder, P.C. and Jackson, A.A. (2000) Undernutrition, infection and immune function. *Nutrition Research Reviews*,**13**, 3-29

Decuypere, J., Dierick, N. and Boddez, S. (1998) The potentials for immunostimulatory substances (b-1,3/1,6 glucans) in pig nutrition. *Journal of Animal and Feed Sciences*, **7**, Supp.1: 259-265

Dritz, S.S., Shi, J., Kielian, T.L, Goodband, R.D., Nelssen, J.L., Tokach, M.D., Chengappa, M.M., Smith, J.E. and Blecha, F. (1995) Influence of dietary beta-glucan on growth performance, nonspecific immunity and resistance to Streptococcus suis infection in weanling pigs. *Journal of Animal Science*, **73**, 3341-3350

Finch, J.M. and Turner, R.J. (1996) Effects of selenium and vitamin E on the immune responses of domestic animals. *Research in Veterinary Science*, **60**, 97-106

Gaskins, H.R. (1996) Development and structure of mucosal defense in the pig intestine. In *Biotechnology in the Feed Industry,Proceedings of Alltech's 12th Annual Symposium*, pp 23-35. Edited by T. Lyons and K. Jacques. Nottingham: Nottingham University Press

Kelley, K.W., Kent, S. and Dantzer, R. ( 1996) Why sick animals don't grow: an immunological explanation. In *Growth of the Pig*, pp 119-132. Edited by G.R.Hollis. Wallingford: CAB INTERNATIONAL

Kim, H.W., Chew, B.P., Wong, T.S., Park, J.S., Weng, B.B., Byrne, K.M., Hayek, M.G., Reinhardt (2000) Dietary lutein stimulates immune response in the canine. *Veterinary Immunology and Immunopathology*, **74**, 315-327

Kolb, E. Vitamins and the immune system. Basel: Hoffmann-La Roche

Langseth, L. (1999) Nutrition and immunity in man. *ILSI Europe Concise Monograph Series*. Brussels: International Life Sciences Institute, ISBN 12-57881-058-2

McCracken, V.J. and Gaskins, H.R. (1999) Probiotics and the immune system. In *Probiotics: A Critical Review,* pp 85-111. Wymondham: Horizon Scientific Press, ISBN 1-898486-15-8

Raa, J. (1996) The use of immunostimulatory substances in fish and shellfish farming. *Reviews in Fisheries Science*, **4**, 229-288

Roitt, I., Brostoff, J. and Male, D. (1985) Immunology. Gower Medical Publishing, London

Sauber, T.E. and Stahly, T.S. (1996) Chronic immune system activation impairs lactational performance of sows. *Feedstuffs*, July 22

Shearer, G.M and Clerici, M. (1997) Vaccine strategies: selective elicitation of cellular or humoral immunity? *Tibtech* ,**15**, 106-109

Snel, J. (1997) Symbiosis between the mouse and segmented filamentous bacteria, a gnotobiotic study. Thesis, University of Nijmegen, ISBN 90-9010578-6

Toussaint, M.J.M., Paboeuf, F., Madec, F., Meijer, J., Gruys, E. (2001) Impact of environmental condition on growth performance and health of pigs: effect of housing and transport on blood indicators of inflammation. *Journal of Animal Science* (Submitted for publication)

Vancaeneghem, S., Cox, E., Deprez, P., Arnouts, S., Goddeeris, B.M. (2000) Beta glucanen als immunostimulantia en als adjuvantia. *Vlaams Diergeneeskundig*

*Tijdschrift*, **69**, 412-421

Van der Stede, Y., Cox, E., Goddeeris, B.M. (2000) 1-25 Dihydroxyvitamine D3, rol in het immuunsysteem.. *Vlaams Diergeneeskundig Tijdschrift*, **69**, 229-234.

Williams, N.H., Stahly, T.S. and Zimmerman, D.R. (1997) Effect of chronic immune system activation on the rate, efficiency, and composition of growth and lysine needs of pigs fed from 6 to 27 kg. *Journal of Animal Science*, **75**, 2463-2471

Williams, N.H., Stahly, T.S. and Zimmerman, D.R. (1997) Effect of chronic immune system activation on body nitrogen retention, partial efficiency of lysine utilization, and lysine needs of pigs. *Journal of Animal Science*, **75**, 2472-2480

Williams, N.H., Stahly, T.S. and Zimmerman, D.R. (1997) Effect of level of chronic immune system activation on the growth and dietary lysine needs of pigs fed from 6 to 112 kg. *Journal of Animal Science*, **75**, 2481-2496

Wills, R.B.H., Bone, K. and Morgan, M. (2000) Herbal products: active constituents, modes of action and quality control. *Nutrition Research Reviews*,**13**, 47-77

*This paper was first published in 2001*

21

# BACTERIOLOGICAL ASPECTS OF THE USE OF ANTIBIOTICS AND THEIR ALTERNATIVES IN THE FEED OF NON-RUMINANT ANIMALS

K. HILLMAN

*Microbiology unit, SAC Aberdeen, Ferguson building, Craibstone, Aberdeen AB21 9YA, UK*

## Introduction

The prophylactic use of antibiotics in animal feeds has made intensive farming possible, and has shown improved feed conversion in these animals. However, the continuous feeding of low levels of antibiotics over many years has resulted in the formation of a gut microflora which is, overall, resistant to these antibiotics. Incoming pathogens may not be, so the inclusion of these antibiotics in feed should still act prophylactically against the spread of many pathogens. When antibiotics are withdrawn, the intensive nature of modern farming could result in the rapid spread of infective agents.

It may be worth mentioning the distinction between the effects of antibiotics on bacteria when these are used as disease therapy or as growth promoters. Many bacterial populations will contain a few individual cells which are resistant to a particular antibiotic, usually by the production of an enzyme which inactivates the antibiotic. Therapeutic dosing is designed to overwhelm this small resistance, so that the resistant cells do not have the opportunity to re-establish as a resistant population. In the presence of low levels of antibiotic, the resistant cells survive and grow, producing an antibiotic-resistant population (Eichner and Gravitz, 2001). As all the cells in this population can now produce the antibiotic-inactivating enzyme, much higher doses of antibiotic are required to overcome the resistance - often, the dose required would be toxic to the animal.

Antibiotics in therapy can also cause serious intestinal problems, particularly when pathogens such as *Clostridium difficile*, which show a natural resistance to many antibiotics, are present. The disruption of the normal microflora by therapeutic doses of antibiotics provides such pathogens with an opportunity to proliferate and infect (Nord and Edlund, 1990).

This chapter intends to examine the influence of antibiotic use on the gut microflora, and the possible effects of some of the alternatives to antibiotics currently available.

## Antibiotic origins

The discovery of antibiotics is credited to Alexander Fleming, although the use of antibiotic-containing preparations (e.g. as "mouldy-bread poultices") on infected wounds dates back much further. The important term here is "discovery", not "invention". Antimicrobials, including antibiotics, are produced by microorganisms as part of the natural competition between species, and it is likely that such compounds were being produced by microorganisms well before the emergence of the human species. When these compounds were discovered, they were already in an advanced stage of development by microbes. Consequently, the mechanisms of resistance must have been around for almost as long. We cannot now say whether the presence of antibiotic resistant bacteria has been brought about by human activity or whether these microbes have been there all along, although human activity has certainly increased the prevalence of resistance.

## Development of resistance

Continued exposure of a population of bacteria to low levels of antibiotics will result eventually in the development of resistance. As an observation, this is entirely correct, although the mechanism of development of resistance is not dependent on the presence of the antibiotic. The bacterial genome is easily mutated, and can be modified by the incorporation of DNA from the environment, processes which occur continuously. Occasionally, mutation, plasmid transfer or incorporation of DNA will result in the acquisition of resistance to an antibiotic. Even if we consider this to be a rare event, perhaps one in a thousand million, the density of the microbial population of the gut exceeds this number of microorganisms per gram of contents. One antibiotic-resistant bacterium in this population is irrelevant in the absence of the antibiotic, but in the presence of a low concentration of the appropriate antibiotic, this one cell can rapidly proliferate. The antibiotic is therefore not involved in the mechanism of development of the resistance, but represents the selective pressure that allows the proliferation of the resistant strains.

As an example, penicillin interferes with cell wall formation in Gram-positive bacteria. If a population contains a few penicillin-resistant individuals, this is normally due to the formation of a penicillin-degrading enzyme (ß-lactamase, penicillinase). Therapeutic doses of penicillin will overwhelm the penicillinase produced by these individuals so that the population is unable to replicate, making it a simple matter for the immune system to remove the infection.

However, if the population is treated with a low continuous dose of penicillin, the enzyme-producers are unaffected and are able to proliferate while the rest of the population is inhibited. Eventually, the entire population is composed of penicillin-resistant individuals. Now, the total production of penicillinase is such that therapeutic doses of penicillin are simply brushed aside. Further, a large population of a penicillin-resistant species in a complex ecosystem such as the gut could effectively "protect" other, normally penicillin-sensitive, pathogens. Antibiotic resistance is not purely a pathogen-linked problem: even where the antibiotic-degrader is a harmless species, the effectiveness of that antibiotic against an infection may be reduced by virtue of its inactivation by the resistant population.

Antibiotic resistant bacteria thrive in environments with constant exposure to antibiotics because the environmental antibiotics effectively remove those bacteria's competitors. Therefore, if we remove the antibiotic from the microbial environment, then the antibiotic resistant species should decline.

## Removal of resistant strains

The occurrence of antibiotic resistant bacteria in pigs in Denmark is now lower than in those countries where antibiotics are still routinely used in feeds. However, antibiotic resistant bacteria are still present in Danish pigs. In the UK, pigs which have been raised organically still retain some antibiotic resistant bacteria within their guts. It is possible to accelerate the decline of antibiotic resistant strains in the gut by the introduction of an antibiotic-sensitive microflora, but it is not currently possible to eradicate resistance altogether. Are the remaining resistant bacteria a residue of the previous, highly resistant population or do they represent a natural gut population? It may not be possible to answer this question, as this would require access to farmed pigs which have not been fed with antibiotics for many generations, and it is unlikely that such pigs currently exist among domesticated herds. It is therefore difficult to establish a baseline level, where we could say that the resistance caused by human intervention has been removed.

## Development and composition of the intestinal microflora

Until the moment of birth, all animals are microbially sterile. However, the animal is quickly colonised by bacteria from its immediate environment, particularly the mother's urinogenital tract and faeces. All skin surfaces, including the gut, will bear a measurable microbial population within a few hours of birth. Close skin and mouth contact between mother and offspring aid the transfer of parental microflora, while the lactose content of mammalian milk encourages the growth of lactic acid bacteria in the neonate intestine.

Selectivity of the neonatal microflora is also enhanced by immunoglobulins in the milk, so that the gut of the newborn effectively remains under the protection of its mother until weaning.

In the case of poultry, the sterile hatchling derives its microflora by pecking at ground contaminated by adult faeces. As poultry do not subsequently undergo the intestinal disruption caused by weaning, the initially derived microflora effectively determines the microbial status of the gut throughout the bird's life (Nurmi and Rantala, 1973). As the gut microflora is derived from the parent animal, it will contain considerable antibiotic resistance from the moment it begins to develop.

In the nonruminant mammal, abrupt weaning results in a sudden change in the composition of the nutrients provided to both the animal and the intestinal microflora. This dramatic change results in equally dramatic effects within the microflora, as the complex population struggles to adapt to the new environment. There are also considerable changes in the structure of villi and crypts over the weaning period (Ewing and Cole, 1994). These physical changes, along with changes in substrate, result in an unstable intestinal microflora over the weaning period as the microflora, like the host animal, change from infant towards adult structure. The reduction in villus height at weaning can also result in reduced absorption from the small intestine, allowing an increase in fermentable carbohydrate reaching the large intestine, with corresponding increase in fermentative microbial activity (Pluske *et al.*, 1996a).

The lactic acid bacteria that dominate the infant gut are gradually overgrown by strictly anaerobic bacteria such as *Bacteroides* (Ewing and Cole, 1994), as the gut lumen enlarges and the feed becomes more solid, allowing the formation of oxygen-free microbial environments. It is notable that the transition from milk-fed to solid-fed microflora is not a smooth one, with wild daily fluctuations in the composition of the microflora for some 7-14 days after weaning (Reid, 1999). Abrupt weaning in piglets may also be associated with a 100-fold drop in the numbers of lactobacilli in the intestine, and a 50-fold increase in the numbers of *Escherichia coli* (Huis in't Veld and Havenaar, 1993). The process of change in the intestinal microflora continues throughout life, albeit more gradually, with the gut tending to favour a higher proportion of strictly anaerobic bacteria as the animal ages. (Maczulak *et al.*, 1989; Piattoni *et al.*, 1996). The disruption of the gut at weaning often results in intestinal infection, requiring treatment with antibiotics which would favour the retention of antibiotic-resistant strains. So, even where the young animal has never been directly fed with antibiotics, it may still harbour a significant antibiotic-resistant microbial population within its gut.

The composition of the intestinal microflora thus depends on the initial colonisation at birth, on the current state of the gut physiology, on the type of feed consumed by the animal, and also on its genetic predisposition to the maintenance of some of the component species. The genetic composition of the host animal has been identified as an important component in certain cases, notably in pigs in susceptibility to the various substrains of *Escherichia coli* K88 (Bijlsma *et al.*, 1982; Vogeli *et al.*, 1992). A less well known example exists in the genetic predisposition to harbouring methane-producing bacteria shown by certain animal species (Hackstein *et al.*, 1995: Hackstein *et al.*, 1996).

More recently, data has been collected which suggests that intestinal lactobacilli with antipathogenic activity are not evenly distributed between pigs: some farms show a high prevalence of these active lactobacilli in pigs, while others show little or no antipathogenic activity within their lactobacilli. A preliminary study (Table 21.1; Hillman and Robertson, 2001) has shown a wide variation in the inherent antipathogenic activity of intestinal lactobacilli in pigs from 19 farms. In this study, the ability of isolated *Lactobacillus* spp to inhibit the growth of *Escherichia coli* K88 was assessed (Hillman and Fox, 1994) and the isolates were grouped by the significance of the difference between the growth rates of *E. coli* in the presence or absence of the lactobacillus. Although only a small part of the total lactobacilli within the intestine could be sampled in this study, those tested were isolated from high dilutions of colonic contents and should therefore represent the predominant groups within the colonic population of these pigs. The data obtained contained examples of both zero and 100% probiotic activity within the colonic *Lactobacillus* population of pigs, with a range of activities detected within the samples from most farms. The implication is that this distribution could affect perceived efficacy of many added antibacterials, particularly probiotics, since adding an antimicrobial to a population with a high indigenous antimicrobial activity is likely to be less effective than adding it to a population which shows little or no such activity. Whether this variation is connected with the genetics of the animals is not known, but the pattern of distribution within herds rather than as a random distribution among individuals suggests that this possibility may be worthy of consideration.

**Table 21.1** NUMBERS OF ISOLATES OF *LACTOBACILLUS* SPP FROM 19 FARMS, GROUPED BY SIGNIFICANCE OF INHIBITION OF *E. COLI* K88

| | *Farm no.* | | | | | | | | | | | | | | | | | | |
|---|---|---|---|---|---|---|---|---|---|---|---|---|---|---|---|---|---|---|---|
| | *1* | *2* | *3* | *4* | *5* | *6* | *7* | *8* | *9* | *10* | *11* | *12* | *13* | *14* | *15* | *16* | *17* | *18* | *19* |
| ns | 6 | 4 | 6 | 4 | 7 | 6 | 3 | 8 | 6 | 3 | | 4 | 8 | 10 | 7 | 10 | 3 | 4 | 39 |
| *P*<0.05 | | | 3 | 2 | 1 | | 2 | 1 | | 1 | | | | | | | 1 | 4 | 4 |
| *P*<0.01 | 4 | 2 | | 2 | | 2 | 4 | 1 | | 3 | 2 | 1 | | | | | 4 | | 9 |
| *P*<0.001 | | 4 | | | | | | | | 3 | 5 | 2 | | | | | 1 | 2 | 2 |
| Total | 10 | 10 | 9 | 8 | 8 | 8 | 9 | 10 | 6 | 10 | 7 | 7 | 8 | 10 | 7 | 10 | 9 | 10 | 54 |

ns, no. of isolates showing no significant inhibitory activity. *P* values, no. of isolates showing significant inhibitory activity at the levels indicated. Total, total no. of isolates per farm. Farm 19 was the SAC Tillycorthie experimental farm, while farms 1-18 were commercial piggeries within Scotland.

Seasonal variation in Campylobacter carriage by poultry has been demonstrated (Wallace *et al.*, 1997), indicating that seasonal effects on the microbial population of the gut may also occur in other cases. Our own studies have produced indications of seasonal changes in the populations of *Lactobacillus* spp, *Bifidobacterium* spp, coliform bacteria and *Clostridium* spp, though not in total anaerobic bacteria or *Bacteroides* spp, in the colonic digesta of pigs (Stefopoulou and Hillman, unpublished). Although the experimental work is currently incomplete, the data obtained so far suggest that the effects of any attempt at gut manipulation may depend on the time of year at which it is applied. This would be particularly true in the case of feed additives which include, or which are intended to affect, the coliform or lactic acid bacteria.

These variations in the intestinal microflora, together with other known sources of variation such as animal age, herd and individual differences and dietary effects, would probably be entirely predictable if their causes were better understood. At the moment, it is not possible to take account of these variabilities within animal trials (more importantly, in comparing data from different trials) because the influence of many of these causes of variation have not been fully studied. It is, however, important to be aware that replication of experimental work will be influenced by all of these factors, and possibly by many other factors not yet identified. It is therefore possible that two separate studies into the effects of a feed additive on the growth of an animal species may give different results, although both datasets would be correct within the current state of all these variables.

## Stability of the intestinal microflora and its importance to health and growth

Where a mixed microbial population is in a state of constant change, opportunities arise for the introduction of new species into the population as niches become temporarily accessible. However, when the same mixed population is stable, *ie* its nutrient supply and environmental conditions do not change rapidly, then all available niches within the system are occupied by one or more species of microorganism. Put simply, this means that any incoming microorganism would have to compete for a niche by displacing its current occupant. For this reason, a stable intestinal microflora is inherently more resistant to pathogenic infection than an unstable one (Van der Waaij *et al.*, 1971; Nurmi and Rantala, 1973; Hill *et al.*, 1986). Much of the resistance of the intestine to invading bacterial species can be attributed to direct competition and inhibition of the invader by the existing microflora (e.g. Wilhelm *et al.*, 1987, Hillman *et al.*, 1994). For the same reasons, an incoming antibiotic-sensitive bacterial species would have to compete with the established antibiotic-resistant strain of the same species in order to remove it. It should be noted that viruses, and many protozoan pathogens, do not take part in the competition for niche and nutrients between the bacteria and so are able to bypass this level of pathogen-resistance.

The health of the gut has a direct bearing on the growth and productivity of livestock animals, since the gut comprises the body's largest organ and represents a considerable part of the animal's protein and energy requirements (Edmunds, Buttery and Fisher, 1980; Murumatsu, Takasu, Furuse, Takaski and Ikumura, 1987). Therefore, an inefficient gut will result in an increased drain on these resources, resulting in less of the feed being converted to muscle tissue. At the same time, a diseased intestine will result in general ill health of the animal, leading to reduced feed intake which would exacerbate the inefficiency of feed conversion. So, providing a stable, disease-resistant microflora within the gut would lead to improved productivity by the animal.

What is actually required in a production system is not a "normal" intestinal microflora, but the development of an "optimal" microflora, which would provide the maximum protection from infection while minimising the microbial use of the animal's feed. There is no reason to suppose that a normal, or wild-type, microflora would be optimised for growth of the animal. In the wild state, animals whose intestines are optimised for disease-resistance would fare better than those optimised for growth, even if enhanced disease-resistance resulted in a higher microbial load for the gut. It is possible that improved growth and improved disease resistance may not be mutually exclusive, although a reduction in numbers or activity of the indigenous microflora would be expected to result in a reduction in its anti-pathogenic activity.

## Alternatives to antibiotics

Developing an alternative to antibiotics is hampered by one important question - what is it that antibiotics do to the gut to improve animal performance? This has never been clear, although some plausible theories have been put forward, such as an improvement in vitamin $B_{12}$ assimilation by reducing the activity of those bacteria which utilise $B_{12}$ while leaving the $B_{12}$-producers unaffected (Postgate, 1992). The idea that antibiotics reduce total bacterial load in the gut is, however, not realistic. While a reduction in total bacteria may be observed within the first few days of treatment, the intestinal bacteria would take very little time to replace the inhibited groups with either new, resistant strains or with bacterial groups which display a natural resistance to the antibiotic. The total bacterial load of any environment is determined by the availability of nutrients and suitable niches for bacterial growth. If we kill one strain of bacteria in an environment like the gut, another will quickly replace it.

So, in the absence of a defined mechanism of action for an antibiotic growth promoter, it is futile to look for something which "works in the same way". Rather, we should look for something that produces the same end result, ie. faster-growing and more cost-efficient animals. Unfortunately, this can only be reliably done by the use of lengthy and expensive animal feeding trials.

It is beyond the scope of this work to provide a comprehensive discussion of all available potential alternatives. The following paragraphs consider a few of the alternatives available, as well as some potentially useful future products which are still at the research stage.

## DIETARY MANIPULATION

Possibly the least controversial method of adjusting the intestinal microflora is by adjusting the composition of the diet: this involves no additives of any kind and can be argued to be a completely "natural" form of controlling gut bacteria. Significant differences in the composition of the gut microflora can be achieved by dietary alterations, which may be as simple as changing the source or treatment of the starch component of the diet (Reid and Hillman, 1999). The amylose/amylopectin content of the starch, the structure of the granule and the degree of pre-feed treatment, influences both the extent of its digestion within the small intestine and the nature of the fermentation of the undigested residue by intestinal bacteria (Reid, 1999; Reid *et al.*, 1998). The effects of three starches, singly and in combination, on the microflora of the piglet colon are shown in Table 21.2 (McFarland, 1998).

**Table 21.2** SELECTED BACTERIAL COUNTS (PER GRAM WET WEIGHT) IN THE PROXIMAL COLON OF WEANED PIGLETS FED MEAL DIETS CONTAINING DIFFERENT STARCHES

| | *Potato* | *Waxy maize* | *Maize* | *Potato/ waxy maize* | *Potato/ maize* | *Maize/ waxy maize* | *SED* |
|---|---|---|---|---|---|---|---|
| Total anaerobes | $9.82^{a}$ | $8.66^{b}$ | $8.88^{b}$ | $10.05^{a}$ | $9.86^{a}$ | $9.56^{ab}$ | 0.43 |
| Coliform bacteria | $1.90^{a}$ | $6.93^{b}$ | $7.88^{b}$ | $6.12^{b}$ | $4.24^{ab}$ | $7.12^{b}$ | 1.81 |
| *Escherichia coli* | $1.73^{a}$ | $6.62^{bc}$ | $7.39^{c}$ | $5.99^{bc}$ | $3.64^{ab}$ | $6.52^{bc}$ | 1.62 |
| *Lactobacillus* spp. | $9.62^{a}$ | $8.62^{b}$ | $8.76^{ab}$ | $9.67^{a}$ | $9.67^{a}$ | $9.17^{ab}$ | 0.42 |
| *Enterococcus* spp. | $5.20^{a}$ | $6.44^{ab}$ | $7.43^{b}$ | $6.11^{ab}$ | $4.69^{a}$ | $6.19^{ab}$ | 0.90 |
| *Bacteroides* spp. | $7.16^{a}$ | $7.43^{ab}$ | $7.16^{a}$ | $8.27^{bc}$ | $8.54^{c}$ | $7.17^{a}$ | 0.44 |

Values within a row bearing different superscript letters differ significantly ($P<0.05$).
Data represent the means of determinations from three piglets on each diet.

In this study, potato starch was found to significantly suppress coliform and *Escherichia coli* numbers in relation to the other two starches. Mixtures of these starches produced intermediate effects in comparison with individual starches, suggesting that this form of manipulation should have the potential to accurately control microbial populations within the gut.

However, there is an important disadvantage in reliance on dietary manipulation. Starch, and other feed components, are natural products, and are therefore inherently variable. In the case of starch, the precise amylose/amylopectin content, granule size and structure, gelatinisation temperature and other factors are dependent on the growing conditions of the plant from which the starch was extracted. Therefore, the effects obtained in this one trial cannot be reliably extrapolated to other situations, because the starches and their effects will vary from one year to the next. Additionally, starches from the same plant species grown in different climates will show differences in response when fermented by intestinal bacteria. Although the general principles should remain consistent (ie, potato starch should result in lower coliform numbers than maize starch), the actual values obtained may show considerable variation. When this is superimposed on other sources of variation inherent in bacteriological studies of the gut (discussed earlier), it is clear that dietary manipulation is currently an imprecise tool in the control of the gut microflora. It is possible that, in the future, accurate and comprehensive chemical analysis of feed components would allow for a more accurate control by dietary manipulation, but at the present time this method is not sufficiently reproducible for commercial application.

## ENZYMES

Although the addition of supplementary enzymes to diets does not directly affect the intestinal bacteria, there is an indirect effect analogous to that observed as a result of dietary manipulation. Feed components such as phytates and non-starch polysaccharides cannot normally be digested by the host animal and therefore become available for fermentation in the colon (pigs) or caeca (birds). Where enzymes are used to render normally indigestible components of the diet susceptible to small intestine digestion, there will be a resultant reduction in the proportions of these components reaching the fermentative bacteria of the lower gut (Ferraz de Oliveira, Hillman and Acamovic, 1994). There may therefore be considerable indirect effects on the intestinal microflora as a result of enzyme treatment of animal diets. Whether or not these effects will all be bacteriologically advantageous is not clear at this time, although a reduction in the concentration of non-starch polysaccharide reaching the lower gut is desirable, as this has been implicated as an initiator of porcine dysentery (Pluske *et al.*, 1998).

## ORGANIC ACIDS

Eidelsburger *et al.* (1992) found that live-weight gain in piglets was increased by the addition of formic acid to the feed, although buffering the feed with sodium bicarbonate reduced this effect. The addition of sodium bicarbonate to a negative control reduced live-weight gain, possibly due to buffering of stomach acids. The improvement in feed conversion ratio obtained with formic acid was not affected by buffering the feed, although the protection against diarrhoea afforded by the acid was abolished.

Feeds with high buffering capacity have adverse effects on animal performance, probably by buffering of stomach acids with a consequent reduction in pepsin activity (Eidelsburger *et al.*, 1992). Reduced stomach efficiency may result in increased feed retention with consequent reduced intake. The reciprocal of this would be that feed acidification would improve the efficiency of digestion in the stomach, resulting in a shorter retention time and improved feed intake.

The most likely mechanisms by which organic acid growth promoting feed additives improve feed conversion efficiency include acidification, either of the feed or of the gut, or selective inhibition of particular intestinal microorganisms. They may also be absorbed directly by the animal, providing an additional nutrient source. The reason for the reported protection from diarrhoea by certain acids is not immediately apparent. Although reduced gut pH would inhibit most pathogens, this effect would be required in the lower gut. Acidification has not been reported to extend this far.

The stomach of the young pig does not secrete sufficient hydrochloric acid to deal with the solid feed it receives at weaning (Ravindran and Kornegay, 1993). Acid secretion in the piglet stomach takes some 3-4 weeks after weaning to reach appreciable levels, so that acidification of feed for weaned piglets may be effective in reducing gastric pH. Inefficient digestion of the feed allows undigested material to reach the colon, and the presence of large quantities of fermentable material in the colon may allow the proliferation of pathogenic microorganisms, resulting in colitis and diarrhoea (Pluske *et al*, 1998). It is therefore possible that the reported reduction in diarrhoea in animals fed acidified feeds is due to a reduction in colonic fermentation, as a consequence of improved digestion in the stomach and small intestine. If this is the case, reducing the proportion of poorly digested carbohydrate in the diet of the piglet would result in a similar reduction in diarrhoea to that observed with acidification.

Although the principal areas of microbial fermentation in the pig are the caecum and colon, there is considerable microbial activity in the small intestine, and bacteria are present throughout the digestive tract of all animals (Ewing and Cole, 1994). In poultry, most microbial activity is found in the caeca. It is difficult to define the role of poultry caecal microflora since surgical removal of these organs seems to have little effect on the health or growth of the bird (Lewis and Swan, 1971). However, Gasaway (1976) suggested that up to 10% of the energy requirements of birds may be provided by volatile fatty acids produced by the microflora of the caeca, while the microbial fermentation in the large intestine of pigs may produce enough volatile fatty acids to account for up to 20% of the maintenance energy requirement for the piglet (Freind *et al.*, 1964). Since a considerable proportion of the energy requirements of birds and pigs can be obtained from the organic acids produced by intestinal microbial fermentation, the possibility that the provision of additional organic acids in the feed may act as a rapidly-absorbed energy source cannot yet be ruled out. Although the increase in growth observed appears out of proportion to the energy content of the added acids, this may be a contributory factor in the observed response.

## PREBIOTICS

Most dietary sugars are digested and absorbed in the small intestine. However, complex oligosaccharides may survive small intestinal digestion and reach the lower gut intact, where they are fermented by intestinal bacteria. With careful selection, oligosaccharides have the potential to selectively enhance specific groups of bacteria.

The term "prebiotic" is used to define those compounds which selectively enhance particular microorganisms in the intestinal tract. The prebiotic may be fed alone, or as a selective substrate in combination with a suitable probiotic bacterium. Normally, compounds are used which are not digested by the host animal, although the use of the term "prebiotic" is occasionally vague, sometimes referring to the prefermentation of food by lactic acid bacteria (Bengmark, 1998) and may also be interchanged with other terms such as "biobiotic" or "synbiotic". The choice of term is perhaps unfortunate, as "prebiotic" has long been used to refer to the chemical soup from which life first developed. This poses considerable difficulties in researching the literature.

Studies *in vitro* have demonstrated the selective enhancement of the growth of certain groups of intestinal bacteria by oligosaccharides, obtained by the hydrolysis of oat beta-glucan and xylan hydrolysates (Jaskari *et al.*, 1998). Fructooligomers increased the growth of *Bacteroides*, *Clostridium* and *Escherichia* as well as *Lactobacillus* and *Bifidobacterium*; while beta-glucooligomers and xylooligomers enhanced the *Lactobacillus* and *Bifidobacterium* strains preferentially but not significantly.

Sucrose caramel, containing a high proportion of oligofructose, can improve growth rate and feed conversion in poultry, and can increase the proportions of *Lactobacillus* and *Bifidobacterium* in the caeca (Manley-Harris and Richards 1994; Orban *et al.*, 1997). However, this caramel had no effect when fed to pigs (Orban, Patterson, Adeola, Sutton and Richards, 1997). Galactosyl-lactose was found to produce improved live-weight gain, comparable to the use of oxytetracycline/neomycin, in week-old calves (Quigley *et al.*, 1997). These sugars appear to work well in both poultry and cattle, although no reports of their successful use in pig diets has been found. It is possible that they act as fermentation-modifiers and are suited more to the low-oxygen environments of the rumen and of the caeca of hens.

In pigs, mannose (mannan)-oligosaccharides have been shown to produce improvements in live-weight gain and feed conversion efficiency comparable to that obtained with olaquindox, or with a combination of Zn-bacitracin and toyocerin (Bolduan *et al.*, 1997). Piglets fed mannan-oligosaccharides in combination with a probiotic (*Enterococcus faecium* M74) showed significant improvements in live-weight gain, feed conversion efficiency and fibre digestibility (Kumprecht and Zobac, 1998). As the surface structures of the intestinal mucosa carry mannose residues which are used as receptors for attachment by many bacteria, and by dietary lectins, mannose and manno-oligosaccharides are important in intestinal toxicity and pathogenicity. Manno-oligosaccharides may therefore directly inhibit the activity of certain lectins by competitive binding (Oda and Tatsumi, 1993) and may also interfere with pathogen attachment.

Since much of the microflora of the intestine cannot currently be isolated and cultured, it is difficult to determine with certainty which species are making use of prebiotic substances. Additionally, making significant alterations to the numbers or activity of one genus of intestinal bacteria may have consequences for many other genera in terms of the substrates used and produced by the enhanced population. For example, the numbers of *Bifidobacterium* spp. can be increased in the gut by the use of inulin - but *Bifidobacterium* has complex nutrient requirements, including a requirement for vitamin K. Therefore, increasing that population 10-fold will result in a 10-fold increase in the requirement for vitamin K within the gut lumen, possibly depriving other genera of this and other nutrients. The gut microflora is a complex system, and the whole system must be considered in attempts at manipulation.

## PROBIOTICS

The intended uses of probiotics are as a prophylactic for the prevention of intestinal disease or to accelerate re-stabilisation of the microflora after illness or antibiotic therapy (Fuller, 1992). They are generally of limited use in the treatment of active infection, since it is difficult for any bacterium to remove an established pathogen. The growth-promoting and other effects reported as a result of probiotic application are outwith the original intention of the products, but may arise as a natural consequence of improvements to the health and efficiency of the gut. Some probiotic preparations have been shown to produce antibiotic-like compounds, which have direct effects on particular groups of bacteria within the gut. Whether these compounds constitute the primary mode of action of the probiotic is unknown; the effects observed under *in vitro* conditions may not correspond exactly with the action of these cultures *in vivo*. It is therefore difficult to assess whether the mode of action of the probiotic growth promoter is similar to that of the antibiotic growth promoter, since little is known of the modes of action of either.

Furthermore, since poultry do not undergo the disruption of weaning, this microflora can persist throughout the life of the bird. The disruption of weaning results in the removal of any probiotic protection which may have been applied to monogastric or ruminant animals at birth, so that continued dosing with large numbers of probiotic bacteria is required throughout the weaning period.

A probiotic preparation may consist of a pure culture of one species, a mixture of known species in known proportions, or an undefined general gut microflora. An example of the latter would be the familiar Nurmi principle, in which the dosing of newly-hatched chicks with a healthy, *Salmonella*-free adult microflora can lead to the establishment of a *Salmonella*-resistant microflora in the adult chickens (Nurmi and Rantala, 1973).

The bacterial species in current use as probiotics for farmed animals comprise principally *Lactobacillus* and *Enterococcus* species, sometimes *Bacillus*, occaisionally *Escherichia* (Goerg and Schlorer, 1998) species. Unusual species have been tried, such as the diatom algae *Scenedesmus* and the cyanobacteria *Spirulina* and *Aphanizomenon* (Kay, 1991) although these do not appear to have found commercial application. Organisms which are to be active in the intestine must be able to survive in that environment, so they require, for example, resistance to bile salts (Chateau *et al.*, 1994) and acid tolerance (e.g. Nemcova *et al.*, 1997) and an ability to inhibit pathogenic bacteria is desirable. They should also prove capable of competing effectively within the gut microflora (e.g. Kontula *et al.*, 1998). Diatoms and cyanobacteria are unlikely to fulfil these requirements.

Yeast and mould probiotics, often using strains of *Saccharomyces cerevisiae* and *Aspergillus oryzae*, can produce improvements in live-weight gain, feed conversion efficiency and milk production in cattle (reviewed by Stewart *et al.*, 1995). Both appear to work by enhancing rumen fermentation. These probiotic fungi do not colonise the rumen, neither are they typical inhabitants of the non-ruminant intestine. It is therefore unsurprising that yeast populations were not maintained in the intestine when a yeast-based probiotic was used in pig feeds (Mathew *et al.*, 1998), although these authors reported an improvement in daily weight gain in pigs with this probiotic. There were no detectable effects on the intestinal microflora.

Yeast-based probiotics do not appear to have significant beneficial effects on the intestinal microflora of the pig, although an effect which may be related to the mechanism of action in the rumen has been observed in the caeca of hens (Andruetto and Doglione, 1993).

**Table 21.3** COMPARISONS OF BACTERIAL PROBIOTICS FOR PIGS WITH ANTIBIOTIC FEED ADDITIVES

| *Additive* | *Growth* | *Feed conversion efficiency* | *Authors* |
|---|---|---|---|
| Virginiamycin | + | - | Harper *et al*, 1983 |
| Freeze-dried *Lactobacillus acidophilus* | - | - | |
| Tylosin | + | + | Pollman *et al*, 1980 |
| ASP-250 | + | + | |
| Lincomycin | + | + | |
| *L. acidophilus* | + | + | |
| *Streptococcus faecium* C68 | - | —* | |
| Furazolidone | + | + | Zani *et al*, 1998 |
| *Bacillus cereus* ("CenBiot") | + | + | |
| Zn-bacitracin | + | ++ | Adami *et al*, 1997 |
| *B. coagulans* | ++ | + | |
| Carbadox | + | | Kreuzer, 1994 |
| *B. licheniformis* + *B. subtilis* ("BioPlus 2B") | + | | |
| Carbadox + BioPlus 2B | ++ | | |
| Zn-bacitracin | + | | Vassalo *et al*, 1997 |
| *B. toyoi* | + | | |
| *L. acidophilus* + *S. faecium* + *Saccharomyces cerevisiae* | + | | |

* In this case, the organism resulted in reduced feed conversion efficiency.

A selection of studies comparing the efficacy of probiotic growth promoters with feed antibiotics in pigs is shown in Table 21.3. These studies are, on the whole, supportive of the use of certain probiotic bacteria as replacements for growth-promoting antibiotics in pig feeds. However, while the results of probiotic administration can equal that of antibiotics, the probiotics appear to be less consistent in activity than antibiotics in both pigs and poultry (reviewed by Thomke and Elwinger, 1998). It is therefore the consistency of activity, rather than the degree of activity, which needs to be improved in the probiotic growth promoters.

A probiotic *Sporolactobacillus* sp. increased apparent absorption of glucose, galactose, and amino-nitrogen in growing pigs. The effects were lost immediately on withdrawal of the supplement, so that the presence of live bacteria was important (Rychen and Nunes, 1993). These same authors later reported that three probiotics (*Sporolactobacillus*, *Bacillus cereus* and a mixture of *Lactobacillus acidophilus*, *Lactobacillus fermentum* and *Lactobacillus brevis*) showed no effect on glucose, galactose or lactic acid absorption, although the absorption of amino-nitrogen was increased (Rychen and Nunes, 1995). So, variable results have been found by the same authors within a single probiotic preparation.

There have been a number of other reports concerning the efficacy of probiotics as growth promoters in pigs, although as these have not included an antibiotic as a positive control so that direct comparison of their effectiveness in relation to a feed antibiotic is not possible (Table 21.4). Most reports show improvements in comparison with a control, but most gains due to probiotic application occur in the first few weeks after weaning.

Studies on probiotics for poultry show results similar to those observed in pigs. Often, the probiotic produces enhancements in growth and/or feed conversion comparable to those observed with an antibiotic (Cavazzoni *et al.*, 1998; Zuanon *et al.*, 1998). These effects are most marked in the first few weeks of growth (Yeo and Kim, 1997; Jin *et al.*, 1998; Istvan *et al.*, 1995). It appears that the benefits of probiotics are restricted to the young animal. It is possible that these improvements, where they occur, are a consequence of improved function in the immature gut. The gut of the fully mature animal may not require the additional protection of extraneous lactobacilli. Additionally, a much larger gut would require a correspondingly larger dose of probiotic in order for any effects to become apparent.

Despite the variability in activity of many probiotic preparations, and the apparent restriction of their utility to the young animal, it is possible that the use of probiotics during early growth may lead to savings on feed due to improved feed conversion efficiency. In the neonate, it is also possible that faster early growth may result in more robust young animals with improved disease resistance.

The overall conclusion must be that while probiotics can be as efficient at growth promotion in pigs as antibiotics, the consistency of their activity seems poor. This may, in part, be due to the wide range of strains and species employed as probiotic strains, and to the variability in the culture conditions used to produce the organisms. It is notable that none of the growth studies with probiotics provide the criteria used for the selection of these strains; in many

**Table 21.4** REPORTED EFFECTS OF PROBIOTIC PREPARATIONS ON PIGLETS

| *Organism(s)* | *Reported effects* | *Authors* |
|---|---|---|
| "LBC" (unidentified lactic acid bacteria) | No beneficial effects on piglet performance, whether fed directly to piglets or to the sow. | Kowarz *et al.* (1994) |
| *Bifidobacterium longum* | No effect on either growth or feed intake of piglets. | Brown *et al.* (1997) |
| *Bif. pseudolongum* | Significant increase in piglet growth, improved FCR and reduced mortality. | Abe *et al.* (1995) |
| *Lactobacillus casei* | Weight gain improved by 10% over 14 days | Danek *et al.* (1991) |
| *L. acidophilus* | Significant increase in piglet growth, improved feed conversion and reduced mortality. | Abe *et al.* (1995) |
| *Enterococcus faecium* M74* | Increased piglet live-weight gain by 5.75%, improved feed conversion. | Kumprecht and Zobac (1998) |
| *Streptococcus faecium* M74* + *L. casei* | Improved weight gain, reduced coliform numbers in the gut. | Tortuero *et al.* (1995) |
| *S. thermophilus* + *L. bulgaricus* | Improved weight gain over the 12-21 days period only. Reduced coliform numbers in the intestine, increased phagocyte activity in the ileal epithelium. | Tortuero *et al.* (1995) |
| *Bacillus* C.I.P. 32 | In weaned piglets, this improved weight gain by 7 to 25%, while reducing feed intake by 8%. Improved crude protein degradation in the intestine. | Kumprecht *et al.* (1994) |

*The genus *Enterococcus* is taxonomically a recent subset of the genus *Streptococcus*, and the two names may be considered to be synonymous for the purposes of this discussion.

cases the authors appear to have used either a randomly selected lactic acid bacterium, or one which has previously been demonstrated to have antipathogenic activity. Relatively few *Lactobacillus* species, or strains of species, exhibit probiotic activity (Hillman and Fox, 1994), so that random selection is unlikely to result in a useful isolate. Further variation may be attributed to the means of dosing; the efficacy of a *Lactobacillus plantarum* at inhibiting the establishment of *Listeria monocytogenes* in an *in vitro* porcine colon simulation was abolished by including the probiotic with the feed (Hillman *et al.*, 1998). A more consistent means of probiotic production, together with an improved understanding of the mechanisms underlying their activity, would lead to more reliable criteria for the selection of potential strains so that consistency in results can be improved. The criteria for selection should also consider the antibiotic resistance profile of the probiotic organism.

## ANTIBIOTIC RESISTANCE IN BACTERIAL PROBIOTICS

In laboratory culture, probiotic *Lactobacillus* spp. were inhibited by as little as 0.4 $\mu g\ ml^{-1}$ of monensin, narasin, lasalocid, salinomycin or maduramycin, but in a mixture of the commercial preparation with water, the lactobacilli were resistant to up to 100 $\mu g\ g^{-1}$ (Marounek and Rada, 1995). As the probiotic proved much more resistant to these antibiotics in a commercial mixture than in laboratory culture, the use of combined probiotic/antibiotic preparations would seem a viable option. Indeed, Mohan *et al.* (1996) showed that using a probiotic in conjunction with an antibiotic provided improved weight gain in poultry in excess of that provided by either the probiotic or antibiotic alone.

However, the principal reason for the removal of antibiotics from animal feeds is the potential for development of resistance to clinical antibiotics in the intestinal microflora. Certainly, antibiotic resistance can develop in a microbial population continually exposed to low doses of the drugs, and the genes coding for resistance can, in many cases, be passed from one bacterium to a related species by conjugation. This feature is not restricted to pathogenic bacteria. Many bacterial species can transfer genes by conjugation, including lactobacilli (Wagner and Balish, 1998; Gabin-Gauthier *et al.*, 1991)

Vancomycin resistance is widespread in some species of *Lactobacillus*, which may indicate a potential for direct transfer of antibiotic resistance to intestinal bacteria. Since many of these vancomycin-resistant *Lactobacillus* species are already present in the intestine, the addition of more of the same may be seen as an insignificant problem. However, the nature of this resistance is currently unclear, as is its potential for transfer. Vancomycin resistance has not been found in *L. acidophilus* or *L. delbrueckii*, but has been found in *L. rhamnosus, L. paracasei, L. plantarum, L. fermentum, L. confusus, L. salivarius* and *L. buchneri*, (Hamilton-Miller and Shah, 1998). Some of these strains are in current use as probiotics and in the preparation of human and animal fermented foods and feeds.

In the absence of antibiotic, resistant strains have no competitive advantage and their numbers reduce. However, continually adding a strain carrying an antibiotic-resistance would increase the potential for transfer of this resistance to other species. Bacteria intended for probiotic use should therefore be screened for antibiotic resistance before the product is released, to avoid the potential carriage of undesirable antibiotic resistance into the intestinal environment (Charteris *et al.*, 1998). Furthermore, the combination of an antibiotic with a probiotic which carries resistance to that antibiotic is, in microbial terms, equivalent to applying a selective pressure while simultaneously providing the genes which confer resistance to that selection.

### FERMENTED LIQUID FEED

Prefermentation of liquid feed for pigs, using *Lactobacillus* spp, has a number of theoretical advantages. The feed is acidified with lactic acid, live and possibly probiotic lactobacilli are continually fed to the animals, and the potential for contamination by pathogenic microorganisms is reduced by virtue of the low pH and high organic acid content of the feed. Unlike grass silage for ruminants, fermented liquid feed for pigs is fed immediately after fermentation. Therefore, much of the microbial population is still active, providing a continuous dosage of active lactic acid bacteria to the animals. This should, in itself, provide a beneficial influence on intestinal fermentation by continuously alleviating the physiological effects of stress on the gut.

## Future possibilities

The long term future of antibiotics as treatments in both veterinary and medical disciplines is in serious doubt. Past overuse of these medications has led to the selection of highly resistant bacterial populations, including bacteria resistant to an array of antibiotics. There is currently little interest in the development of new antibiotics, and no new antibiotics active against Gram-negative pathogens are being developed (Mor, 2000). In response, there has been considerable research into alternative chemotherapeutic agents which could ultimately replace the antibiotic as the mainstay of medicine.

As is often the case, the natural world can provide the basis for new therapeutic agents. Antibacterial agents called “defensins” operate in a similar manner to gramicidin, by causing membrane perforation and ion loss from the cytoplasm. These peptide antimicrobials kill cells within seconds, unlike conventional antibiotics which are normally bacteriostatic (Mor, 2000). Within this group are the dermaseptins (secreted in the skin of frogs), and cecropin and mellitin (manufactured by moths and bees respectively). These have existed in these natural systems for some considerable time, and are still effective at preventing infections in these animals (Otvos, 2000). It is possible that the development of microbial resistance is limited by the extremely rapid activity of these compounds, and by the nature of their action. There may be insufficient time for a microorganism to produce enzymes capable of degrading these antibacterials, and the site of action is the cell membrane, a site which is difficult to alter without adversely affecting its functions. Mellitin has been found to be highly effective against spirochaetes (Lubke and Garon, 1997), while a synthetic peptide based on magainin has been demonstrated to rapidly kill *Escherichia coli* O157 (Appendini and Hotchkiss, 1999). Unfortunately, like gramicidin, the defensins would currently be suitable only for surface applications in human or veterinary medicine as they are also damaging to eukaryotic cells, particularly mammalian red blood cells.

A similar mechanism has been developed artificially using self-assembling organic nanotubes. These can be formulated in a range of diameters, and can perforate cell membranes in a similar manner to the defensins (Buriak and Ghadiri, 1997). These peptide nanotubes are formed not from helices, as are the defensins, but from stacked rings. The rings can be made stable in solution, forming tubes only when they enter cell membranes (Hartgerink *et al.*, 1996). These structures can now be used to form highly effective ion channels in cell membranes (Clark *et al.*, 1998) and are now being developed into specifically antibacterial compounds, so that their medicinal use should soon be realised.

If bacteria prove unable to develop resistance to these compounds, they may eventually replace antibiotics in medicine. It will be some time before they could become sufficiently cost-effective for use in animals, but the relatively simple mechanism of action and the ease with which the structures of these compounds can be manipulated would open enormous possibilities for manipulation of the intestinal microflora with highly specific antibacterials.

A further possibility for manipulation of the microflora may lie in the domain of bacterial quorum sensing, or cell-density-dependent gene expression. Originally discovered in marine bioluminescent bacteria in the 1960s (Strauss, 1999), the term relates to the activation or deactivation of certain metabolic processes within bacteria, as a direct response to the size of the population. The mechanism relies, in Gram-negative bacteria, on the production of acylated homoserine lactones (AHL; Eberhard, Burlingame *et al.*, 1981), and the concentration of these chemicals within individual cells is dependent on the number of AHL-producing cells present. A similar mechanism occurs in Gram-positive bacteria but this makes use of peptide pheromones (Kleerebezem *et al.*, 1997) rather than AHLs. This communication mechanism has been shown to be important in the virulence of infectious pathogens such as *Staphylococcus aureus* (Kleerebezem *et al*, 1997) and in enteropathogenic *E. coli* (Sperandio *et al.*, 1999). Therefore, interfering with this extracellular communication system has the potential for control of the infective capability of these and other pathogens.

## Conclusion

Reports of effective growth-promoting substances, which have included microbiological investigation of the gut microflora, show that improved gut health is linked to an increase in the numbers of lactic acid bacteria and/or a decrease in the numbers of coliform bacteria. As the coliform bacteria typically comprise about 1% of the total microbial population of the intestine, while *Lactobacillus* species account for more than 90% of the population (Khaddour *et al.,* 1998; Reid and Hillman, 1999), it is not immediately apparent why a reduction in numbers of coliforms, or an increase in lactobacilli, should make much difference to the absorption of digested material by the gut?

The reason may lie in both the formation of lactic acid by lactobacilli and the sugar-utilising qualities of coliforms. The principal product of metabolism of sugars by *Lactobacillus* spp. is lactic acid, which may be absorbed and used by the animal. The degradation of feed in the gut by lactobacilli, therefore, need not result in a great deal of energy loss to the animal. On the other hand, the coliform bacteria use oxygen, which is present at appreciable quantities in the piglet intestine (Hillman *et al.*, 1993). The coliform bacteria have a complete set of tricarboxylic acid cycle enzymes, so that the products of aerobic sugar breakdown by coliforms will be carbon dioxide and water, resulting in complete loss of the feed energy.

In this scenario, any reduction in the numbers and/or activity of coliform bacteria would be beneficial to the animal. Additionally, any increase in lactic acid bacteria in relation to the total bacterial load could also prove beneficial, since these bacteria are unable to extract more than a small fraction of the available energy from the feed. Acidification as a result of the activity of *Lactobacillus* spp. may also assist digestion by chemical hydrolysis of certain feed components, and would inhibit the activity of coliform pathogens.

Many alternatives to antibiotics are currently being made available but there seems to be little confidence in these among producers, as the efficacy of these products is considered, at best, highly variable. In fact, the efficacy of many feed antibiotics as growth promoters can be just as variable as, for example, that seen with probiotic preparations. The prophylactic effect of feed antibiotics (an effect which none of the alternatives can claim) is what really makes the antibiotics important in current production systems. The removal of antibiotics may force animal production into less intensive, more "organic" systems with a consequent reduction in productivity, at least in the short term. Unfortunately, the abrupt manner in which antibiotics are being removed from feeds means that the development of a reliable replacement is likely to take longer than the time that is left for the antibiotic feed additives.

## Acknowledgements

Much of the work described was supported by SERAD or MLC

## References

Abe, F., Ishibashi, N. and Shimamura, S. (1995) Effect of administration of bifidobacteria and lactic acid bacteria to newborn calves and piglets. *Journal of Dairy Science*, **78**, 2838-2846.

Adami, A., Sandrucci, A. and Cavazzoni, V. (1997) Piglets fed from birth with the probiotic Bacillus coagulans as additive: Zootechnical and microbiological aspects. *Annali di Microbiologica ed Enzimologia*, **47**, 139-149.

Andruetto, S. and Doglione, L. (1993) Modifications of poultry enteric microflora after feeding with feed containing live yeast. In *Prevention and Control of Potentially Pathogenic Microorganisms in Poultry and Poultry Meat Processing; FLAIR no. 6, Probiotics and Pathogenicity*, pp 73-76. Edited by J.F. Jensen, M.H. Hinton and R.W.A.W. Mulder, Het Spelderholt, The Netherlands.

Appendini, P. and Hotchkiss, J.H. (1999) Antimicrobial activity of a 14-residue peptide against *Escherichia coli* O157:H7. *Journal of Applied Microbiology*, **87**, 750-756.

Bengmark, S. (1998) Immunonutrition: Role of biosurfactants, fiber, and probiotic bacteria. *Nutrition,* **14**, 585-594.

Bijlsma, I.G.W., de Nijs, A., van der Meer, C. and Frik, J.F. (1982) Different pig phenotypes affect adherence of *Escherichia coli* to jejunal brush borders by K88ab, K88ac and K88ad antigens. *Infection and Immunity*, **73**, 891-894.

Bolduan, G., Schuldt, A. and Hackl, W. (1997) Diet feeding in weaner piglets. *Archiv für Tierzucht - Archives of Animal Breeding,* **40**, 95-100.

Brown, I., Warhurst, M., Arcot, J., Playne, M., Illman, R.J. and Topping, D.L. (1997) Fecal numbers of bifidobacteria are higher in pigs fed *Bifidobacterium longum* with a high amylose cornstarch than wih a low amylose cornstarch. *Journal of Nutrition*, **127**, 1822-1827.

Buriak, J.M. and Ghadiri, M.R. (1997) Self-assembly of peptide-based nanotubes. *Materials Science and Engineering C- Biomimetic Materials Sensors and Systems*, **4**, 207-212.

Cavazzoni, V., Adami, A. and Castrovilli, C. (1998) Performance of broiler chickens supplemented with *Bacillus coagulans* as probiotic. *British Poultry Science,* **39**, 526-529.

Charteris, W.P., Kelly, P.M., Morelli, L. and Collins, J.K. (1998) Antibiotic susceptibility of potentially probiotic *Lactobacillus* species. *Journal of Food Protection,* **61**, 1636-1643.

Chateau, N., Deschamps, A.M. and Sassi, A.H. (1994) Heterogeneity of bile-salts resistance in the lactobacillus isolates of a probiotic consortium. *Letters in Applied Microbiology,* **18**, 42-44.

Clark, T.D., Buehler, L.K. and Ghadiri, M.R. (1998) Self-assembling beta(3)-peptide nanotubes as artificial transmembrane ion channels. *Journal of the American Chemical Society*, **120**, 651-656.

Danek, P., Novak, J., Semradova, H. and Diblikova, E. (1991) Administration of the probiotic *Lactobacillus casei* CCM-4160 to sows - its effects on piglet efficiency. *Zivocisna Vryoba*, **36**, 411-415.

Edmunds, B.K., Buttery, P.J. and Fisher, C. (1980) Protein and energy metabolism in the growing pig. In *Energy Metabolism*, pp 129-133. Edited by L.E. Mount, Butterworths, London,

Eidelsburger, U., Roth, F.X. and Kirchgessner, M. (1992) Influence of formic acid, calcium formate and sodium hydrogen carbonate on daily weight gain, feed intake, feed conversion rate and digestibility. *Journal of Animal Physiology and Animal Nutrition - Zeitschrift fur Tierphysiologie Tierernahrung und Futtermittelkunde*, **67**, 258-267.

Eidelsburger, U., Kirchgessner, M. and Roth, F.X. (1992) Influence of formic acid, calcium formate and sodium hydrogen carbonate on dry matter content, pH value, concentration of carbonic acids and ammonia in different segments of the gastrointestinal tract. *Journal of Animal Physiology and Animal Nutrition - Zeitschrift fur Tierphysiologie Tierernahrung und Futtermittelkunde*, **68**, 20-32.

Eberhard, A., Burlingame, A.L., Eberhard, C., Kenyon, G.L., Nealson, K.H. and Oppenheimer, N.J. (1981) Structural identification of autoinducer of *Photobacterium fischeri* luciferase. *Biochemistry*, **20**, 2444-2449.

Eichner, D. and Gravitz, B. (2001) The effects of under-usage of antibiotics on bacteria. http://www.sidwell.edu/~bgravitz/bio/bio.html

Ewing, W.N. and Cole, D.J.A. (1994) *The Living Gut*, Context, Northern Ireland.

Ferraz de Oliveira, M.I., Hillman K. and Acamovic, T. (1994). The effects of enzyme treated and untreated lupins and their alkaloids on poultry gut microflora. In *Plant-associated toxins; Agricultural, Phytochemical and Ecological aspects*, pp 195-199. Edited by S.H. Colegate and P.R. Dorling, CAB International, Oxon, UK.

Freind, D.W., Nicholson, J.W.G. and Cunningham, H.M. (1964) Volatile fatty acid and lactic acid content of pig blood. *Canadian Journal of Animal Science*, **44**, 303-308.

Fuller, R. (1992) History and development of probiotics. In *Probiotics- the scientific basis*, pp 1-8. Edited by R. Fuller, Chapman and Hall, London,

Gabin-Gauthier, K., Gratadoux, J.J. and Richard, J. (1991) Conjugal plasmid transfer between lactococci on solid surface matings and during cheese making. *FEMS Microbiology Ecology,* **85**, 133-140.

Gasaway, W.C. (1976) Volatile fatty acids and metabolizable energy derived from cecal fermentation in the willow ptarmigan. *Comparative Biochemistry and Physiology*, **53A**, 115.

Goerg, K.J. and Schlorer, E. (1998) Probiotic treatment of pseudomembranous colitis: combination of intestinal lavage and oral administration of *Escherichia coli. Deutsche Medizinische Wochenschrift,* **123**, 1274-1278.

Hackstein, J.H.P., van Alen, T.A., op den Camp, H., Smits, A. and Mariman, E. (1995) Intestinal methanogenesis in primates - a genetic and evolutionary approach. *Deutsche Tierarztliche Wochenschrift*, **102**, 152-154.

Hackstein, J.H.P., Langer, P. and Rosenberg, J. (1996) Genetic and evolutionary constraints for the symbiosis between animals and methanogenic bacteria. *Environmental Monitoring and Assessment*, **42**, 39-56.

Hamilton-Miller, J.M.T. and Shah, S. (1998) Vancomycin susceptibility as an aid to the identification of lactobacilli. *Letters in Applied Microbiology,* **26**, 153-154.

Harper, A.F., Kornegay, K.L., Bryant and Thomas, H.R. (1983) Efficacy of virginiamycin and a commercially available Lactobacillus probiotic in swine diets. *Animal Feed Science and Technology*, **8**, 69-76.

Hartgerinck, J.D., Granja, J.R., Milligan, R.A. and Ghadiri, M.R. (1996) Self-assembling peptide nanotubes. *Journal of the American Chemical Society*, **118**, 43-50.

Hill, M.J., Fadden, K., Fernandez, F. and Roberts, A.K. (1986) Biochemical basis for microbial antagonism in the intestine. In *Natural Antimicrobial Systems, FEMS symposium no. 35*, pp 29-39. Edited by G.W. Gould, M.E. Rhodes-Roberts, A.K. Charnley, R.M. Cooper and R.G. Board, Bath University Press, Bath,

Hillman, K., Whyte, A.L. and Stewart, C.S. (1993). Dissolved oxygen in the porcine gastrointestinal tract. *Letters in Applied Microbiology*, **16**, 299 - 302.

Hillman, K., Murdoch, T.A., Spencer, R.J. and Stewart, C.S. (1994) Inhibition of enterotoxigenic *Escherichia coli* by the microflora of the porcine ileum, in an *in vitro* semicontinuous culture system. *Journal of Applied Bacteriology*, **76**, 294-300.

Hillman, K. and Fox, A. (1994). The effects of porcine faecal lactobacilli on the rate of growth of enterotoxigenic *Escherichia coli* O149:K88:K91. *Letters in Applied Microbiology*, **19**, 497-500.

Hillman, K., Khaddour, R. and Fenlon, D.R. (1998) Inhibition of *Listeria monocytogenes* by *Lactobacillus plantarum* is abolished by food intake, in an *in vitro* simulation of the porcine colon. *Proceedings of the British Society for Animal Science 1998*, p. 164.

Hillman, K. and Robertson, S.M. (2001) Distribution of potentially probiotic *Lactobacillus* spp. in pig farms. *Proceedings of the British Society of Animal Science* 2001, abstract no. 100.

Huis in't Veld, J.H.J. and Havenaar, R. (1993) Selection criteria for microorganisms for probiotic use. In *Prevention and Control of Potentially Pathogenic Microorganisms in Poultry and Poultry Meat Processing; FLAIR no. 6, Probiotics and Pathogenicity*, pp 11-19. Edited by J.F. Jensen, M.H. Hinton and R.W.A.W. Mulder, Het Spelderholt, The Netherlands.

Istvan, T., Zoltan, K., Dalma, M. and Laszlo, C. (1995) Effect of probiotic treatment on the body-mass gain and Salmonella excretion of growing geese. *Magyar Allatorvosok Lapja,* **4**, 197-200.

Jaskari, J., Kontula, P., Siitonen, A., Jousimies-Somer, H., Mattila-Sandholm, T. and Poutanen, K. (1998) Oat beta-glucan and xylan hydrolysates as selective substrates for *Bifidobacterium* and *Lactobacillus* strains. *Applied Microbiology and Biotechnology*, **49**, 175-181.

Jin, L.Z., Ho, Y.W., Abdullah, N., Ali, M.A. and Jalaludin, S. (1998) Effects of adherent Lactobacillus cultures on growth, weight of organs and intestinal microflora and volatile fatty acids in broilers. *Animal Feed Science and Technology,* **70**, 197-209.

Kay, R.A. (1991) Microalgae as food and supplement. *Critical Reviews in Food Science and Nutrition,* **30**, 555-573.

Khaddour, R., Reid, C-A. and Hillman, K. (1998) Maintenance *in vitro* of the microflora and fermentation patterns of the porcine intestine. *Pig News and Information*, **19**, 111N-114N.

Kleerebezem, M., Quadri, L.E.N., Kuipers, O.P. and deVos, W.M. (1997) Quorum sensing by peptide pheromones and two-component signal-transduction systems in Gram-positive bacteria. *Molecular Microbiology*, **24**, 895-904.

Kontula, P., Jaskari, J., Nollet, L., DeSmet, I., vonWright, A., Poutanen, K. and Mattila-Sandholm, T. (1998) The colonization of a simulator of the human intestinal microbial ecosystem by a probiotic strain fed on a fermented oat bran product: effects on the gastrointestinal microbiota. *Applied Microbiology and Biotechnology,* **50**, 246-252.

Kowarz, M., Lettner, F. and Zollitsch, W. (1994) Use of a microbial growth promotor in feeding sows and piglets. *Bodenkultur*, **45**, 85-97.

Kreuzer, M. (1994) Probiotic-antibiotic interactions in performance, intestinal fermentation and manure properties of piglets using a Bacillus (Bacillus licheniformis Bacillus subtilis) preparation and Carbadox. *Agribiological Research - Zeitschrift fur Agrarbiologie Agrikulturchemie Okologie*, **47**, 13-23.

Kumprecht, I., Zobac, P. and Robosova, R. (1994) The effect of administration of Bacillus CIP-5832 on some physiological parameters and performance of piglets after weaning. *Zivocisna Vyroba*, **39**, 331-342.

Kumprecht, I. and Zobac, P. (1998) Study of the effect of a combined preparation containing *Enterococcus faecium* M-74 and mannan-oligosaccharides in diets for weanling piglets. *Czech Journal of Animal Science,* **43**, 477-481.

Lewis, D. and Swan, H. (1971) The role of intestinal microflora in animal nutrition. In *Microbes and Biological Productivity, Society for General Microbiology Symposium 21*, pp 149-175. Edited by D.E. Hughes and A.H. Rose, Cambridge University Press, Cambridge.

Lubke, L.L. and Garon, C.F. (1997) The antimicrobial agent mellitin exhibits powerful *in vitro* inhibitory effects on the Lyme disease spirochaete. *Clinical Infectious Diseases*, **25**, S48-S51, Suppl. 1.

Maczulak, A.E., Wolin, M.J. and Miller, T.L. (1989) Increase in colonic methanogens in aging rats. *Applied and Environmental Microbiology,* **55,** 2468-2473.

Manley-Harris, M. and Richards, G.N. (1994) Thermolysis of sucrose for food-products - a sucrose caramel designed to maximize fructose oligosaccharides for beneficial moderation of intestinal bacteria. *Zuckerindustrie,* **119**, 924-928.

Marounek, M. and Rada, V (1995) Susceptibility of poultry lactobacilli to ionophore antibiotics. *Journal of Veterinary Medicine series B - Zentralblatt für Veterinarmedizin Reihe B- Infectious Diseases and Veterinary Public Health,* **42**, 193-196.

Mathew, A.G., Chattin, S.E., Robbins, C.M. and Golden, D.A. (1998) Effects of a direct-fed yeast culture on enteric microbial populations, fermentation acids and performance of weanling pigs. *Journal of Animal Science,* **76**, 2138-2145.

McFarland, S.P. (1998) The influence of dietary starches on the microflora and fermentation pattern of the porcine colon. M.Sc. thesis, SAC/University of Aberdeen.

Mohan, B., Kadirvel, R., Natarajan, A. amd Bhaskaran, M. (1996) Effect of probiotic supplementation on growth, nitrogen utilisation and serum cholesterol in broilers. *British Poultry Science,* **37**, 395-401.

Mor, A. (2000) Peptide-based antibiotics: A potential answer to raging antibiotic resistance. *Drug Development Research*, **50**, 440-447.

Murumatsu, T., Takasu, O., Furuse, M., Takaski, I. and Ikumura, J. (1987) Influence of the gut microflora on protein synthesis in tissues and in the whole body of chicks. *Biochemical Journal,* **246**, 475-479.

Nemcova, R., Laukova, A., Gancarcikova, S. and Kastel, R. (1997) In Vitro studies of porcine lactobacilli for possible probiotic use. *Berliner und Munchener Tierarztliche Wochenschrift,* **110**, 413-417.

Nord, C.E. and Edlund, C. (1990) Impact of antimicrobial agents on human intestinal microflora. *Journal of Chemotherapy*, **2**, 218-237.

Nurmi, E. and Rantala, M. (1973) New aspects of *Salmonella* infection in broiler production. *Nature,* **241**, 210-211.

Oda, Y. and Tatsumi, Y. (1993) New lectins from bulbs of Crocus-sativus. *Biological and Pharmaceutical Bulletin,* **16**, 978-981.

Orban, J.I., Patterson, J.A., Sutton, A.L. and Richards, G.N. (1997) Effect of sucrose thermal oligosaccharide caramel, dietary vitamin-mineral level and brooding temperature on growth and intestinal bacterial populations of broiler chickens. *Poultry Science,* **76**, 482-490.

Orban, J.I., Patterson, J.A., Adeola, O., Sutton, A.L. and Richards, G.N. (1997) Growth performance and intestinal microbial populations of growing pigs fed diets containing sucrose thermal oligosaccharide caramel. *Journal of Animal Science,* **75**, 170-175.

Otvos, L. (2000) Antibacterial peptides isolated from insects. *Journal of Peptide Science*, **6**, 497-511.

Piattoni, F., Demeyer, D.I. and Maertens, L. (1996) *In vitro* study of the age-dependent caecal fermentation pattern and methanogenesis in young rabbits., *Reproduction Nutrition Development*, **36**, 253-261.

Pluske, J.R., Williams, I.H. and Aherne, F.X. (1996a) Maintenance of villous height and crypt depth in piglets by providing continuous nutrition after weaning. *Animal Science*, **62**, 131-144.

Pluske, J.R., Pethick, D.W. and Mullan, B.P. (1998) Differential effects of feeding fermentable carbohydrate to growing pigs on performance, gut size and slaughter characteristics. *Animal Science*, **67**, 147-156.

Pollman, D.S., Danielson, D.M. and Peo, E.R. (1980) Effects of microbial feed additives on performance of starter and growing-finishing pigs. *Journal of Animal Science*, **51**, 577-581.

Postgate, J. (1992) *Microbes and Man, Third Edition.* Cambridge University Press, Cambridge.

Quigley, J.D., Drewry, J.J., Murray, L.M. and Ivey, S.J. (1997) Body weight gain, feed efficiency and fecal scores of dairy calves in response to galactosyl-lactose or antibiotics in mik replacers. *Journal of Dairy Science,* **80**, 1751-1754.

Ravindran, V. and Kornegay, E.T. (1993) Acidification of weaner pig diets: a review. *Journal of the Science of Food and Agriculture,* **62**, 313-322.

Reid, C-A. (1999) Fermentation of resistant starch: implications for colonic health in the monogastric animal. PhD. Thesis, Robert Gordon University, Aberdeen.

Reid, C-A., Hillman, K. and Henderson, C. (1998) The effect of retrogradation, pancreatin digestion and amylose/amylopectin ratio on the fermentation of starch by *Clostridium butyricum* (NCIMB 7423) *Journal of the Science of Food and Agriculture*, **76**, 221-225.

Reid, C-A. and Hillman, K. (1999) The effects of retrogradation and amylose/amylopectin ratio of starches on carbohydrate fermentation and microbial populations in the porcine colon. *Animal Science*, **68**, 503-510.

Rychen, G. and Nunes, C.S. (1993) Effects of a microbial probiotic (*Sporolactobacillus* P44) on postprandial porto-arterial concentration differences of glucose, galactose and amino-nitrogen in the growing pig. *Reproduction Nutrition Development*, **33**, 531-539.

Rychen, G. and Nunes, C.S. (1995) Effects of 3 microbial probiotics on postprandial porto-arterial concentration differences of glucose, galactose and amino-nitrogen in the young pig. *British Journal of Nutrition*, **74**, 19-26.

Sperandio, V., Mellies, J.L., Nguyen, W., Shin, S. and Kaper, J.B. (1999) Quorum sensing controls expression of the type III secretion gene transcription and protein secretion in enterohaemorrhagic and enteropathogenic *Escherichia coli. Proceedings of the National Academy of Sciences of the United States of America*, **96**, 15196-15201.

Stewart, C.S., Hillman, K. and Maxwell, F. (1995) Effects of probiotics on the gut microbiology of animals. In *Medical and dental aspects of anaerobes*, pp 109 - 120. Edited by B.I. Duerden, W.G. Wade, J.S. Brazier, A. Eley, B. Wren and M.J. Hudson, Science Reviews Press, Northwood,

Strauss, E. (1999) A Symphony of Bacterial Voices. *Science*, **284**, 1302-1304.

Thomke, S. and Elwinger, K. (1998) Growth promotants in feeding pigs and poultry III. Alternatives to antibiotic growth promotants. *Annales de Zootechnie*, **47**, 245-271.

Tortuero, F., Rioperez, J., Fernandez, E. and Rodriguez, M.L. (1995) Response of piglets to oral administration of lactic acid bacteria. *Journal of Food Protection*, **58**, 1369-1374.

Van der Waaij, D., Berghuis de Vries, J.M. and Lekkerkerk van der Wees, J.E.C (1971) Colonization resistance of the digestive tract in conventional and antibiotic treated mice. *Journal of Hygeine (Cambridge)*, **69**, 405-411.

Vassalo, M., Fialho, E.T., de Oliveira, A.I.G., Teixeira, A.S. and Bertechini, A.G. (1997). Probiotics for piglets from 10 to 30 kg of life weight. *Revista da Sociedade Brasileira de Zootechnica - Journal of the Brazilian Society of Animal Science*, **26**, 131-138.

Vogeli, P., Kuhn, B., Kuhne, R., Obrist, R., Stranzinger, G., Huang, S.C., Hu, Z.L., Hasler-Rapacz, J. and Rapacz, J. (1992) Evidence for linkage between the swine L blood group and the loci specifying the receptors mediating adhesion of K88 *Escherichia coli* pilus antigens. *Animal Genetics*, **23**, 19-29.

Wagner, R.D. and Balish, E. (1998) Potential hazards of probiotic bacteria for immunodeficient patients. *Bulletin de l'Institut Pasteur*, **96**, 165-170.

Wallace, J.S., Stanley, K.N., Currie, J.E., Diggle, P.J. and Jones, K. (1997) Seasonality of thermophilic *Campylobacter* populations in chickens. *Journal of Applied Bacteriology*, **82**, 219-224.

Wilhelm, M. P., Lee, D.T. and Rosenblatt, J.E. (1987) Bacterial interference by anaerobic species isolated from human feces. *European Journal of Clinical*

*Microbiology*, **6**, 266-270.

Yeo, J. and Kim, K.I. (1997) Effect of feeding diets containing an antibiotic, a probiotic, or yucca extract on growth and intestinal urease activity in broiler chicks. *Poultry Science*, **76**, 381-385.

Zani, J.L., daCruz, F.W., dos Santos, A.F. and GilTurnes, C. (1998) Effect of probiotic CenBiot on the control of diarrhoea and feed efficiency in pigs. *Journal of Applied Microbiology*, **84**, 68-71.

Zuanon, J.A.S., Fonseca, J.B., Rostagno, H.S. and Silva, M.D.E. (1998) Effects of growth promoters on broiler chickens performance. *Revista Brasileira de Zootechnica - Brazilian Journal of Animal Science*, **27**, 999-1005.

*This paper was first published in 2001*

22

# TRACING MODES OF ACTION AND THE ROLES OF PLANT EXTRACTS IN NON-RUMINANTS

C. KAMEL
*Technical and Business Development Manager, IQF Group, Tarragona, Spain*

## Introduction

Global population is steadily increasing. In 25 years time, there will be almost 9 billion inhabitants on Earth (United States Census Bureau, 1998; FAOSTAT, 1998) expecting enough food to meet their daily nutritional needs. This objective can only be met by a 2% increase per year in world food production, which is expected for pigs and poultry in the next 20-25 years (FAOSTAT, 1998).

At the same time, there is a growing consumer consciousness about the necessity of food safety. This is no doubt due in part to serious issues in recent decades, such as the use of hormones and beta-agonists in animal nutrition, the presence of heavy metals in fish, the overuse of sludge, the presence of pesticides in fruit, the dioxins in meat, the use of antibiotics in animal feed, the production of genetically modified organisms, and Bovine Spongiform Encephalopathy.

"Let your food be your first medicine" (Hippocrates, 377 BC) was probably the first time that the link was made between nutrition and well-being. This old aphorism has come back into fashion in human and animal nutrition over the last few years as global markets have returned to a more "natural" source. In the animal feed industry, most diets can provide the diverse blend of nutrients needed for growth, maintenance and overall well-being. In some instances, however, diet formulation alone may not supply adequate amounts of the required nutrients, or the animal may not be in a state to make proper use of it, as is the case with ageing, during pregnancy and lactation, or under stress or disease challenge. During the twentieth century, much work was directed towards elucidating the biochemical structures and physiological roles of many nutritional additives, especially the routine inclusion of in-feed antibiotic growth promoters in pig and poultry diets over the last 50 years. These have proven to be an effective method of both enhancing animal performance and reducing digestive disorders that often presented themselves as scouring, particularly in weaner pigs. At the same time, increased concerns over food safety, environmental contamination and general health risks have made "natural" the norm, promoting the trend toward alternative strategies to manage and feed young animals without reliance on antibiotics. In response to this void in the marketplace, a new generation of alternative products has vied to take their place, many of which present more questions than answers. These have been defined by Rosen (1996) as "microfeedingstuffs used orally in a relatively small amount to improve the intrinsic value of the nutrient mix in the animal diet." Whether labelled under the name of 'adaptogens', 'dietetics', 'neutraceuticals', 'neutricines' or 'multi-functional additives', these are marketed for their benefits to animal nutrition. They include natural plant extracts; much research has focused on the specific beneficial effects of these as feed micro-ingredients, but this is by no means exhaustive. In particular, it remains unclear if a particular action, e.g. antioxidant, antiseptic, immunomodulator, can be associated with a specific molecule; this is complicated even more because one active substance may have multiple actions. In some cases, while searching for the "magic bullet", what results is more of a "dietary machine gun." Nonetheless, the elucidation of well-defined modes of action will provide the scientific basis for establishing the efficacy and safety of these additives to develop a long-term strategy for their use in specific diet formulations and other feed supplements. Only then will the industry and consumer feel confident about the potential of these products and embrace them as part of standard practice, as once they did with the antibiotic growth promoters.

## Historical overview

One generation of productivity enhancers includes additives based on natural plant extracts and their intrinsic active principles. The use of plants and their respective extracts dates back some thousands of years to the ancient Egyptians, Chinese, Indians and Greeks. Even Christopher Columbus discovered America while looking for a shortcut to many of the herbs and spices found today in practically everyone's kitchen in one form or another. In addition, many natural extracts have provided the basis for modern medications, such in the case of digoxin from the digitalis plant, ephedrine from the Chinese herb ma huang, and common aspirin from willow. Clearly, much can be learnt from history, but the empirical knowledge of plants has risen to another level, due largely to modern technologies that have led to the systematic isolation and characterisation of active principles contained in these plant sources. As summarised in Table 22.1, many of the current extracts have beneficial multi-

**Table 22.1** SUMMARY TABLE REPRESENTING COMMON PLANT EXTRACTS, THEIR UTILISED PARTS, MAIN ACTIVE SUBSTANCES AND REPORTED PROPERTIES (RICHARD, 1992; CHARALAMBOUS, 1994)

| *Vegetal form* | *Utilised parts* | *Main Compounds* | *Reported properties* |
|---|---|---|---|
| *Aromatic spices* | | | |
| Nutmeg | Seed | Sabinene | Digestion stimulant, antidiarrhoeic |
| Cinnamon | Bark | Cinnamaldehyde | Appetite and digestion stimulant, antiseptic |
| Clove | Cloves | Eugenol | Appetite and digestion stimulant, antiseptic |
| Cardamom | Seed | Cineol | Appetite and digestion stimulant |
| Coriander | Leaf, seed | Linalol | Digestion stimulant |
| Cumin | Seed | Cuminaldehyde | Digestive, carminative, galactagogue |
| Anise | Fruit | Anethol | Digestion stimulant, galactagogue |
| Celery | Fruit, leaf | Phtalides | Appetite and digestion stimulant |
| Parsley | Leaf | Apiol | Appetite and digestion stimulant, antiseptic |
| Fenugreek | Seed | Trigonelline | Appetite stimulant |
| *Pungent spices* | | | |
| Capsicum | Fruit | Capsaicin | Antidiarrhoeic, anti-inflammatory, stimulant, tonic |
| Pepper | Fruit | Piperine | Digestion stimulant |
| Horseradish | Root | Allylisothio-cyanate | Appetite stimulant |
| Mustard | Seed | Allylisothio-cyanate | Digestion stimulant |
| Ginger | Rhizome | Zingerone | Gastric stimulant |
| *Aromatic herbs and spices* | | | |
| Garlic | Bulb | Allicin | Digestion stimulant, antiseptic |
| Rosemary | Leaf | Cineol | Digestion stimulant, antiseptic, antioxidant |
| Thyme | Whole plant | Thymol | Digestion stimulant, antiseptic, antioxidant |
| Sage | Leaf | Cineol | Digestion stimulant, antiseptic, carminative |
| Bay laurel | Leaf | Cineol | Appetite and digestion stimulant, antiseptic |
| Peppermint | Leaf | Menthol | Appetite and digestion stimulant, antiseptic |

functional aspects that derive from their specific bioactive components. However, this represents only a fraction of the phytogenic elements known to man. To date, more than 10,000 species of plants known in the modern world remain undiscovered, and 90% of the molecules that account for many of the actions remain a mystery. Through the integration of current knowledge, these molecules will become easier to find, identify and characterise. Furthermore, information regarding dose-response, metabolism, toxicity and maximum residue levels (MRL) should also be accumulated, with the intention of establishing an international database of information available to feed experts and consumers alike.

## Back to basics

### RELATING STRUCTURE TO FUNCTION

Plant extracts contain a vast source of different molecules that have intrinsic bioactivities on animal physiology and metabolism. One example is the phenolic compounds, a diverse series of either single (simple phenolic) or multiple (polyphenolic) aromatic rings differing principally in their respective side chains (Figure 22.1). In this sense, the phytogenic active components share something in common with organic acids, which also represent a non-homologous group, varying in the numbers of carboxy groups, hydroxy groups and carbon-carbon double bonds at the molecular level. These structural differences confer different stabilities to polyphenolic compounds over a standard pH range of 3-11. A funded project is ongoing at TEKTRAN (Technology Transfer Automated Retrieval System) of the United States Department of Agriculture Research Service to investigate the family of phytogenic phenolic compounds. In this programme, series of structurally well-defined phenolic compounds are being tested for their stability coefficients by changes in the ultraviolet absorption spectra of the phenolic compounds left standing in different pH buffers for several periods up to 72 hours. The results of this screening have suggested that the stability of the phenolic compounds strongly depended on the structure of the compound, the pH and length of storage buffer time (Friedman and Jurgens, 1999).

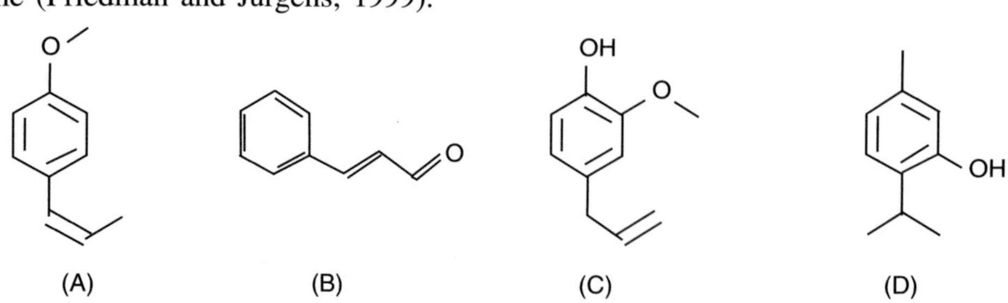


**Figure 22.1** Chemical structures and molecular weights (MW) for common plant active substances. (A) anethol, MW 148.2; (B) cinnamaldehyde; MW 132.2; (C) eugenol, MW 164.2; (D) thymol, MW 150.2.

Principal Components Analysis (PCA), performed at the Department of Microbiology at the University of Auvergne Faculty of Medicine, Clermont-Ferrand, France, has also been used to study the properties of a preliminary screening panel of plant extracts. The pH distribution of this panel (data not shown) ranged from pH 4.3 (cinnamon extract) to pH 6.7 (ginger extract). This analysis continues to support the theory that not all extracts are created equal, but are representative of a group of structurally and chemically distinct molecules.

In addition, previous work has shown that, like organic acids, these chemical properties may correspond structurally to the incidence of polar groups, the number of double bonds, molecular size, and solubility in non-polar matrices. This, in turn, may dictate the activities observed *in vitro*: for example, antiseptic (Hammer *et. al.,* 1999), antifungal (Apisariyakul *et. al.,* 1995); antioxidant (Aeschbach *et. al.,* 1994); as well as *in vivo*: for example, stimulation of feed intake (Petit *et. al.,* 1993), stimulation of digestive enzymes (Platel and Srinivasan, 1996).

## NATURAL PLANT EXTRACTS SHOW STRUCTURE-SPECIFIC $MIC_{50}$ SPECTRA

The antiseptic effects of natural plant extracts are incontrovertable. The scientific literature is filled with work supporting the minimum inhibitory concentration ($MIC_{50}$) and minimum bacteriocidal concentration ($MBC_{50}$) of these substances. What has remained unclear is the relationship between structure of the active substances found in plant sources and their effects. Preliminary work carried out in collaboration with the University of Auvergne Department of Microbiology has confirmed that different extracts do indeed have different $MIC_{50}$ spectra when screened against a diverse bacterial panel (Tabel 22.2).

**Table 22.2** $MIC_{50}$ VALUES (PPM) FOR SELECTED PLANT EXTRACTS AGAINST A PANEL OF GRAM-POSITIVE, GRAM-NEGATIVE AND ANAEROBIC BACTERIA (PERFORMED IN COLLABORATION WITH THE DEPARTMENT OF MICROBIOLOGY, UNIVERSITY OF AUVERGNE, CLERMONT-FERRAND, FRANCE). NE: NO EFFECT

| *$MIC_{50}$ values* | *E. coli H7:O157* | *S. typhimurium* | *C. coli* | *C. perfringens* |
|---|---|---|---|---|
| Capsaicin | NE | NE | NE | 50 |
| Cinnamaldehyde | 1,000 | 1,000 | 1,000 | 1,000 |
| Eugenol | 500 | 500 | 500 | 500 |
| Allicin | NE | NE | NE | 100 |
| Carvacrol | 500 | 500 | 500 | 500 |
| Cineol | 50,000 | 50,000 | 50,000 | 50,000 |

From these studies, romarin showed very little effect against gram-negative micro-organisms. Cinammon, clove and oregano showed moderate and wide-spectra efficacy against the panel. The spice extracts, capsicum and garlic, showed specific efficacy against *Clostridium sp.* alone. These differences in efficacy at the *in vitro* level can be clearly linked to the level of their active substances, with purity of the plant extract playing a critical role (C. Forestier, University of Auvergne: personal communication). While their *in vitro* effects are well documented, the mode of action by which these substances exhibit their effect on bacteria is currently being investigated. On-going work seems to confirm that these substances, like antiseptic agents in general, exert their effects by disrupting the microbe at the cellular membrane. The effect of natural plant extracts on the hydrophobicity of an *E. coli* strain of post-weaning pig origin was determined by the salt aggregation test, a measure of the aggregative (binding) properties of strains of bacteria. The preliminary panel included extracts from St. John's Wort, cassia, cinnamon and thyme, which showed $MIC_{50}$ values at 250 ppm or more on *E. coli sp.* The results shown indicate a strong increase (40-60%) in hydrophobicity of the microbial species by the addition of St. John's Wort and cassia. Cinnamon and thyme showed more moderate effects (Table 22.3). These differences in hydrophobicity correlated strongly with the $MIC_{50}$ values for the extracts investigated (data not shown). Therefore, one of the probably and potentially important action mechanisms of certain plant extracts may be their ability to influence the surface characteristics of microbial cells and thereby their putative virulence properties. This has interesting implications in the animal gut, where the adhesion of microbes to host cells is of fundamental importance in the development of Gram-negative, microbe-induced infections, and which is influenced strongly by the surface hydrophobicity of the microbial cell (Mbwambo *et al.*, 1996).

**Table 22.3** HYDROPHOBICITY OF E. COLI (SUIS STRAIN 4596) IN THE PRESENCE OF ST. JOHN'S WORT, CASSIA, CINNAMON OR THYME. VALUES EXPRESSED AS PERCENTAGE AGGREGATION BY THE SALT AGGREGATION TEST

| *Aggregation* | *St. John's wort extract* | *Cassia extract* | *Cinnamon extract* | *Thyme extract* |
|---|---|---|---|---|
| *E. coli* (suis 4596) | 58%[c] | 42%[b] | 23%[a] | 28%[a] |

Values on the same row with different supercripts are significantly different.

## The role of complementary *in vitro* modelling techniques

The feed industry, and nutrition of the young animal in particular, is shifting into a phase of intensified research and development. Few companies, however, have adequate manpower or resources to put into place and follow long-term research programmes. On the other hand, public institutions often have difficulty finding the financial support necessary for project funding, given the dwindling government-sponsored funding programmes available. While this has become the norm in human nutrition and medical research, the possibilities are just beginning in the animal feed industry for a pooling of resources from the public and private sectors to work jointly toward one or more common objective(s).

One example where this may be most easily realised in the immediate future is in the development and validation of complementary *in vitro* systems modelled after various aspects of animal behaviour and physiology. There is a growing need for the development of systems which will be able to complement the information obtained through classical *in vivo* animal testing, while adding a dimension toward understanding small yet significant mechanisms, benefits or constraints which may remain hidden due to internal or external variability. Research and development on new feed-additive products has been, and will continue to be, one area where *in vitro* modelling operates at its best. Probably the greatest advantages of these models lie in qualities that are not so obvious. Trials with most systems are neither time nor labour intensive and cost only a fraction of comparable live animal trials. There are also advantages in the case of animal welfare considerations, as no live animals are directly involved.

These models are tools for innovative feed-additive companies whose goal is to aid nutritionists and feed compounders in the difficult, time-consuming challenge of evaluating products and their combinations within a range of diet formulations and production practices. Using these models, it has been possible to screen a "library" of plant extracts to investigate their effects on many aspects of bioavailability, normal digestion and gut flora mechanics, environmental and animal impact as it pertains to traceability and residues.

## *IN VITRO* STUDIES: GASTRIC ACID SECRETION

It is proposed that acidification of the diet may provide a prophylactic measure similar to that provided by feed antibiotic growth promoters. While antibiotics are designed to inhibit growth in general, the acidifier would cause the beneficial rather than the harmful microorganisms to dominate in the gastro-intestinal tract. Supplementation of the diet for weanling pigs with acidifying agents has been shown, in many cases, to increase live-weight gain and feed conversion ratio, and to reduce the incidence of diarrhoea. However, the performance response to supplementation with dietary acidifiers is often variable. This has led to investigation of the possible modes of action of the acidifying agents but, although several hypotheses have been proposed, the exact mechanisms remain unclear. It is generally considered that feed acidifiers lower gastric pH, resulting in increased gastric proteolytic enzyme activity, and improved gastric emptying. Furthermore, acids entering the duodenum stimulate the exocrine pancreas to secrete bicarbonates. Therefore, it was expected that feed acidifiers would increase exocrine pancreatic secretion. The hypothesis that lowering dietary pH with feed acidifiers reduces gastro-intestinal pH has been tested in several studies. However, only a few have shown that dietary acidification significantly decreased gastric pH.

One way to understand the mechanisms behind different classes of products is by using *in vitro* modelling systems, which allow animal variability to be eliminated.

One such system is the non-ruminant intestinal model, developed by Drs. Robert Haavenar and Mans Minekus at the TNO Institute in Zeist, Netherlands. Briefly, this accurate "mechanical" model provides continuous monitoring of the natural parameters of digestion and its by-products. This can in turn determine the traceability of ingested feed components as well as their possible effects on the animal and their impact on the environment (Kamel, 1999). Certainly any type of digestion modelling has its limits, but this model has provided clear in-roads into the modes of action of various plant extracts and their possible usage in combination with other alternatives such as organic acids. Feeds that included certain plant extracts demonstrated effects in the gastric compartment similar to those observed with specific organic acids (Figure 22.2). Specifically, some extracts exerted an acid-sparing effect when included in a feed whose basic pH nature could compromise production of gastric acid, which can result in poor feed digestibility and potential overgrowth of pathogenic bacteria. Using a weaning porcine gastro-intestinal model, 200g diet samples were added to the gastric compartment and the amount of acid needed to maintain the pH at a level of pH 3.0 during a 6-hour period was recorded. The samples were taken from three groups of a piglet field trial (performance results shown in Table 22.4). The feed samples were based on a diet of wheat and soya, with no enzyme supplement, differing only in the micro-supplementation with either plant extracts at 2 g/kg, or formic acid (85%) at 10 g/kg and a combination of both. The results are summarised in Figure 22.2.

In general, responses confirm previous observations that the addition of certain plant phenols can act as an acid-sparing agent against the highly basic components found in a wheat and barley based weaning diet. Preliminary evidence suggests that the addition of an acid with a low pKa (i.e. formic or lactic acid) intensifies this effect as early as 60 minutes post-digestion. Whether extract and acid act alone or together to reduce gastric pH significantly, and whether this brings about influences on performance parameters (such as feed utilisation), remains to be seen.

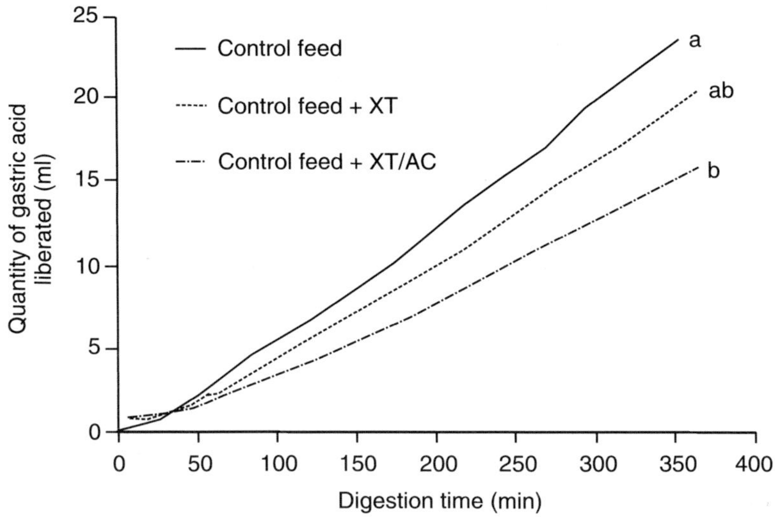


**Figure 22.2.** Experimental means for gastric acid secretion required to maintain a gastric pH of 3.0 for three different feed formulations in a porcine gastro-intestinal model. The three feeds are: Control (neutral) feed with no additive; control feed with XT (plant extracts based on cinnamaldehyde, thymol and capsaicin; and control feed with XT + AC (formic acid 85%).

*In vivo* animal studies comparing the performance benefits of plant extracts and organic acids either alone or in combination

For many years, feed additives have been used in young animal diets where digestion problems at weaning lead to scouring and a growth check. The slow, uneven acidification of the stomach contents of young animals plays a major role in the classic over-proliferation *of E. coli*, which then leads to enterotoxaemia in weaned piglets. The nutritional effectiveness of organic acids in piglet and broiler production has resulted in their routine use in young animal diets. However, raw material changes and evidence for "acid-resistant" micro-organisms, such as *E. coli H7:O157*, have led many nutritionists to use acid blends or a combination of acids with other alternatives, such as enzymes or probiotics. Early research into the modes of action of certain plant extracts and phytogenic active substances indicates that a synergism may occur between this class of compounds and organic acids. Development using many of the before-mentioned laboratory and *in vitro* modelling systems have shown promise in optimising the actions of these products alone and in combination with each other. A series of post-weaning pig trials is underway to confirm the promising combinations studied. One such trial was conducted on a commercial farm in Switzerland in pigs weaned at 21 days of age. The results (Table 22.4) show the benefits of inclusion of a precise combination of plant extracts on both live-weight gain (DWG, + 7.3% compared with control) and feed conversion (FCR, + 5.9% compared with control). The addition of formic acid to the plant extracts potentiated the observed effects even more dramatically, as well as having a significant effect on the incidence of diarrhoea. The evidence that this strategy may be useful in reducing stress associated with early-weaning programmes is currently being studied at several levels to determine the underlying mechanisms *in vivo*.

**Table 22.4** MEANS FOR DAILY FEED INTAKE (DFI), DAILY LIVE-WEIGHT GAIN (DLWG), FEED CONVERSION RATIO (FCR) AND DIARRHOEA SCORES OF POST-WEANING PIGS FED FROM 21 TO 70 DAYS ON DIETS EITHER CONTAINING XT (PLANT EXTRACTS BASED ON CINNAMALDEHYDE, THYMOL AND CAPSAICIN), FA85 (FORMIC ACID 85%) OR A COMBINATION OF XT AND FA85

| *Parameter* | *Negative control group Neutral feed* | *Experimental group 1 Neutral feed + XT* | *Experimental group 2 Neutral feed + XT/FA85* |
|---|---|---|---|
| Number of animals | 28 | 28 | 28 |
| Start weight (kg) | 6.90 | 6.92 | 6.90 |
| End weight (kg) | 21.21[b] | 22.36[ab] | 23.32[a] |
| DLWG (g/d) | 292[b] | 315[ab] | 335[a] |
| DFI (g/d) | 491[b] | 503[b] | 530[a] |
| FCR (kg/kg) | 1.68[b] | 1.58[a] | 1.52[a] |
| Diarrhoea Score | 39.0[b] | 33.8[ab] | 28.5[a] |

Values on the same row with different supercripts are significantly different.

From the above trial in weaning pigs, it can be clearly seen that a diet based on wheat and barley gives particularly poor performance results in the absence of exogenous feed enzymes. This is due to the presence of anti-nutrients in wheat (pentosans) and barley (beta-glucans). The addition of beta-glucanases can improve diet digestibility. In addition, wheat and barley exhibit particularly high acid-binding coefficients. Therefore, the addition of plant extracts XT alone, but particularly in combination with organic acid FA85, improves digestibility, as evidenced by improved feed conversion ratios and higher live weights. This follows previous work in a number of published works showing the benefits of specific spice principles in enhancing the activities of non-ruminant digestive enzymes (Platel and Srinivasan, 1996). In addition, the combination also leads to a lower incidence of diarrhoea (27% lower than the control group), probably due to the reduction in volume of digesta, which can often act as a substrate for pathogenic bacterial growth.

## ESTABLISHING REPRODUCIBLE METHODS OF DETECTION FOR NEW ALTERNATIVE PRODUCTS

Traceability and residues are probably two of the "hottest" topics of discussion in the modern global feed industry. The need to be able to follow the course of a product and its active ingredients from start to finish is seen as a fundamental requirement. Reliable detection techniques found in most analytical laboratories, such as GC (gas chromatography), LC (liquid chromatography), MS (mass spectrophotometry) and HPLC (high-pressure liquid chromatography) as well as their combinations, are necessary to realise this objective. Early work has shown that the phenolic compounds (Figure 22.3) can be identified and quantified, with detection systems reaching the sensitivity levels of picograms of material depending on the system in place (1 picogram is $10^{-12}$g). These analytical techniques will be vital for implementing programmes of feed traceability, as well as establishing minimum residue levels (MRL) in carcass, egg and milk evaluation programmes for these categories of products.

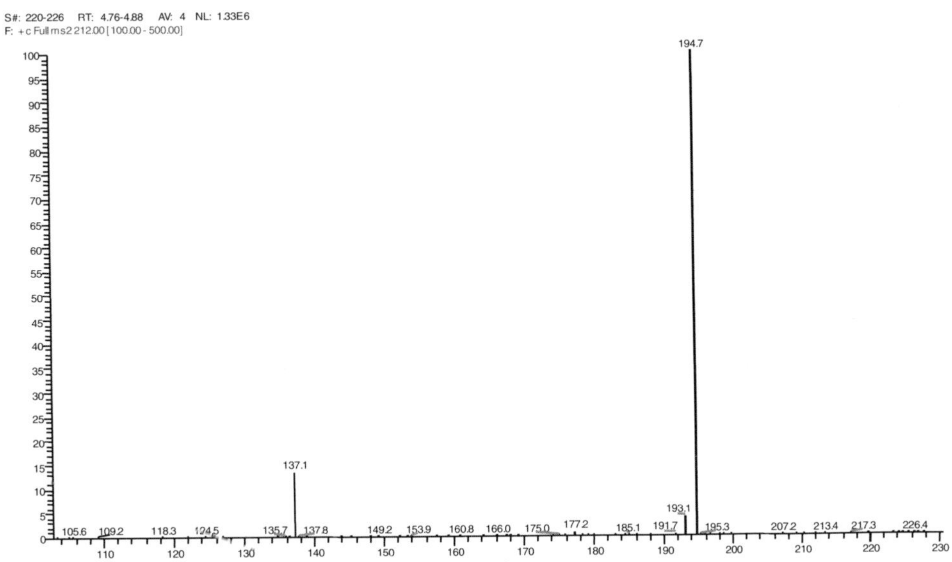


**Figure 22.3** Sample extract representing 50 picograms of zingerone, from Zingiber officinale Roscoe, analysed by electrospray ionisation in LC-MS

## *In vitro* intestinal epithelium cell culture systems

The first step in any traceability approach is to determine what level of the compound crosses the intestinal epithelium. If the substance in question and its respective metabolites remain intraluminal and are finally excreted in the urine or faeces, there is little need to check for its deposition in internal depots. In this regard, immortalised epithelium cell systems (e.g. Caco-2 cell line), or certain primary pig intestinal cell lines, will figure as an important tool in tracking these new substances (Figure 22.4). Indeed, there is an extensive database of several thousand scientific publications relating to these cells, making them an extremely well-characterised research and development tool for many areas of scientific research. Their use has been quite extensive in the area of pharmacology, especially since there is a high degree of correlation between the permeability to pharmacological agents and the absorption of these same compounds in live subjects. This demonstrates only one value of the system in predicting potential bioavailability and absorbability of active compounds. In addition, it can be used to screen for detrimental effects of novel compounds following ingestion. The potential of this system in the traceability, safety and toxicity studies in the elucidation of plant extracts and their intrinsic active substances is exciting. Preliminary screening of panels of extracts and their active components has shown that these substances can be traced to different intracellular, as well as transcellular, destinations. The differences seen among phytochemicals may be due to the cellular sorting signals that are found deep in their molecular structure.

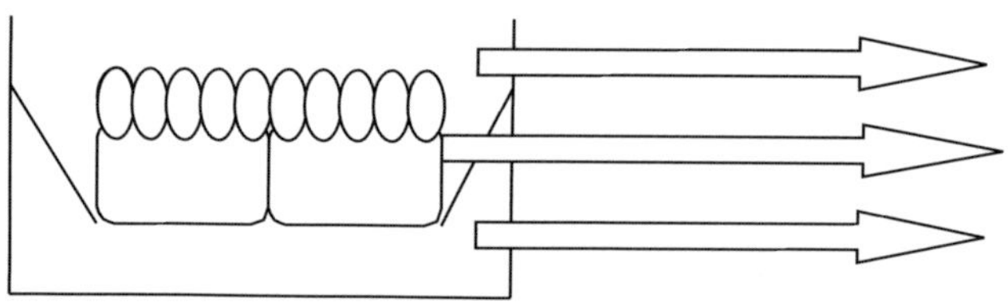


**Figure 22.4.** Schematic representation of a primary intestinal cell culture system illustrating its two interfaces: apical (luminal) and basolateral (blood). Substances added at the apical side are monitored over time along the cell transport system.

The future of this approach will lie in the full characterisation of these natural active substances on a molecule-by-molecule basis in an effort to associate families of compounds with specific activities and targeting routes. Indeed, research supports the idea that that not all extracts are created equal, but represent a group of structurally and chemically distinct molecules with specific and quantifiable activities, some of which are synergistic in nature. Based on preliminary screening experiments, synergistic combinations of plant active principles have been shown to provide benefits in the field (Table 22.5). Their cost-effective benefits in broilers, for example, can approach the results seen with antibiotic growth promoters still available in the marketplace.

One general observation in the majority of these trials is the evidence of an improved uniformity within the experimental groups fed on a diet supplemented with plant extracts. Clearly, one of the problems encountered in current "all-in/all-out" programmes is birds that fall behind the main group. These "laggers" can present significant problems to handlers in additional costs for prolonged finishing, floor utilisation, or extra care and treatment. Many natural plant extracts, due to their beneficial effects on feed efficiency and friendly gut flora populations, appear to optimise performance within the genetic framework of the bird. Therefore, their use may yield more important benefits, leading to a more uniform, cost-effective output.

**Table 22.5** SUMMARY OF UNIVERSITY, INSTITUTE AND FIELD TRIALS, CARRIED OUT IN WESTERN EUROPE, CENTRAL EUROPE AND SCANDINAVIA, ILLUSTRATING THE EFFECTS ON BROILER PERFORMANCE OF USING PLANT EXTRACTS BASED ON CAPSAICIN AND POLYPHENOLS AT A FINAL FEED INCLUSION LEVEL OF 200 PPM

| *Parameter* | *Control feed No additive* | *Plant extracts XT 200 ppm* |
|---|---|---|
| Number of trials | 6 | 6 |
| Average trial duration (days) | 37 | 37 |
| Number of animals | 31,756 | 49,756 |
| Initial weight (g) | 39.4 | 39.4 |
| Final weight (g) | 1770 | 1849 |
| Live-weight gain (g/d) | 46.8 | 48.9 |
| Feed intake (g/d) | 81.9 | 85.1 |
| Feed conversion ratio | 1.78 | 1.74 |

Individual trial reports available upon request from the author.

Current research is taking account of public concern in investigating the advantages from the programmed administration of these phytogenic additives on the animal carcass. Only recently has the industry come to appreciate some of the many factors involved in determining meat quality and composition. One of those most obvious is the area of genetics, where work over the last few years in the United Kingdom has shown that certain exotic genes, such as those pertaining to the Duroc breed, can influence eating characteristics of meat. However, despite the excellent research being carried out by hybrid companies in generating pigs that grow faster and are leaner and more efficient than their predecessors, there have been costs in terms of meat quality. Colour and drip loss have worsened in recent years and the level of marbling fat has deteriorated, with the associated effect on eating quality. While the majority of studies have focused on raw material changes in the diet, supplements such as those based on plant extracts may also contribute to meat colour and drip loss, reduction in intermuscular fat stores, and shifts in fatty acid content and profile. Until now, the benefits from inclusion of plant extracts as a diet supplement have been measured largely on body composition. This includes several independent European university and trial station studies that have shown significant benefits in carcass backfat and lean characteristics, all in the absence of quantifiable residue deposition of these phytogenic substances in meat, fat or soft organ tissue (Table 22.6).

**Table 22.6** TRIALS 1485 AND 1602: EFFECT OF INCLUSION OF A MICRO-ADDITIVE BASED ON NATURAL PLANT EXTRACTS IN WHEAT AND BARLEY DIETS ON SLAUGHTER CHARACTERISTICS IN 128 GROWING AND FINISHING PIGS

| | *Trial 1485* | | *Trial 1602* | |
|---|---|---|---|---|
| *Parameter* | *Control feed No additive* | *Natural extracts XT* | *Control feed No additive* | *Natural extracts XT* |
| Carcass weight (kg) | 82.0 | 81.3 | 83.6 | 84.2 |
| Dressing percentage (%) | 59.9 | 60.7 | 54.9 | 55.7 |
| Backfat thickness P1 (mm) | $18.0^{b}$ | $16.7^{a}$ | 18.9 | 19.1 |
| Muscle depth (LD, mm) | 52.4 | 52.8 | $52.2^{b}$ | $54.8^{a}$ |
| *Meat quality* | | *% Distribution* | | |
| European Meat Classification Scheme | | S | 0b | 10a |
| | | E | 50b | 42a |
| | | U | 50 | 48 |

Values on the same row with different superscripts are significantly different

The inclusion of plant extracts as micro-supplements in current formulations for non-ruminant diets appears to yield improvements in certain carcass characteristics. At the moment, however, there are more questions than answers, as the framework within which these promising benefits operate needs to be better defined. In particular, more information must be obtained with respect to the specific class of phytochemicals responsible for these effects, their dose-response, their effects in combination with different commercial feed formulations, as well as the contribution of animal genetics and rearing conditions, in order to better explain the processes involved. Furthermore, the effects on carcass yield must be studied in relation to effects on carcass quality (i.e. meat structure and composition) in order to get a more complete picture.

## Conclusions

Plant extracts represent one of a myriad of alternatives in response to the void created by the ban on antibiotic growth promoters in Europe. These substances have been in use since the beginning of recorded history, but little is known about the mechanisms that lead to the benefits seen in both man and animals. Furthermore, the supplier of feed additives will be responsible for a "checklist" of issues surrounding these components, such as: (i) composition identification; (ii) technical and performance efficacy; (iii) toxicity analysis; (iv) feed traceability; (v) residue analysis; and (vi) exposure and handling risks. Although this will be an arduous task for many, it will represent a responsible, informed approach within the feed industry and towards the consumer.

## References

Aeschbach R., Löliger, J. Scott, B.D., Murcia, A., Butler, J. Halliwell, B and Aruoma, O.I. (1994). Antioxidant actions of thymol, carvacrol, 6-gingerol, zingerone and hydroxytyrosol. *Food Chemistry and Toxicology,* 32(1), 31-6.

Apisariyakul A., Vanittanakom, N., Buddhasukh, D. (1995). Antifungal activity of turmeric oil extracted from Curcuma longa (Zingiberaceae). *Journal of Ethnopharmacology*, 49(3), 163-9.

Charalambous, G. (ed) (1994). *Spices, Herbs and Edible Fungi.* Elsevier, London.

Friedman, M. and Jurgens H. (1999). Effect of pH on the stability of plant polyphenols. *U.S. Agriculture Research Report*, United States Department of Agriculture.

Kamel, C. (1999). Novel tools to test new feed additives. *Feed International,* 20(8), 22-26.

Mbwambo, Z.., Luyengi, L. and Kinghorn, D. (1996). Phytochemicals: A glimpse into their structural and biological variation. *International Journal of Pharmacognosy*, 34(5), 335-343.

Petit, P., Sauvaire, Y., Ponsin, G., Manteghetti, M. Fave, A. and Ribes, G. (1993). Effects of a fenugreek seed extract on feeding behaviour in the rat: Metabolic-endocrine correlates. *Pharmacology Biochemistry and Behavior*, 45, 369-74.

Platel, K. and Srinivasan K. (1996). Influence of dietary spices or their active principles on digestive enzymes of small intestinal mucosa in rats. *International Journal of Food Science and Nutrition*, 47(1), 55-9.

Richard, H. (ed) (1992). *Spices and Aromats.* Lavoisier, Paris.

Türii, M., Türi, E., Koljalg, S., and Mikelsaar, M. (1997). Influence of aqueous extracts of medicinal plants on surface hydrophobicity of *Escherichia coli* strains of different origin. *APMIS,* 105, 956-62.

*This paper was first published in 2001*

23

# THE EFFECT OF COMMERCIAL-SCALE PROCESSING ON THE DEGREE OF DNA FRAGMENTATION IN ANIMAL FEEDS

N. Smith[1], E.R. Deaville[2], W.S. Hawes[3] and G.C. Whitelam[3]
[1]*ADAS Rosemaund, Preston Wynne, Hereford, HR1 3PG*
[2]*ADAS Nutritional Sciences Research Unit, Alcester Road, Stratford-on-Avon, CV37 9RQ*
[3]*Department of Biology, The University of Leicester, Leicester, LE1 7RH*

## Introduction

A key question in assessing new genetically modified (GM) crops is whether it is possible for novel genetic material present in animal feed to transfer to animal tissues or bacteria in the gastro-intestinal (GI) tract of animals fed such material. Of particular concern has been the introduction of antibiotic-resistance genes to some GM crops and the potential for these to cause an increase in the levels of antibiotic-resistant human pathogens. The Advisory Committee on Novel Foods and Processes (ACNFP, 1996) has concluded that the likelihood of transfer is low, but cannot be ruled out altogether.

If a foreign gene is to transfer to a bacterium and express a functional protein product, it is a requirement that the feed material contain fragments of DNA large enough to contain the potentially functional gene. The varied feed ingredients included in the diets of animals may be subjected to a range of physical and/or chemical processes, which could have the effect of fragmenting feed DNA. This chapter describes recent work carried out to assess the degree of DNA fragmentation in various animal feeds as a result of commercial-scale processing.

Introduction of foreign DNA into plant genomes during the generation of GM crops has led to concerns over the safety of such plants. Of particular concern is the presence of antibiotic-resistance genes in some plants, the integration of which can occur in two ways. Firstly, during the initial phases of constructing the foreign DNA to be added to the plant, it is necessary to select the DNA in bacterial cells. An efficient method for achieving this uses an antibiotic-resistance gene which, when incorporated into the DNA, will confer resistance to the antibiotic later used to kill other bacterial cells lacking the gene, thereby selecting only bacteria containing the DNA of interest. Unless steps are taken to remove the antibiotic-resistance gene, it will remain as part of the foreign DNA added to the plant cell and can therefore become integrated into the plant genome along with the gene of interest. Secondly, once foreign DNA has been added to plant cells, those cells that have received the DNA must be selected from those that have not. This can be achieved by adding an antibiotic-resistance gene on the same piece of DNA containing the gene of interest. When the plant cells are treated with the appropriate antibiotic, those that contain the resistance gene and gene of interest will survive and continue to grow, whereas those that lack the gene will die.

## CIBA-GEIGY BT MAIZE

The product initiating concern over antibiotic-resistance genes in plants was Ciba-Geigy (now Novartis) Bt Maize. Submitted to the EC for marketing consent to cultivate the product for the production of seed, silage and grain for animal feed and grain for industrial processing, the product contains a number of foreign genes including the *bla* gene, which confers resistance to ß-lactam antibiotics such as ampicillin. The main worry is that antibiotic genes present in animal feed might be capable of being taken up by bacteria present in the GI tract of animals fed such material, which could lead to the development of antibiotic-resistant human pathogens and ultimately compromise clinical treatment of serious infections.

It is thought that the widespread use of antibiotics in animal feed and for clinical use has already led to high levels of antibiotic-resistant bacteria that infect humans. Would an increase in the number of antibiotic-resistant bacteria, as a result of transfer from animal feeds, cause a significant risk to human health and welfare? In the assessment of Ciba-Geigy (now Novartis) Bt maize, the risk was deemed negligible and a qualified majority vote by Member States resulted in the product receiving marketing consent in February 1997.

## CROPS SUBMITTED FOR MARKETING CONSENT

To date ten GM food-crop products have received EC marketing consent. The number of applications pending for EC marketing consent totals 18 (Table 23.1). Three of these applications did not receive a qualified majority decision, which leaves them to be considered by the Council of Ministers. An application for a potato product has been withdrawn and the remaining products are at various stages of the application process. Amongst those crops already submitted for marketing consent are some containing genes that confer resistance to the antibiotics: streptomycin and spectinomycin, which are becoming increasingly clinically important, kanamycin and ß-lactams such as ampicillin.

**Table 23.1** APPLICATIONS FOR EC MARKETING CONSENT

| *Crop* | *Total Applications* | *Approved* |
|---|---|---|
| Chicory | 2 | 1 |
| Cotton | 2 | |
| Fodder Beet | 1 | |
| Linseed Flax | 1 | |
| Maize | 10 | 4 |
| Oilseed Rape | 8 | 4 |
| Potato | 2 | |
| Soyabean | 1 | 1 |
| Tomato | 1 | |

## ASSESSMENT OF RISK

In order for foreign DNA to transfer from animal feed and become expressed in a bacterium, the following must occur:

(i) DNA in animal feed must be in fragment sizes large enough to hold complete and therefore potentially functional genes
(ii) DNA must survive conditions in the GI tract
(iii) bacteria in the GI tract must be capable of physically taking up the DNA
(iv) once inside the bacterium, to prevent the DNA from being degraded by bacterial enzymes it would need to be incorporated into a plasmid or chromosomal DNA, or else form a plasmid itself
(v) for the gene to be expressed, it would have to bring with it the necessary DNA sequences to facilitate expression in a bacterium. Alternatively, if integrated at an appropriate location in the host's DNA, it is possible that the foreign DNA could become expressed through the influence of endogenous regulatory mechanisms.

The likelihood of all of these criteria culminating to facilitate expression of an antibiotic-resistance gene in a bacterium is probably low, but not impossible. The factors that might be involved in facilitating such a phenomenon have been comprehensively reviewed by Forano and Flint (1998). The work described in the current chapter serves to answer questions related to the first requirement for transfer to occur: that foreign DNA in animal feeds must be present in fragment sizes large enough to contain potentially functional genes.

## Experimental approach

The application of chemicals, heat, pressure and enzymes to DNA can result in changes in the physical structure of the DNA, including breaking of the molecule into smaller fragments. One could reasonably expect therefore, that industrial processing of plant material in the production of animal feeds might serve to fragment DNA substantially. The types of feed material under examination in this study are illustrated in Figure 23.1. They have been taken from various sources and include unprocessed material, material from sequential points within the processing system and finished products.

| Unprocessed Material | | Processed Material |
|---|---|---|
| Soya bean | ⇨ | Soyabean Meal / Soya Hulls |
| Maize Grain | ⇨ | Maize Gluten Feed / Maize bran |
| Rapeseed | ⇨ | Rapeseed Meal |
| Rice | ⇨ | Rice Bran |
| | ⇨ | Wheat Feed |
| | ⇨ | Sunflower Meal |
| | ⇨ | Palm Kernel Meal |
| | ⇨ | Distillers' Grains |
| | ⇨ | Cotton Seed Meal |

**Figure 23.1** Animal feed ingredients proposed for study

DNA fragment size in the feeds is being examined using established DNA extraction techniques, followed by separation and visualisation of the resulting DNA using electrophoresis in agarose gels and ethidium bromide staining. In instances where the DNA cannot be visualised using this method, the samples are subject to analysis by Polymerase Chain Reaction (PCR) to determine whether fragments large enough to contain potentially functional genes are present.

DNA is purified from the feed material using a technique that involves freezing and grinding the tissue in liquid nitrogen, lysing the nuclei and digesting any RNA present. Precipitating and removing proteins and other unwanted substances and finally precipitating the DNA and resuspending in a small volume of buffer. The DNA is then separated according to size by electrophoresis in an agarose gel. The gel is a solid matrix through which DNA can travel. Once the sample has been placed into the gel and an electrical current applied, the DNA, being negatively charged, will move toward the positive electrode. Smaller molecules move through the matrix more easily than larger molecules, so in any given time smaller DNA molecules will move further than larger molecules, thus separating the DNA on the basis of it's size. To visualise the DNA, it is stained using ethidium bromide, a chemical that intercalates between the double strands of the DNA molecule in a 1: 1 ratio. When the gel is placed in UV light and photographed, the ethidium bromide fluoresces and the DNA appears white on a black background.

## Interim results

### PRELIMINARY STUDY

The wide range of feed samples to be examined in this study necessitated identification of a DNA-extraction method capable of producing sufficient yields of good quality DNA from the majority of samples. In order to achieve this, a preliminary study was carried out using four feed samples representing diverse chemistries and processing methods. The feeds chosen were whole maize grains, maize gluten feed, whole soya beans and extracted soyabean meal. Six commercially available DNA extraction kits were evaluated. In our hands, two of the kits gave consistently low DNA yields. Three kits gave inconsistently higher yields of DNA, but the samples were usually visibly contaminated with impurities that had co-precipitated with the DNA during the extraction procedure. Such impurities would undoubtedly have adversely affected attempts to PCR from such samples. In contrast, however, the Promega Wizard® Genomic DNA Purification Kit produced consistently higher yields of DNA compared with other kits, with less visible contamination from co-precipitating substances. Furthermore, purified DNA from these samples was used as a template to amplify specific fragments of DNA successfully using PCR.

Typical DNA yields extracted from the four feeds used in the preliminary study to evaluate the DNA extraction process are illustrated in Figure 23.2. For each sample half of the total DNA yield from 30mg of starting tissue has been loaded on to the gel and in each case duplicate extractions have been performed (all gels illustrating results of DNA extractions in this chapter, show loadings representing half the total yield of DNA from 30 mg of feed material). DNA purified from both the whole maize grains and whole soya beans indicates that it is present in fragments of approximately 23kbp. This is the expected size of DNA from plant tissue that has not undergone treatment other than the extraction procedure itself. The DNA purified from the maize gluten feed and extracted soyabean meal appear, however, to have undergone some form of degradation during the processing of the products. The DNA purified from the extracted soyabean meal appears to consist of fragments of DNA ranging from 12000bp - 100bp. The nucleic acid from the maize gluten feed appears as a band of less than 400bp in length. Further experiments performed on the sample of maize gluten feed established that the bright 400bp band consists mostly, if not entirely of RNA. In this particular instance, digestion of RNA into its constituent ribonucleotides to remove it from the gel, and therefore prevent it from interfering with the DNA results, was not very efficient. Although no DNA can be seen from the maize gluten feed sample this does not mean that there is no DNA present. It may simply be that DNA is present but not in sufficient quantity for visualisation. In order to establish whether DNA is present in the sample, PCR was employed.

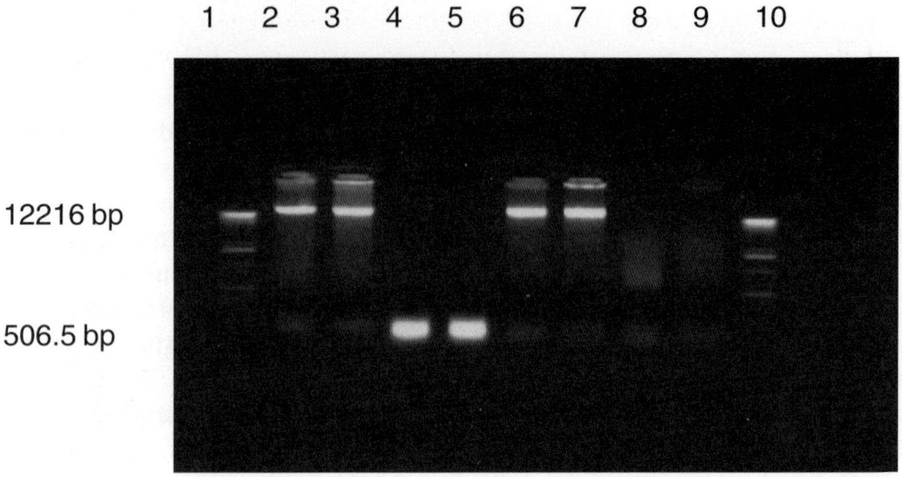


**Figure 23.2** DNA extraction from samples of maize and soya using Promega Wizard® Genomic Purification Kit. 1, 1 kb DNA ladder; 2-3, whole maize grains; 4-5, maize gluten feed; 6-7, whole soyabeans (A); 8-9, extracted soyabean meal (A); 10, 1 kb DNA ladder.

## POLYMERASE CHAIN REACTION (PCR)

PCR is an *in vitro* technique that generates many copies of a specific short piece of DNA lying between two regions of known DNA sequence. Short single-stranded DNA primers flank the target sequence that is then repeatedly replicated by a thermostable DNA polymerase enzyme in a series of heating and cooling cycles. These cycles include (i) denaturation of the double-stranded DNA into it's component single strands, (ii) annealing of the synthetic single-stranded primers to their complementary sequence on the now single-stranded DNA and (iii) generation of new DNA by extension from the synthetic primers using DNA polymerase and the single-stranded full-length DNA as a template. PCR can generate thousands of copies of the same piece of DNA from just a few starting molecules, thus providing sufficient DNA for visualisation.

In order to establish whether or not the DNA extraction technique could provide template DNA of sufficient purity to facilitate the amplification of PCR products, PCR primers were designed to amplify DNA fragments of varying sizes from the four feed samples in the preliminary study. These primers amplify regions of two endogenous genes, one found in maize and the other in soyabean, encoding ribulose-1,5-bisphosphate carboxylase small subunit. The results of PCR using primers designed to amplify a 554 bp and

221 bp product from whole soya beans (sample A) and extracted soyabean meal (A) are illustrated in Figure 23.3. The results indicate that the DNA template from each of the extractions is of sufficient purity to facilitate amplification of the expected PCR product (although not visible on the photograph of the gel, it was possible to see a band of 221bp in lane 3). Similar PCR reactions were also performed using template DNA from the maize DNA extractions and PCR primers specific for maize ribulose-1,5-bisphosphate carboxylase small subunit gene.

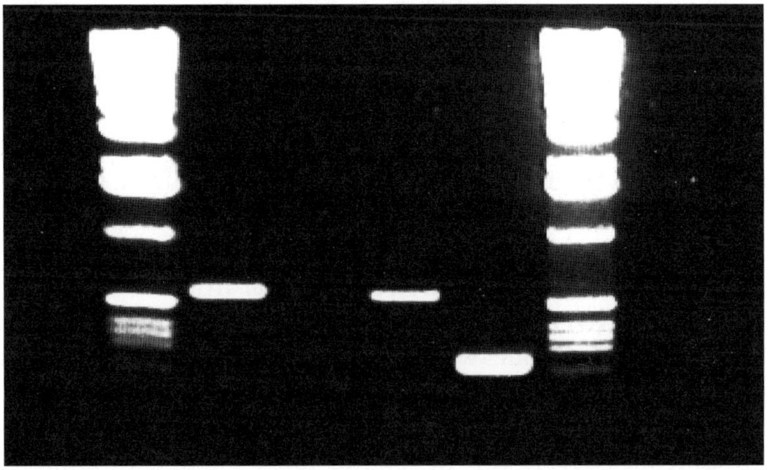


**Figure 23.3** PCR amplification of 554 bp and 221 bp fragments from samples of soyabean feed. 1, 1 kb DNA ladder; 2, whole soyabeans (A) -554bp fragment; 3, whole soyabeans (A) - 221 bp fragment; 4, extracted soyabean meal (A) - 554bp fragment; 5, extracted soyabean meal (A) - 221 bp fragment; 6, 1 kb DNA ladder.

To date, 533bp and 266bp DNA fragments have been amplified from the whole maize grains, but not from the sample of maize gluten feed (results not shown). The question therefore remains as to whether or not the maize gluten feed contains DNA of sufficient size to contain potentially functional genes. Although DNA has not been detected in this sample, it is likely that there is DNA present. Investigations are being conducted to see whether the problem can be resolved by: (i) performing larger-scale DNA extractions using a greater mass of starting material, essentially to create a DNA sample (that can be loaded on to an agarose gel) that contains a potentially higher concentration of DNA, and/or (ii) modification of the chosen DNA extraction procedure, which may be unsuitable for this particular sample.

In some instances it is possible for DNA to be present in a sample and for PCR to fail to amplify any piece of DNA repeatedly from that sample. This might occur for a number of reasons, but is usually the result of inhibitory substances from the plant that have co-precipitated with the DNA.

## SOYABEAN FEED SAMPLES

Once the preliminary study had been completed, further feed samples were analysed using the techniques established and optimised during the initial phase of the work. DNA extracted from two sources of whole soya beans (B and C) and a sample of full-fat soyabean meal (A) are illustrated in Figure 23.4. As expected, the two samples of whole soya beans contain DNA of approximately 23kbp in length, large enough to contain numerous potentially-functional genes. In contrast however, the sample of full-fat soyabean meal appears to contain no DNA. Figure 23.5. illustrates DNA extracted from other processed soyabean products including soya cake, two different samples of extracted soyabean meal (A and B) and full-fat soyabean meal (B). These results are interesting because they highlight differences between equivalent feed samples sourced from different locations, which perhaps suggests that differences in the production of feed material may affect the amount of DNA present in a sample and the degree to which it has been degraded. In Figure 23.4. the DNA extraction from full fat soyabean meal (A) produced no visible DNA, however in Figure 23.5. DNA extraction from a different source of full fat soyabean meal (B) resulted in visible high molecular weight DNA. Likewise, the DNA extractions from two different sources of extracted soyabean meal, shown in Figure 23.5., resulted in visibly high molecular weight DNA in one sample and no visible DNA in the other. The sample of soya cake produced DNA fragments over 12kbp in length, large enough to contain potentially functional genes. Again, PCR was performed using several of the soyabean samples to determine whether or not DNA was present in the samples from Figures 23.4 and 23.5 which showed no visible DNA. The results of the PCR experiments with soyabean samples are illustrated in Figure 23.6. In all samples, including the samples of full-fat (A) and extracted soyabean meal (A) that lacked visible DNA in the agarose gels, a PCR product of 554bp was amplified. This indicates that there is DNA in these samples of sufficient length to contain potentially functional genes. (The mobility of the DNA in lanes 2-8 has been affected slightly by the high concentration of salt in these samples).

## OILSEED RAPE FEED SAMPLES

Figure 23.7 illustrates DNA extracted from three oilseed rape samples: whole rapeseed, rapeseed meal expelled and rapeseed meal extracted. The whole rapeseed, as expected, resulted in the extraction of DNA fragments of approximately 23kbp. DNA extracted from the expelled rapeseed meal, which had undergone some degree of processing, also yielded large fragments of

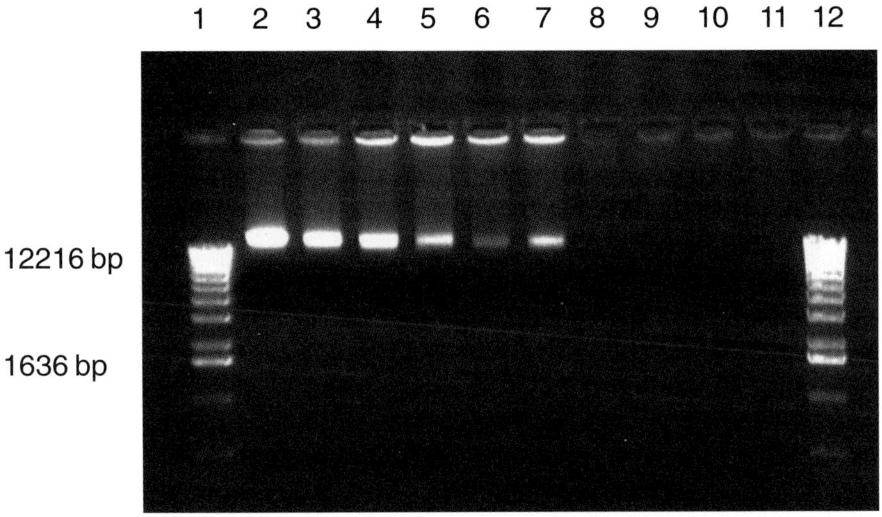


**Figure 23.4** DNA extracted from samples of soyabean feed. 1, 1 kb DNA ladder; 2-4, whole soya beans (B); 5-7, whole soya beans (C), 8-10, full-fat soyabean meal (A); 11, water control; 12, 1 kb DNA ladder.

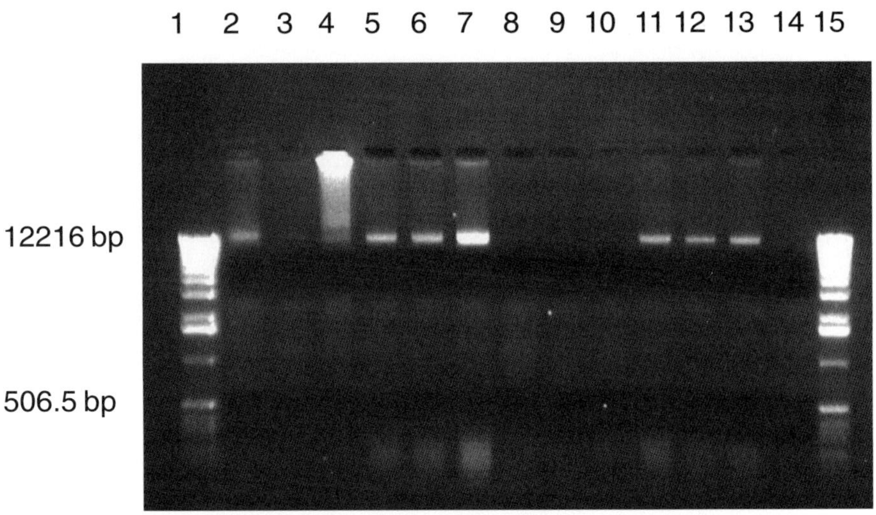


**Figure 23.5** DNA extracted from samples of processed soyabean feed. 1, 1 kb DNA ladder; 2-4, soya cake; 5-7, extracted soyabean meal (B); 8-10, extracted soyabean meal (A); 11-13, full-fat soyabean meal (B); 14, water control; 15, 1kb DNA ladder.

DNA approximately 12kbp in length, but more extensive fragmentation had also occurred resulting in a visible range of DNA fragments from approximately 12000bp to 100bp. The DNA sample purified from extracted rapeseed meal, like some of the other processed samples, showed no visible DNA in any of the extractions performed. To establish whether DNA was present in this

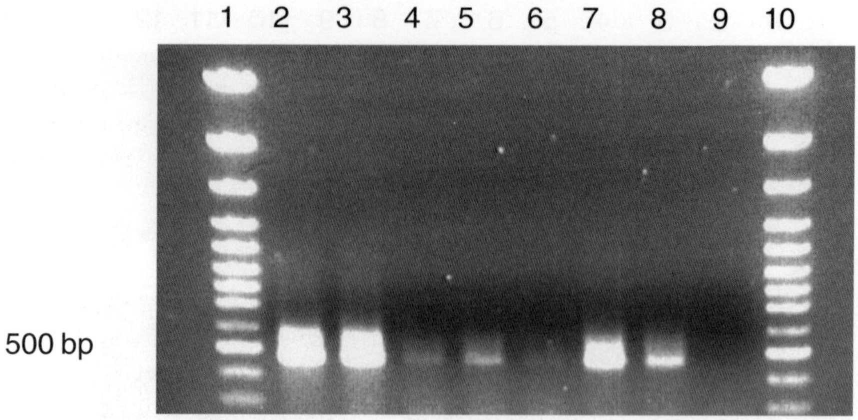


**Figure 23.6** PCR amplification of a 554 bp fragment from samples of soya bean feed. 1, 100 bp DNA Ladder Plus; 2, whole soya beans (B); 3, whole soya beans (C); 4-6, full-fat soyabean meal (A); 7, whole soyabeans (A); 8, soyabean meal extracted (A); 9, water control; 10, 100 bp DNA Ladder Plus.

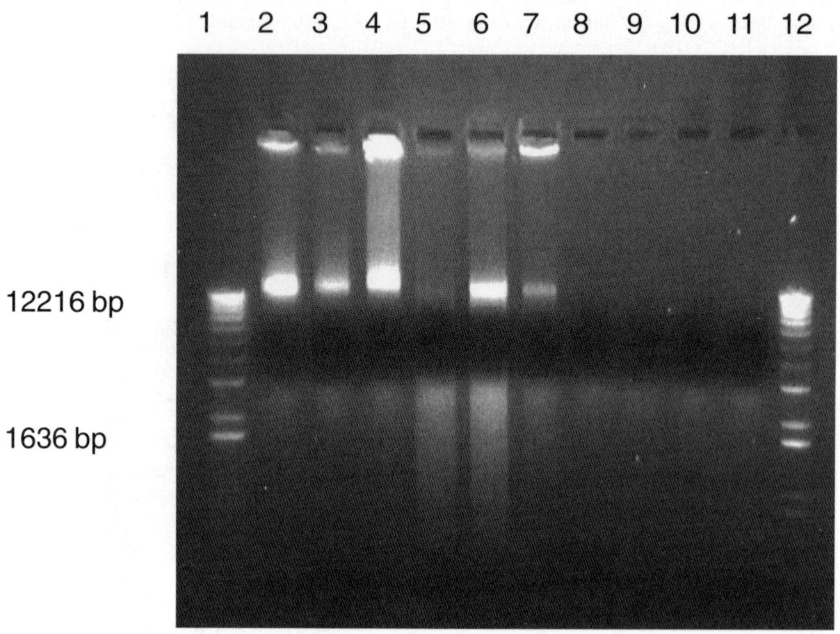


**Figure 23.7** DNA extracted from samples of oilseed rape feed. 1, 1 kb DNA ladder; 2-4, whole rapeseeds; 5-7, rapeseed meal expelled; 8-10, rapeseed meal extracted; 11, water control; 12, 1 kb DNA ladder.

sample, PCR was performed to amplify a 532bp region of an endogenous ribulose-1,5-bisphosphate carboxylase small subunit gene. Using DNA from the whole rapeseed and expelled rapeseed meal extractions as positive controls, the expected PCR products were obtained for both positive controls but not the extracted rapeseed meal (Figure 23.8). This negative result could be indicative of DNA fragments smaller than 532bp. A second PCR reaction was designed to amplify a fragment of 186bp. Again, the expected PCR products were obtained for the positive controls, whole rapeseed and expelled rapeseed meal DNA, but a negative result was obtained for the extracted rapeseed meal (Figure 23.9).

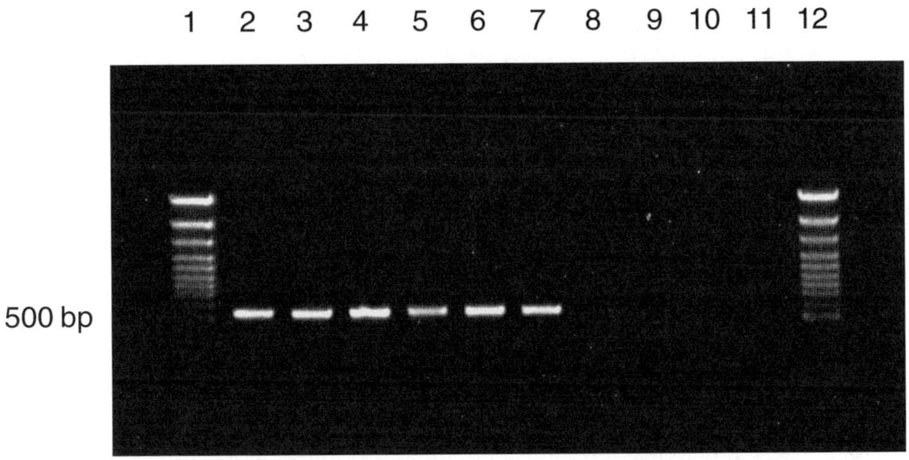


**Figure 23.8** PCR amplification of a 532 bp fragment from samples of oilseed rape feed. 1, 100bp DNA Ladder Plus; 2-4, whole rapeseed; 5-7, rapeseed meal expelled; 8-10, rapeseed meal extracted; 11, water control; 12, 100bp DNA Ladder Plus.

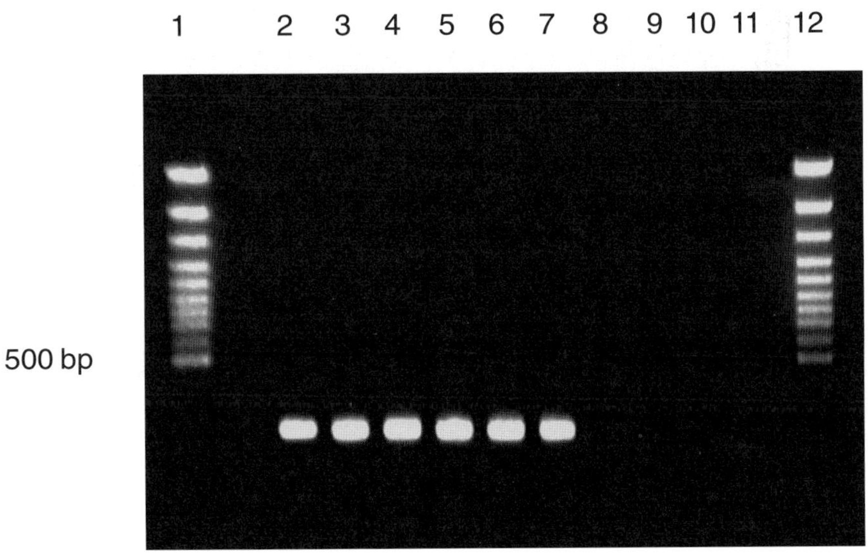


**Figure 23.9** PCR amplification of a 186 bp fragment from samples of oilseed rape feed. 1, 100bp DNA Ladder Plus; 2-4, whole rapeseed; 5-7, rapeseed meal expelled; 8-10, rapeseed meal extracted; 11, water control; 12, 100bp DNA Ladder Plus.

## Conclusions

Our interim results show that extraction of DNA from unprocessed soyabean, maize and oilseed rape material yields DNA fragments of approximately 23kbp in length. This is shorter than the DNA present in plant cells because the extraction process itself fragments the DNA to some extent. However, 23 kbp is the typical length of DNA yielded from undamaged plant cells. This inherent fragmentation by the extraction process does not affect our results in any way because we are interested in establishing which feed samples do and do not contain DNA fragments large enough to contain a potentially functional gene. Any fragment of DNA smaller than 500bp is very unlikely to contain a functional gene.

Processed samples of soyabean and oilseed rape have produced a variety of results including samples containing unfragmented DNA, visibly fragmented DNA, no visible DNA and DNA fragments of at least 500bp detected only by the use of PCR. It is interesting that different sources of the same feed ingredient have produced different results, which may reflect different processing regimes during the production of these products.

Where DNA extraction and/or PCR analysis has failed to detect DNA in the maize gluten feed and extracted rapeseed meal samples, work is continuing to ensure the results obtained are correct.

Antibiotic-resistance genes were used widely in the production of the first generation of GM crops. Although they appear to be the focus of attention at the moment, the development of new selectable marker genes and methods for the removal of unwanted genes from transgenic plants mean that their use and integration into plant genomes is now being avoided wherever possible (Malik and Saroha, 1999). The completed results from this project will provide background information on DNA fragment size in animal feeds. Such information will be valuable in the safety assessment of new products by expert advisory committees.

## Acknowledgements

The authors would like to thank the Ministry of Agriculture, Fisheries and Food for their financial support of this project and the feed industry for providing appropriate feed samples.

## References

Advisory Committee on Novel Foods and Processes (1996) The use of antibiotic resistance markers in genetically modified plants for human food,

Clarification of principles for decision making. ACNFP Secretariat, MAFF, London.

Forano, E. and Flint, H.J. (1999) Genetically modified organisms: consequences for ruminant health and nutrition. *Proceedings of the European Conference Ruminant Nutrition, human health and environment,* cité des Sciences et de l'Industrie, Paris, 30 November 1999, 25pp.

Malik, V.S. and Saroha, M.K. (1999) Marker gene controversy in transgenic plants. *Journal of Plant Biochemistry and Biotechnology*. **8**, 1-13

*This paper was first published in 2000*

24

# FEED COMPOSITION AND ENVIRONMENTAL POLLUTION

MARTIN VERSTEGEN AND SEERP TAMMINGA
*Department of Animal Sciences, Animal Nutrition Group, Wageningen University and Research Centre, The Netherlands*

## Introduction

Animal production has always been closely related to the interchange of minerals and nutrients between soil, animals and plants. In some countries and parts of the world intensive animal production systems have evolved with high animal numbers on a relatively small land surface. This has led to a burden for the soil, water and air. The soil and water have been enriched with minerals, with concomitant consequences for the ecosystem. This has brought awareness that this excessive burden is undesirable. In addition, emissions into the air are becoming increasingly important because some greenhouse gases are produced as a consequence of agricultural activities. Causes of the problem can be related to the intensity of production and to extensify this again may be part of the solution of the problem. The other part of the solution may be found in technical approaches. For example, in the Netherlands legislation in the 1980s and 1990s was mostly aimed at reducing the surplus of phosphorus (P) on the land back to equilibrium with its uptake by plants and some unavoidable losses. The consequence of this was that research focussed on reducing P excretion, especially by pigs and poultry. This was mainly achieved by nutritional means; e.g. selecting feedstuffs with higher P digestibility or adding phytase and by adjusting P in diet to the needs of the animals. This has led to a drastic reduction in P excretion per animal, as shown in Table 24.1 (Jongbloed, 2001). The surplus of minerals and greenhouse gases produced by agriculture has led to legislation, which in most countries is based on restoring the equilibrium between emission by the animals on the one hand, and uptake by the crop and inevitable losses on the other. In other countries, additional solutions are used, with the aid of technology, to reach the desired equilibrium.

This chapter will focus on a few aspects that are related to nutrition and environment, and some aspects of legislation

**Table 24.1** EXCRETION OF PHOSPHORUS (P) BY A GROWING-FINISHING PIG FROM 25 TO 110 kg IN THE NETHERLANDS

| *Year* | **Feed P (g/kg)* | *Feed/Gain* | *Excretion P (kg)* |
|---|---|---|---|
| 1973 | 7.4 | 3.37 | 1.62 |
| 1983 | 6.2 | 3.08 | 1.18 |
| 1988 | 6.0/5.0* | 2.96 | 0.88 |
| 1992 | 5.5/4.9 | 2.87 | 0.80 |
| 2000 | 5.3/4.7 | 2.60 | 0.62 |

* starter/grower-finisher diet (from Jongbloed 2001)

## Legislation

The subject of animal nutrition and environmental pollution in farm animals under Dutch conditions has been reviewed several times (Tamminga, 1992; Tamminga and Verstegen, 1992; Tamminga, 1996). For about 15 years, the Dutch government has developed and introduced various pieces of legislation to reduce mineral surpluses and ammonia volatilisation (Siemes, 2000). These measures comprise a mineral accounting system called MINAS, the necessity for farmers to have manure disposal contracts and levies for losses that exceed the loss standards. In 2002 standard losses for nitrogen (N) are 180 and 100 kg/ha for grassland and arable land respectively; for phosphate ($P_2O_5$) they are 20 kg/ha for both grass and arable land.

It is important to note that the EU plans to standardise allowances of, for example, N in manure. EU Nitrate Directive standards are based on an equilibrium between production and discharge of manure. This is done by allowing maximum deposits per hectare and by having a system of manure contracts. It is not yet certain how much the minimum deposits will be. The general EU standards in 2002 will probably be 170 kg N/ha/year. The Netherlands is applying for a more flexible standard for grassland (e.g. 250 kg N/ha/year)

It is foreseen that maximum levels for Cu and Zn in diets for different categories of animal will be as shown in Table 24.2 (Jongbloed 2001)

For each category of farm animal, a standard N excretion per animal per year has been established. This comprises an estimate of N production in urine and faeces (Table 24.2; Tamminga *et al.*, 2000), corrected for losses considered inevitable (Oenema *et al.*, 2000). These latter losses comprise those from farmhouses, during manure storage and during the application of manure to the land. An equally detailed system for controlling input and output of N was developed in Denmark (Damgaard Poulsen and Kristensen, 1998). Other Scandinavian countries have also introduced legislation to control N and a comparison of the different figures in the different countries is shown in Table 24.3.

**Table 24.2** EXPECTED MAXIMUM LEVELS OF CU AND ZN IN FEEDS mg/kg (JONGBLOED 2001)

| | | *Currently* | *EU-2002?* |
|---|---|---|---|
| Cu | Pigs | 35/175 | 25 |
| | Sheep/fish | 15 | 15 |
| | Calves | 30-50 | 10-15 |
| | Other | 35 | 20 |
| Zn | Pigs/poultry | 250 | 120 |
| | Ruminants | 250 | 100 |

**Table 24.3** STANDARD N EXCRETIONS IN DIFFERENT COUNTRIES (TAMMINGA *et al.*, 2000)

| | *Netherlands* | | *Denmark* | | *Norway* | | *Sweden* | |
|---|---|---|---|---|---|---|---|---|
| | *kg N/yr* | *eq.*[a] | *kg N/yr* | *eq.*[a] | *Animal units* | *eq.*[a] | *Animals/ ha* | *eq.*[a] |
| Dairy cow | 129 | 1.00 | 128 | 1.00 | 1 | 1.00 | 1.6 | 1.00 |
| Suckler cow | 86.9 | 1.48 | 73.3 | 1.75 | 1.5 | 1.50 | 2.3 | 1.44 |
| Heifer (1-2 yr) | 82.9 | 1.56 | 45.0 | 2.84 | 3 | 3.00 | 4.6 | 2.88 |
| Calf (<1yr) | 40.5 | 3.19 | 39.6 | 3.23 | | | 5.8 | 3.63 |
| Sheep | 13.3 | 9.70 | 20.0 | 6.40 | 7 | 7.00 | 15 | 9.38 |
| Goats | 14.2 | 9.08 | 20.0 | 6.40 | 7 | 7.00 | 15 | 9.38 |
| Sow | 28.1 | 4.59 | 36.7 | 3.49 | 2.5 | 2.50 | 2.2 | 1.38 |
| Fattening pig | 11.7 | 11.0 | 10.2 | 12.6 | 18 | 18.0 | 10.5 | 6.56 |
| Laying hen | 0.676 | 191 | 0.742 | 173 | 80 | 80 | 100 | 63 |
| Pullet | 0.325 | 397 | 0.285 | 449 | 550 | 550 | 250 | 156 |
| Broiler | 0.543 | 238 | 0.494 | 259 | 1400 | 1400 | 470 | 294 |
| Turkey | 1.92 | 67 | 1.90 | 67 | 40 | 40 | 140 | 88 |
| Duck | 1.10 | 117 | 1.41 | 91 | | | | |
| Horse | | | 50.0 | 2.56 | 2 | 2.00 | 3.0 | 1.88 |
| Mink | 1.30 | 99.2 | 0.879 | 146 | 40 | 40 | 50 | 31 |

[a]: number of animals equivalent to 1 dairy cow

On the basis of these standard excretions, farmers in The Netherlands had to demonstrate by January 2002 that they have access to sufficient land, so that surpluses above allowed levels could be avoided. This land can either be part of the farm, or contracted from others to dispose of manure within the nitrogen application limits. By 2003, the maximum application of N with manure will be 250 kg N/ha on grassland and 170 kg N/ha on arable land; the latter including land used to grow maize. Surpluses will be charged with a levy that, from 2003 onwards, will amount to €9.09 per kg surplus phosphate/ha and €1.14 per kg surplus N/ha.

A second important aspect is preventing ammonia emissions. To prevent these losses on grassland, manure injection has to be used, rather than spreading. On arable land spreading manure is still allowed, but it has to be ploughed in right away. In addition, manure application is restricted to the growing season, roughly between February 15 and October 15. Storage outside livestock housing is only allowed in covered manure stores.

## Nitrogen balances in dairy farms and possible interventions

The vast majority of N losses to the environment by ruminants are caused by dairy farms which, in the Netherlands, are largely based on grassland. About half of the 2 million ha available for farming is permanent grassland. Important inputs of N are through the use of high levels of inorganic N-fertiliser and to a lesser extent through concentrates. Monitoring ruminal N losses at farm level seems possible by monitoring the urea content in milk at farm level (Hof et al., 1997). Various ways exist to reduce N inputs in dairy farms. Most of them have an impact on or are related to nutrition.

### USE OF INORGANIC N FERTILISER

Since 1985 the use of inorganic fertiliser has declined by about 20% and seems set to stabilise at around 200 kg N/ha/yr. An important reason for this decline has been a better utilisation of N as fertiliser in animal manure (Siemes, 2000). A further reduction seems feasible, as shown by Valk *et al.* (2000). Reducing N fertilisation significantly reduced the N-content in grass (Figure 24.1) without showing negative effects on milk production.

Reducing N-fertilisation from 450 kg to 300 kg/ha/yr increased the days of re-growth by 4%; a further reduction to 150 kg/ha/yr caused an increase in the days of re-growth of 12%. At the lowest level of fertilisation, the crude protein content of the grass, when harvested at 2000 kg DM/ha, ranged between 130 and 180 g/kg Dry Matter (DM). At this level, N losses from the rumen were slightly negative to moderately positive. If necessary, a further reduction in rumen losses is possible by supplementing grass with products that have surplus energy, in relation to their CP content. Both roughages and concentrates can be used.

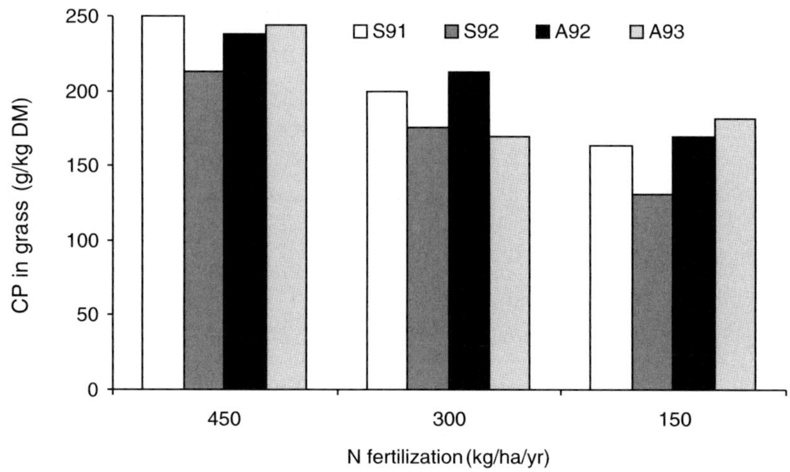


**Figure 24.1** Effect of N fertilisation on Crude Protein (CP) content of fresh grass in different seasons and years (Valk *et al.*, 2000)

## USE OF MAIZE SILAGE

An important development in the last ten years has been the supplementation of grass and grass-silage based diets with maize silage. The area of grass has declined by 0.9% per year, whereas the area of maize has grown by 2% per year. A wide range of maize varieties is available, varying in digestibility of the vegetative part, notably cell walls, as well as varying in starch content.

## USE OF CONCENTRATES

Supplementation with concentrates can be performed by designing concentrates with a relatively low N content, or by designing concentrates with a higher than average ratio between the protein value (PDI, DVE, Metabolizable Protein, AAT) and crude protein (Nx6.25) content. Concentrates with a low N content will have a surplus of energy, which can be used to capture the surplus of protein in grass. It should be realised, however, that of each g of N captured in microbial protein, about one third is lost either in faecal excretion of undigested N or in urinary excretion of purine derivatives originating from microbial nucleic acids.

To increase the protein value/crude protein content of concentrates, a variety of processing methods is available. As an example, the effects of pressure toasting for different lengths of time are shown in Table 24.4 (Goelema, 1999).

**Table 24.4** EFFECT OF PRESSURE TOASTING ON THE RATIO BETWEEN SMALL INTESTINAL DIGESTIBLE PROTEIN (DVE) AND CRUDE PROTEIN (CP) IN LEGUME SEEDS (GOELEMA 1999)

| *Temp (°C)* | *Time (s)* | *Faba beans* | *Peas* | *Lupins* | *Soya beans* |
|---|---|---|---|---|---|
| Control | | 0.349 | 0.429 | 0.409 | 0.346 |
| 100 | 7 | 0.393 | 0.478 | 0.521 | 0.425 |
| 100 | 15 | 0.398 | | 0.585 | 0.483 |
| 100 | 30 | 0.431 | 0.520 | 0.596 | 0.532 |
| 118 | 3 | 0.438 | 0.536 | 0.598 | 0.537 |
| 118 | 7 | 0.464 | 0.578 | 0.612 | 0.553 |
| 118 | 15 | 0.501 | 0.620 | 0.666 | 0.572 |
| 118 | 30 | 0.519 | 0.645 | 0.672 | 0.557 |
| 136 | 3 | 0.555 | 0.673 | 0.698 | 0.548 |
| 136 | 7 | 0.608 | 0.722 | 0.680 | 0.581 |
| 136 | 15 | 0.667 | 0.773 | 0.718 | 0.590 |

## SYNCHRONISATION OF RUMEN FERMENTATION

An imbalance between the quantity of carbohydrates and protein degraded in the rumen is an important cause of N losses from the rumen. A lack of synchronisation between the rate at which carbohydrates and proteins are degraded may also contribute to N-losses from the rumen. For instance, the rapid degradation of CP of immature grass is not synchronised with the degradation of structural carbohydrates, creating an imbalance. If necessary, imbalances between energy and protein can be reduced by supplementing the grass. Options are supplementation with low protein roughages, such as maize silage, or with low protein concentrates (Van Vuuren et al., 1993), either high in starch, present in most grains, or high in rapidly degradable structural carbohydrates, such as beet pulp, citrus pulp, soya hulls or coconut expeller.

Synchronisation can be expressed on a daily and on an hourly basis. Experiments *in vitro* (Hoover and Stokes, 1991; Newbold and Rust, 1992) have shown positive effects of synchronisation on microbial protein synthesis. The results of *in vivo* experiments (McCarthy *et al.*, 1989; Herrera-Saldana *et al.*, 1990; Kolver *et al.*, 1998) have rarely shown positive production responses. Sinclair *et al.* (1993, 1995) tested a variety of diets with sheep, which were formulated to be either synchronised or asynchronised with respect to their hourly supply of energy and N. It was concluded that the diets formulated to be synchronous, based on *in situ* degradation characteristics of the ingredients, could alter microbial growth and efficiency positively compared with the a-synchronous diet. Sinclair *et al.* (1995) concluded that most experiments reported in the literature were based on matching the daily supply of energy and N to rumen microbes, and have therefore failed to establish a positive effect of the rate of energy and protein supply on the efficiency of microbial protein synthesis. It was also pointed out that many experimental and practical diets, which are formulated on rate of supply rather than hourly supply, incorrectly estimate the supply to rumen microbes. The positive results obtained by Sinclair *et al.* (1995) in sheep were based on an hourly release of energy and N in the rumen using *in situ* degradation characteristics of raw materials, providing evidence that synchronisation can improve the efficiency of microbial protein synthesis. To calculate the ratio between energy and protein as an estimate of synchronisation, Sinclair (1992) calculated a synchrony index to express the hourly ratio between N and organic matter. In this system a synchrony index of 1.0 represents perfect synchrony between N and energy supply throughout the day. Less than 1.0 indicates a degree of asynchrony.

Blank *et al.* (1998) reviewed the methods used to measure degradation and questioned whether synchrony of carbohydrate and crude protein could be a new variable for diet formulation. They concluded that the lack of direct evidence for positive effects of synchronisation could be partly due to the low number of trials that were conducted with high-producing ruminants and also with the low level of standardisation of methods that were used for characterisation of synchronous and asynchronous nutrient degradation. Furthermore, when too much starch is fed in a synchronised supply of carbohydrates and protein this could cause a lower microbial synthesis due to the acidic rumen environment. Therefore, synchronisation could only be an additional variable in diet formulation and not the main criterion. In their review, Sauvant and Van Milgen (1995) also concluded that the microbial protein synthesis of diets that were synchronised was not different from that with diets that were not synchronised.

## FEEDING BELOW RECOMMENDED PROTEIN LEVELS

In the Dutch DVE system, as well as in the French PDI system, recommended protein levels are fixed at an efficiency of utilisation of 0.65. Reducing DVE input to about 0.80 of these recommendations improved the efficiency of utilisation of DVE from 0.65 to 0.75 without dramatic negative effects on milk production and milk protein content (Hof *et al.*, 1994). Furthermore, no signs of an impaired feed intake due to a shortage of rumen degradable protein was observed, but the DVE/CP ratios in these experiments were relatively low and ranged only between 0.46 and 0.59 (Hof and Tamminga, 1994).

IMPROVING PROTEIN QUALITY

Supplementing dairy diets with rumen-protected lysine and methionine has been shown to improve milk protein output and lower the N output in urine and faeces (Rulquin and Verité, 1993). Effects are however marginal.

## N balances in pigs and poultry

Until recently, the emphasis in nutrition and in nutritional studies was on maximising the synthesis of body components from ingested nutrients. Kornegay and Verstegen (2001) discussed this topic. The approach has usually led to systems that maximised protein output in body and in animal products from absorbed dietary amino acids. In order to have a good protein requirement system, it is worthwhile, according to Moughan (1999), to distinguish between processes of maintenance and those associated with the growth of new body tissue. The knowledge of the amino acid requirements for different parts (or pools) of the body is used in mechanistic modelling. This can lead to new systems. At zero N growth there are still processes associated with protein metabolism at maintenance level. In a producing animal feed protein is involved both in the processes of maintenance and growth. Animals retain protein in their body in relation to their potential growth and feed availability (Black 1995; Black *et al.*, 1995). There is considerable genetic variation in growth characteristics of animals, particularly in the retention of protein in relation to energy deposition. This varies with genotype of the animal but also with physiological age, body weight and also with the diet. Black *et al.* (1986) concluded that the relationship between potential protein deposition and body weight varies considerably between strain and sex. Thus each strain will have its own protein deposition level and, as a consequence, its own optimum protein level in the diet. In poultry, different strategies are also applied for different strains of chicken for efficiency reasons and, in addition, for health reasons (Scheele *et al.,* 1999). In practice, animals are kept for production and various strategies are applied currently to reduce the amount of surplus N related to production and dietary intake.

The first group of possibilities concerns the reduction in amounts of N consumed relative to output in the animal. This can be done in various ways:

- Reduce surplus N-intake by not having a safety margin. For feed formulation this means that only minor errors can be tolerated in feed preparation and in the estimation of actual N content of raw materials from which the feed is prepared. It also means that reliable and accurate data on AA composition, or preferably AA availability, should be known.

Knowledge and use of data on ileal digestible, or preferably available, amino acids in the diet is a possible means of increasing accuracy of diet composition. De Lange *et al.* (1999) argued that, by the use of standardised true digestible amino acids of each feedstuff, one could add up the different values. With the exception of phosphorus and amino acids, however, estimates of the available nutrient requirements of pigs are not published and generally are not known. For those that are known, the use of more precise data on composition and nutrient availability of feed ingredients, and the use of better defined requirements, will allow nutritionists to formulate balanced diets to meet the needs of animals at various stages of production.

A portion of the N excreted by pigs is a direct result of feeding excessive levels of N; the greater the excess, the greater the portion of N excreted. Results of surveys of the nutrient composition of diets indicate that diets commonly contain excess amounts of certain nutrients, such as total AAs. These excesses are called "safety factors", and are included in the diet to allow for the variability of nutrient composition of feed ingredients, or to compensate for uncertainty about the availability and requirements of the nutrients. The average range of university recommendations was 110 to 120% of the National Research Council (1998) recommendations, whereas the average range of industry recommendations was 120 to 130% of these requirements (Kornegay and Verstegen, 2001). The excess for sows was somewhat lower than for finishing pigs. Other surveys have reported similar findings and, for poultry, a safety margin is also included. Furthermore, phase feeding can considerably reduce N-output through reduced N input, as shown in Table 24.5.

**Table 24.5** EFFECT OF FEEDING STRATEGY DURING THE GROWING-FINISHING PERIOD (25 TO 105 kg) ON N OUTPUT IN PIGS [a]

| *CP (g CP/kg)* | *Single-feed* *170* | *Two-feeds*[b] *170-150* | *Three-feeds*[c] *170-150-130* |
|---|---|---|---|
| N output, g/d | 31.9 | 29.0 | 26.7 |
| Percentage of two-feed strategy | 110 | 100 | 92 |

[a]Adapted from Henry and Dourmad (1993).
[b]Crude protein changed at 55 kg body weight
[c]Crude protein changed at 50 and 75 kg body weight

- A second way to reduce the amount of ingested N, whilst maintaining that available for the animals, is by inclusion of feedstuffs with a high apparent digestibility of N in feed components. This determines how much appears in the faecal matter. FEFANA (1992) estimated that nutrient excretion in waste could be reduced by about 5% through selecting highly digestible ingredients (see also Van Heugten and Van Kempen (1999)). This means that feedstuffs are used that have low levels of antinutritional factors and/or feedstuffs in which these have been reduced through processing.

- A third way to reduce N input relative to utilisation can be by optimising amino acid intake. Utilisation of amino acids is mainly determined by the availability of the most limiting amino acid. Any excess of AAs over what is needed is degraded and the surplus N will be excreted as urea or uric acid depending on the animal species. In a maize soyabean diet, about 25 % of the protein consists of unbalanced amino acids. It has been estimated that about 50 % of N in excreta of pigs, for example, can be attributed to non-optimal amino acid balance (De Lange *et al.*, 1999). If a balanced AA level is the limiting factor, e.g. a low protein diet (below that for maximum protein gain) with a sufficiently high energy level, about 15-20 % of absorbed protein is catabolysed (Kyriazakis and Emmans, 1992).
- A further improvement can be achieved by adding crystalline amino acids to diets, in order to balance amino acid composition further and match requirements for maintenance and growth. A simple means of correcting an imbalance is to replace some of the protein with crystalline amino acids, e.g. L-lysine, L-threonine, DL-methionine and L-tryptophan in the diets of animals. Ten Doeschate (1995) showed that the ratio of essential to non-essential amino acids is also important.

  This has been tested many times in pigs and poultry and the results show that it is a very effective way of reducing N-input and also N surplus by optimising dietary amino acid levels while maintaining production level (see as example Table 24.6 from Nonn and Jeroch 2000).

**Table 24.6** IMPACT OF ADDED AMINO ACIDS ON N EXCRETION IN PIGS IN g N PER ANIMAL PER DAY (NONN AND JEROCH 2000)

| *Weight range* | *Controls* | | *Added amino acids* | |
|---|---|---|---|---|
| | *Females* | *Castrates* | *Females* | *Castrates* |
| 25-60 kg | 40.1 | 33.7 | 25.0 | 19.9 |
| 60-85 kg | 44.5 | 59.2 | 29.5 | 37.3 |
| 85-110 kg | 36.2 | 43.9 | 22.6 | 28.2 |
| 25-110 kg | 39.8 | 43.3 | 25.4 | 26.6 |

Lysine supplementation of cereal grain-plant protein based diets has been widely used, and it has generally led to a decrease in dietary crude protein of approximately 20 g/kg, which results in a 17 to 22% reduction in N excretion (Gatel and Grosjean, 1992; Henry and Dourmad, 1993; Van der Honing *et al.*, 1993; Cromwell, 1994; Gatel, 1994). A further reduction in N excretion was obtained when the crude protein level was reduced by 40 g/kg and diets were supplemented with three or four of the following amino acids: lysine, threonine, tryptophan, or methionine (Bridges *et al.*, 1995; Kerr and Easter, 1995; Kephart and Sherritt, 1990; Carter *et al.,* 1996). Reductions in total N excretion ranged from 28 to 40%, and most of the decrease in Table 24.6 was in urinary N excretion; there was only a small change in faecal N losses.

Based on a review of several review papers Kerr and Easter (1995) suggested that, for each 10g/kg reduction in dietary crude protein, combined with amino acid supplementation, total N losses (faecal and urinary) could be reduced by approximately 8%. According to these authors, the use of added amino acids (often-crystalline AA) can reduce N-excretion via manure in pigs by about 35 %. Although the application of crystalline amino acids in practical situations is generally straightforward, it is recognised that there will be limits to their use, compared with intact dietary protein. For example, N retained may sometimes be lower when amino acids are supplemented to a high degree, especially when three or more amino acids replace 40 g CP/kg or more. In poultry there is also an abundance of literature on reduction of protein levels with simultaneous addition of amino acids. Studies by Summers *et al* (1992), Fancher and Jensen (1989) and Holsheimer and Janssen (1991) reported impaired weight gain in broilers with low protein and extra amino acids. Other studies by Moran *et al* (1992) and Aletor *et al* (2000) found similar performances in broilers with low dietary protein levels and extra-added amino acids. If changes occurred, these were likely to result in more abdominal fat in the body. In addition, Aletor *et al* (2000) found increased fat when protein in broiler diets was reduced to 153g/kg and the diet was fortified with extra amino acids. About 41 % less N was excreted, compared with the non-fortified diet.

- In addition to the above-mentioned approach, there are other possibilities to reduce N in excreta. One method is optimising output instead of using maximising input. Gahl *et al.* (1995) demonstrated that the most economical daily weight gain does not occur when daily weight gain is maximised, and the optimum would change as feedstuffs and input costs change. They further discussed the principle of diminishing returns. Previously, it has not been clear what exactly is meant by optimised production. It can be argued that, by maximising various subsystems, the main system will also incorporate these. The optimum will probably be at such a level that marginal efficiency is still considerable, but no longer approaching zero, as is often the case currently. The principle of diminishing returns in response to nutrient input is not new. Heady *et al.* (1954) reported that, in 14 out of 16 years, pig diets formulated using the diminishing return concept would have produced greater profits than diets formulated for maximum gain. In animal production, the larger proportion of ingested N is excreted as waste in faeces and urine. This surplus is then dispersed to the environment in water, soil and air.

There is ample evidence that the efficiency with which absorbed AAs can be used by an animal can increase considerably from current levels, provided that a correct level of essential AAs, a proper level of total AAs, and a proper amino acid/ energy ratio are supplied.

## Phosphorus

According to Van der Meer and Van der Putten (1995), inputs in intensive dairy farms originate mainly from purchased feeds (59%) and to a lesser extend from inorganic fertiliser (26%). Phosphorus requirements for dairy cows contain a fairly high safety margin. In the feed-animal part of a dairy production system, this results in a low efficiency of utilisation and a high loss of P to the soil-plant part of the system. In intensive dairy farms the high P losses also result in a low efficiency of utilisation in the soil-plant part of the system. Phosphorus excretion in ruminants and prospects for minimising P excretion by dietary manipulation in ruminants were reviewed by Valk *et al.* (2000).

### AVAILABILITY OF P

For unknown reasons, availability of P from dried forages appears to be lower than from fresh forages and concentrates. Considerable variation has been observed between P sources used as supplements in dairy diets. Significant amounts of P in ruminant diets may originate from by-products, such as soyabean meal or rapeseed meal. In such ingredients, a significant proportion of P is present in phytate. It is generally accepted that, unlike in non-ruminant animals, phytates are normally completely hydrolysed in ruminants because of the presence of microbial phytase in the rumen. However, it has recently been shown that methods that successfully reduce protein degradation in the rumen, such as heat treatment or treatment with formaldehyde, also negatively affect the availability of P (Konishi *et al*, 1999; Park *et al.,* 1999), because the treatments also protect phytate against microbial degradation.

### PHOSPHORUS REQUIREMENTS

Recommendations differ considerably between countries. For a 600 kg non-pregnant cow, eating 20 kg DM and producing 30 kg of milk, Valk *et al.* (2000) showed recommendations to vary between 59 and 85 g/day. The main causes of this variation were net requirements for maintenance, ranging between 7.2 and 22.1 g P/day, and the true absorption coefficient of P, ranging between 0.5 and 0.7. Requirements in the Netherlands were 70 g/day, but long-term experiments (Valk and Šebek, 1999) showed that even those requirements could be considerably reduced without negative effects on feed intake, milk production and body weight.

In pigs and poultry, the availability of phosphorus can be expressed in various ways (Jongbloed, 1987; Jongbloed and Henkens, 1996; Crenshaw, 2001). Environmental concerns have led to drastic changes in dietary P content and the use of phytase in the Netherlands, with some results in pigs as given in Table 24.1. Reduction in P content needs to be undertaken with knowledge of available or digestible P content (Jongbloed 2001).

## NEGATIVE P BALANCE

Like other dietary components (energy, protein) phosphorus in dairy cows is a dynamic nutrient in that to some extend the cow can adapt its metabolism to different levels of supply. In an extensive long-term study of over 100 weeks, covering two lactations and two dry periods, Valk *et al* (2002) fed three groups of multiparous dairy cows of six, nine and nine animals each, at either 100%, 80% or 67% of recommended Dutch P requirements. At nine time points in this period, the distribution of P between faecal excretion, excretion in urine and in milk and P deposition in the body were measured (Figure 24.2).

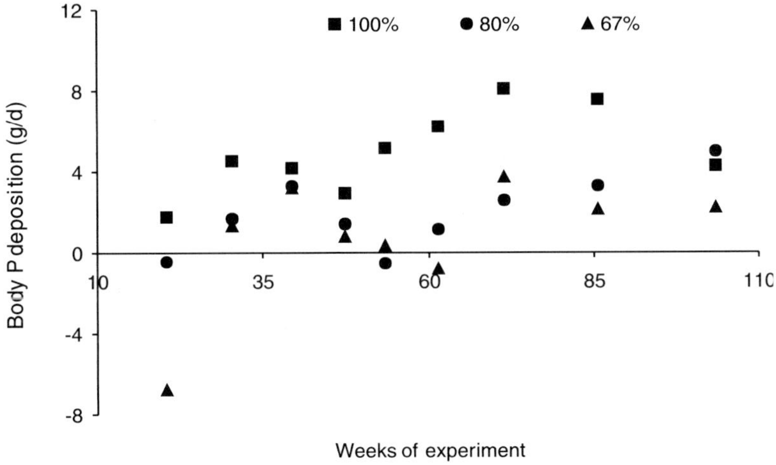


**Figure 24.2** Phosphorus balance in dairy cows fed at 100 %, 80% and 67 % of Dutch requirements

The results show that in early lactation, when fed low amounts of P in the diet (1.9 g P/kg DM), P is mobilised. However, not only was P mobilised, N excretion in milk, faeces and urine was also reduced. At the lowest level, milk production was reduced, but at the level of 80% of requirement (2.6 g P/kg DM) no negative effects were observed on feed intake, milk production, health and fertility. The authors concluded that, without much risk, P requirements could be reduced by 20%, which would significantly contribute to the desired reduction of P excretion to the environment.

## Composition of manure

Manure is a mixture of excreta (urine and faecal matter). It is composed of undigested dietary components, endogenous components and fermentation end products from endogenous microorganisms and the biomass of those microorganisms themselves. Recently, increased interest in composition of manure has developed because of its environmental impact and its value as fertiliser. In addition, there is a difference in suitability as organic fertiliser in relation to soil quality. It is thought that a high carbon to nitrogen (C/N) ratio in manure may increase its value for the soil. There is an abundance of recent evidence showing that nutrition can alter manure composition with regard to non-N, while maintaining the same total N excretion and protein gain (Canh *et al.*, 1997). Composition is related to the quality of manure and it will undoubtedly become more important in the future. Some developments already show this. It is well known that by allowing proper microbial fermentation in the large intestine, more microbial biomass will be present in the excreta of pigs. This results in apparently lower amounts of faecal digestible N. However, ileal digestible N may be at a similar level. The other consequence is that there is a different partitioning of surplus N between faecal matter and urine, as shown by Jongbloed (2001), who summarised a number of trials (Figure 24.3). An additional advantage of proper fermentable carbohydrates may be that many of them may be beneficial for gut health. However, according to Houdijk (1998), this is only true if fermentation continues in the large intestine of pigs.

Canh *et al.* (1997) showed that the excreta originating from pigs with higher levels of fermentable carbohydrates in their diet emitted considerably less ammonia than with low levels (Figure 24.4). This would also limit the release of $NH_3$ into the air (Aarnink, 1997).

## Conclusion

From the previous data and discussion it is clear that nutrition and pollution are closely associated. It is also clear that, despite the progress made in adjusting

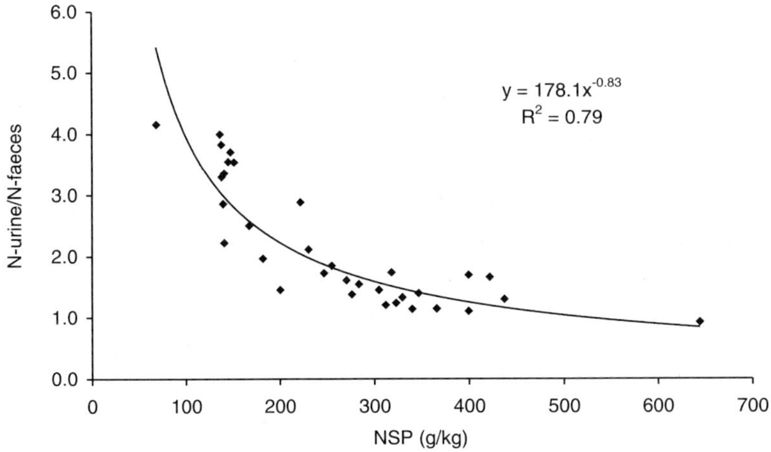


**Figure 24.3** Non Starch Polysacharide (NSP) content (oos) in the diet and the ratio of N-urine/N-faeces, Jongbloed (2001)

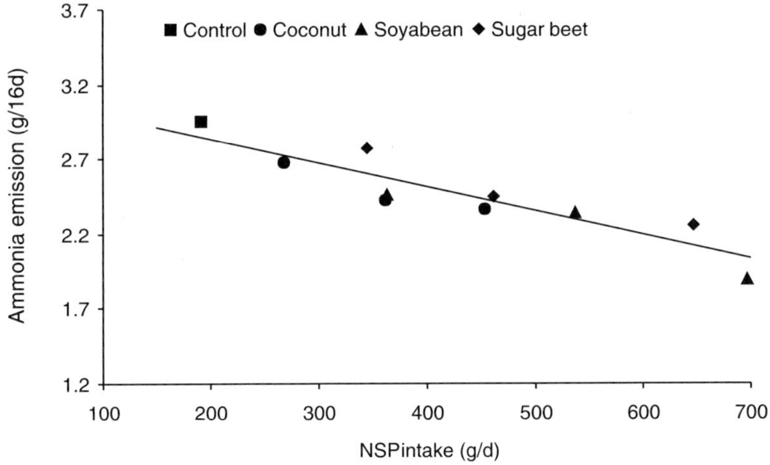


**Figure 24.4** Ammonia emission from slurry as affected by daily intake of Non Starch Polysaccharides (NSP) (Canh *et al.*, 1997)

nutrition to the needs of animals, considerable progress can be made. Legislation introduced in several countries of the EU will further stimulate research and application of techniques to reduce N and P surpluses. In addition, possibilities to limit emission of ammonia into the air from manure have not yet been fully exploited.

## References

Aarnink, A. J. A. (1997). Ammonia emission from houses for growing pigs as affected by pen design, indoor climate and behaviour. Ph.D. thesis Agricultural University, Wageningen.

Aletor V.A., I.L. Hamid, E. Niess and E. Pfeffer (2000). Low-protein amino acid-supplemented diets in broiler chickens: effects on performance, carcass characteristics, whole body composition and efficiency of nutrient utilisation *Journal of the Science of food and Agriculture* **80**:547- 554.

Black J.L., R.G. Campbell, I.H. Williams, K.J. James and G.T. Davis (1986). Simulation of energy and amino acid utilisation in the pig. *Research and development in agriculture* **3**: 121-145.

Black, J.L., G.T. Davies, H.J. Bray, L.R. Giles and R.P. Chapple (1995). Modelling the effects of genotype environment and health on nutrient utilisation. In Danfaer A and O. Lescoat eds. *Proceedings of the IV International Workshop on Modelling Nutrient Utilisation in Farm Animals*. National Institute of Animal Science Denmark, p. 85-105.

Black, J.L. (1995). Modelling energy metabolism in the pig – critical evaluation of a simple reference model p 87-102. In: P.J. Moughan, M.W.A. Verstegen, M.I. Visser-Reijneveld (Eds.). *Modelling growth in the pig*, Wageningen Press, The Netherlands.

Blank, R., K-H. Südekum, I. Immig,. and J. Kleinmans, (1998). Synchroner abbau von Kohlenhydraten und Rohprotein in den Vormägen-eine neue variable für die Rationsgestaltung? *Ubers. Tierernährg.* **26**:157-188.

Bridges, T.C., L.W. Turner, G.L. Cromwell, and J.L. Pierce (1995). Modeling the effects of diet formulation on nitrogen and phosphorus excretion in swine waste. *Appl. Eng. Agric.* **11**:731.

Canh, T. T., M.W.A. Verstegen, A.J.A. Aarnink, and J.W. Schrama (1997). Influence of dietary factors on nitrogen partitioning and composition of urine and feces of fattening pigs. *J. Anim. Sci.* **75**:700.

Carter, S. D., G.L. Cromwell, M.D. Lindemann, L.W. Turner, and T.C. Bridges (1996). Reducing N and P excretion by dietary manipulation in growing and finishing pigs. *J. Anim. Sci.* **74** (Suppl. 1):59 (Abstr.).

Crenshaw T. (2001). Calcium, phosphorus, vitamin D and vitamin K in Swine Nutrition. In (.A.J. Lewis and L.L. Southern eds.) *Swine Nutrition* CRC Press Boca Raton p 187-212

Cromwell, G.L. (1994) Feeding strategies urged as techniques to decrease pollution from hog manure. *Feedstuffs*, July 25, p 9,27

Damgaard Poulsen, H. and V.F. Kristensen (1998) Standard values for farm manure. Ministry of Food, Agriculture and Fisheries, Danish Institute of Agricultural Science, DIAS report 7: 1-160

De Lange, C.F.M., M. Nyachotti and S. Birkett (1999). Manipulation of diets to minimize the contribution to environmental pollution in: *advances in pork production.* 10th Banff pork seminar p 173-186

De Lange, C.F.M. and M.F. Fuller. (2000). Advances in feed evaluation for pigs, p. 221-241 In P.J. Moughan, M.W.A.Verstegen, M.I.Visser-Reyneveld. Eds. *Feed Evaluation, Principles and Practice.* Wageningen Press The Netherlands

Fancher B.I. and L.S. Jensen (1989). Dietary protein level and essential amino acid content: Influence upon female broiler performance during the grower period. *Poultry Science* **68**:897-908.

FEFANA – Federation Europeenne des Fabricants d'Adjuvants pour la Nutrition Animale 1992. Improvements in the environments: possibilities for the reduction of nitrogen and phosphorus pollution caused by animal production. Belgium.

Gahl, M.J., T.D. Crenshaw, and N.J. Benevenga (1995). Diminishing returns in weight, nitrogen, and lysine gain of pigs fed six levels of lysine from three supplemental sources. *J. Anim. Sci.* **73**:3177.

Gatel, F. (1994). Low protein, amino acid supplemented diets for pigs. *Feed Mix* **2**:32.

Gatel, F. and F. Grosjean (1992). Effect of protein content of the diet on nitrogen excretion by pigs. *Livest. Prod. Sci.* **31**:109.

Goelema, J.O. (1999). Processing of legume seeds: effects on digestive behaviour in dairy cows. PhD Thesis Wageningen University.

Heady, E.O., R. Woodworth, D.R. Catron, and G.C. Ashton (1954). New procedures in estimating feed substitution rates and in determining economic efficiency in pork production. In *Agric. Exp. Sta. Res. Bull.* Iowa State College, Ames, p 893.

Henry, Y., and J.Y. Dourmad (1993). Feeding strategies for minimizing nitrogen outputs in pigs. In *Nitrogen flow in pig production and environmental consequences.* Proc. First Intern. Symp. on Nitrogen flow in Pig Production and Environmental Consequences. EAAP Publication No. 69, p 137.

Holzheimer P.J. and W.M.M.A Janssen (1991). Limiting amino acids in low protein Maize-soybean meal diets fed to broiler chicks from 3 to 7 weeks of age. *British Poultry Science* **32**: 151-158.

Herrera-Saldana, R., R. Gomez-Alarcon, M. Torabio, J.T. Huber (1990). Influence of synchronizing protein and starch degradation in the rumen on nutrient utilization and microbial protein synthesis. *J. Dairy Sci.* **73**:142-148.

Hof, G., and S. Tamminga. (1994). Feeding management to reduce nitrogen losses in dairy cows. In: E.A. Huisman, J.W.M. Osse, D. van der Heide, S. Tamminga, B.J. Tolkamp, W.G.P Schouten, C.E. Hollingworth, and G.L. van Winkel (Eds.). *Biological basis of sustainable animal production.* p 149. Wageningen Pers, Wageningen, The Netherlands.

Hof, G., S. Tamminga, and P.J. Lenaers. (1994). Efficiency of protein utilization in dairy cows. *Livest. Prod. Sci.* **38**:169-178

Hof, G., M.D. Vervoorn, J.P. Lenaers and S. Tamminga (1997). Milk urea nitrogen as a tool to monitor the protein nutrition of dairy cows. *J. Dairy Sci.*, **80**:3333.

Hoover, W.H., and S.R. Stokes (1991). Balancing carbohydrate and proteins for optimum rumen microbial yield. *J. Dairy Sci.* **74**:3630.

Houdijk, J.G.M. (1998). Effects of non-digestible oligosaccharides in young pig diets. Ph.D. thesis Wageningen, The Netherlands.

Jongbloed, A.W. (1987). Phosphorus in the feeding of pigs: Effect of diet on the absorption and retention of Phosphorus by growing pigs. PhD thesis Wageningen University, the Netherlands.

Jongbloed, A.W. (2001). Lecture at postgraduate course on pig nutrition. New Developments and practice in Dutch. December 2001

Jongbloed, A. W., and C. H. Henkens (1996). Environmental concerns of using animal manure – The Dutch case. *In Nutrient Management of Food Animals to Enhance and Protect the Environment.* Kornegay, E.T., Ed. CRC, Boca Raton p 315.

Kephart, K.B., and S.P. Sherrit (1990). Performance and nutrient balance in growing swine fed low-protein diets supplemented with amino acids and potassium. *J. Anim. Sci.* **68**:1999.

Kerr, B. J., and R.A. Easter (1995). Effect of feeding reduced protein, amino acid-supplemented diets on nitrogen and energy balance in grower pigs. *J. Anim. Sci.* **73**:3000.

Kolver E., L.D. Muller, G.A. Varga and T.J. Cassidy (1998). Synchronization of ruminal degradation of supplemental carbohydrate with pasture nitrogen in lactating dairy cows. *J. Dairy Sci.* **81**:2017-2028.

Konishi, C., T. Matsui, W. Park, H. Yano and F. Yano (1999). Heat treatment of soybean meal and rapeseed meal suppresses rumen degradation of phytate phosphorus in sheep. *Anim. Fd. Sci. Technol.*, **80**:115-122.I.

Kyriazakis and G. C. Emmans (1992) , Effects of varying protein and energy intakes on the growth and body composition of pigs 2. Effect of varying both energy and protein intake *British Journal of Nutrition* **68**: 615-625.

Kornegay E.T. and M.W.A. Verstegen (2001) Swine nutrition and pollution and odor control. In (A.J. Lewis and L.L. Southern eds.): *Swine nutrition.* CRC Press Boca Raton p 609-630.

McCarthy, R.D., T.H. Klusmeyer, J.L. Vicini, J.H. Clark and D.R. Nelson (1989). Effects of source of protein and carbohydrate on ruminal fermentation and passage of nutrients to the small intestine of lactating cows. *J. Dairy Sci.* **72**:2002-2016.

Newbold, J.R. and S.R. Rust (1992). Effect of asynchronous nitrogen and energy supply on growth of ruminal bacteria in batch culture. *J. Anim. Sci.* **70**:538-546.

Moran, E. T. Jr., R.D. Bushony and S.F. Bilghi (1992). Reducing dietary crude protein for broilers chicks while satisfying amino acid requirements by least cost formulation: live performance, litter composition and yield of fast food carcass cuts at six weeks. *Poultry Science* **71**:1687-1694.

Moughan, P.J. Protein metabolism in the growing pig. In: I. Kyriazakis ed . A *Quantitative Biology of the pig*. CABI International Wallingford, UK p 299-332.

Nonn, H. and H. Jeroch (2000). Zur reduzierten Futterung von Mastschweine bei Einsatz freier Amino Sauren. *Archiv für Tierzucht, Dummerstorf* **43**:179-191.

NRC (1998). Nutrient requirements of swine. National Research Council, (10th Ed.). National Academy Press, Washington, DC.

Oenema, O., G.L. Velthof, N. Verdoes, P.W.G. Groot Koerkamp, G.J. Monteny, A. Bannink, H.G. van der Meer and K.W. van der Hoek (2000). Forfaitaire waarden voor gasvormige stikstofverliezen uit stallen en mestopslagen. [Standard values for gaseous nitrogen losses from animal houses and manure stores], *Report Alterra*, **107**:1-185.

Park, W-Y, T. Matsui, C. Konishi, S-W. Kim, F. Yano and H. Yano, H. (1999). Formaldehyde treatment suppresses ruminal degradation of phytate in soybean meal and rapeseed meal. *Br. J. Nutr.* **81**:467-471.

Rulquin, H. and R. Verité, R. (1993) Amino acid nutrition off ruminants. In: P.C. Garnsworthy and D.J.A. Cole (eds.). *Recent advances in animal nutrition*. Nottingham University Press, Sutton Bonington, UK, pp. 55-77.

Sauvant, D. and J. van Milgen, (1995). Consequences of kinetics of ruminal degradation on ruminal metabolism and zootechnical performances. *INRA Prod. Anim.* **8**:353-367.

Scheele, C.W., M.W.A. Verstegen, R.P. Kwakkel, R.A. Dekker and C. Kwakernaak (1999). Towards a new net energy system for poultry in The Netherlands. Proceedings 12th European Symposium on poultry Nutrition, Veldhoven, The Netherlands Branch of WPSA 399-407.

Summers J.D., D. Spratt and J.L. Atkinson (1992). Broiler weight and carcass composition when fed diets varying in amino acid balance, dietary energy and protein level. *Poultry Science* **71**:263-273

Siemes, H., Ed. (2000). Manure and the environment. Department of Agriculture, Ministry of Agriculture, Nature Management and Fisheries, the Netherlands.

Sinclair, L.A. (1992). Energy and nitrogen synchronization and its effect on rumen metabolism in sheep. Ph.D. Thesis University of Nottingham.

Sinclair, L.A., P.C. Garnsworthy, J.R. Newbold and P.J. Buttery (1993). Effects of synchronizing the rate of dietary energy and nitrogen release on rumen fermentation and microbial protein synthesis in sheep. *J. Agric. Sci. Camb.* **120**:251-263.

Sinclair, L.A., P.C. Garnsworthy, J.R. Newbold and P.J. Buttery (1995). Effects of synchronizing the rate of dietary energy and nitrogen release in diets with similar carbohydrate composition on rumen fermentation and microbial protein synthesis in sheep. *J. Agric. Sci. Camb.* **124**:463-472.

Tamminga, S. (1992) Feeding management for dairy cows as a means to contribute to environmental pollution control. *J. Dairy Sci.*, **75**:345-357.

Tamminga, S. (1996). A review on environmental impacts of nutritional strategies in ruminants. *J. Anim. Sci.* **74**(1996):3112-3124.

Tamminga, S., A.W. Jongbloed, M.M. van Eerdt, H.F.M. Aarts, F. Mandersloot, N.J.P. Hoogervorst and H. Westhoek (2000). De forfaitaire excretie van stikstof door landbouwhuisdieren [The standard excretion of nitrogen by farm animals], Report ID-Lelystad, 00-2040R:1-71.

Tamminga, S. and M.W.A. Verstegen (1992). Implications of nutrition of animals on environmental pollution. In: *Recent Advances in Animal Nutrition* (P.C. Garnsworthy, W. Haresign & D.J.A. Cole, eds.), Butterworth\Heinemann, London, p. 113-129.

Ten Doeschate R.H.M. (1995). Towards a new feeding strategy for protein in broilers. PhD thesis Wageningen University The Netherlands p 1-237.

Valk, H., I.E. Leusink-Kappers and A.M. van Vuuren (2000). Effect of reducing N fertiliser on grassland on grass intake, digestion and milk production of dairy cows. *Livest. Prod. Sci.* **63**:27-38.

Valk, H. and L.B.J. Šebek (1999). Influence of long term feeding of limited amounts of phosphorus on dry matter intake, milk production, and body weight of dairy cows. *J. Dairy Sci.*, **82**:2157-2163.

Valk, H., J.A. Metcalf and P.J.A. Withers (2000). Prospects for minimizing phosphorus excretion in ruminants by dietary manipulation. *J. Environ. Qual.*, **29**:28-36.

Valk, H., L.B.J. Šebek and A.C. Beynen (2002). Influence of phosphorus intake on phosphorus excretion and phosphorus concentrations of blood plasma and saliva in dairy cows. *J. Dairy Sci.* (in press).

Van der Meer, H.G. and A.H.J. van der Putten (1995). Reduction of nutrient emissions from ruminant livestock farms. In: G.E. Pollott. (ed) *Grassland into the 21st century: Challenges and opportunities*. British Grassland Society. p.118-134.

Van der Honing, Y., A.W. Jongbloed and N.P. Lenis (1993). Nutrition management to reduce environmental pollution by pigs. *VII World Conf. on Anim. Prod.*, Edmonton, Alberta (Abstr.).

Van Heugten, E., and T. van Kempen (1999). Methods may exist to reduce nutrient excretion. *Feedstuffs* (April 1:6).

Van Vuuren, A.M., C.H. van der Koelen, H. Valk, and H. de Visser (1993). Effects of partial replacements of ryegrass by low protein feeds on rumen fermentation and nitrogen loss by dairy cows. *J. Dairy Sci.* **76**: 2982-2993

*This paper was first published in 2002*

# INDEX